WHAT TO EXPECT®
WHEN YOU'RE EXPECTING

5TH EDITION

Also Available from What to Expect®

What to Expect® the First Year

What to Expect® the Second Year

Eating Well When You're Expecting

What to Expect® Before You're Expecting

*The What to Expect® When You're Expecting
Pregnancy Journal & Organizer*

*Qué puedes esperar® cuando estás esperando
(What to Expect® When You're Expecting—Spanish Edition)*

*Qué puedes esperar® en el primero año
(What to Expect® the First Year—Spanish Edition)*

The What to Expect® Baby-Sitter's Handbook

WHAT TO EXPECT®
WHEN YOU'RE EXPECTING

5TH EDITION

By Heidi Murkoff
and Sharon Mazel

Foreword by Charles J. Lockwood, MD
Professor of Obstetrics and Gynecology and Public Health
Dean, Morsani College of Medicine, University of South Florida

Workman Publishing • New York

To Erik, my everything

*To Emma and Wyatt for making me a mom,
and Lennox for making me a grandmom*

*To Arlene, my first partner in What to Expect and my most important one.
Your legacy of caring, compassion, and integrity lives on forever;
you'll always be loved and always be remembered.*

*To moms, dads, and babies everywhere—
and to all those who care for and about them*

....

Library of Congress Cataloging-in-Publication Data

Names: Murkoff, Heidi Eisenberg, author. | Mazel, Sharon, author.
Title: What to expect when you're expecting / by Heidi Murkoff and Sharon
    Mazel ; foreword by Charles J. Lockwood, MD, Senior Vice President, USF
    Health, and Dean of the Morsani College of Medicine.
Description: Fifth edition. | New York : Workman Publishing, [2016]
Identifiers: LCCN 2015044527 | ISBN 978-0-7611-8748-6 (alk. paper)
Subjects: LCSH: Pregnancy. | Childbirth. | Postnatal care.
Classification: LCC RG525 .M87 2016 | DDC 618.2--dc23 LC record available at
http://lccn.loc.gov/2015044527

ISBN 978-0-7611-8748-6 (PB)
ISBN 978-0-7611-8924-4 (HC)

Book design: Lisa Hollander and Barbara Peragine
Interior illustrations: Karen Kuchar
Cover design: Vaughn Andrews
Cover photographs: © mattbeard.com
Cover quilt: Lynette Parmentier, Quilt Creations
Cover quilt photography: Davies + Starr

Workman books are available at special discounts when purchased in bulk for premiums and
sales promotions as well as for fund-raising or educational use. Special editions or book excerpts
can also be created to specification. For details, contact the Special Sales Director at the address
below or send an email to specialmarkets@workman.com.

Workman Publishing Co., Inc.
225 Varick Street
New York, NY 10014-4381
workman.com

WHAT TO EXPECT is a registered trademark of What to Expect LLC
WORKMAN is a registered trademark of Workman Publishing Co., Inc.

Printed in the United States of America
First printing April 2016

10 9 8 7 6 5 4 3 2

Thanks and More Thanks

So, it's time for another delivery. And if delivering a book is anything like delivering a baby—and it is, in many ways (you nurture, nurture, nurture, stress, stress, stress, try to breathe, breathe, breathe, and then you push, push, push)—I have a whole lot of birth attendants to thank:

First, always and forever, the father of What to Expect, Erik—the man who made me a mom to Emma and Wyatt, a mom to What to Expect, and the happiest woman on the planet. My 24/7 partner in life, love, work, parenting, and (best of all) grandparenting.

Suzanne Rafer, editor and friend, who has helped me birth more baby books than I can count, and has been there since What to Expect was first conceived (and who actually named our first baby): tirelessly coaching, cheering, and policing my puns (with limited success—that's what erasers were made for).

Peter Workman, who created the house I've delivered all my babies in, and whose legacy lives on in them.

Everyone else at Workman who contributed to this baby: Jenny Mandel, Emily Krasner, Suzie Bolotin, Dan Reynolds, Page Edmunds, Selina Meere, Jessica Wiener, and Sarah Brady.

Matt Beard, who had us covered, cover-to-cover, bringing beautiful images of Lennox before and after. Karen Kuchar for bringing moms and babies to life with her lovely illustrations. Lisa Hollander and Vaughn Andrews for putting it altogether artfully in such a pretty package, Beth Levy, Claire McKean, Barbara Peragine, and Julie Primavera for masterfully producing and managing the seamless sausage-making.

Sharon Mazel, who has nurtured, stressed, breathed (and reminded me to breathe), and pushed alongside me for the last 15 years of birthing What to Expect babies—without ever asking for an epidural—while somehow managing to raise 4 amazing daughters and staying happily married to the second most patient man on earth, Jay.

Dr. Charles Lockwood (who appropriately played the role of ob in *What to Expect When You're Expecting*, 4th and 5th editions!), our intrepid medical advisor—always ready to tackle any topic on the minds of moms (even those perhaps best left on the fringe), to bring his enormous reserves of knowledge, experience, wisdom, caring, and compassion to help deliver our latest baby safe and sound (as in sound advice). Dr. Stephanie Romero for her incredibly insightful contributions. Dr. Howie Mandel, for delivering compassionate care—and Lennox.

ACOG, for being tireless advocates for moms and babies everywhere, and to all the doctors, midwives, nurses, childbirth educators, doulas, and lactation consultants around the world who literally nurture the nurturers among us, helping deliver the healthiest start in life for every baby and the healthiest future for all of us. The experts and advocates at the CDC—an organization passionately devoted to the health and wellbeing of our global family, especially when it comes to our most vulnerable—for your shared mission and commitment, for being an invaluable partner in spreading important health messages (and preventing the spread of disease!).

Our other partners in mom and baby health and #BumpDay: International Medical Corps (internationalmedicalcorps.org), humanitarians, first responders, and trainers of healthcare heroes (like my personal midwife hero from South Sudan, Tindilo Grace Losio, aka Amazing Grace). 1,000 Days™, for believing that a healthy future depends on a healthy (and well-fed) beginning. The UN Foundation's Universal Access Program, for their passionate support of women and girls and their reproductive rights, health, and wellbeing.

Our partners in Special Delivery, the USO, and the amazing military mamas around the world I've had the honor to hug and have yet to hug (more hugs coming!).

Our incredible WhatToExpect.com team, fearlessly led by Michael Rose, Diane Otter, and Kyle Humphries, for their endless energy, enthusiasm, innovation, integrity, creativity, conviction, passion, and shared purpose (and for believing in the power of purple).

For inspiration and love, our beautiful "children": Wyatt, Emma, and Russell, and of course, Lennox. Howard Eisenberg, Abby and Norm Murkoff, Victor Shargai, and Craig Pascal.

Contents

Foreword to the Fifth Edition

By Charles J. Lockwood, MD

Professor of Obstetrics and Gynecology and Public Health
Dean, Morsani College Medicine, University of South Florida

This fifth edition of *What to Expect When You're Expecting* continues an amazing legacy of bringing expectant moms (and their partners) the most accurate, up-to-date information available, as well as sound, practical medical advice. And it does it with a wonderful mix of compassion and practicality. I have recommended the book for years and for good reason—it's comprehensive and packed with the kind of information you would expect to hear from your favorite doctor or healthcare provider. That is, one who's wise but with a good sense of humor, thorough but practical, experienced but enthusiastic, organized but empathetic. All the key issues most expectant parents will likely face are covered in just the right amount of detail. The diet and nutrition, exercise, and mental health recommendations are incredibly helpful, and the discussions of labor and birth live up to the high standards I've come to expect from Heidi. Exciting and new for this edition is that the advice specifically for dads-to-be is carefully woven into each chapter, underscoring the fact that dads are an integral, important part of pregnancy.

In short, the book is literally packed with the latest in medical, genetic and obstetrical advances all presented in a clear, interesting and comprehensible fashion. As a high-risk obstetrician who has delivered thousands of babies, often to mothers with very complicated medical and obstetrical conditions, I know that a well-informed patient is the cornerstone to a successful outcome. This book could not be better at providing that much-needed information. It is no accident that *What to Expect* has become the standard by which other pregnancy books are judged. Put your feet up and enjoy the read. Best wishes for a wonder-filled pregnancy.

Introduction
to the Fifth Edition

Maybe you know the story (I tell it a lot) of how *What to Expect When You're Expecting* was born. Or, really, how it was conceived, because that's exactly how it happened. I conceived a baby, and then I conceived a book. And let's just say, I didn't expect either.

So, first, the baby. It was an "oops" pregnancy—as in, Erik and I got married and just 3 months later, oops . . . I was pregnant. Pregnant and completely clueless. Clueless about how I'd gotten pregnant (beyond the basic biology—I had that down, but I was pretty sure I wouldn't be able to conceive) and clueless about what to do now that I was. I searched in books (the only way we could back in the days before search engines) for answers to my questions, reassurance from my worries, a hand to hold, a shoulder to cry on, a voice to talk me down and cheer me on through the exciting but bewildering pregnancy journey Erik and I were headed on. I read and I read, but I couldn't find what both of us desperately needed to know: what to expect when you're expecting. So, I wrote a book—delivering the proposal for *What to Expect When You're Expecting* just two hours before I went into labor with the baby who inspired it all, Emma.

And the rest would be history, except that history doesn't get rewritten (or at least, it shouldn't), and pregnancy books do (or should, and often). After all, while some things about pregnancy never change (it's still 9 months long, give or take, and you still get bloated, queasy, and constipated), many others do change. A lot.

With those changes in mind—and with the incredible insight and suggestions I receive online and in person from moms and dads around the world, hands down my most valuable resource—I've delivered again . . . for the fifth time.

What's new in this fifth edition? Plenty, from cover to cover (including the covers—more about that later). You'll find new "For Fathers" boxes integrated throughout the book that speak to dads' unique concerns as partners in pregnancy, childbirth, and parenting (and also speak to partners who are other mothers, not fathers). All the medical bases are completely covered and completely updated, of course: The latest on prenatal screening and diagnosis, the safety of medications during pregnancy (including antidepressants), cord blood banking options, complementary and alternative therapies, and a brand new section on postpartum birth control are here. Lifestyle trends get their due, too: from gender reveals to push presents, from overcaffeinating at the coffee bar or sipping an occasional glass of wine or puffing on an e-cigarette or nibbling on a weed edible, to the wisdom of oversharing on social media, and much more. Pregnancy eating is on the expanded menu, including raw and Paleo diets, juicing, grass-fed, organic, and health foods (and supposed super foods), GMOs—even why eating peanuts and other nuts can actually help baby-to-be avoid allergies. The greening of pregnancy is covered, as well, including how to avoid BPA and phthalates. There's skin care, hair care, cosmetics and cosmetic procedures, and spa treatment guidelines for the expectant set. There's simply a boatload of information for everyone who's expecting: expanded advice on multiple pregnancy, back-to-back pregnancy (including breastfeeding while you're expecting). IVF pregnancy, pregnancy after weight loss surgery. More birthing options, too: water and home births,

delayed cord blood clamping, VBAC, and gentle cesareans, laboring down, and pushing positions.

And remember the covers I was telling you about? Well, there you'll find a couple of special surprises: On the front, Emma, the baby who started it all, pregnant with her first baby (and our first grandchild), Lennox. And on the back, who else? Lennox.

Just another couple of things I didn't expect when I was expecting—and way more than I ever could have expected . . . or dreamed possible.

May all your greatest expectations come true!

Big hugs,

heidi

About the What to Expect Foundation

Every mom should be able to expect a healthy pregnancy, a safe delivery, and a healthy, happy baby. That's why we created The What to Expect Foundation, a nonprofit organization dedicated to making that mission a reality for moms and babies in need around the world. Our programs include Baby Basics, Special Delivery baby showers for military moms-to-be (in partnership with the USO), and a global midwife training initiative (in partnership with International Medical Corps). For more information and to find ways you can help, please visit our website at whattoexpect.org.

First Things First

CHAPTER 1

Are You Pregnant?

M aybe your period's only a day overdue. Or maybe it's going on 3 weeks late. Or maybe your period isn't even slated to arrive yet, but you've got a gut feeling (literally, in your gut) that something's cooking—like a brand new baby bun in your oven! Maybe you've been giving baby making everything you've got for 6 months or longer. Or maybe that hot night 2 weeks ago was your very first contraceptive-free love connection. Or maybe you haven't been actively trying at all, and still managed to succeed. At least, you think you did. No matter what the circumstances that have brought you to this book, you're bound to be wondering: Am I pregnant? Well, read on to find out.

What You May Be Wondering About

Early Pregnancy Signs

"My period isn't even due yet, but I already feel pregnant. Is that possible?"

T he only way to be positively positive that you're pregnant—at least this early on—is to produce a positive pregnancy test. But that doesn't mean your body is staying mum on whether you're about to become a mom. In fact, it may be offering up plenty of conception clues. Though many women never feel any early pregnancy symptoms at all (or don't feel them until weeks into pregnancy), others get lots of hints that there's a baby in the making. Experiencing any of these symptoms or noticing any of these signs may be just the excuse you need to run to the store for a home pregnancy test:

Tender breasts and nipples. You know that tender, achy feeling you get in your breasts before your period arrives?

That's nothing compared with the breast tenderness you might be feeling postconception. Tender, full, swollen, tingly, sensitive, and even painful-to-the-touch breasts are some of the first signs many (but not all) women notice after sperm meets egg. Such tenderness can begin as soon as a few days after conception (though it often doesn't kick in until weeks later), and as your pregnancy progresses, it could get even more pronounced. Make that a lot more pronounced. How can you tell PMS breasts from pregnant ones? Often, you can't right away—adding to the guesswork.

Darkening areolas. Not only might your breasts be tender, but your areolas (the circles around your nipples) may be getting darker—something that doesn't typically happen before a period. They may even begin to increase in diameter. You can thank the pregnancy hormones already surging through your body for these and other skin color changes (much more about those in the coming months).

Bumpy areolas. You may have never noticed the tiny bumps on your areolas, but once they start growing in size and number (as they typically do early in pregnancy), they'll be hard to miss. These bumps (called Montgomery's tubercles) are actually glands that produce oils to lubricate your nipples and areolas—lubrication that'll certainly be welcome protection when baby starts suckling. Another sign your body is planning ahead—way ahead, in fact.

Spotting. Up to 30 percent of brand new mamas-to-be experience spotting when the embryo implants in the uterus. Such so-called implantation bleeding will likely arrive earlier than your expected monthly flow (usually around 6 to 12 days after conception) and will probably appear light to medium pink in color (rarely red, like a period).

Fatigue. Extreme fatigue. Make that exhaustion. Complete lack of energy. Super sluggishness. Whatever you call it, it's a drag—literally. And as your body starts cranking up that baby-making machine, it'll only get more draining. See page 130 for reasons why.

Urinary frequency. Has the toilet become your seat of choice lately? Appearing on the pregnancy scene fairly early (usually about 2 to 3 weeks after conception) may be the need to pee with surprising frequency. Curious why? See page 138 for all the reasons.

Nausea. Here's another reason why you might want to consider setting up shop in the bathroom, at least until the first trimester is finished. The nausea and vomiting of pregnancy—aka morning sickness, though it's often a 24/7 kind of thing—can strike a newly pregnant woman fairly soon after conception, though it's more likely to begin around week 6. For a host of reasons why, see page 132.

Smell sensitivity. Since a heightened sense of smell is one of the first changes some newly pregnant women report, pregnancy might be in the air if your sniffer's suddenly more sensitive—and easily offended.

Bloating. Feeling like a walking flotation device? That bloated feeling can creep up (and out) on you very early in a pregnancy—though it may be difficult to differentiate between a preperiod bloat and a pregnancy bloat. It's definitely too soon to attribute any swelling to your baby's growth, but you can chalk it up to those hormones again.

Rising temperature. If you've been using a special basal body thermometer to track your first morning temperature, you might notice that it rises around 1 degree when you conceive and continues to stay elevated throughout your pregnancy. Though not a foolproof sign (there are other reasons why you may notice a rise in temperature), it could give you advance notice of big—though still very little—news.

Missed period. It might be stating the obvious, but if you've missed a period (especially if your periods generally run like clockwork), you may already be suspecting pregnancy—even before a pregnancy test confirms it.

Diagnosing Pregnancy

"How can I find out for sure whether I'm pregnant or not?"

Aside from that most remarkable of diagnostic tools, a woman's intuition (some women "feel" they're pregnant within days—even moments—of conception), modern medical science is still your best bet when it comes to diagnosing a pregnancy accurately. Luckily, there are many ways to find out for sure if you've got a baby on board:

The home pregnancy test. It's as easy as 1-2-pee, and you can do it all in the privacy and comfort of your own bathroom. Home pregnancy tests (HPTs) are not only quick and accurate, but you can even start using most brands before you've missed your period (though accuracy will get better as you get closer to P-day).

All HPTs measure urinary levels of human chorionic gonadotropin (hCG), a (developing) placenta-produced hormone of pregnancy. HCG finds its way into your bloodstream and urine almost immediately after an embryo begins implanting in the uterus, between 6 and 12 days after fertilization. As soon as hCG can be detected in your urine, you can (theoretically) get a positive reading. But there is a limit to how soon

Testing Smart

The home pregnancy test is probably the simplest test you'll ever take. You won't have to study for it, but you should read the package instructions carefully before you take the test (yes, even if you've taken HPT tests before, since different brands come with different instructions). A few other things to keep in mind:

- You don't need to use first-of-the-morning urine. Any-time-of-the-day pee will do.

- Most tests prefer you use midstream urine. And since your practitioner will prefer that you use this in your monthly urine samples, too, you might as well master the technique now if you haven't before: Start peeing for a second or two, stop, hold the flow, and then put the stick you're supposed to pee onto or the cup you're supposed to pee into in position to catch the rest of the stream (or as much as needed).

- Any positive read, no matter how faint, is a positive. Congratulations—you're pregnant! If the result isn't positive, and your period still hasn't arrived, consider waiting a few days and testing again. It may have just been too soon to call.

these HPTs can work—they're sensitive, but not always that sensitive. One week after conception there's hCG in your urine, but it's not enough for the HPT to pick up—which means that if you test 7 days before your expected period, you're likely to get a false negative even if you're pregnant.

Just can't wait to pee on that stick? Some tests promise 60 to 75 percent accuracy 4 to 5 days before your expected period. Not a betting woman? Wait until the day your period is expected, and you'll have up to a 99 percent chance (depending on the brand's claim) of scoring the correct result. Whenever you decide to take the testing plunge, the good news is that false positives are much less common than false negatives—which means that if your test is positive, you can be, too. (The exception: if you've recently had fertility treatments; see box, page 6.)

Some HPTs can tell you not only that you're pregnant but also approximately how far along you are in your pregnancy, displaying along with the word "pregnant" the estimated weeks since ovulation—either 1 to 2 weeks, 2 to 3 weeks, or 3 or more weeks since your tiny egg was fertilized by your partner's sperm. Operative word "approximately"—so don't use this reading to calculate your official estimated due date. Also on the market: an HPT that's app-compatible.

No matter what type of HPT you use (from budget brand basic to super high-tech) you'll get a very accurate diagnosis very early in pregnancy—and that early heads-up can give you an early head start on taking the best possible care of yourself. Still, medical follow-up to the test is essential. So if the result is positive, it's time to call your practitioner and book that first prenatal appointment.

Testing for the Irregular

So your cycles don't exactly run on schedule? That'll make scheduling your HPT testing date a lot trickier. After all, how can you test on the day that your period is expected if you're never sure when that day will come? Your best testing strategy if your periods are irregular is to wait the number of days equal to the longest cycle you've had in the last 6 months (hopefully you've been keeping track on an app)—and then test. If the result is negative and you still haven't gotten your period, repeat the test after a week (or after a few days if you just can't wait).

The blood test. The more sophisticated blood pregnancy test can detect pregnancy with virtually 100 percent accuracy as early as 1 week after conception, using just a few drops of blood. It can also help approximately date the pregnancy by measuring the exact amount of hCG in the blood, since hCG values change as pregnancy progresses (see page 144 for more on hCG levels). Many practitioners order both a urine test and a blood test to be doubly certain of the diagnosis.

The medical exam. Though a medical exam can be performed to confirm the diagnosis of a pregnancy, today's accurate HPTs and blood tests make the exam—which looks for physical signs of pregnancy such as enlargement of the uterus, color changes in the vagina and cervix, and a change in the texture of the cervix—almost beside the point. Still, getting that first exam and beginning regular prenatal care isn't (see page 8).

Pregnancy Testing and Fertility Treatments

Every hopeful mama-to-be is on pins and needles (and the edge of her toilet seat) waiting for the moment when she'll finally be able to pee on a stick to confirm that she's pregnant. But if you've been undergoing certain fertility treatments, the wait for a positive pregnancy test can be even more nerve-racking, especially if you've been told to skip the HPT and hold off until a blood test can be done (which, depending on your fertility clinic, may be a week to 2 weeks after conception or embryo transfer). But there's a very good reason why most fertility specialists prescribe this approach: HPTs can provide unreliable results for fertility patients. That's because hCG, the hormone tested for in an HPT, is often used in fertility treatments to trigger ovulation and may remain in your system (and show up in your urine) even if you're not pregnant.

Usually, if the first blood test given by your fertility specialist is positive, it will be repeated in 2 to 3 days. Why the repeat blood test? Your doctor will not only be looking to see that there's hCG in your system, but also making sure the level of hCG increases by at least two-thirds (indicating that all is going well so far). If it has increased, another blood test will be ordered 2 to 3 days later, when the hCG level should have increased by two-thirds or more again. These blood tests will also measure hormones (like estrogen and progesterone) to make sure they are at the level they should be to sustain a pregnancy. If all 3 blood tests point to a pregnancy, then an ultrasound is scheduled around 5 to 8 weeks of pregnancy to look for the heartbeat and a gestational sac (see page 170).

A Faint Line

"I used a cheaper HPT instead of the more expensive digital kind, but when I took it, it showed a faint line. Am I pregnant?"

The only way a home pregnancy test can give you a positive result is if you have a detectable level of hCG in your urine. And the only way you'll have a detectable level of hCG in your urine (unless you've been receiving fertility treatments) is if you're pregnant. Which means that if your test is showing a line, no matter how faint it is—you can be positive that you're pregnant.

Just why you're getting a faint line instead of that loud-and-clear line you were hoping for may have to do with the sensitivity of the test you've

used. To figure out how sensitive your pregnancy test is, look for the milli-international units per liter (mIU/L) measurement on the packaging. The lower the number, the better (20 mIU/L will tell you you're pregnant sooner than a test with a 50 mIU/L sensitivity). Not surprisingly, the more expensive tests usually have greater sensitivity.

Keep in mind, too, that the farther along in your pregnancy you are, the higher your levels of hCG. If you're testing very early on in your pregnancy (before your expected period), there might not be enough hCG in your system yet to generate a no-doubt-about-it line. Give it a couple of days, test again, and you'll likely see a line that'll erase your doubts once and for all.

No Longer Positive

"My first HPT was positive, but a few days later I took another one and it was negative. And then I got my period. What's going on?"

Unfortunately, it sounds like you may have experienced what's known as a chemical pregnancy—when an egg is fertilized, but for some reason never completes implantation. Instead of turning into a viable pregnancy, it ends in a period. Though experts estimate that up to 70 percent of all conceptions are chemical, the vast majority of women who experience one don't even realize they've conceived (certainly in the days before HPTs, women didn't have a clue they were pregnant until much later). Often, a very early positive pregnancy test and then a late period (a few days to a week late) are the only signs of a chemical pregnancy, so if there's a downside to early testing, you've definitely experienced it.

Medically, a chemical pregnancy is more like a cycle in which a pregnancy never really occurred than a true miscarriage. Emotionally, for women like you who tested early and got a positive result, it can be a very different story. Though it's not technically a pregnancy loss, the loss of the promise of a pregnancy can also be understandably upsetting for both you and your partner. Reading the information on coping with a pregnancy loss in Chapter 20 can help you with those emotions. And keep in mind that the fact that conception did occur once for you means that it'll more than likely occur again soon, and with the happier result of a healthy pregnancy.

A Negative Result

"My period's late and I feel like I'm pregnant, but I've done 3 HPTs and they were all negative. What should I do?"

If you're experiencing the symptoms of early pregnancy and feel, test or no test—or even 3 tests—that you're pregnant, act as though you are (by taking prenatal vitamins, eating well, cutting back on caffeine, not drinking or smoking, and so on) until you find out definitely otherwise. Even the best HPTs can slip up, producing a false negative result, especially when they're taken very early. You may well know your own body better than a pee-on-a-stick test does. To find out if your hunch is more accurate than the tests, wait a week and then try again—your pregnancy might just be too early to call. Or ask your practitioner for a blood test, which is more sensitive in detecting hCG than a urine test is.

It is possible, of course, to experience all the signs and symptoms of early pregnancy and not be pregnant. After all, none of them alone—or even in combination—is absolute proof positive of pregnancy. If the tests continue

---

Turning a Negative Into a Positive

If it turns out you're not pregnant this time, but you'd like to become pregnant soon, start making the most of the preconception period by taking the steps outlined in *What to Expect Before You're Expecting*. Good preconception prep before you start trying to conceive will help ensure the best possible pregnancy outcome when sperm and egg do meet up. Plus, you'll find tons of tips on how to boost your chances of conceiving—and conceiving faster.

to be negative but you still haven't gotten your period, be sure to check with your practitioner to rule out other physiological causes of your symptoms (say, a hormonal imbalance). If those are ruled out as well, it's possible that your symptoms may have emotional roots. Sometimes, the mind can have a surprisingly powerful influence on the body, even generating pregnancy symptoms when there's no pregnancy, just a strong yearning for one (or fear of one).

Making the First Appointment

"The home pregnancy test I took was positive. When should I schedule the first visit with my doctor?"

Good prenatal care is one of the most important ingredients in making a healthy baby. So don't delay. As soon as you have a positive HPT result, call your practitioner to schedule an appointment. Just how soon you'll be able to come in for that appointment may depend on office traffic and policy. Some practitioners will be able to fit you in right away, while some very busy offices may not be able to accommodate you for several weeks or even longer. At certain offices, it's routine to wait until a woman is 6 to 8 weeks pregnant for that first official prenatal visit, though some offer a "pre-ob" visit to confirm a pregnancy as soon as you suspect you're expecting (or have the positive HPT results to prove it).

But even if your official prenatal care has to be postponed until midway through the first trimester, that doesn't mean you should put off taking care of yourself and your baby. Regardless of when you get in to see your practitioner, start acting pregnant as soon as you see that positive readout on the HPT. You're probably familiar with many of the basics, but don't hesitate to call your practitioner's office if you have specific questions about how best to get with the pregnancy program. You may even be able to pick up a pregnancy packet ahead of time (many offices provide one, with advice on everything from diet do's and don'ts to prenatal vitamin recommendations to a list of medications you can safely take) to help fill in some of the blanks. Of course, you'll also find plenty of pregnancy advice in this book.

In a low-risk pregnancy, having the first prenatal visit early on isn't considered medically necessary, though the wait can be hard to handle. If the waiting's stressing you out, or if you feel you may be a high-risk case (because of a chronic condition or a history of miscarriages, for instance), check with the office to see if you can come in earlier. (For more on what to expect at your first prenatal visit, see page 125.)

Your Due Date

"I just got a positive result on my pregnancy test. How do I calculate my due date?"

Once the big news starts to sink in, it's time to reach for the calendar and mark down the big day: your due date. But wait—when are you due? Should you count 9 months from today? Or from when you might have conceived? Or is it 40 weeks? And 40 weeks from when? You just found out you're pregnant, and already you're confused. When is this baby coming, anyway?

Take a deep breath and get ready for pregnancy math 101. As a matter of convenience (because you need some idea of when your baby will arrive) and convention (because it's important to have benchmarks to measure your baby's growth and development against), a pregnancy is calculated as 40 weeks long—even though only about 30 percent of pregnancies actually last precisely 40 weeks. In fact, a full-term pregnancy is considered to be anywhere from 39 weeks to 41 weeks long (a baby born at 39 weeks isn't "early" any more than one born at 41 weeks is "late").

But here's where things get even more confusing. The 40 weeks of pregnancy are not counted from the day (or passionate night) your baby was conceived—they're counted from the first day of your last menstrual period (or LMP). Why start the clock on pregnancy before sperm even meets egg (and before your ovary even releases the egg)? The LMP is simply a reliable day to date from. After all, even if you're pretty positive about ovulation day (because you're a master of cervical mucus or an ovulation predictor pro), and definitely sure about the day or days you had sex, you probably can't pinpoint the moment egg and sperm got together (aka conception). That's because sperm can hang out and wait for an egg to fertilize up to 3 to 5 days after they've arrived through the vagina, and an egg can be fertilized up to 24 hours after it's been released— leaving a wider window than you might think.

So instead of using an uncertain conception date as a start date for pregnancy, you'll use a sure thing: your LMP, which (in a typical cycle) would have occurred about 2 weeks before your baby was conceived. Which means you'll have clocked in 2 of those 40 weeks of pregnancy by the time sperm and egg actually meet, and 4 weeks by the time you miss your period. And when you finally reach that 40-week mark, your baby bun will have been baking for just 38 weeks.

Still confused by the system? That's not surprising—it's a confusing system.

Happily, you don't have to understand the system to work it. To arrive at a due date (called an EDD, or estimated due date, because it's always an estimate), you can just do this simple calculation: Subtract 3 months from the first day of your last menstrual period (LMP), then add 7 days. For example, say your last period began on April 12. Count backward 3 months, which gets you to January 12, and then add 7 days. Your due date would be January 19. Don't feel like doing any math at all? No need to. Just plug your LMP date into the What To Expect app and—baby bingo!—your EDD will be calculated for you, you'll find out the week of pregnancy you're in, and your week-by-week countdown will begin.

Keep in mind that if you have irregular cycles, you may have difficulty calculating your due date with the LMP method. And even if your cycles are regular, your practitioner might give you a different date than you arrived at by using the LMP method or an app. That's because the most accurate way of estimating a due date is through an early ultrasound, usually done at about 6 to 9 weeks, which reliably measures the size of the embryo or fetus (measurements done by ultrasound after the first trimester aren't as accurate).

Though most practitioners will rely on the ultrasound-plus-LMP method to officially date your pregnancy, there are also other physical signs that may be used to back it up, including the size of your uterus and the height of the fundus (the top of the uterus, which will be measured at each prenatal visit after the first trimester and will reach your navel at about week 20).

All signs point to the same date? Remember, even the most reliable EDD is still just an estimate. Only your baby knows for sure when his or her birth date will be . . . and baby's not telling.

ALL ABOUT:
Choosing and Working with Your Practitioner

Everybody knows it takes two to conceive a baby. But it takes a minimum of three—mom, dad, and at least one health care professional—to make that transition from fertilized egg to delivered infant a safe and successful one. Assuming you and your partner have already taken care of conception, the next challenge you both face is selecting that third member of your pregnancy team and making sure it's a selection you can live with—and labor with.

Obstetrician? Family Practitioner? Midwife?

Where to begin your search for the perfect practitioner to help guide you through your pregnancy and beyond? First, you'll have to give some thought to what kind of medical credentials would best meet your needs.

The obstetrician. Are you looking for a practitioner who is trained to handle every conceivable medical aspect of pregnancy, labor, delivery, and the postpartum period—from the most obvious question to the most obscure complication? Then you'll want to consider an obstetrician, or ob. An ob can not only provide complete obstetrical care, but can also take care of all your non-pregnancy female health needs (Pap smears, contraception, breast exams, and so on). Some also offer general medical care, acting as your primary care physician as well.

If yours is a high-risk pregnancy, you will very likely need and want to seek out an ob. You may even want to find a specialist's specialist, an ob who specializes in high-risk pregnancies and is certified in maternal-fetal medicine. These physicians spend an extra 3 years training to care for women with high-risk pregnancies beyond the typical 4 years of ob-gyn residency training. If you've become pregnant with the help of an infertility specialist, you'll probably start your prenatal care with him or her, then "graduate" to a general ob or midwife (typically toward the end of the first trimester, though possibly sooner)—or, if your pregnancy turns out to be high-risk, a maternal-fetal medicine specialist.

More than 90 percent of women select an ob for their care. If you've been seeing an ob-gyn you like, respect, and feel comfortable with for your gynecological care, there may be no reason to switch now that you're pregnant. If your regular gyn care provider doesn't do ob, or if you're not convinced this is the doctor you'd like to have caring for you during pregnancy or while delivering your baby, it's time to start shopping around.

The family physician. Family physicians (FP) provide one-stop medical service. Unlike an ob, who has had post–medical school training in women's reproductive and general health as well as surgery, the FP has had training in primary care, maternal care, and pediatric care after receiving an MD. If you decide on an FP, he or she can serve as your internist, ob-gyn, and, when the time comes, pediatrician. Ideally, an FP will become familiar with the dynamics of your family and will be interested in all aspects of your health, not just your obstetric ones. If your pregnancy takes a turn for the complicated,

Paging Dr. Google?

Visit those pregnancy websites and apps, by all means, but search (and research) with care. Realize that you can't believe everything you read, especially online—and, emphatically—on social media. Before you consider following any of Dr. Google's prescriptions and guidelines, always get a second opinion from your real practitioner—usually your best source of pregnancy information, particularly as it applies to your individual pregnancy.

an FP may send you to an ob for consultation or for more specialized care, but will remain involved in your care for comforting continuity.

The certified nurse-midwife. If you're looking for a practitioner who will put more caring into your ob care, take extra time with you at prenatal visits, be as attentive to your emotional wellbeing as your physical condition, offer more detailed nutritional advice and comprehensive breastfeeding support, be open to more complementary and alternative therapies and more birth options, and be a strong advocate of unmedicated childbirth, then a certified nurse-midwife (CNM) may be right for you (though, of course, many doctors fit that profile, too). A CNM is a medical professional—an RN (registered nurse) or a BSN (bachelor of nursing science) who has completed graduate-level programs in midwifery and is certified by the American College of Nurse-Midwives. A CNM is thoroughly trained to care for women with low-risk pregnancies and to deliver uncomplicated births. In some cases, a CNM may provide continuing routine gyn care and, sometimes, newborn care. Most midwives work in hospital settings, and others deliver at birthing centers and/or do home births. Ninety-five percent of births with CNMs are in hospitals or birthing centers. Though CNMs have the right in most states to offer pain relief, as well as to

prescribe labor-inducing medications, a birth attended by a CNM is less likely to include such interventions. On average, midwives have much lower cesarean delivery rates (performed by their affiliated obs) than physicians, as well as higher rates of vaginal birth after cesarean (VBAC) success—in part because they're less likely to turn to unnecessary medical interventions, and in part because they care only for women with low-risk pregnancies, who are less likely to end up needing a surgical delivery. Studies show that for low-risk pregnancies, deliveries by CNMs are as safe as those by physicians. Something else to keep in mind, if you'll be paying some or all of your costs out-of-pocket: The cost of prenatal care with a CNM is usually less than that with an ob.

If you choose a certified nurse-midwife (about 9 percent of expectant moms do), be sure to select one who is both certified and licensed (all 50 states license nurse-midwives). Most CNMs use a physician as a backup in case of complications, and many practice with one or with a group that includes several. For more information about CNMs, look online at midwife.org.

Direct-entry midwives. These midwives are trained without first becoming nurses, though they may hold degrees in other health care areas. Direct-entry midwives are more likely than CNMs to do home births, though some also

Division of Labor

What happens if your ob is away on the day you deliver? Some obstetricians and hospitals turn to laborists—obs who work exclusively in the hospital (which is why they may also be called hospitalists), only attending labors and delivering babies. These laborists don't have an office and don't follow patients through pregnancy, but are there to help your baby come into the world if your ob (perhaps because he's on vacation or because she's attending a conference) isn't available.

If you're told that a laborist may be delivering your baby, ask your practitioner if he or she and the hospital laborists have worked closely together in the past. Also ask whether their philosophies and protocols are similar. You might also want to call the hospital to ask if you can meet the staff docs before labor, so that you're not being attended by a complete stranger during childbirth. Make sure, too, that you arrive at the hospital with your birth plan (if you have one; see page 323) in hand, so whoever is attending you is familiar with your wishes even if he or she isn't familiar with you.

If you're uncomfortable with the whole arrangement, think about switching practices sooner rather than later. Remember, though, that if you're with a multiple-doc practice already, there's a good chance your "regular" ob won't be on call the day you go into labor anyway. Keep in mind, too, that because hospitalists focus solely on deliveries, they're extra-prepared to give the best possible care during labor. And extra-rested, also, because they work on shifts instead of around the clock.

---

deliver babies in birthing centers. Those who are certified through the North American Registry of Midwives are called certified professional midwives (CPMs)—other direct-entry midwives are not certified. Licensing for direct-entry midwives is also offered in certain states, while in other states, direct-entry midwives can't practice legally. It's important to know that the training CPMs receive falls short of most international standards, and many wouldn't qualify as midwives in other developed countries. Less than half of 1 percent of births in the U.S. are attended by a direct-entry midwife. For more information, contact the Midwives Alliance of North America at mana.org.

Types of Practice

You've settled on an obstetrician, a family practitioner, or a midwife. Next you've got to decide which kind of medical practice you would be most comfortable with. Here are the most common kinds of practices and their possible advantages and disadvantages:

Solo medical practice. Searching for a doctor who's one of a kind, literally? Then you might want to look for a solo practice—in which the doctor of your choosing works alone, relying on another doctor to cover when he or she is unavailable. An ob or a family physician might be in solo practice, while a midwife must work in a collaborative practice with a physician in most states. The major advantage of a solo practice is that you'll see the same doctor at each visit—familiarity that can definitely breed comfort, especially when it comes time for delivery. You'll also receive consistent advice, instead of being consistently confused by seeing different practitioners sharing different (and sometimes conflicting) points of view. The major disadvantage is that if your one-of-a-kind doctor is out of town, sick, or otherwise unavailable on the day (or night) your baby decides to arrive, a backup practitioner you don't know (in some cases, a laborist; see box, facing page) may deliver your baby. Arranging to meet the covering practitioner ahead of time can help you feel more comfortable about that possibility. A solo practice may also be a problem if, midway through the pregnancy, you find that your one-of-a-kind doctor really isn't the one you were hoping for after all. If that happens and you decide to switch practitioners, you'll have to start from scratch, searching for one who fits your patient profile.

Partnership or group practice. In this type of practice, two or more doctors in the same specialty care jointly for patients, often seeing them on a rotating basis (though you usually get to stick with your favorite through most of your pregnancy and start rotating only toward the end of your pregnancy, when you're having more frequent office visits). Again, you can find both obs and family physicians in this type of practice. The advantage of a group practice is that by seeing a different doctor each time, you'll get to know them all—which means that when those contractions are coming strong and fast, there's sure to be a familiar face in the room with you. The disadvantage is that you may not like all of the doctors in the practice equally, and you usually won't be able to choose the one who attends your baby's birth. Also, hearing different points of view from the various partners may be an advantage or a disadvantage, depending on whether you find it reassuring or head-spinning.

Combination practice. A group practice that includes one or more obs and one or more midwives is considered a combination practice. The advantages and disadvantages are similar to those of any group practice. There is the added advantage of having the extra time and attention a midwife may offer at some of your visits and the extra medical know-how of a physician's extensive training and expertise at others. You may have the option of a midwife-attended delivery, plus assurance that if a problem develops, a doctor you know is in the wings.

Maternity center or birthing center practice. In these practices, certified midwives provide the bulk of the care, and obs are on call as needed. Some maternity centers are based in hospitals with special birthing rooms, and others are stand-alone facilities. All maternity centers provide care for low-risk patients only.

The benefits of this type of practice are obviously great for moms-to-be who prefer a CNM as their primary practitioner. Another possibly sizable advantage may be the bottom line: CNMs and birthing centers usually charge less than obs and hospitals. That can be a key consideration, since while your health insurance is required to cover maternity and delivery care, you may need to foot part of the bill, depending on the type of insurance you have, your deductible, and whether you go in or out of network. A potential disadvantage of this kind of care: If a complication arises during pregnancy, you may have to switch your care to an ob and start developing a relationship all over again. Or, if a complication comes up during labor or delivery, you may need to be delivered by the doctor on call—someone you may never have met before. And finally, if you are delivering at a freestanding maternity center and complications arise, you may have to be

Centering Pregnancy

Looking for an alternative to the traditional model of prenatal care? Maybe Centering Pregnancy is for you. Instead of booking appointments for monthly checkups, you'll join a group of 8 to 12 other moms-to-be (and their partners) with due dates close to yours, usually for about 10 sessions over your pregnancy and early postpartum (babies attend, too!). You'll get your monthly assessments by your practitioner, as you would with individual care, but you'll also spend about 2 hours at each session getting your questions answered, sharing experiences with the other parents-to-be, and discussing topics ranging from pregnancy nutrition to birthing options.

Think Centering Pregnancy might be just the care you're looking for? Go to centeringhealthcare.org to learn more, and to see if there's a site near you.

transported to the nearest hospital for emergency care.

Independent CNM practice. In the states in which they are permitted to practice independently, CNMs offer women with low-risk pregnancies the advantage of personalized pregnancy care and a low-tech natural delivery (sometimes at home, but more often in birthing centers or hospitals). An independent CNM should have a physician available for consultation as needed and on call in case of emergency—during pregnancy, childbirth, and postpartum. Care by an independent CNM is covered by most health plans, though only some insurers cover midwife-attended home births or births in a facility other than a hospital.

Finding a Candidate

When you have a good idea of the kind of practitioner you want and the type of practice you prefer, where can you find some likely candidates? The following are all good sources:

- Your gyn or family physician (if he or she doesn't do deliveries) or your internist, assuming you're happy with his or her style of practice. Doctors tend to recommend others with philosophies similar to their own.

- Friends, coworkers, or pals from your local group on WhatToExpect.com who've recently given birth and whose personalities and childbirth philosophies are similar to yours.

- Your insurance company, which can give you a list of names of in-network physicians who deliver babies, along with information on their medical training, specialties, special interests, type of practice, and board certification.

- The American Medical Association (ama-assn.org; click on "Doctor Finder") can help you search for a doctor in your area.

- The American Congress of Obstetricians and Gynecologists (ACOG) Physician Directory has the names of obstetricians and maternal-fetal specialists. Go to acog.org and click on "Find an ob-gyn."

- The American College of Nurse-Midwives, if you're looking for a CNM. Go to midwife.org (click on "Find a Midwife").

- The local La Leche League, especially if breastfeeding support is a priority for you.

- A nearby hospital with facilities that are important to you—for example, birthing rooms with whirlpool tubs, rooming-in for both baby and dad, or a NICU (neonatal intensive care unit)—or a local maternity or birthing center you'd like to deliver in. Ask for the names of attending physicians and midwives.

Making Your Selection

Once you've secured a prospective practitioner's name, call to make an appointment for a consult. Go prepared with questions that'll help you figure out if your philosophies are in sync and your personalities mesh comfortably. (Don't expect that you'll agree on everything.) Be observant, too, and try to read between the lines at the interview: Is the doctor or midwife a good listener? A patient explainer? Equally responsive to both you and your partner? Does he or she have a sense of humor, if that's a must for you? Does he or she seem to take your emotional concerns as seriously as your physical ones? Now's the time to find out this candidate's positions on issues that you feel strongly about: unmedicated childbirth versus pain relief as needed or wanted, breastfeeding, induction of labor, use of continuous fetal monitoring or routine IVs, VBAC, water birth, or anything else that's important to you. Knowledge is power—and knowing how your practitioner practices will help ensure there won't be unhappy surprises later.

Almost as important as what the interview reveals about your potential practitioner is what you reveal about yourself. Speak up and let your true patient persona shine through. You'll be able to judge from the practitioner's reaction whether he or she will be comfortable with—and responsive to—you, the patient.

You will also want to consider the hospital or birthing center the practitioner is affiliated with, and whether it provides features that are important to you. Though your delivery preferences clearly shouldn't be your only criteria in picking a practitioner, they should certainly be on the table. Ask about any of the following features and options that are important to you (keeping in mind that no firm birthing decisions can be made until further into your pregnancy and many can't be finalized until the delivery itself): Does the hospital or birthing center offer a tub to labor in, a squat bar for pushing, a comfortable place for dad to room-in, plenty of space for family and friends to hang out in, a NICU? Is there flexibility about rules or procedures that concern you (say, eating or drinking during labor or routine IVs)? Is there an on-call anesthesiologist so you won't have to wait for an epidural if you want one? Is VBAC encouraged (see page 357) if that applies to you? Are "gentle" cesareans offered (see page 353)? Are siblings allowed at delivery? Does the hospital have a Baby-Friendly designation or has it implemented breastfeeding- and baby-friendly policies (such as making skin-to-skin contact right after birth a priority)? Is there round-the-clock breastfeeding support from lactation consultants (or support if you choose not to breastfeed)? See page 323 for more on birth choices and options.

Before you make a final decision, think about whether your potential practitioner inspires trust. Pregnancy is one of the most important journeys you'll ever make, so you'll want to secure a copilot you have faith in.

Where Will You Give Birth?

Absolutely set on giving birth in a hospital? Wondering if a delivering in a birthing center is more your speed? Hoping for a home birth? Pregnancy and childbirth are full of personal choices—often including where you'll be welcoming your brand new baby into the world:

In a hospital. Don't think cold and clinical. The birthing rooms at nearly all hospitals are cozy and family-friendly, with soft lighting, comfy chairs, soothing pictures on the walls, and beds that almost look like they came out of a furniture showroom instead of a hospital supply catalog. Medical equipment is usually stowed out of sight inside home-like cabinetry. The back of the birthing bed can be raised to support a laboring mom in a comfortable position, and the foot of the bed snaps off to make way for the birthing attendants. After delivery, there's a change of sheets, a few flipped switches, and presto, you're back in bed. Many hospitals also offer showers and/or whirlpool tubs in or adjacent to the birthing rooms, both of which can offer hydrotherapy relief during labor. Tubs for water birth are also available in some hospitals (see box, page 326 for more on water birth). Most birthing rooms have sleeper sofas for your coach and other guests.

Most birthing rooms are used just for labor, delivery, and recovery (LDRs), which means you and your baby will most likely be moved from the birthing room to a postpartum room after an hour or so of largely uninterrupted family togetherness.

If you end up needing a c-section, you'll be moved from the birthing room to the operating room, and afterward to a recovery room—but you'll be back in a nice postpartum room as soon as the business of birthing your baby is done.

At a birthing center. Birthing centers, usually freestanding facilities (often just minutes from a hospital, although they may also be attached to—or even located in—a hospital), offer a cozy, low-tech, and personalized place for childbirth, with softly lit private rooms, showers, and whirlpool tubs for labor and water birth. A kitchen may also be available for family members to use. Birthing centers are usually staffed by midwives, but many have on-call obs. And though birthing centers generally do not use interventions such as fetal monitoring, they do have medical equipment on hand so emergency care can be started as needed while waiting for transfer to a nearby hospital. Still, only women with low-risk pregnancies are good candidates for delivery in birthing centers. Something else to consider: Unmedicated childbirth is the focus in a birthing center, and though mild narcotic medications are available, epidurals aren't. If you end up wanting an epidural, you'll have to be transferred to the hospital.

At home. Only about 1 percent of the deliveries in the U.S. are home births. The upside of delivering at home is obvious: Your newborn arrives amid family and friends in a warm and loving atmosphere and you're able to labor and deliver in the familiar comfort and privacy of your own home, without hospital protocols and personnel getting in the way. The downside is that if something unexpectedly goes wrong, the facilities for an emergency cesarean delivery or resuscitation of the newborn will not be close at hand.

Statistics show that there is a slightly higher risk to the baby in a home birth attended by a midwife compared to a hospital birth attended by a midwife. According to the American College of Nurse-Midwives, if you are considering a home birth, you should be in a low-risk category, be attended by a CNM with a consulting physician available, and have transportation readily available and live within 30 miles of a hospital.

CHAPTER 2

Your Pregnancy Profile

T he HPT is positive and the news has (sort of) sunk in: You're having a baby! Excitement is growing, and so are your questions. Many, no doubt, have to do with those wild and crazy symptoms you might already be experiencing. But others may have to do with your personal pregnancy profile. What's a pregnancy profile? No, it's not something you'd post on social media (or that bump selfie you were planning on taking every week). It's actually a compilation of your medical, gynecological, and obstetrical (if you're not a first-timer) histories. In other words, your pregnancy backstory—which may actually impact the pregnancy story that's about to unfold.

Keep in mind that much of this chapter may not apply to you—that's because your pregnancy profile (like the baby you're expecting) is unique. Read what fits your profile and skip what doesn't.

Your Gynecological History

Birth Control During Pregnancy

"I got pregnant while using birth control pills. I kept taking them for over a month because I had no idea I was pregnant. Will this affect my baby?"

I deally, once you stop using oral contraception, you'd have at least one normally occurring menstrual cycle (that is, one that's triggered by your own hormones) before you tried to become pregnant. But conception doesn't always wait for ideal conditions, and while it's pretty uncommon (less than a 1 in 100 chance when used with

A Book for All Families

A family is a family—no matter what its makeup, it's the love that matters most. But as you read *What to Expect When You're Expecting*, you'll notice references to traditional family relationships. These references definitely aren't meant to exclude expectant moms (and their families) who don't mold neatly into that traditional family form—for example, those who are single by choice or by circumstances, who have same-sex partners, or who have chosen not to marry their live-in partners. Rather, the use of a term like "spouse" or "partner" is a way of avoiding phrases (for instance, "your husband or significant other") that are more inclusive but also a mouthful to read. Ditto the use of "dad" instead of "dad or other mom" in referring to the not-pregnant parent. Please mentally edit out any phrase that doesn't fit and replace it with one that's right for you and your loving family.

Are you a couple expecting with a surrogate? This is your pregnancy, too—and your book. Use it to keep track of your surrogate's progress, and your baby's.

perfect consistency), it is possible to become pregnant on the Pill. In spite of warnings you've probably read on the package insert, there's no reason for concern. There's just no good evidence of an increased risk to a baby when mom has conceived while on oral contraception. Need more reassurance? Talk the situation over with your practitioner—you're sure to find it.

You'll likely get the same reassurance from your practitioner if you conceived while using the ring, patch, injections, or implants. These forms of birth control use the same hormones that are in the Pill, which means that just like there's no evidence of an increased risk to a baby when mom has conceived using the Pill, there's also no evidence of increased risk while using other forms of hormonal birth control.

"I conceived while using a condom with spermicides and kept using spermicides before I knew I was pregnant. Should I be worried?"

No need to worry if you got pregnant while using a condom (or diaphragm, cap, or sponge) with spermicides, a spermicide-coated condom, or just plain spermicides. The reassuring news is that there is absolutely no known connection between the use of spermicides and birth defects. So relax and enjoy your pregnancy, even if it did come a little unexpectedly.

"I've been using an IUD as birth control and just discovered that I'm pregnant. Will I be able to have a healthy pregnancy?"

Getting pregnant while using birth control is always a little unsettling (wasn't that why you were using birth control in the first place?), but it does occasionally happen. The odds of its happening with an IUD are pretty low—about 1 in 1,000.

Having beaten the odds and managed conception with an IUD in place leaves you with two options, which you should talk over with your practitioner as soon as possible: leaving the IUD in place or having it taken out. Which of these options is best in your situation will depend on whether or not your practitioner can see the removal cord protruding from your cervix. If the cord isn't visible, the pregnancy has a very good chance of proceeding uneventfully with the IUD in place—even if the IUD is the hormone-releasing kind. It will simply be pushed up against the wall of the uterus by the expanding amniotic sac surrounding the baby and, during childbirth, it will usually deliver with the placenta. If, however, the IUD string is visible early in pregnancy, the risk of an infection developing is increased. In that case, the chances of a safe and successful pregnancy are greater if the IUD is removed as soon as feasible, once conception is confirmed. If it isn't removed, there is a significant risk of miscarriage, but the risk drops to only 20 percent when the IUD is removed. If that doesn't sound all that reassuring, keep in mind that the rate of miscarriage in all known pregnancies is estimated to be about 15 to 20 percent.

If the IUD is left in, be especially alert for bleeding, cramping, or fever during the first trimester, because having an IUD in place puts you at higher risk for early pregnancy complications. Notify your practitioner of such symptoms right away.

Fibroids

"I've had fibroids for several years, and they've never caused me any problems. Will they now that I'm pregnant?"

Chances are your fibroids won't stand between you and an uncomplicated pregnancy. In fact, most often these small nonmalignant growths on the inner walls of the uterus don't affect a pregnancy at all.

Sometimes, a mom-to-be with fibroids notices abdominal pressure or pain, though it's usually nothing to worry about. Still, report it to your practitioner. Reduced activity or modified bed rest for 4 or 5 days along with a safe pain reliever usually brings relief.

Very occasionally, fibroids can slightly increase the risk of such complications as abruption (separation) of the placenta, preterm birth, and breech birth. Since every case of fibroids—like every expectant mom—is different, talk yours over with your practitioner so you can find out more about the condition in general and the risks, if any, in your particular case. If your practitioner suspects that the fibroids could interfere with a safe vaginal delivery, he or she may opt to deliver by c-section. In most cases, however, even a large fibroid will move out of the baby's way as the uterus expands during pregnancy.

"I had a couple of fibroids removed a few years ago. Will that affect my pregnancy?"

In most cases, surgery for the removal of small uterine fibroid tumors (particularly if the surgery was performed laparoscopically) doesn't affect a subsequent pregnancy. Extensive surgery for large fibroids could, however, weaken the uterus enough so that it wouldn't be able to handle labor. If your practitioner decides this might be true of your uterus, a c-section will be planned. Become familiar with the signs of early labor in case contractions begin before the planned surgery, and have a plan in place for getting to the hospital quickly if you do go into labor.

Endometriosis

"After years of suffering with endometriosis, I'm finally pregnant. Will I have problems with my pregnancy?"

Endometriosis is typically associated with two challenges: problems becoming pregnant, and pain. Becoming pregnant means that you've overcome the first of those challenges (congratulations!). And the good news gets even better. Being pregnant may actually help with the second challenge.

Endometriosis causes pain in the pelvic area because tissue from the uterine lining (called the endometrium) grows outside the uterus and reacts to the hormonal changes of the menstrual cycle by thickening, breaking down, and bleeding (as the uterine lining normally does). During pregnancy, when ovulation and menstruation take a hiatus and progesterone increases, these so-called endometrial implants become smaller and less tender, often inducing a bit of remission from the pain endometriosis causes. In fact, many moms-to-be are symptom-free or nearly so during the entire pregnancy—though some may start to feel discomfort as baby grows and begins packing a stronger punch, particularly if those punches and kicks reach tender areas.

The less happy news is that pregnancy provides only a break from the symptoms of endometriosis, not a cure. After pregnancy and breastfeeding (and sometimes earlier), the symptoms usually return. The other less happy news is that women with endometriosis do face an increased risk of ectopic pregnancy (so be sure to be alert for associated signs; see page 588), as well as preterm birth. Because of these increased risks, your practitioner will likely monitor your pregnancy more frequently (with more frequent ultrasounds, for instance). Finally, in the very unlikely case that you've had uterine surgery for your condition, your practitioner will probably opt to deliver via c-section.

Colposcopy

"A year before I got pregnant, I had a cervical biopsy and a LEEP to remove some abnormal cells. Does this put my pregnancy at any risk?"

Happily, probably not. The cervical biopsy itself definitely isn't a concern, since the sampling of cells taken is tiny. The LEEP (loop electrocautery excision procedure, which cuts away abnormal cervical tissue using an electrical current) is also very unlikely to have any impact on a future pregnancy—in fact, the vast majority of women who have a LEEP are able to have completely normal pregnancies. Ditto for women who had their abnormal cells treated with cryosurgery (when the abnormal cells are frozen). Some women, however, depending on how much tissue was removed during either type of treatment, may be at a somewhat increased risk for certain complications, such as cervical insufficiency (sometimes called incompetent cervix) and preterm delivery. Make sure your prenatal practitioner knows about your cervical history so that your pregnancy can be more closely monitored.

If abnormal cells are found during a routine Pap smear during your first prenatal visit, your practitioner may opt to perform a colposcopy for a closer look, but biopsies or further procedures are usually delayed until after the baby is born.

Previous Abortions

"I've had two abortions. Will that have any impact on this pregnancy?"

Multiple first-trimester abortions aren't likely to have an effect on future pregnancies. So if the abortions were performed before the 14th week, chances are there's no cause for concern. Multiple second-trimester abortions (performed between 14 and 27 weeks), however, may slightly increase the risk of premature delivery. In either case, be sure your practitioner knows about the abortions. The more familiar

Other STDs and Pregnancy

Not surprisingly, most STDs can affect pregnancy. Fortunately, most can be easily and safely treated, even during pregnancy. But because women are often unaware of being infected, the CDC recommends that all expectant mothers be tested early in pregnancy for the STDs most likely to pose a serious risk to mom and baby. These include:

Gonorrhea. Gonorrhea has long been known to cause conjunctivitis, blindness, and serious generalized infection in a baby delivered through an infected birth canal. An expectant mom who tests positive for gonorrhea will be treated immediately with antibiotics. Treatment is followed by another culture to be sure the mom is infection-free. As an added precaution, an antibiotic ointment is squeezed into the eyes of every newborn at birth.

Syphilis. Because this STD can cause a variety of birth defects as well as stillbirth, testing is routine at the first prenatal visit. Antibiotic treatment of infected pregnant women before the 4th month, when the infection usually begins to cross the placental barrier, almost always prevents harm to the fetus. The very good news is that mother-to-baby transmission of syphilis is rare.

Chlamydia. More common than syphilis or gonorrhea and occurring most often in sexually active women under age 26 (especially those who have had multiple partners), chlamydia is the most common infection passed from mother to baby, and is considered a potential risk to both. Because half of women infected with chlamydia don't have symptoms (which means it's possible to have picked it up at some point and not know it), routine screening is important.

The best time to treat chlamydia is before pregnancy. But prompt treatment with antibiotics (usually azithromycin) during pregnancy can prevent transmission of the infection to baby (in the form of pneumonia, which fortunately is usually mild, and eye infection, which is occasionally severe) at delivery.

he or she is with your complete reproductive history, the better care you and your baby will get.

HPV (Human Papillomavirus)

"Can having genital HPV affect my pregnancy?"

Genital HPV is the most common sexually transmitted virus in the U.S., though thanks to the HPV vaccine, the numbers of those affected are declining. Most people who become infected with it never know, because most of the time, HPV causes no obvious symptoms and usually resolves on its own within 6 to 10 months.

There are some times, however, when HPV does cause symptoms. Some strains cause cervical cell irregularities (detected on a Pap smear), and other strains can cause genital warts (in appearance they can vary from a barely visible lesion to a soft, velvety "flat" bump or a cauliflower-like growth; colors range from pale to dark pink) that will show up in and on the vagina, vulva, and rectum. Though usually painless, genital warts may occasionally burn, itch, or even bleed. In most cases,

The antibiotic ointment routinely used at birth protects the newborn from chlamydial, as well as gonorrheal, eye infection.

Trichomoniasis. The symptoms of this parasite-caused STD (also referred to as trichomonas infection, or "trich") are a greenish, frothy vaginal discharge with an unpleasant fishy smell and, often, itching. About half of those affected have no symptoms at all. Though the disease does not usually cause serious illness or pregnancy problems (or affect a baby whose mom is infected), the symptoms can be irritating. Generally, expectant moms with symptoms of trichomoniasis are tested, and if found positive for the infection, are treated safely with antibiotics.

HIV infection. ACOG recommends (and most states require) that all pregnant women be counseled about and screened for HIV as early as possible during each pregnancy unless they decline the test (so-called "opt out testing"). That's because infection in pregnancy by the HIV virus, which causes AIDS, is a threat not just to the expectant mom but to her baby as well. About 25 percent of babies born to untreated mothers will develop the infection (testing will confirm it in the first 6 months of life). Fortunately, the treatments that are now available offer plenty of hope for infected moms and their babies-to-be. Treating an HIV-positive pregnant woman with AZT (also known as ZDV or Retrovir) or other antiretroviral drugs can dramatically reduce the risk of her passing the infection on to her baby, without any harmful side effects. For women with a high amount of HIV in their body, delivering by elective c-section (before contractions begin and before membranes rupture) can reduce the risk of transmission even more.

If you're not sure whether you've been tested for STDs, check with your practitioner. Testing is a vital precaution to take in pregnancy, even if you're pretty certain you couldn't be infected with an STD. If a test does turn out to be positive, treatment (for both you and your partner, if necessary) will protect not only your health, but that of your baby-to-be.

the warts clear without treatment within a couple of months.

How does having an active case of genital HPV affect a pregnancy? Luckily, it's unlikely to affect it at all. Occasionally, however, the hormonal changes of pregnancy can cause the warts to multiply or get larger. If that's the case with you, and if the warts don't seem to be clearing on their own, your practitioner may recommend treatment during pregnancy—especially if the warts get so big that they obstruct your birth canal. The warts can be safely removed by freezing, electrical heat, or laser therapy. If they're not impacting your pregnancy, this treatment may be delayed until after delivery.

If you do have HPV, your practitioner will also check your cervix to make sure there are no cervical cell irregularities. But even if abnormalities are found, any necessary cervical biopsies to remove the abnormal cells will likely be postponed until after your baby arrives.

Worried about whether your baby can catch your HPV infection? Don't be. HPV transmission to babies is very low—and even in the unlikely case that a baby does get the HPV virus, it typically clears without treatment.

HPV can be prevented with the HPV vaccine, which is recommended for all girls and boys beginning at age 11 or 12 but can also be given through age 26 if it wasn't previously. The vaccine is given in a series of 3 doses, and if you started the series and then became pregnant before completing it, you'll need to hold off on the remaining doses until after your baby is born.

Herpes

"I have genital herpes. Can my baby catch it from me?"

The chances are excellent that your baby will arrive safe, sound, and completely unaffected by herpes, particularly if you and your practitioner take protective steps during pregnancy and delivery. Here's what you need to know.

First of all, infection in a newborn is rare. A baby has a less than 1 percent chance of contracting the condition if a mom has a recurrent infection (that is, she's had herpes before) during pregnancy. Second, though a primary infection (one that appears for the first time) in pregnancy increases the risk of miscarriage and premature delivery, that kind of infection is uncommon, since pregnant women and their partners are far less likely to participate in at-risk behaviors (such as having unprotected sex with a new partner). Even for babies at greatest risk—those whose moms have their first herpes outbreak as delivery nears (again, a very unlikely scenario)—there is an up to 50 percent chance that they will arrive infection-free. If you haven't had genital herpes before, and show any signs of a primary infection (fever, headache, fatigue, and achiness for 2 or more days, accompanied by genital pain, itching, pain when urinating, vaginal and urethral discharge, and tenderness in the groin, as well as lesions that blister and then crust over), call your practitioner.

If you picked up your herpes infection before pregnancy, the risk to your baby is very low. To lower it even more, your practitioner will probably give you antiviral meds beginning at week 36 of your pregnancy—even if you don't have active lesions. If you end up having active lesions when labor starts, you'll probably have a c-section to protect your little one from infection in the birth canal. In the unlikely event a baby is infected, he or she will be treated with an antiviral drug.

After delivery, the right precautions can allow you to care for—and breast-feed—your baby without passing along the virus, even during an active infection.

Your Obstetrical History

In Vitro Fertilization (IVF)

"I conceived my baby through IVF. How different will my pregnancy be?"

Some well-deserved congratulations on your IVF success! With all you've been through to get to pregnancy, you've earned some smooth sailing—and happily, you're likely to get it. The fact that conception took place in a lab instead of in your fallopian tube shouldn't impact your pregnancy all that much, at least once the first trimester is over. The same is true for a baby conceived via other fertility treatments (such as ICSI or GIFT). Early on, however, there will be some differences in your pregnancy and your care.

Because a positive test doesn't necessarily mean that a pregnancy will stick (particularly since IVF pregnancies are usually confirmed by blood tests super-early on), because trying again can be so emotionally and financially draining, and because it's not known right off how many of the transferred embryos are going to develop into fetuses, the first 6 weeks or so of an IVF pregnancy are usually more nerve-racking than most. Expect to spend more time in your fertility specialist's office—for repeat blood work and ultrasounds. Sex and other physical activities may be restricted, and you might even be put on modified bed rest (though studies show that bed rest doesn't seem to help boost odds of IVF success). And as an added precaution, the hormone progesterone (and possibly baby aspirin) will likely be prescribed to help support your developing pregnancy during the first 2 to 3 months.

But once this extra-cautious period is past (and once you've graduated to your regular prenatal practitioner, usually at about 8 to 12 weeks), you can expect that your pregnancy will be pretty much like everyone else's—unless it turns out that you have multiple baby passengers on board, as more than 40 percent of IVF moms do. If you do, see Chapter 15.

The Second Time Around

"This is my second pregnancy. How will it be different from the first?"

Since no two pregnancies are exactly alike, there's no predicting how different (or how similar) these 9 months will be from the last. There are some generalities, however, about second and

---

Do Tell

Whatever's in your past, now's not the time to try to put it behind you. In fact, your sexual, reproductive, and medical history are more important (and relevant) than you might think. Previous pregnancies (and any complications), miscarriages, abortions, surgeries, STDs, or other infections may or may not have an impact on what happens in this pregnancy, but be sure to share any information you have about them—or any aspect of your history—with your practitioner (all will be kept confidential). Share, too, any history of depression or other mental illness, as well as any history of eating disorders. The more your practitioner knows about you, the better he or she will be able to care for you and your baby-to-be.

---

subsequent pregnancies that hold true at least some of the time (like all generalities, none will hold true all of the time):

- You'll probably "feel" pregnant sooner. Like most second-timers, you'll probably be more attuned to the early symptoms of pregnancy and more apt to know them when you feel them.

- You'll likely have a repeat when it comes to pregnancy symptoms. In general, your first pregnancy is a pretty good predictor of future pregnancies, all things being equal. That said, all pregnancies, like all babies, are different—and that could mean that your symptoms in this pregnancy may be different, too. Some symptoms may seem less noticeable because you're too busy to pay attention to them (or in the case of fatigue, you're already so tired, who can tell?). Some may appear

Room for Improvement?

Have every symptom in the book the first time around? Or even a complication or two? That doesn't necessarily mean you won't have better luck (and smoother sailing) this time. In fact, if there was room for improvement in your first pregnancy, now's your chance to make some of the tweaks that might reduce your chances of bumps along the way to baby 2, including: gaining weight at a steady rate and keeping the gain within the recommended guidelines (see page 177), eating well (see Chapter 4 to find out how), getting enough and the right kind of exercise (see page 229 for guidelines), and finding ways to relax if you're a stress mama. Having older children can often exacerbate pregnancy symptoms; see the box on the facing page for tips on minimizing pregnancy symptoms when you're combining the work of being a mom and a mom-to-be.

sooner (like urinary frequency) and some may appear later or not at all. And some symptoms—like food cravings and aversions, breast enlargement and sensitivity—are typically (but not universally) less pronounced in second and subsequent pregnancies due to a body that's been there and done that. You may worry less, too, especially if you did a lot of worrying in your first pregnancy.

- You'll "look pregnant" sooner. Thanks to abdominal and uterine muscles that are more lax (there's no gentler way to put that), you're likely to "pop" much sooner than you did the first time. You may notice, too, that your baby-number-2 bump looks different from your bump with baby number 1. Baby number 2 (or 3 or 4) is liable to be larger than your firstborn, too, so you may have a heavier load to carry around. Another potential result of those loosened-up abs: Pregnancy back and hip aches may be more of a pain—and may appear earlier.

- You'll probably feel movement sooner. Something happy to thank those looser muscles for—chances are you'll be able to feel baby kicking much sooner this time around, possibly as early as 16 weeks (maybe even sooner, maybe later). You're also more likely to know it when you feel it, having felt it before. Of course, placenta placement can make a difference in when those first kicks are noticed, even in second or subsequent pregnancies.

- You may not feel as excited. That's not to say you aren't happy to be expecting again. But you may notice that the excitement level isn't quite as over-the-top. This is a completely normal reaction (again, you've been here before) and in no way reflects on your love for your baby-to-be. Keep in mind, too, that you're preoccupied (physically and emotionally) with the little one who's already here.

- You will probably have an easier and faster labor and delivery. Here's the really good part about those laxer muscles. All that loosening up (particularly in the areas involved in childbirth), combined with your body's prior experience, may help ensure a speedier exit for baby number 2. Though there are no sure bets in the birthing room, just about every phase of labor is likely to be shorter, and pushing time will probably be significantly reduced—second babies often pop out in a matter of minutes.

Keeping Up with the Kids

For some second-time mamas-to-be, keeping up with a little one (or little ones) keeps them so busy that they barely have time to notice pregnancy discomforts, major or minor. For others, all the running around that comes with running after kids tends to aggravate pregnancy symptoms. For example, morning sickness and heartburn can increase during times of stress (the getting-to-school or the getting-dinner-on-the-table rush, for instance). Fatigue can (big duh) be even more draining because there doesn't seem to be any time to rest. Backaches can be an extra pain if you're doing a lot of tot toting. Even constipation becomes more likely if you never have a chance to use the bathroom when the urge strikes. You are also more likely to come down with colds and other illnesses, courtesy of older germ-spreading kids.

It's not realistic to always put your pregnant body first when you've got another little body clamoring for care (the days of pampered pregnancy almost certainly ended with your first delivery). But taking more time to take care of yourself—putting up your feet while you read that story, napping (instead of vacuuming) while your toddler naps, getting into the healthy snack habit even when there's no time for sit-down meals, and taking advantage of help whenever it's available— can help lighten the load your body's carrying, minimizing those pregnancy miseries.

"I had some complications with my first pregnancy. Will this one be just as rough?"

One complicated pregnancy definitely doesn't predict another one. While some pregnancy complications can repeat, most don't repeat routinely—and some are extremely unlikely to strike twice (for instance, a complication that was triggered by a onetime event, like an infection). You're also less likely to have a repeat of complications that were caused by lifestyle habits you've since improved (say, not eating well or not getting any exercise). If the cause was a chronic health problem, such as diabetes, controlling the condition before you become pregnant can greatly reduce the risk of repeat complications. Also keep this in mind: Even if the complications you faced last time have a chance of repeating no matter what prevention steps you take, earlier detection and treatment (because you and your practitioner will be on the lookout for a repeat) can make a big difference.

Discuss with your practitioner the complications you had last time and what can be done to prevent them from repeating. No matter what the problems or their causes (even if no cause was ever pinpointed), the tips in the box on the facing page can help make your pregnancy more comfortable and safer for both you and your baby.

Back-to-Back Pregnancies

"I got pregnant again just 10 weeks after delivering my first baby—and while we're happy about it, let's just say we didn't plan it that way. Does becoming pregnant again so soon put any added risk on me or the baby?"

Repeat Miscarriages

When you've had recurring miscarriages (defined as 2 or 3 in a row), it's understandably hard for you to believe that a healthy pregnancy and a healthy baby can be in your future, as much as you hope for it. But it can be—especially with the right care and the right management.

The causes of repeated early miscarriages are sometimes unknown, but there are tests that may shed light on why the miscarriages took place— even if they each had a different cause. Trying to determine the cause of a single loss usually isn't worthwhile, but a medical evaluation and testing will probably be recommended if you've had 2 or more consecutive miscarriages.

Recurrent miscarriage was once a mystery far more often than not, but much progress has been made in uncovering its causes. Many tests can now pick up risk factors for pregnancy loss, and there are more effective strategies for preventing a future one. So talk to your practitioner to discuss the options in your case, which might include referral to a maternal-fetal specialist.

Some of the tests you may be offered after your repeat miscarriages include:

- A karyotyping blood test for both you and the baby's father to see if either of you carries a balanced translocation—an altered chromosome arrangement, which may be the cause of the miscarriages

- A blood test for antiphospholipid antibodies (antibodies that attack a woman's own tissues, causing blood clots that can clog the maternal blood vessels that feed the placenta)

- An ultrasound before pregnancy where saline is infused into the uterus to check for anatomical problems

- An analysis of the chromosomal makeup of the miscarried embryo or fetus, which can help determine a cause for the miscarriages

- Tests for vitamin deficiencies

- Tests of hormone levels

Once you know the cause, or causes, you can talk to your practitioner about what kind of treatment or treatments might best protect your next pregnancy. In some instances, patients with a history of early or late miscarriages can benefit from hormone therapy: progesterone for women who appear to be producing too little of this important pregnancy hormone, or a medication to reduce levels of the hormone prolactin in the mother's blood if tests show that excess prolactin is the cause. If a thyroid problem is detected, it can be treated easily.

Even if a cause can't be identified and treated, you still have a good chance of sustaining a successful pregnancy. But that may be hard for you to believe or even to hope for. It will be important to find ways of managing any understandable fear that being pregnant again will mean you'll miscarry again. Yoga, meditation, visualization techniques, and deep-breathing exercises can help with the anxiety, and support can come from other women who've suffered similar losses (you'll find plenty of sharing going on in the WhatToExpect.com Grief and Loss forum). Communicating your feelings openly with your partner may also help. Remember, you're in this together.

For more on miscarriage, see Chapter 20, starting on page 582. For more on detailed information on preventing a repeat pregnancy loss, see *What to Expect Before You're Expecting.*

Expanding your family (and your belly) again a little sooner than expected? Starting another pregnancy before you've fully recovered from the last one can be hard enough without adding stress to the mix. So first of all, relax. Though closely spaced pregnancies can take their physical toll on a mom-to-be who just became a mom, there are lots of things you can do to help your body better handle the challenge of back-to-back (or bump-to-bump) baby making, including:

- Getting the best prenatal care, starting as soon as you think you're pregnant. Very closely spaced pregnancies (when there's less than 12 months between pregnancies) increases the risk for preterm birth, though getting good prenatal care from the get-go can help reduce that risk.

- Eating as well as you can (see Chapter 4). Your body probably hasn't had a chance to rebuild the stores of vitamins and nutrients that were tapped to make your last baby, and that can put you at a nutritional disadvantage, particularly if you're still breastfeeding. You may need to overcompensate nutritionally to be sure both you and the baby you're currently carrying don't get shortchanged. Continue taking your prenatal vitamins, of course (or start them up again if you already quit), but don't stop there. Try not to let lack of time or energy (you'll have little of both, that's for sure) keep you from eating enough or well enough. Healthy grazing may help you fit those much-needed nutrients into your busy schedule, so stock up on wholesome, ready-to-grab munchables like cheese sticks, almonds, freeze-dried fruit, and mini bags of baby carrots to dip in ready-to-serve hummus.

- Gaining the right amount of weight. Your brand new baby boarder doesn't care whether or not you've had time to shed the extra pounds his or her sibling just finished putting on you—which means you'll probably have to shelve any plans to drop that baby weight until you deliver this baby. Talk over a sensible weight gain goal with your practitioner (which might be the same, lower, or higher than last time). Focus on the quality of the food you eat (always important during pregnancy, but especially important when you're going back-to-back), but also keep an eye on the scale.

- Fair-share feeding. If you're breastfeeding your newborn, you can continue as long as you want to and feel up to it (see box, page 30).

- Resting up. You need more rest than may be humanly (and new-motherly) possible. Getting close to that rest quota will require not only your own determination but help from your spouse and others as well. Set priorities, too: Let less important chores or work go undone, and force yourself to nap (or at least put your feet up) when your baby is napping. If you're not breastfeeding, daddy can take over night feedings. If you are, he can do the baby-fetching at 2 a.m.

- Exercising. Getting through a day (and a night) with a newborn might seem workout enough—especially now that you've added the around-the-clock demands of baby growing to your exhausted body's to-do list. Still, the right amount and the right kind of exercise can boost your energy level when you need that boost most—plus, boost your odds of a healthier and more comfortable pregnancy. If you can't seem to find the time for a regular pregnancy workout routine, build physical activity into your day with your baby—a couple of 15-minute

Breastfeeding While Pregnant

Still breastfeeding your precious bundle, but just discovered there's another baby bun baking away? Breastfeeding and pregnancy are usually perfectly compatible—which means there's probably no need to retire your breasts for the next 9 months if you don't want to.

Have concerns that the oxytocin that's released during breastfeeding might cause contractions that could lead to miscarriage or early labor? Not to worry. In a low-risk pregnancy, the mild contractions triggered by nursing aren't a problem. In fact, until your uterus is ready to switch from baby-boarding to baby-birthing mode (usually around 38 weeks), oxytocin doesn't seem to have much effect on the uterus at all.

Having a hard time keeping anything down, never mind eating well enough to fuel both baby growing and milk production (a combo that can require upward of 800 extra calories per day)? Morning sickness can be a drain, literally—and that can deplete you of the nutrients and fluids necessary to nourish the baby that's already here and the one that's on the way. If nausea and vomiting are especially severe, and if you're losing weight early on, discuss this challenge with your practitioner. You both might come to the conclusion that the best choice for all three of you (mom, baby, and baby-to-be) is to wean your firstborn. But if your morning sickness is manageable and you're not losing weight—and if your practitioner supports you—you can ride out the first few months and use the remaining 2 trimesters to further bump up your pregnancy weight gain and reestablish those depleted nutrient stores. That way you can be sure you, your baby, and your baby-to-be are getting all the calories and nutrients necessary.

Concerned that the pregnancy hormones circulating in your system might find their way into your milk? Happily, your breast milk is just as safe now that you're pregnant, and experts say pregnancy hormones don't pass easily to breast milk.

Wondering whether your breast milk supply might start slowing down once the demands of pregnancy start picking up? It probably will, but usually not until midpregnancy. Your breastfeeding baby may or may not notice any slowdown in milk production. Another thing your breastfeeding baby may or may not notice: changes in the consistency or taste of your milk supply once colostrum starts being produced (again, usually midway through pregnancy).

Some little ones decide to self-wean at some point in mom's pregnancy (either because of the decreased milk supply or the changes in taste), while others never miss a breastfeeding beat, even after the arrival of a new nurser. In fact, assuming you and your milk supply are still going strong after you've delivered your latest bundle, you can breastfeed both your newborn and your older baby (tandem nursing).

If your baby does opt to wean, or if you just don't feel up to breastfeeding while you're expecting (or you're too sick or tired to continue), don't feel guilty about calling it quits. You've already provided your little (if soon-to-be-older) one with many of the benefits of breastfeeding, and those continued cuddles and kisses will keep the bond between you as tight as ever. Another option if you aren't up to full-time breastfeeding but you're also not ready to fully wean: do the combo (supplement with formula as needed or wanted).

walks will do the trick. Or enroll in a pregnancy exercise class or swim at a club or community center that offers babysitting services. Or let baby watch from the infant seat while you bop to the *What to Expect When You're Expecting Pregnancy Workout* DVD.

Having a Big Family

"I'm pregnant with my sixth child. Does this put me or the baby at any extra risk?"

The more, the merrier in your home? Then here's another reason to celebrate: Adding to your family for a sixth (or more) time doesn't come with added risks. In fact, beyond a small jump in the incidence of multiple births (twins, triplets, and so on—which could mean that your large brood could potentially grow even larger still), a mom of many is as likely to have an uncomplicated pregnancy as a mom of 1 or 2. Just make sure that caring for this pregnancy (and yourself) doesn't take a backseat to caring for all the little ones you already have in the backseat (of your probably extra large minivan). See box, page 27 for tips.

Preterm Birth

"I had a preterm delivery in my first pregnancy. I've done everything I can to lower my risk, but I'm still worried about a repeat."

Congratulations on doing everything you can to make sure your pregnancy is as healthy as possible this time around—and to give your baby the very best chances of staying on board until term. That's a great first step. Together with your practitioner, there are probably even more steps you can take to minimize the chances for a repeat preterm labor.

If you had a previous spontaneous preterm birth, ask your practitioner if you're a good candidate for progesterone shots. Research shows that giving the hormone progesterone as weekly shots starting at 16 weeks of pregnancy and continuing through week 36 reduces the risk for preterm birth in women who've delivered early before and who are carrying only one baby.

Your practitioner might also offer you a fetal fibronectin (fFN) screening test, which looks for signs of preterm labor in women who have risk factors for having a premature baby (such as a previous preterm delivery). Fetal fibronectin is the glue your body makes to hold your baby in your uterus. If the test—which is done in your practitioner's office—comes back negative (meaning the fFN hasn't started to break down yet and therefore isn't detectable), it means the odds of delivering within the next 2 weeks are less than 1 percent (so you can breathe easy). If it's positive, your risk of going into preterm labor is significantly higher, and your practitioner may take steps to prolong your pregnancy and prepare your baby's lungs for an early delivery.

Another screening test for preterm labor in women who have had a prior one is cervical length. The length of your cervix is measured via ultrasound, and if there are any signs that the cervix is short, your practitioner may prescribe a daily progesterone gel—it comes in a tampon-like applicator that you place in your vagina—starting at week 20 of pregnancy and continuing until 37 weeks. If you're already on progesterone shots due to a prior premature birth and ultrasound shows that your cervix has shortened midway through pregnancy, your practitioner may recommend cerclage (stitching the cervix). See the next question to learn more.

Also ask about a new type of blood test given at 20 weeks that may help predict the risk of preterm labor.

Your Pregnancy Profile and Preterm Birth

Just about 12 percent of births are considered premature, or preterm—that is, occurring before completion of the 37th week of pregnancy. And around half of these occur in women who are known to be at high risk for premature delivery, including the ever-multiplying percentage of moms-to-be of multiples.

Is there anything you can do to help prevent preterm birth if your pregnancy profile puts you at higher risk for it? In some cases, there isn't: Even when a risk factor is identified (and it won't always be), it can't necessarily be controlled. But in other cases, the risk factor or factors that might lead to an early birth can be controlled or at least minimized. Eliminate any that apply to you, and you may up the chances that your baby will stay put until term. Here are some known risk factors for premature labor that can be controlled:

Too little or too much weight gain. Gaining too little weight can increase the chances your baby will be born early, but so can packing on too many pounds. Conceiving at your ideal body weight and gaining just the right number of pounds for your pregnancy profile can provide your baby with a healthier, more nurturing uterine environment and, ideally, a better chance of staying safely ensconced until term. So set an ideal weight-gain goal with your practitioner—and then try your best to meet it.

Not enough nutrients. Giving your baby the healthiest start in life isn't just about gaining the right number of pounds—it's about gaining them on the right types of foods. A diet that lacks necessary nutrients (especially folate, the dietary version of folic acid) increases your risk for premature delivery, while a diet that's nutrition packed decreases that risk.

Too much standing or heavy physical labor. Definitely no need to sit out pregnancy—in fact, staying active is just what the doctor (or midwife) orders for most moms-to-be. And everyday kind of standing—like when you're shopping at the mall or in line at the movies—isn't a problem in a normal pregnancy. But if your job involves long hours on your feet every day—especially if it involves heavy physical labor or lifting—check with your practitioner to see if you should cut back or request a change in work duties, especially late in pregnancy.

Extreme emotional stress. Some studies have shown a link between extreme emotional stress (not your everyday, life-in-the-fast-lane, my-work-is-never-done stress) and premature labor. What's the difference between a normal stress level and extreme stress? Normal stress may keep you on your toes—let's face it, even on the run—but it's manageable, and you can thrive on it. Extreme stress, on the other hand, is unhealthy—it drains and debilitates you, keeps you from sleeping well, keeps you from eating well, keeps you from enjoying life. Sometimes the cause of such excessive stress can be eliminated or minimized (by quitting or cutting back at an unhealthily high-pressure job, for example), and sometimes it's unavoidable (as when a lost job leaves you with a pile of unpaid bills, or there's been an illness or a death in the family). Still, many kinds of stress can be reduced with relaxation techniques, a healthy diet, a balance of exercise and rest, and by talking over the problems that are getting you down with your spouse or friends, your practitioner, or a therapist.

Alcohol and drug use. Moms-to-be who use alcohol and illegal drugs increase their risk of having a premature delivery.

Smoking. Smoking during pregnancy may be linked to an increased risk of premature delivery. Quitting before conception or as early as possible in pregnancy is best, but quitting at any time in pregnancy is definitely better than not quitting at all.

Gum infection. Some studies show that gum disease is associated with preterm delivery. Researchers suspect that the bacteria that cause inflammation in the gums can get into the bloodstream, reach the fetus, and initiate early delivery. Another proposed possibility: The bacteria that cause inflammation in the gums can also trigger the immune system to produce inflammation in the cervix and uterus, triggering early labor. Regularly brushing and flossing and staying up to date on dental cleanings and other dental care can prevent infections. Treating existing infections before pregnancy may also help lower the risk for a variety of complications, including preterm labor.

Cervical insufficiency. The risk of premature delivery as a result of an incompetent cervix—in which a weak cervix opens early—can possibly be reduced by stitching the cervix closed (cerclage) and/or by closely monitoring the length of the cervix via ultrasound (see page 34 for more).

History of preterm birth. Your chances of a preterm birth are higher if you've had one in the past. Your practitioner may prescribe progesterone shots or gels during this pregnancy to avoid a repeat preterm birth.

The following risk factors aren't controllable, but in some cases they can be somewhat modified. In others, knowing they exist can help you and your practitioner best manage the risks, as well as greatly improve the outcome if an early birth becomes inevitable:

Multiples. The optimal time for the delivery of twins is at 38 weeks. But many moms of twins (and more) deliver earlier. Good prenatal care, optimal nutrition, and the elimination of other risk factors, along with restriction of activity and more time spent resting in the last trimester, may help prevent a too-early birth. See Chapter 15.

Premature cervical shortening. In some moms-to-be, for reasons unknown and apparently unrelated to cervical insufficiency, the cervix begins to shorten mid-pregnancy, putting them at increased risk for preterm birth. A routine ultrasound of the cervix mid-pregnancy may uncover that increased risk. Treatment with progesterone gels or suppositories may be prescribed in some cases to try to prolong pregnancy.

Pregnancy complications. Gestational diabetes, preeclampsia, and excessive amniotic fluid, as well as problems with the placenta, such as placenta previa or placental abruption, can make an early delivery more likely. Managing these conditions as best as possible may help pregnancy reach term.

Chronic maternal illness. Chronic conditions, and heart, liver, or kidney disease, may raise the risk for preterm delivery, but good care may help prevent complications.

General infections. Certain infections (some STDs, urinary, cervical, vaginal, and kidney infections) can increase the risk for preterm labor. When the infection is one that could prove harmful to the fetus, early labor may be the body's way of attempting to rescue the baby from an unhealthy environment. Preventing the infection or promptly treating it may prevent a too-soon birth.

Age. Teen moms-to-be are often at a higher risk for preterm delivery. Older moms (over age 35) are also more likely to give birth early. Good nutrition and prenatal care can help reduce the risk.

Cervical Insufficiency

"I had a miscarriage in the 5th month of my first pregnancy, due to cervical insufficiency. I just had a positive pregnancy test, and I'm worried that I'll have the same problem again."

The good news (and there is good news here) is that it doesn't have to happen again. Now that your cervical insufficiency (also known as incompetent cervix) has been diagnosed as the cause of your past pregnancy loss, your doctor should be able to take steps to prevent it from causing another loss. With proper treatment and careful watching, the odds of your having a healthy pregnancy and a safe delivery this time around are very much in your favor.

An incompetent cervix, one that opens prematurely under the pressure of the growing uterus and fetus, is estimated to occur in 1 or 2 of every 100 pregnancies, and it is believed responsible for 10 to 20 percent of all second-trimester miscarriages. It's usually diagnosed when a woman miscarries in the second trimester after experiencing progressive painless effacement (shortening and thinning) and dilation of the cervix without apparent uterine contractions or vaginal bleeding. While it's unclear precisely what causes cervical insufficiency, it may be the result of genetic weakness of the cervix, extreme stretching of or severe lacerations to the cervix during one or more previous deliveries, an extensive "cone" biopsy done for precancerous cervical cells, or cervical surgery or laser therapy. A multiple pregnancy can also lead to cervical insufficiency (due to the extra weight of an extra baby pressing on the cervix), but if it does, the problem will not usually recur in a later single-baby pregnancy.

To help protect this pregnancy, your ob may perform cerclage—a simple procedure to stitch up the opening of the cervix—when you're in your second trimester (anywhere from 12 to 22 weeks). Cerclage is done through the vagina under local or epidural anesthesia. Twelve hours after surgery, you'll be able to resume normal activities, though sex may not be allowed for the rest of your pregnancy, and you may need more frequent prenatal exams. Usually the sutures are removed a few weeks before the estimated due date. In some cases, they may not be removed until labor begins, unless there is infection, bleeding, or premature rupture of the membranes.

However, there's a lot of controversy about how effective cerclage is and whether it should be performed routinely on women who have cervical insufficiency. Some doctors will perform it only on a woman with a prior history of preterm birth (one that occurred before 34 weeks) when ultrasound done before 24 weeks shows that the cervix is shortening or opening. Others will perform cerclage as a preventive measure between weeks 13 and 16 in women who have had one or more second-trimester losses, even if there's no evidence of cervical weakness or shortening. Cerclage is not currently recommended for a woman who has a short cervix in the second trimester but hasn't had a prior pregnancy loss—in this case vaginal progesterone gel is recommended. Cerclage is not performed in a multiple pregnancy, either.

Whether or not you have a cerclage placed this time, your history means you'll have to be alert for signs of an impending problem in the second or early third trimester: pressure in the lower abdomen, bloody discharge, unusual urinary frequency, or the sensation of a lump in the vagina. If you experience any of these, call your doctor right away.

Rh Incompatibility

"My doctor said my blood tests show I am Rh negative. What does that mean for my baby?"

Fortunately, it doesn't mean much, at least now that both you and your doctor know about it. With this knowledge, simple steps can be taken that will effectively protect your baby from Rh incompatibility.

What exactly is Rh incompatibility, and why does your baby need protection from it? A little biology lesson can help clear that up quickly. Each cell in the body has numerous antenna-like structures, called antigens, on its surface. One such antigen often present on the surface of red blood cells is the Rh factor. Most people inherit the Rh factor (making them Rh positive), while other people lack it (making them Rh negative)—and whether you're Rh positive or Rh negative doesn't much matter, except when it comes to pregnancy. When an Rh-negative mom is carrying a baby who's Rh positive (having inherited the Rh factor from an Rh-positive dad), mom's red blood cells don't match up with baby's. If the Rh-positive fetal blood cells enter the Rh-negative mom's circulation, her immune system may view them as "foreign"—and may mobilize armies of antibodies to attack the foreigner who's generating those cells (her baby) in a normal immune response. This is known as Rh incompatibility.

All pregnant women are tested for the Rh factor early in pregnancy, usually at the first prenatal visit. If a mom-to-be turns out to be Rh positive, as 85 percent of the population is, the issue of incompatibility isn't an issue at all. That's because whether the baby is Rh positive or Rh negative, there are no foreign antigens on fetal red blood cells to cause mom's immune system to mobilize against them.

When the mother is Rh negative, the baby's father is tested to determine whether he is Rh positive or negative. If you are Rh negative and your spouse also turns out to be Rh negative, your baby will be Rh negative, too (since two "negative" parents can't make a "positive" baby), which means that your red blood cells and baby's are compatible, and there's no potential for a problem. But if your spouse is Rh positive, there's a significant possibility that the baby will inherit the Rh factor from him, creating an incompatibility between you and your little one.

This incompatibility is usually not a problem in a first pregnancy because there aren't yet antibodies to the baby's Rh factor. But once a mom's natural protective immune response kicks in and produces antibodies during her first pregnancy or delivery (or abortion or miscarriage), they stay in her system—which isn't a concern until she becomes pregnant again with another Rh-positive baby. During the subsequent pregnancy, these antibodies could potentially cross the placenta into the baby's circulation and attack the fetal red blood cells, causing very mild (if maternal antibody levels are low) to very serious (if they are high) anemia in the fetus.

Prevention of the development of Rh antibodies is the key to protecting the baby when there is Rh incompatibility. Most practitioners use a two-pronged strategy. At 28 weeks, an Rh-negative expectant mom is given a vaccine-like injection of Rh-immune globulin, known as RhoGAM, to prevent the development of antibodies. Another dose is administered within 72 hours after delivery if blood tests show her baby is Rh positive. If the baby is Rh negative, no treatment is required.

Expecting Deployment

If you're married to the military—with a spouse who's often deployed—being separated from your partner for major life events (like anniversaries, holidays, and graduations) is just a part of everyday life. And you've probably come to accept that, if not exactly embrace it (especially at those times when you could really use an embrace).

But what about when you're expecting—and he's expecting to be deployed? How do you stay connected when you're separated during the ultimate life event, pregnancy—and even separated at your baby's birth? With a little creativity—and a lot of technology. Here are some ideas to get you started:

- **Document your bump.** Start every morning with a bump selfie. It may not seem to change much from day to day, but getting a daily bump update in his inbox will make his day, every day. Plus you'll both get a kick out of looking back on your tummy transformation from flat to fabulously round later on. As you close in on delivery, consider splurging on a maternity photo shoot meant just for him.

- **Decorate your bump.** Ready to unleash your inner artist—while keeping close during holidays? Send holiday greetings on your bump: Mark July 4th with a flag, Halloween with a pumpkin, Thanksgiving with a turkey, Christmas with a tree.

- **Follow along together.** Start a long-distance baby book club—get him a matching copy of this book, and later, *What to Expect the First Year*, so you can read along together. Download the What To Expect app together, so you can watch the videos and share the updates on your baby's progress—as well as help him understand all those crazy symptoms you've been venting about. Play the name game, too—share a baby name app and toss around contenders.

- **Take him to checkups.** If time zones and schedules permit, try to book some of your prenatal checkups when he can attend via videochat (and make sure he gets a chance to ask any questions he has). Same for any ultrasound appointments. If he can't videochat in for the appointments, try to get a selection of ultrasound stills or video clips to send him. And for his listening pleasure, try recording baby's heartbeat.

- **Connect over cravings.** Can't get enough black olive and peanut butter sandwiches? Bananas for bananas? Create a cravings care package so he can get a taste of home—and a taste for what you're craving. Find substitutes for items that won't travel well (like the bananas—you can send him a bag of the freeze-dried kind). Or send him a photo of the extreme sundae baby had you building at 2 a.m. last night.

RhoGAM should also be administered after a miscarriage, an ectopic pregnancy, an abortion, CVS (chorionic villus sampling), amniocentesis, vaginal bleeding, or physical trauma during pregnancy. Giving RhoGAM as needed at these times can head off problems in future pregnancies.

What if an Rh-negative mom-to-be has already developed levels of Rh antibodies capable of causing anemia in an Rh-positive fetus? First, the baby's father will be tested for the Rh factor, if he hasn't already been. If he is Rh positive, then baby's blood type will be checked. This can be done through amniocentesis or a noninvasive blood test (though not all insurance

- Do a long-distance gender reveal. If you're planning to find out your baby's sex when he (or she) reveals it at your 20-week ultrasound or via an elaborate gender-reveal party, make sure daddy's able to join in. Videochat during the reveal, or have the friend or relative who's gotten the gender 411 pack up matching boxes of pink or blue confetti or candy to send to him and give to you, to be opened via videochat at the same time.

- Get him bonding with baby. From about the 6th month on, a baby's sense of hearing is well developed. So put it to good use—and let the bonding begin. Whenever you're videochatting or on the phone, put the audio close enough to your bump so baby can hear the sound of daddy's voice—which will already be music to your little one's ears. That way, baby will recognize daddy's voice right from the start. Another way to bond: Put together a highlights reel to send to him of baby's hiccups, pokes, and squirms once they're visible from the outside.

- Go shopping together. So maybe he doesn't have the time to scroll through pages of cribs, strollers, and monitors (and maybe he's just as happy that way), but he'd probably like to vote on the finalists once you've narrowed the nursery and gear field a bit. Same for paint colors and theme choices for baby's room. Take step-by-step pictures as you remodel baby's room or nook (make sure you're not doing the painting and

heavy lifting). And sign up for your online baby registry together online.

- Find the support you need. Every mom-to-be needs a strong support system—a shoulder to cry on, someone to vent to, someone to cheer her on or share special moments with. You need it—and deserve it—even more. Connect with other military moms-to-be, online or on base, supporting each other and sharing resources. The local U.S.O. can provide support and programs that bring moms together, too, as well as help with resources. Enlist a friend or relative to be your stand-in coach if your partner won't be home for delivery (hopefully, you'll be able to videochat every step of the way), and take childbirth classes (and breastfeeding classes, and infant CPR classes) together. Also consider adding a doula to your birthing team (see page 328). Many doulas offer services free or at a discounted rate to military moms, especially those who have a partner deployed. And if you feel you need more than a friend to talk to—if you're feeling depressed or anxious, having trouble eating or sleeping or taking care of yourself, ask your practitioner for help. Professional counseling, possibly combined with a support group, can help immeasurably.

- Get Centered. If there's a Centering Pregnancy program at your base, consider signing up for the extra support and camaraderie it offers. See page 14 for more.

companies will cover the blood test, since it's pricey). If the fetus is Rh negative, mother and baby have compatible blood types and there's no cause for concern or treatment. If the fetus is found to be Rh positive, and the mother's antibody levels have reached a critical level, a special ultrasound test will be performed every week or two

to assess the baby's condition and rule out anemia. If at any point anemia has developed, a transfusion of Rh-negative blood to the fetus may be necessary. This is done through a small needle placed in the fetal umbilical cord under ultrasound guidance. Such fetal transfusions are very effective and associated with excellent outcomes.

Fortunately, the use of RhoGAM has greatly reduced the need for transfusions in Rh-incompatible pregnancies to less than 1 percent.

A similar incompatibility can arise with other factors in the blood, such as the Kell antigen, though these are less common than Rh incompatibility. If the mother doesn't have the antigen and the father does, there is again potential for problems. A standard screening, part of the first routine blood test, looks for the presence of circulating antibodies in the mother's blood. If these antibodies are found, the baby's father is tested to see if he is positive, in which case the management is the same as with Rh incompatibility.

Your Medical History

Obesity

"I'm about 60 pounds overweight. Does this put my baby and me at higher risk during pregnancy?"

Most overweight moms (and even those who are obese, defined as someone whose weight is 20 percent or more over ideal weight), have completely safe pregnancies and completely healthy babies. Still, carrying a lot of extra weight while you're carrying a baby does increase the possibility of certain pregnancy complications, including miscarriage, birth defects, stillbirth, preterm birth, high blood pressure, and gestational diabetes (GD). Being overweight poses some practical pregnancy problems, too. The extra layers of fat may make it trickier for a practitioner to determine a fetus's size and position (as well as make it harder for you to feel those first kicks). And a prolonged labor and difficult delivery can result if a baby is much larger than average, which is often the case when mom is obese (particularly if she's diabetic, and even if she hasn't gained too much weight during pregnancy). And if a cesarean delivery is necessary, obesity can complicate both the surgery and recovery from it.

Then there's the issue of pregnancy comfort, or rather discomfort—and unfortunately, as the pounds multiply, so do those uncomfortable pregnancy symptoms. Extra pounds (whether they're pounds you already had or pounds you added during pregnancy) can spell extra backache, varicose veins, swelling, heartburn, and more.

Discouraged? Don't be. There's plenty you and your practitioner can do to minimize the extra risks of those extra pounds (as well as the extra discomforts)—it'll just take some extra effort. On the medical side, you may be monitored more closely than the typical average-weight woman (for instance, you may be screened for GD earlier and more often, and have extra ultrasounds to check your baby's size).

As for your part, good self-care can make a big difference. Eliminating all pregnancy risks that are within your control—such as drinking and smoking—will be particularly important for you. Keeping your weight gain on target will be, too—and it's likely that your target will be smaller than the average expectant mom's and monitored by your doctor more closely. ACOG recommends that overweight women gain 15 to 20 pounds and obese women gain no more than 15 pounds, though your practitioner's recommendations may differ. In fact, some practitioners recommend that obese women pack on no extra pounds at all during pregnancy—but again, stick to the plan your doctor or midwife has mapped out for you.

Even with a scaled-down bottom line to stick to, your daily diet should be packed with foods that are concentrated sources of vitamins, minerals, and protein (see the Pregnancy Diet, starting on page 84). Focusing on the quality of the calories you choose will make them count—and will help your baby get the most nutritional bang from every bite you take. Taking your prenatal vitamin faithfully will provide extra insurance. Getting regular exercise, within the guidelines recommended by your practitioner, will allow you to eat more of the healthy foods you and your baby need without packing on too many pounds. Combine regular exercise, the right amount of weight gain, and a healthy diet, and you'll also lower your risk of developing GD.

Wondering whether you can keep your pregnancy weight gain down by popping supplements and sipping beverages that claim to suppress appetite? These can be dangerous during pregnancy, so stay away from them—even if they're marketed as "natural."

For your next pregnancy, if you are planning on one, try to get as close as possible to your ideal weight before you conceive. It will make everything about pregnancy a lot easier—and less potentially complicated.

Underweight

"I've always been skinny—I have a hard time gaining weight. Will being underweight have any impact on my pregnancy?"

Pregnancy's definitely a time for eating well and gaining weight—for both the skinny and the not-so-skinny. But if you've come into pregnancy on the super-skinny side (with a BMI of 18.5 or less; see page 178 for how to calculate yours), you'll have to be filling up your plate even more. That's because there are some potential risks (such as having a small-for-date baby and preterm birth) associated with being pregnant and extremely underweight, particularly if you're also undernourished (this is far less likely if you're a healthy eater who just happens to be naturally thin). But any added risk can be eliminated by eating well (getting plenty of calories and nutrients), taking a prenatal vitamin, and gaining enough weight. Depending on where you started out on the scale, your practitioner may advise you to gain a little extra—possibly 28 to 40 pounds, instead of the 25 to 35 pounds recommended for the average-weight woman. If you've been blessed with a speedy metabolism that makes putting on pounds tricky, see page 192 for some tips. As long as your weight gain stays on track, though, your pregnancy shouldn't encounter any other bumps (besides that belly bump).

An Eating Disorder

"I've been bulimic for almost 10 years. I thought I'd be able to stop now that I'm pregnant, but I can't seem to. Will it hurt my baby?"

Not if you get the right kind of help right away. The fact that you've been bulimic (or anorexic) for a number of years means your nutritional reserves are probably low, putting your baby and your body at a disadvantage right off the bat. Fortunately, early in pregnancy the need for nourishment is less than it will be later on, so you have the chance

Pregnancy After Weight Loss Surgery

Have you lost weight thanks to bariatric surgery? Chances are you were told to hold off on becoming pregnant until 12 to 18 months after your surgery—the time of the most drastic weight loss and potential for malnutrition. But now that you've passed that benchmark and are growing a baby, it's time for a double congratulations— you've lost a whole lot of weight, and you're about to gain a baby! Pat yourself on the back (and rub yourself on the belly), because having lost all that weight (no matter how it happened— gastric sleeve, lap band, or gastric bypass) gives you an even better chance of having a healthy pregnancy and healthy baby. You've lowered your risk for gestational diabetes, preeclampsia, and having a too-big baby. How's that for a win-win?

Still, there are some extra precautions you will need to take as a mom-to-be who's had weight loss surgery:

- Keep your weight loss surgeon on your team (now, Team Baby). He or she will be best able to advise your ob or midwife on some of the specific needs of a weight loss surgery patient.

- Keep those vitamins coming. You'll need to keep up with your recommended vitamin supplementation while you're expecting—after all, you're nourishing for two now. A prenatal vitamin is a good start, but you may need more iron, calcium, folic acid, vitamin B_{12}, and vitamin A because of certain malabsorption issues. So discuss your supplement needs with both your prenatal practitioner and your surgeon.

- Keep your eye on the scale. You're used to watching your weight, of course—but lately, you're used to watching it go down. Now that there's a baby on board, you'll probably watch it go up. Your job will be to keep to that weight-gain goal—gaining too few pounds or too many can put your pregnancy and your baby at unnecessary risk. Keep in mind that there's an increased chance of having a too-small baby after bariatric surgery, but that gaining the right number of pounds can help ensure a healthy bottom line for your baby at birth.

- Keep an eye on your eating. Eating for two is more challenging when your stomach space has been downsized by weight-loss surgery. You may find the challenges multiply, too, as your uterus and your baby start to grow, crowding out your stomach even more. Since the quantity of food you can comfortably eat is limited, you'll need to focus on quality. Try not to waste space (or calories) on foods that don't satisfy nutritional requirements, and instead try to choose foods that efficiently pack the most nutrients into the smallest volume.

- Keep an eye on your symptoms. If you're experiencing excessive vomiting or nausea, or if you notice any unusual abdominal pain, call your pregnancy practitioner and your bariatric surgeon right away. The symptoms could be pregnancy-related—or they could be something more serious related to your surgery, in which case they would require immediate medical attention.

to make up for your body's nutritional shortfall before it can hurt your baby.

Very little research has been done in the area of eating disorders and

pregnancy, partly because these disorders often disrupt the menstrual cycle, which means few women suffering from these problems become pregnant in the first place. But the studies that have been done suggest that bingeing and purging during pregnancy (in other words, active bulimia) seems to increase the risk of miscarriage and premature birth, as well as postpartum depression. Active anorexia during pregnancy increases the risk of miscarriage, preeclampsia, preterm delivery, and cesarean delivery. Taking laxatives, diuretics, appetite suppressants, and other drugs sometimes used by bulimics and anorexics can also be harmful during pregnancy. They draw off nutrients and fluids from your body before they can be used to nourish your baby (and later to produce milk), and may lead to multiple serious problems, including possible birth defects, if used regularly. And not gaining enough weight during pregnancy can lead to a number of problems, including preterm delivery and a baby who is born small for his or her gestational age.

Happily, the studies also suggest that if you put those unhealthy habits behind you now, you're just as likely to have a healthy baby as anyone else, all other things being equal. If you're having trouble eating normally and well, having a hard time distinguishing between morning sickness and bulimia, or if you're hiding your bulimia under the cover of morning sickness, make sure you get the help you need. Start by telling your prenatal practitioner about your eating disorder—not only so he or she can help make sure it doesn't affect your baby or your pregnancy, but also so you'll get the supportive care you need to get healthy and stay healthy. Your practitioner may be able to refer you to a therapist who is experienced in treating eating disorders. Professional counseling is always smart when you've been battling anorexia or bulimia, but it's really essential when you're trying to eat well for two. You may also find

support groups helpful (check online, or ask your practitioner or therapist for a recommendation).

Just being committed to conquering your eating disorder, so that you can start nurturing that beautiful baby of yours, is the first and most important step. It will also help to put the dynamics of pregnancy weight gain in perspective. Keep in mind:

- The pregnant shape is universally viewed as healthy and beautiful. Its roundness is normal, a sign that you're growing a baby. Celebrate those curves! Embrace your pregnant self!

- You're supposed to gain weight during pregnancy. The right amount of weight (as recommended by your practitioner), gained at the right time, on the right foods is vital to your baby's growth and wellbeing in utero and beyond (some of the extra fat you lay down during pregnancy will be used after delivery to help you breastfeed your baby). And this sensible strategy isn't just baby-friendly, it's mom-friendly, too. It will help ensure a healthier, more comfortable pregnancy and a speedier return to your prepregnancy shape postpartum. If you're uneasy watching the numbers on the scale climb as you gain that vital weight, let your practitioner do the watching. Hide your bathroom scale so you won't be tempted to check your weight yourself, and close your eyes during your checkup weigh-ins (ask the nurse to note the number in your chart without announcing it first).

- You can (and should!) stay in shape when you're expecting. Exercise can help guide to the right places the extra pounds you need to gain (primarily, your baby and baby by-products).

If You Have a Chronic Condition

Anyone who's lived with a chronic condition knows that life can get pretty complicated—between medications to take and extra doctor's appointments to make (not to mention, new therapies and treatments to keep up with). Add pregnancy into the mix, and you've got your plate even fuller. Happily, with some extra precautions, extra effort, and extra care, most chronic conditions are completely compatible with pregnancy. Here are some general recommendations for moms-to-be with a few common chronic conditions (but be sure to follow your doctor's orders, since they've probably been tailored to your specific needs):

Diabetes. The key to managing a diabetic pregnancy successfully—whether the diabetes is Type 1 (in which the body doesn't produce insulin) or Type 2 (in which the body doesn't respond as it should to insulin)—is achieving normal blood glucose levels before conception and maintaining them throughout the 9 months after it. You'll be able to do that with a carefully designed diet (it will probably be similar to the Pregnancy Diet, containing few sugary sweets and refined grains and plenty of fiber-rich food and healthy snacks), regular exercise, careful monitoring of your blood sugar, and the right medication (insulin, if necessary). You also will be given a pregnancy weight-gain goal, which will be especially important to stick to since gaining too much weight can put you at risk of pregnancy complications.

To make sure all is going well, you'll be watched carefully during pregnancy. Along with regular tests for blood sugar levels you'll also have urine tests (to check kidney function) and eye exams (to check your retinas), and your baby will be checked with a fetal echocardiogram (to make sure his or her heart is developing without problems). Your doctor will also watch you closely for early signs of preeclampsia (page 550) and gestational diabetes (page 548), since diabetics are at somewhat higher risk for both those conditions.

Because babies of diabetics sometimes grow very large, even if mom's weight is on target, your baby's growth will be monitored more closely using ultrasound. Heavier babies make delivery more difficult (there's a higher chance of childbirth complications and/or cesarean delivery when baby is very large). Early delivery may be necessary if problems develop late in pregnancy, but your medical team will ensure that baby's lungs are sufficiently mature before inducing labor or performing a c-section.

Finally, if you're planning to breastfeed, try to get started as soon as possible after birth (ideally within 30 minutes) and feed every 2 to 3 hours to prevent hypoglycemia (low blood sugar). To play it safe, babies of diabetic moms are usually not discharged from the hospital until they are maintaining blood glucose levels and feeding well.

Hypertension. If you have chronic hypertension your pregnancy will be considered high risk. But with the right medical care and self-care, you're likely to have the best payoff of all—a safe pregnancy and a healthy baby. You'll have to keep track of your blood pressure at home, exercise regularly (which lowers blood pressure), reduce stress (through relaxation exercises, mediation, and other CAM therapies, such as biofeedback), eat well, stay hydrated, and keep your weight gain on track. Pregnancy-safe medication, as needed, will also help ensure that your blood pressure stays under control. Medical monitoring will be stepped up, too, to make sure you don't develop preeclampsia (see page 550).

Irritable bowel syndrome. It's hard to pinpoint the effect of pregnancy on

IBS—and vice versa—because bowels are often impacted (sometimes literally) by pregnancy. Expectant women are more prone to constipation (a symptom of IBS) and/or looser stools (also a symptom of IBS). Same for gas and bloating, which typically worsen when you're expecting, whether or not you have IBS.

To keep your symptoms manageable, stick to the techniques you're used to using to combat IBS during other times in your life: Eat smaller, more frequent meals, stay well hydrated, avoid excess stress, and steer clear of foods or drinks that make your symptoms worse. If you're on the FODMAP diet, check with your practitioner to make sure you're getting the right balance of nutrients for pregnancy. And if you're on medication for help with IBS symptoms, check with your prenatal practitioner to make sure it's pregnancy safe—not all are. You might also want to consider adding some probiotics. They're surprisingly effective in regulating bowel function.

Sickle cell anemia. This condition puts pregnancy at high risk, but with the right care moms with sickle cell disease—even those with complications like heart or kidney disease—have a good chance of having a safe pregnancy and delivery and a healthy baby. Preeclampsia and hypertension are more common in women with sickle cell anemia, and many women with sickle cell anemia find themselves hospitalized at least once during their 9 months. Complications such as miscarriage, preterm delivery, and fetal growth restriction are also more common.

Though it's not certain whether it's beneficial or not, it's possible that you'll be given a blood transfusion at least once or even periodically throughout pregnancy as well as in early labor or just before delivery.

Thyroid disease. If you're hypothyroid (your thyroid doesn't produce enough thyroxine), it's important to keep taking your thyroid pills (they're not only pregnancy safe but can be pregnancy essential). You'll also need to have your thyroid levels monitored more closely to be sure the dose you're taking is meeting your needs and your baby's (and if you've had a thyroid condition in the past but since stopped taking meds, let your practitioner know so your levels can be tested again now). Untreated hypothyroidism increases the chances of miscarriage. What's more, babies who don't get enough maternal thyroid hormones in the first trimester can develop neurological problems and, possibly, deafness. (After the first trimester, the fetus makes its own thyroid hormones and is protected even if mom's levels are low.) Low thyroid levels are also linked to maternal depression during pregnancy and postpartum—another compelling reason to continue treatment.

Iodine deficiency, which is becoming more common among women of childbearing age in the U.S. because of reduced iodized salt consumption, can interfere with the production of the thyroid hormone, so be sure you are getting adequate amounts of this trace mineral.

Untreated moderate to severe Graves disease (aka hyperthyroidism—when the thyroid gland produces excessive amounts of thyroid hormones) can lead to serious complications for both you and your baby, including miscarriage and preterm birth, so appropriate treatment is necessary. Happily, when the disease is treated properly (in pregnancy the treatment of choice is the antithyroid medication propylthiouracil, or PTU, in the lowest effective dose), the outcome is likely to be good for both mom and baby.

Don't see the chronic condition you're dealing with listed here? You'll find asthma on page 219, scoliosis on page 255, and information on other chronic conditions, including cystic fibrosis, epilepsy, fibromyalgia, chronic fatigue syndrome, lupus, multiple sclerosis, PKU, physical disability, and rheumatoid arthritis at WhatToExpect.com.

But make sure any exercise you do is pregnancy-appropriate and practitioner-approved. If you've always used strenuous workouts as a way to burn off extra calories you've eaten, it's time to trade in that strategy for a healthier approach. Also avoid any exercise that raises your temperature excessively, which isn't safe during pregnancy (saunas and hot yoga are out).

- You will lose a lot of the pregnancy pounds at delivery, but far from all of them. It can take several months to lose the rest, and realistically longer to get back into shape. For this reason, women with eating disorders sometimes find that negative feelings about their body image cause them to slip back into bingeing and purging or starving during the postpartum period. Because these unhealthy habits could interfere with your ability to recover from childbirth, to parent effectively, and to produce enough milk if you choose to breastfeed, it's important that you continue professional counseling postpartum with someone experienced in the treatment of eating disorders. Support groups (in your community or online) can also help.

The most important thing to keep in mind: Your baby's wellbeing depends on your wellbeing during pregnancy. If you're not well nourished, your baby won't be, either. Positive reinforcement can definitely help, so try putting pictures of cute babies on the fridge, in your office and car, anywhere you might need a reminder of the healthy eating you should be doing. Visualize the food you eat making its way to your baby (and your baby happily gobbling up those healthy meals).

If you can't seem to stop bingeing, vomiting, using diuretics or laxatives, or practicing semistarvation during pregnancy, discuss with your physician the possibility of hospitalization until you get your disorder under control. There's never been a better reason to get—and stay—healthy.

Depression

"I was diagnosed with depression a few years ago, and I've been on an antidepressant ever since. Now that I'm pregnant, should I stop taking the meds?"

Around 15 percent of women of childbearing age battle bouts of depression, so you're far from alone. Luckily for you and all the other expectant moms who share your condition, there's a sunny forecast: With the right treatment, women with depression can have perfectly normal pregnancies—and happy ones, too. Deciding what that treatment should consist of during pregnancy is a delicate balancing act, however, when it comes to the use of medications. Together with your mental health care provider and your prenatal practitioner, you'll need to weigh the risks and benefits of taking such meds—and not taking them—while you're growing a baby.

Maybe it seems like a simple decision to make, at least at first glance. After all, could there ever be a good reason to put your emotional wellbeing over your baby's physical wellbeing? But the decision is actually a lot more complicated than that. For starters, pregnancy hormones can do a number on your emotional state. Even women who've never had an encounter with mood disorders, depression, or any other psychological condition may experience wild emotional swings when they're expecting—but women with a history of depression are at greater risk of having depressive bouts during pregnancy and are more likely to suffer from postpartum depression. And this is especially true for moms-to-be who stop taking their antidepressants during pregnancy.

What's more, untreated depression isn't likely to affect only you (and those you're close to)—it's also likely to affect your baby's health. Depressed moms-to-be may not eat or sleep well or pay as much attention to their prenatal care, and they may be more likely to turn to unhealthy lifestyle habits, like drinking or smoking. Any or all of those factors, combined with the debilitating effects of excessive anxiety and stress, have been linked in some studies to an increased risk of preterm birth, low birthweight, and a lower Apgar score for babies. Treating depression effectively, however—and keeping it under control during pregnancy—allows a mother-to-be to nurture her body and her developing baby.

So what does all this mean for you? It means you should think twice before you consider tossing your antidepressants. But it also means that you should consult both with your prenatal practitioner and the doctor and/or therapist who has been treating you for depression before you decide what your next medication move should be, if any. Certain meds are safer than others during pregnancy, and some aren't recommended for pregnancy use at all—which means that the med (or meds) you used preconception might not be the right choice now. Or that your dose may need to be changed.

Your prenatal practitioner (in conjunction with your mental health care provider) can give you the most up-to-date and accurate information on the safety of antidepressant drugs during pregnancy, because it's ever changing—as well as often misinterpreted or misreported on the internet. Another reason to look to professional guidance (instead of search engines): Research so far has been conflicting, with some studies showing increased risk for autism, cardiac defect, and low birthweight in babies whose moms took certain antidepressants during pregnancy, and other studies showing no correlation at all. What is known right now is that the SSRIs (selective serotonin re-uptake inhibitors) Celexa, Prozac, and Zoloft are generally considered good options during pregnancy (Paxil, another SSRI, is not, because it's associated with a small increase in fetal heart defects). SNRIs (serotonin and norepinephrine re-uptake inhibitors) such as Cymbalta and Effexor XR, are also among the treatment options for expectant moms. Wellbutrin isn't considered a first choice medication during pregnancy but can be used if a woman isn't responding to the other options.

Here's the important thing to keep in mind as you and your practitioner weigh your options: Though taking any kind of medicine during pregnancy—including antidepressants—isn't without risks, experts believe these risks shouldn't keep pregnant women from taking antidepressants if their depression can't be treated effectively in other ways. That's because untreated depression carries its own risks, many with long-term effects. Choosing the safest medication possible, prescribing it at the safest dose possible, and taking it at the safest time during pregnancy as possible will help mitigate the risks of both the depression and the medications.

Also remember that there are non-drug treatments for depression that can be quite effective, either on their own (in some cases, allowing a mom with mild depression to avoid medication altogether) or when used in conjunction with medication (allowing a mom to take a lower dose of a medication or switch to a safer med). These treatments include psychotherapy (talk therapy), bright light therapy, and complementary and alternative medicine (CAM) approaches, such as acupuncture and possibly neurotherapy. Exercise (for its release of feel-good endorphins), meditation (which can help you manage stress), and diet (keeping blood sugar up with regular healthy meals and snacks) can also be beneficial additions to a treatment program. Talk to your practitioner and mental health care provider to see if these options have a place in yours.

ADHD

"I was diagnosed with ADHD as a teenager and have been taking daily medication for it ever since. Do I have to stop taking my meds during pregnancy?"

Plenty of adults take amphetamines like Adderall or methylphenidates like Concerta or Ritalin to help stay focused and functioning socially and at work—and that includes plenty of women who ultimately become pregnant. The problem is, there isn't much known about the safety of these drugs during pregnancy since they haven't been well studied in humans, only in animals. At this point, they've been categorized as medications that haven't been shown to be harmful to a fetus but haven't been proven harmless, either.

So what's a human mom-to-be to do? First, talk to your pregnancy practitioner as well as to the doctor who prescribed the medication. Ask about the latest on the safety of stimulant medications during pregnancy, and discuss whether you should continue using them or not (or whether you should stop using them during the first trimester and resume use during the second). Any potential risk of taking the medications during pregnancy will, of course, have to be balanced against the potential risks of letting your ADHD go untreated. Ask, too, about nondrug treatments for ADHD (such as cognitive behavioral therapy or clinical coaching) that could act as alternatives to the use of stimulants during pregnancy, or as supplements to a lower dose of those medications. Finally, remember that no matter what treatment you end up with, pregnancy can do a number on your focus, concentration, and functioning—and that a hormone-induced fog settles on just about every expectant mom.

Having a Baby After 35

"I'm 38 and thrilled to be pregnant for the first time—but I wonder what my age means for my pregnancy and my baby."

Being over 35 and pregnant with your first baby means you're in good—and steadily growing—company. Also growing: the number of moms over 40 having baby number 1.

And your good company shares good news. The risks of pregnancy are very small to begin with, and rise only slightly and gradually as you get older. Most of the risks that do rise can be reduced, or even eliminated.

So first, the risks. The major reproductive risk faced by a woman over 35 (an age group perhaps unfairly referred to as "advanced maternal age," or AMA) is that she might not become pregnant at all due to the slight and very gradual decline in fertility that begins once a woman has exited the optimum fertility window of her early 20s (so it's not downhill overnight at age 35). Now that you've got conception covered (congrats!), you face a somewhat increased chance of having a baby with Down syndrome. Here, again, it's a relatively low risk that increases gradually as mom gets older: 1 in 1,250 for 25-year-old moms,

Older Dads

Throughout most of history, it was believed that a father's responsibility in the reproductive process was limited to fertilization. Only during the 20th century (too late to help those queens who lost their heads for failing to produce a male heir) was it discovered that a father's sperm holds the deciding genetic vote in determining his child's gender. And only in the last few decades have researchers started realizing that an older father's sperm might also contribute increased risks for his baby, too. Like the older mother's eggs, the older father's spermatocytes (undeveloped sperm) have had longer exposure to environmental hazards and might be more likely to contain altered or damaged genes or chromosomes. What does that mean for an older dad's baby-to-be? Researchers have found that, regardless of the mom's age, a couple's risk of miscarriage increases as the dad's age increases, as does the incidence of Down syndrome once he's over 50 or 55 (again, no matter what mom's age). There also seems to be a somewhat increased risk of autism or mental health issues when a dad is over age 40.

Wondering whether your older age will mean more diagnostic tests for your partner and your baby? Genetic counselors don't recommend invasive tests like amnio or CVS based only on a dad's age—and happily, the screening tests that are offered routinely to every mom-to-be (no matter how old she or her partner is) can rule out most chromosomal problems.

The bottom line if you're an older dad, as it is for older moms: The risks are very small—and the benefits of having a baby at the time in your life that's right for you are clearly great. Really, really great. So relax and enjoy this pregnancy adventure together—it'll be worth the wait.

about 3 in 1,000 for 30-year-old moms, 1 in about 300 for 35-year-old moms, and 1 in 35 for 45-year-old moms. It's speculated that the gradual rise in this and other chromosomal abnormalities is most often linked to an older woman's older eggs (women are born with a lifetime supply of eggs that gradually age along with her). That said, because an estimated minimum 25 percent of Down syndrome cases and other chromosomal abnormalities are the result of a defect in an older dad's sperm—and because older moms are often married to older dads—it's not always clear whether it's mom's age or dad's age that's implicated.

A handful of other pregnancy risks increase slightly with age. One may not sound like a risk at all, but a benefit:

Older moms are more likely to conceive twins (even if they've conceived naturally), thanks to an age-related predisposition to releasing more than one egg at a time. In general, increasing age also increases the risk of miscarriage (because of an older mom's older eggs), preeclampsia, gestational diabetes, and preterm labor. Labor and delivery, on average, are longer and slightly more likely to be complicated (often because the pregnancy is higher-risk to begin with), with c-section rates higher in older moms, too.

But even though the risks of pregnancy at your age are slightly elevated, they are still low—and of course, they're nothing when compared to the reward you're eagerly anticipating. Best of all,

Not for Fathers Only

Happy expectant families come in all packages. Maybe you're two mommies expecting a baby that one of you is carrying. Or two daddies expecting through a surrogate or planning an open adoption—and you'd both like to stay emotionally and physically connected to the woman who's expecting your precious bundle. Or maybe you're a single mom without an involved (or traditional) partner, but with friends and family standing by to provide the support he otherwise might. No matter what family package you're coming to parenthood with, this entire book is for you but so are the For Fathers boxes sprinkled throughout are for your family, too. Edit them any way you like, take from them what applies, and use them to help your family make that momentous transition to life with baby.

pregnancy complications that are more common in older moms can sometimes be prevented, and if not, they can usually be well controlled. The right combination of medical management and medications can help forestall preterm labor, and breakthroughs continue to decrease risks in the birthing room. And though Down syndrome isn't preventable, it can be identified in utero through a variety of screening and diagnostic tests. Better still, today's essentially noninvasive first-trimester screenings (see page 53), which are recommended for all pregnant women regardless of age (so don't worry, mama—you're not being picked on!), are much more accurate than in the past. Moms who pass these screens don't necessarily have to proceed to more invasive diagnostic tests (amnio or CVS) as was once routine, even if they've passed their 35th birthday. This saves time, money, and—most important—stress.

But as much as obstetrical science can do to help you have a safe pregnancy and delivery and a healthy baby, it's nothing compared to what you can do yourself through exercise, eating well, sensible weight gain, and regular prenatal care. Just being older doesn't necessarily put you in a high-risk category, but an accumulation of many individual risks can. Eliminate or minimize as many risk factors as you can, and you'll be able to take years off your pregnancy profile—making your chances of delivering a healthy baby virtually as good as those of a younger mother. Yes, maybe even better.

So relax, enjoy your pregnancy, and be reassured. There's never been a better time to be over 35 and expecting a baby.

Genetic Screening

"I keep wondering if I might have a genetic problem that I don't know about. Should I get genetic screening?"

Just about everyone carries a gene for at least one genetic disorder—even if it has never shown up in family history. But fortunately, because most disorders require a matched pair of genes, one from mom and one from dad, they're not likely to show up in their children. One or both parents can be tested for some of these disorders before (which is preferable) or during pregnancy, thanks to genetic testing. In most cases, testing is recommended for one parent—testing the second parent becomes necessary only if the first tests positive.

Official recommendations on who should be tested and for what have

Immunizations in Pregnancy

Since just about all vaccine-preventable diseases can cause pregnancy problems, being up to date on your immunizations is especially important when you're expecting. Most immunizations using live viruses are not recommended during pregnancy, including the MMR (measles, mumps, and rubella) and varicella (chicken pox) vaccines, which is why it's smart to catch up on these, as necessary, before conceiving. Other vaccines, according to the CDC, shouldn't be given routinely but can be given if they're needed. These include the hepatitis A and pneumococcal vaccines. You also can be immunized safely against hepatitis B when you're expecting.

In the must-have department during pregnancy: The CDC recommends that every woman who is pregnant during flu season (generally October through April) receive a flu vaccine and that every pregnant woman get the Tdap vaccine (which protects the baby from diphtheria, tetanus, and pertussis) between 27 and 36 weeks of pregnancy (see page 328 for more on the Tdap).

For more information on vaccines, check with your practitioner and see page 534.

---

been, until recently, based on ethnic or geographical background and limited to just a few disorders. For example, Jewish couples whose ancestors came from Eastern Europe (Ashkenazi) should be tested for Tay-Sachs, Canavan disease, and possibly for other disorders (contact victorcenters.org or jscreen.org to learn more). Tay-Sachs has also been noted in other ethnic groups, including Southern Louisiana Cajuns, French Canadians, and the Pennsylvania Dutch, so getting tested is something to consider if your family has these roots. Similarly, African American couples should be tested for the sickle cell anemia trait, and those of Mediterranean and Asian descent for thalassemia (a hereditary form of anemia).

But because it's harder and harder to assign a single ethnic or geographical profile to anyone in today's multiethnic and far-flung society, the basis for these recommendations has become far less reliable. Case in point: While Caucasians of European descent have long been told of the importance of testing for cystic fibrosis (CF) since they have about a 1 in 25 chance of being a carrier of the condition, blended backgrounds have expanded the pool of carriers. As a result, the guidelines for CF screening have expanded, too. It's now recommended that all couples, regardless of their ethnicity, be screened for CF.

Should the guidelines for screening genetic disorders be expanded even further? Many believe so. And now, new advances in genetic testing are enabling all couples—regardless of their ethnic or geographical profile—to test for a broad array of genetic conditions before conceiving. Such so-called expanded carrier screening can screen for the carrier gene of more than 300 diseases, and it gives you the power of knowing whether you and your partner are at risk of passing along any of these genetic conditions to a baby you conceive together. If you both test positive as carriers for a condition (again, no need to test dad if mom tests negative), further genetic counseling and testing can be used to screen your baby or future

Uninsured, Mama?

Having a baby these days can definitely be an expensive proposition—and that's before you even purchase onesie number one. Still, no expectant mother needs to go through pregnancy and childbirth without the prenatal care she and her baby need. And luckily, there are ways to get that care.

Affordable Care Act (ACA). The ACA requires private insurance companies to cover preexisting conditions, including pregnancy. If your employer or your spouse's doesn't offer insurance or you're unemployed, you may be able to apply for a plan through the Health Insurance Marketplace. However, you must enroll during the open-enrollment period (which happens on an annual basis) unless you're eligible for special enrollment for a qualifying life event. Pregnancy itself is not considered a qualifying life event, but marriage, divorce, and moving count—and you can usually add the baby to your coverage, or change to coverage that also covers your baby within 60 days of the birth, even outside the open-enrollment period. Find out more, including how to get in touch with a local marketplace representative, at healthcare.gov.

Medicaid and CHIP. Even if you haven't qualified in the past, many states increase their income eligibility levels during pregnancy to help more pregnant women get coverage through Medicaid. The Kaiser Family Foundation (kff.org) has a list of each state's income limits, and the U.S. Department of Health and Human Services also has a useful fact sheet (medicaid.gov). Or call your local Health Insurance Marketplace representative at 800-318-2596 to ask whether you're eligible.

In all states, the Children's Health Insurance Program (CHIP) provides low-cost health coverage to children in families that earn too much money to qualify for Medicaid. In some states, CHIP also covers pregnant women. To find out if you're eligible for CHIP's prenatal coverage, fill out your state's marketplace application or visit insurekidsnow.gov.

COBRA. If you or your spouse are recently unemployed and previously had health insurance, you may be able to get coverage for up to 36 months through a program called COBRA. Unfortunately, COBRA premiums are usually very high since they don't include employer contributions, but it

babies for the condition. What's more, knowing in advance that they carry a significant risk of having a baby with a genetic disorder gives couples the choice of using new reproductive techniques (like IVF with preimplantation genetic diagnosis to screen embryos for the diseases before implantation), or to consider sperm donation and other nontraditional routes to starting a family.

While many experts are calling for guidelines that would make expanded carrier screening routine for all couples, ACOG isn't yet on board with that position. For now they recommend that expanded carrier screening be done mainly on the basis of family history and ethnicity (as unreliable as self-reporting of ethnicity might be), with routine screening limited to the cystic fibrosis gene.

Even so, ACOG and the American College of Medical Genetics and Genomics (ACMG) agree that all couples should be offered the option of may be a good compromise until you or your spouse gets a new job with insurance benefits (contact your former employer's human resources department for more information). Before you commit to COBRA, it may be worth comparing the costs and benefits of it against a plan through the health insurance marketplace if you're within an open-enrollment period or you qualify for special enrollment. Marketplace coverage can be less expensive than the COBRA option, especially if you're eligible for subsidies under the ACA.

Your parents. Under the ACA, if you're under 26 years old and one of your parents has a health plan, they should be able to add you as a dependent—even if you don't live with them, whether you're married or not, and regardless of whether they've declared you as a dependent on their taxes. The catch? You may have to wait for an open-enrollment period to be added, and many health care plans do not cover maternity services for dependents.

Clinics. If you can't afford any health plan and don't qualify for coverage through Medicaid and CHIP, you may be able to get low-cost health care at a nearby community health center or clinic. Find one at findahealthcenter.hrsa.gov or call 800-311-BABY.

Discounts. If you've investigated the other insurance options and it turns out you still have to pay out of pocket for your care, call your health care providers—they may be able to help. Many doctors and hospitals will give you a discount, sometimes as much as 20 or 30 percent, if you're paying cash. They also usually offer payment plans that give you the option of paying the bill over time, but check to see if they charge interest for this arrangement. Check, too, before signing up for a health care financing credit card offered by a medical practice to cover the cost—you could pay interest rates of 20 percent or higher. Another possibility: health care discount services or discount cards, which negotiate price cuts on health care services for a monthly fee. Do read the fine print to make sure your health care providers and services are covered and that there are no hidden fees.

Other ways to save if you're paying out of pocket: If you're healthy, at low risk for complications, and want an unmedicated childbirth for your bundle of joy, you can save a bundle by delivering at a birthing center instead of a hospital. At a birthing center, the average unmedicated vaginal birth with no complications usually costs less than what a hospital charges. Choosing a midwife will save you more, too, even if you opt for a hospital delivery.

having carrier screening, if they choose, before they start trying to conceive. But to reduce the potential emotional downside of screening, experts recommend that it be accompanied by counseling with an ob or geneticist who can explain exactly which disorders the expanded carrier screening panels test for, so couples can opt out of receiving test results they don't want to know about. ACMG adds that the carrier screen should test only for disorders that would be relevant for reproductive

decision making, and not include disorders that are adult onset (some of the conditions in the 300-disease carrier screen are only adult onset)—unless the couple provides specific consent to screen for them all.

The best way to decide how to approach genetic screening—regardless of the current recommendations—is to talk it over with your practitioner. That way you and your partner can decide what's best for you and your soon-to-be-growing family.

Pregnancy and the Single Mom

Are you a single mom-to-be? Just because you don't have a partner doesn't mean you have to go it alone during pregnancy. The kind of support you'll need (and every mom needs) can come from sources other than a partner. A friend or a relative you feel close to and comfortable with can step in to hold your hand, emotionally and physically, throughout pregnancy. That person can, in many ways, play the partner role during the 9 months and beyond— accompanying you to prenatal visits and childbirth education classes, lending an ear (and a shoulder), helping you get both your home and life ready for the new arrival, and acting as coach, cheerleader, supporter, and overall advocate during labor and delivery. And since no one will know better what you're going through than another single mom, you might also consider joining (or starting) a support group for single mothers or finding an online support group (check out the single moms' message board at WhatToExpect.com). Also consider adding a doula to your birth team, as well as to your postpartum team (see page 328). Or, if the option is open locally, choose a Centering Pregnancy program for your prenatal care, since the group approach means you're never alone at checkups (see page 14). If you're going solo during pregnancy because your partner is deployed or working far from home for weeks or months at a time, see page 36.

Just as happy to go it alone, and maybe even happier? That's an option some single moms take, happily.

"My partner and I didn't have genetic testing done before pregnancy. Should we see a genetic counselor now?"

Since most couples are, happily, at such low risk for passing along a genetic disorder, most don't need to see a genetic counselor—and chances are, you're in that majority. To ease your mind, talk over your specific situation with your prenatal practitioner and see whether you'll need to take genetic counseling to the next level. Usually, referral to a genetic counselor or a maternal-fetal-medicine specialist is limited to those who need extra expertise:

- Couples whose blood tests and/or expanded carrier screen show they are carriers of a genetic disorder that they might pass on to their children

- Couples who have already had 1 or more children with genetic birth defects

- Couples who have experienced 2 or more consecutive miscarriages

- Couples in which the woman is over age 35 and/or the man is over age 40

- Couples who know of a hereditary disorder on any branch of either of their family trees. In some cases (as with cystic fibrosis or certain thalassemias), DNA testing of the parents before pregnancy makes interpreting later testing of the fetus much easier.

- Couples in which 1 partner (or their parent or sibling or older child) has a congenital defect (such as congenital heart disease)

- Pregnant women who have had a positive screening test for a chromosomal defect

- Closely related couples, since the risk of a genetic disease in offspring is greatest when parents are close relatives (for example, 1 in 8 for first cousins)

The best time to see a genetic counselor (and to consider expanded screening) is before getting pregnant. A genetic counselor is trained to give couples the odds of their having a healthy child based on their genetic profiles and can guide them in deciding whether or not to have children. But it's not too late even after pregnancy is confirmed. The counselor can suggest appropriate prenatal testing based on the couple's genetic profile, and if testing uncovers a serious defect in the fetus, a genetic counselor can outline for the expectant parents all the options available and help them decide how to proceed. Genetic counseling has helped countless high-risk couples avoid the heartbreak of giving birth to children with serious problems while helping them realize their dreams of having completely healthy babies.

ALL ABOUT:
Prenatal Diagnosis

Is it a boy or a girl? Will baby have blond hair or brown? Green eyes or blue? Mom's mouth and dad's dimples? Dad's musical talent and mom's knack for numbers . . . or the other way around?

Babies definitely keep their parents guessing (and placing friendly bets) long before they actually arrive—sometimes before they're conceived. But the one question that expectant parents wonder about the most is also the one they hesitate most to talk about, or even think about: "Will my baby be healthy?"

Time was, that question could be answered only after birth. Today, it can be answered as early as the first trimester, through a very wide variety of prenatal screening and diagnostic tests. What screens can you expect to have during your 40 weeks? Will diagnostic tests be part of your pregnancy plan? With the field ever-growing and recommendations ever-changing, you'll need to rely on your practitioner to help guide you to the choices that are right for you and your pregnancy. But it will also help to read ahead, so you're in the know about the most common screening and diagnostic tests.

Screening Tests

Most expectant moms (even those considered at low risk of having a baby with a defect) undergo several screening tests during their 40 weeks. That's because screening tests are noninvasive and increasingly accurate. They pose no risk to mom (except maybe to your nerves) or baby—but can provide a lot of beneficial reassurance. An easy way to breathe easy.

Prenatal screening tests use a blood draw and/or ultrasound to identify whether you're at an increased risk of having a baby with a genetic disorder like Down syndrome or a neural tube defect like spina bifida. They can't diagnose such conditions—only a diagnostic test can do that—but they can determine the likelihood that your baby is affected, with anywhere from 80 to 99 percent accuracy. Here's what you need to know about each of them.

Noninvasive prenatal screening (after 9 weeks). Did you know that pieces of your baby's DNA circulate in your bloodstream? The noninvasive prenatal screening test (NIPT, or NIPS) involves a simple blood screening any time after 9 weeks that analyzes DNA (it's called cell-free fetal DNA, or cfDNA) to pinpoint baby's risk for a number of genetic disorders, including Down syndrome. NIPT is a screening test, which means it can only tell you the likelihood of your baby having a disorder (with the added bonus of letting you know your baby's sex—if you want to find out, that is)—not if your baby definitely has (or doesn't have) a disorder. The companies that perform these new screening tests say that NIPT creates far fewer false positives than standard blood screenings (like the quad screening; see page 56). The results can help you and your practitioner decide next steps, including whether invasive diagnostic tests—which are even more precise but carry some risk—are worth that risk.

Because NIPT involves only a quick blood draw with a needle and syringe, all you'll need to do is offer up your arm at the practitioner's office or a lab—so it's perfectly safe for you and baby. Your sample is then sent off to a lab, which will check the DNA in your blood for signs of an elevated risk of abnormalities.

Once the results of your NIPT are back, your practitioner will likely pair them with the results of your first-trimester ultrasound or nuchal translucency screening (see below) to determine whether more testing is needed. If it's positive, your practitioner will recommend following up with amniocentesis (see page 59) or CVS (see page 58) to confirm the result and check for other problems NIPT can't detect, such as neural tube defects.

Because NIPT is relatively new, it's not FDA approved. Currently, ACOG recommends that NIPT be offered only to women at higher risk of carrying a baby with a chromosomal abnormality (such as moms-to-be who are 35 or older or those who previously had a child with a genetic disorder, or who have a family history of a genetic disorder), not to low-risk women. NIPT is not recommended at all for women carrying multiples or those who are using a donor egg.

Before you schedule NIPT, check with your insurance plan to find out if the test is fully covered (most plans do cover it)—and if not, what it will cost you.

Nuchal translucency screening (10 to 13 weeks). The nuchal translucency (NT) screening test—basically a specialized ultrasound—lets you know if you're at an increased risk for having a baby with a chromosomal problem such as Down syndrome. Unlike diagnostic tests, however, the NT screening can't give you a definitive answer about whether your baby has a genetic abnormality—instead, it gives the statistical likelihood of one. With that information in hand, you and your practitioner can then decide if further (more invasive, but conclusive) diagnostic testing, such as amniocentesis or CVS, is necessary.

What exactly does NT measure? It focuses on a small, clear space in the tissue at the back of a growing baby's neck called the nuchal fold. Experts have found that this spot tends to accumulate fluid and, as a result, expands in size in babies who have genetic abnormalities like Down syndrome (caused by an extra copy of chromosome 21, one of the 23 pairs of chromosomes that contain a human's genetic code), trisomy 18 (an extra copy of chromosome 18), and trisomy 13 (an extra number 13 chromosome).

NT screening, which must be performed between 10 and 13 weeks of pregnancy (after that, the tissue gets so thick that it is no longer translucent, making test results inconclusive), is done with a highly sensitive ultrasound machine (but like a standard ultrasound, is considered safe). A sonographer will first measure your baby to confirm his or her gestational age before zooming in on the nuchal fold and measuring its thickness on the screen. Those measurements, plus your age and baby's gestational age, will be entered into an equation that calculates the probability of a chromosomal abnormality.

An NT screen is often part of routine prenatal testing during the first trimester and recommended for all women. While it's widely available, some areas—especially rural ones—may not have the machine and technicians with the expertise to perform the procedure.

Because increased NT measurements are also associated with fetal heart defects, your practitioner might suggest a fetal echocardiogram at around 20 weeks to screen for heart defects if your levels are high. Increased NT measurements may also be linked to a very slightly higher risk of preterm birth, so you may be monitored for that as well if your NT results are high.

Combined screening (11 to 14 weeks). Because NT results by themselves have an accuracy rate of just 70 to 75 percent (meaning that the test misses 25 to 30 percent of babies with Down syndrome), your practitioner might offer what's referred to as a combined screening, in which the NT ultrasound results are combined with 1 or 2 blood tests that measure and compare your levels of 2 hormones, hCG and PAPP-A (pregnancy-associated plasma protein A), which are produced by the fetus and passed into the mother's bloodstream.

Knowing the Negatives of False Positives

You undergo screening tests for the reassurance you hope they'll provide—and ultimately the results are usually reassuring. But it's important to start off the screening process with an open discussion with your practitioner so you can learn about the negatives of false positives (test results that come back positive for an increased risk of a disorder when in fact baby's just fine): what it really means if you get a positive result, which tests have a high rate of false positives (like the quad screen or the NT alone), and which tests have a lower rate of false positives (like NIPT). What you'll hear is that more than 90 percent of moms who get a positive screen will end up having perfectly normal and healthy babies. Talk about positive!

By combining these blood tests with the NT screening, the accuracy of detection rates for Down syndrome rises dramatically to between 83 and 92 percent.

If your combined screening test shows that your baby may be at an increased risk of having a chromosomal defect, a test such as CVS or amniocentesis will be offered. If the screening test doesn't show an increased risk, your practitioner might recommend that you take the integrated screening test in the second trimester (see page 56) to rule out neural tube defects as well.

Remember, this screen doesn't directly test for chromosomal problems, and it can't diagnose a specific condition. Rather, the results provide your baby's statistical likelihood of having a problem. An abnormal result on the combined screening test definitely doesn't mean that your baby has a chromosomal problem, just that he or she has an increased risk of having one—making follow-up diagnostic testing advisable. In fact, most women who have an abnormal result on their screening test go on to have a perfectly normal baby. At the same time, a normal result isn't an absolute guarantee that your baby is normal, but it does mean that it is extremely unlikely that your baby has a chromosomal defect.

Integrated screening (first and second trimesters). Another screening test option that you may be offered combines measurements of the hormone PAPP-A and (possibly) NT from the first trimester with the measurements of the 4 hormones tested for in the second trimester quad screening (see below). Combining the first and second trimester measurements gives a bit more sensitivity to the screening.

Quad screening (14 to 22 weeks). Quad screening is a blood test that measures the levels of 4 substances produced by the fetus and passed into the mother's bloodstream: alpha-fetoprotein (AFP), hCG, estriol, and inhibin-A. High levels of AFP may suggest the possibility (but by no means the probability) that a baby is at higher risk for a neural tube defect. Low levels of AFP and abnormal levels of the other markers may indicate that the developing baby may be at higher risk for a chromosomal abnormality, such as Down syndrome. The quad screening, like all screening tests, can't diagnose a birth defect—it can only indicate a higher risk. Any abnormal result simply means that follow-up testing is needed.

Your doctor may recommend a quad screen instead of NIPT screening because NIPT may not be available in your area or may not be covered by your insurance. This screening is also less accurate than the NT screen combined with first-trimester blood work, so it's usually recommended only for moms-to-be who are already in their second trimester.

When an abnormality actually exists, the quad screen is pretty good at detecting an increased risk of it—picking it up in approximately 85 percent of neural tube defect cases, nearly 80 percent of Down syndrome cases, and 80 percent of trisomy 18 cases. But the false-positive rate for the independent quad screen is very high. Only 1 or 2 out of 50 women with abnormal readings eventually prove to have an affected fetus—in all the rest, further testing shows that no abnormality exists after all. Sometimes, it turns out that hormone levels tested outside of the normal range because there's more than one baby, other times it's because the EDD is off (the fetus is either a few weeks older or younger than expected), and still other times it's because the test results were inaccurate or misinterpreted. If you get a positive result, you're carrying a single baby, and your ultrasound shows your dates are correct, you'll be offered amniocentesis as followup. But before you consider taking this or any action on the basis of a quad screening, be sure a genetic counselor or a doctor experienced in interpreting these types of screening tests has evaluated and verified the results.

One other thing to consider when getting your quad screening results: Studies indicate that women who receive abnormal results on their quad screen but receive normal results on follow-up testing such as amniocentesis may still be at very slightly increased risk of certain pregnancy complications, such as a small-for-gestational-age fetus, preterm delivery, or preeclampsia. Talk to your practitioner about whether this might apply to you.

Level 2 ultrasound (18 to 22 weeks). Even if you had an ultrasound in your first trimester to date your pregnancy (see page 170), you'll probably also get a screening ultrasound in your second trimester. This level 2 scan (also called an anatomy scan; see box, page 262) is much more detailed and focuses closely on fetal anatomy to make sure everything is growing and developing as it should. It also can be a lot more fun to look at, because it gives a far clearer picture of your baby-to-be than that first fuzzy one you got way back in trimester 1.

A level 2 scan also checks for hard and soft markers, characteristics that may indicate an increased risk of a chromosomal abnormality. Important to know before you head in for your scan: Very few babies showing soft markers (choroid plexus cyst, echogenic foci, or pyelectasia, to name an unpronounceable few) end up having an abnormality. In fact, these markers are spotted on as many as 11 to 17 percent of all healthy babies—good reason not to worry if one is spotted on your baby's scan. Your practitioner will let you know whether any follow-up testing is necessary (it often isn't).

As with any ultrasound, a wand (transducer) is placed on your belly that sends sound waves through your body. The waves bounce off internal organs and fluids, and a computer converts those echoes into a 2-dimensional image (or a cross-sectional view) of the fetus on a screen. Sometimes 3D or even 4D technology is used instead of 2D.

During your level 2 ultrasound, you may be able to spot your baby's beating heart, the curve of the spine, and the face, arms, and legs. You may even catch sight of your baby sucking a thumb.

Usually, the genitals can be seen and the sex determined, although with less than 100 percent reliability and depending on baby's cooperation (if you'd like to keep the sex a surprise until delivery, make sure you let your practitioner or technician know this in advance).

Diagnostic Tests

While just about every expectant mom will sign up for screening tests, going a step further to definitive diagnostic tests isn't for everyone. Many parents—particularly those whose screening tests come back negative—can continue to play the waiting game, with the happy assurance that the chances are overwhelming that their babies will arrive completely healthy.

But if you receive a positive result on a screening test, your practitioner may recommend following up with a diagnostic test to see if an abnormality actually exists, which it most often doesn't. Other reasons why a mom-to-be might consider having prenatal diagnostic testing: having a family history of and/or being a carrier of a genetic condition, having had a baby with a birth defect, or having been exposed to an infection or substance that could possibly cause harm to a developing baby.

Unlike screenings, diagnostic tests, like chorionic villus sampling (CVS) and amniocentesis (amnio), analyze the genetic material in cells collected from baby's placenta or amniotic fluid. These tests are more accurate in detecting chromosomal abnormalities like Down syndrome and, in the case of amnio, neural tube defects, because they directly test for problems—not just signs that possibly point to problems. You might want to consider speaking to a genetic counselor before taking diagnostic tests, just so you are armed with accurate information going in.

Mistakes Happen

As far as prenatal diagnosis has come, it's still important to remember that it's far from infallible. Mistakes happen, even in the best labs and facilities, even with the most skilled professionals wielding the most high-tech equipment—with false positives being much more common than false negatives. That's why further testing and/or consultation with additional professionals should always be used to confirm a result that indicates there is something wrong with the fetus—and if that's confirmed, what the prognosis for your baby will be.

Why go through diagnostic testing if there's some risk involved? The best reason is the reassurance it usually brings. Most of the time, diagnostic tests diagnose a perfectly healthy baby—which means that mom and dad can stop worrying and start enjoying their pregnancy.

Chorionic villus sampling (10 to 13 weeks). CVS is a first-trimester prenatal diagnostic test that involves taking a small tissue sample from the finger-like projections of the placenta called the chorionic villi and testing the sample to detect chromosomal abnormalities. Because CVS is performed in the first trimester, it can give results (and most often, reassurance) earlier in pregnancy than amniocentesis, which is usually performed after the 16th week. CVS can detect (with 98 percent accuracy) a number of disorders, including Down syndrome, Tay-Sachs disease, sickle cell anemia, and most types of cystic fibrosis. CVS can't test for neural tube and other anatomical defects. Testing

for specific genetic diseases (other than Down syndrome) is usually done only when there is a family history of the disease or the parents are known to be carriers.

CVS is most often performed by a maternal-fetal medicine specialist in an ultrasound suite. Depending on the location of the placenta, the sample of cells is taken via the vagina and cervix (transcervical CVS) or via a needle inserted in the abdominal wall (transabdominal CVS). Neither method is entirely pain-free, and the discomfort can range from very mild to moderate. Some women experience cramping (similar to menstrual cramps) when the sample is taken. Both methods take about 30 minutes, start to finish, though the actual withdrawal of cells takes no more than a minute or two.

In the transcervical procedure, you'll lie on your back with your feet in stirrups while a long, thin tube is inserted through your vagina into your uterus. Guided by ultrasound imaging,

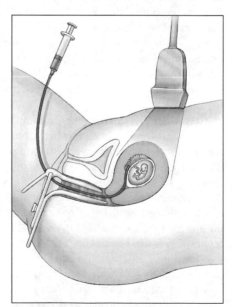

Transcervical CVS testing

the doctor positions the tube between the uterine lining and the chorion, the fetal membrane that will eventually form the fetal side of the placenta. A sample of the chorionic villi is then snipped or suctioned off for diagnostic study.

In the transabdominal procedure, you'll also lie flat, tummy-up. Ultrasound is used to determine the location of the placenta and to view the uterine walls. Then, with continued ultrasound guidance, a needle is inserted through your abdomen and the uterine wall to the edge of the placenta, and the cells to be studied are drawn up through the needle.

Because the chorionic villi are of fetal origin, examining them can give a clear picture of the genetic makeup of the fetus. Test results are available in 1 to 2 weeks.

CVS is safe and reliable. The procedure carries a miscarriage rate equal to that of amnio—less than half a percent. Choosing a testing center with a good safety record and waiting until right after your 10th week can further reduce the risks associated with the procedure.

Some vaginal bleeding can occur after CVS and shouldn't be cause for concern, though it should be reported. You should also let your doctor know if the bleeding lasts for 3 days or longer. Since there is a very slight risk of infection with CVS, report any fever that occurs in the first few days after the procedure. If you're Rh negative, you'll be given an injection of Rh-immune globulin (RhoGAM) after the CVS to be sure the procedure doesn't result in Rh problems later on (see page 35).

Amniocentesis (16 to 20 weeks). In this diagnostic test, which is usually done between weeks 16 and 18 of pregnancy, a long, thin, hollow needle is inserted through your abdomen, through the

It's a . . . Surprise!

Diagnostic testing (and some screening tests like NIPT or second-trimester ultrasound) can determine whether your bundle of joy is a boy or a girl. But unless it's a necessary part of the diagnosis, you'll have the option of either learning baby's sex when you receive the testing results (or when you cut into a pink or blue cake at the gender-reveal party) or waiting to find out the old-fashioned way, in the birthing room. Just make sure your practitioner knows about your decision ahead of time so your surprise won't be inadvertently spoiled.

wall of the uterus, and into the fluid-filled amniotic sac. Ultrasound is done at the same time, so your baby doesn't get accidentally poked by the needle (see illustration, page 60). You'll feel the prick and might experience some mild pain and cramping. About 1 to 2 tablespoons of the fluid are drawn out (don't worry, it will be quickly replenished) and sent to the lab for analysis. The fluid contains cells that your baby has sloughed off, plus chemicals. By analyzing this baby brew, your practitioner can assess the health of your fetus and look for certain medical conditions (such as Down syndrome) caused by abnormalities in the chromosomes. The entire procedure—including prep time and ultrasound—will usually take about 30 minutes, start to finish (though the actual withdrawal of amniotic fluid takes no more than a minute or 2). If you're Rh negative, you'll be given an injection of Rh-immune globulin (RhoGAM) after the amniocentesis to be sure the procedure does not result in Rh problems (see page 35).

If a Problem Is Found

In the vast majority of cases, prenatal diagnosis yields the results that parents hope for—that all is well with their baby-to-be. But when the news isn't happy—when something does turn out to be wrong—the information provided by such a heartbreaking diagnosis can still be valuable to parents. Teamed with expert genetic counseling, it can be used to make vital decisions about this and future pregnancies.

Following positive results on definitive diagnostic testing, you'll get (or you should ask for) a referral to experts, such as genetic counselor and/or a doctor specializing in your baby's condition, so you can learn about your options (including whether or not you might want to repeat the testing just to be sure the diagnosis is correct). You can also do your own research. After all, the more you know about your baby's condition and what you're facing as a family, the better prepared you can be

(both emotionally and practically) for what lies ahead—whether it's receiving a child with special needs or coping with the inevitable loss of a baby. You'll also be able to begin working through the reactions (denial, resentment, guilt) that can come with discovering that your dreams of a perfectly healthy baby aren't coming true. Joining a condition-specific support group—even one online—can help make coping somewhat easier, providing both answers and community.

Depending on your baby's condition, it may be recommended that you give birth at a specialized hospital, if possible. A specialized birth facility for labor and delivery can better address your specific needs or recommend medical interventions that, if performed immediately after birth, can improve your baby's quality of life. What's more, many of the hospitals that cater to high-risk births already have support groups

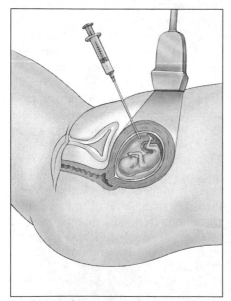

Amniocentesis

Amnio and CVS diagnose nearly all chromosomal disorders, including Down syndrome, with 99 percent accuracy, with at least 90 percent accuracy for several hundred other genetic diseases (such as sickle cell anemia) when they're specifically checked for. It does not, however, detect every kind of abnormality, including cleft lip or palate, and it can't determine the severity of the problem. Unlike CVS, amnio can also rule out neural tube defects (such as spina bifida).

Amnio is usually recommended if you're at high risk of certain abnormalities, had a previous child with a birth defect, have a family history of genetic conditions (unless you've been screened and found that you're not a carrier), and/or have received a positive in their community outreach programs as well as specialized NICUs (neonatal intensive care units) that can provide the best care for your baby if necessary. Lining up a pediatrician with specialized training while you're still pregnant guarantees care specific to your little one's condition from the day he or she arrives.

In some cases, an abnormality can be addressed prenatally. If your baby has a serious heart condition or spina bifida, for example, you may be able to opt for a prenatal procedure to correct it, if necessary, rather than waiting until after your baby is born. Be sure to ask your practitioner whether your baby is a candidate for prenatal surgery. Early interventions—such as therapy and other medical treatment—performed as soon as baby is born may also go a long way toward improving the prognosis for your little one, as well as his or her quality of life.

If you've been told your baby likely won't make it to term (since a fetus with certain chromosome disorders often won't survive a pregnancy) or may not live very long after birth, it may be possible to donate one or more healthy organs to an infant in need. Some parents find that this provides some consolation for their own loss. A maternal-fetal specialist (or neonatologist) may be able to provide helpful information in such a situation and can help you prepare physically and emotionally for it. There are also numerous hospitals, hospices, and clinics that provide perinatal hospice and palliative care support for families who wish to continue their pregnancies with babies who likely will not live long after birth.

If testing suggests a defect that will be fatal or extremely disabling, and retesting and interpretation by a genetic counselor confirms the diagnosis, some parents may make the agonizing decision, in consultation with their practitioner or other experts, to terminate the pregnancy. If you do, allow yourself time and space to grieve in the same way that moms-to-be who experience any kind of pregnancy loss need to.

result on a screening like NT, NIPT, combined screen, or quad screen and you've missed the first-trimester window for CVS (or opted not to get a CVS because that test can't detect neural tube defects). Test results are usually back in 10 to 14 days.

Although most of the conditions detected by amniocentesis can't be cured, the test can let parents know about their baby's abnormality in advance. This gives them time to become informed about a condition, as well as make decisions about their baby's future health care or make the difficult decision to not continue the pregnancy.

The news is rarely bad, however. More than 95 percent of the time amnio will find nothing but a healthy baby. (And if you'd like to know the sex of your baby, amnio will give you that news, too.)

After the procedure you'll be able to drive yourself home (some doctors recommend you have someone else drive you just to be on the safe side) and you'll probably be told to rest in bed for a few hours to a full 24 hours. You'll need to avoid sex, heavy lifting, strenuous exercise, and flying for the next 3 days. You might experience minor cramping, but if cramps become severe or persistent, call your practitioner. Also call if you notice leaking amniotic fluid or spotting, or if you develop a fever.

Complications from amnio are rare, but you should discuss them with your practitioner when considering the procedure.

CHAPTER 3

Your Pregnancy Lifestyle

Of course you're expecting to make some adjustments in your everyday life now that you're expecting (goodbye baby tees, hello baby-on-board tees). But you might also be wondering just how drastically your lifestyle will have to change now that you're living for two. How about that pre-dinner cocktail—will it have to wait until post-delivery? Those regular dips in the hot tub—are those washed up, too? Can you wipe your bathroom sink with that effective (but smelly) disinfectant? And what's that you heard about cat litter? Does being pregnant really mean you have to think twice about all those things you've never given a second thought to—from letting your best friend smoke in your living room to zapping your dinner in the microwave? In a few cases, you'll find, the answer is an emphatic yes (as in "No wine for me, thanks"). But in many others, your expectant self will be able to continue doing business—and pleasure—as usual, with maybe just a side of caution ("Honey, it's your turn to change the cat litter—for the next 9 months!").

What You May Be Wondering About

Working Out

"Can I keep up with my regular workout now that I'm pregnant?"

Workouts are not only a can-do for most pregnant women, but a definite should-do. In fact, the vast majority of workouts work well with the vast majority of pregnancies, which means you can almost certainly count on continuing your usual routine through your 9 months. Just to be sure, check in with your practitioner for the all-clear on your current workout regimen, and ask before beginning a new one (pregnancy isn't the time to take on an extreme sport). Also, remember this mama-to-be mantra: Listen to your body. Don't exercise until you drop . . . or until it hurts. Instead, make moderation your pregnancy workout MO. See page 231 for more.

Caffeine

"I drink coffee to keep me going all day. Do I have to give up caffeine while I'm pregnant?"

No need to surrender your Starbucks card entirely—though you may have to start pulling it out a little less often. Most evidence suggests that drinking up to about 200 mg of caffeine a day is perfectly safe for your little bean. What does that break down to, exactly? Possibly not as much as you'd hope—about 12 ounces of brewed coffee (2 small cups or 1 "tall") or about 2 shots of espresso. Which means you're good to go—and fuel your get-up-and-go—if you're a light to moderate coffee drinker. But you'll have to reassess your intake if you've got a more serious java jones (for instance, you're a member in good standing of the 5-shot Americano club).

Why go so low? Well, for one thing, you share that coffee—like everything you eat and drink when you're expecting—with your baby. Caffeine (found most famously, abundantly, and arguably deliciously in coffee but also available in other foods and beverages) does cross the placenta—though to what extent (and at what dose) it affects a fetus is not completely clear. The latest information indicates that heavier caffeine intake early in pregnancy slightly increases the risk of miscarriage.

But there's more to the caffeine story, at least when you overdo the stuff. Sure, caffeine has impressive pick-me-up powers, but in large doses it can block the absorption of iron. It can also act as a diuretic, causing calcium and other key pregnancy nutrients to be washed out of your system before they can be thoroughly absorbed—not to mention, increasing urinary frequency (something you've likely found is plenty frequent enough). It can be irritating to your bladder, too, which is already under plenty of pressure (literally) during pregnancy. Need more motivation for cutting down? Too much caffeine mixed with pregnancy hormones can make an especially intense brew for many expectant moms—the perfect storm for even more volatile mood swings. It can also prevent you from getting the rest your body's craving more than ever, especially if you drink it after noon (caffeine can stay in your system, keeping your engine revved, for at least 8 hours).

Different practitioners have different recommendations on caffeine consumption, so check in with yours for a bottom line on your coffee quota. When calculating your daily intake, keep in mind that it's not necessarily as easy as counting cups (especially because those cups vary so much in size and strength). Caffeine isn't found just in coffee—it's also in caffeinated soft drinks (too many Mountain Dews are a Mountain Don't), coffee ice cream and yogurt, many varieties of tea, energy bars and drinks, and chocolate (the darker the chocolate, the more caffeine it packs). You'll need to know, too, that dark brews poured at coffee bars contain far more caffeine than homemade. Likewise, instant coffee contains less than drip does (see box, page 64).

How do you cut down on a hefty caffeine habit (or cut it out altogether if you choose)? That depends on what's in the caffeine for you. If it's a part of your day (or many parts of your day) you're not excited about parting with, there's

Caffeine Counter

How much caffeine do you get per day? It may be more—or less—than you think (and more or less than that approximate limit of 200 mg). Check out this handy list, so you can do the math before you belly up to the coffee bar . . . or the chocolate bar:

- 1 cup brewed coffee (8 ounces) = 135 mg

- 1 cup instant coffee = 95 mg

- 1 cup decaf coffee = 5 to 30 mg

- 1 shot espresso (or any drink made with 1 shot) = 90 mg

- 1 cup tea = 40 to 60 mg (green tea has less caffeine than black tea)

- 1 can cola (12 ounces) = about 35 mg

- 1 can diet cola = 45 mg

- 1 can Red Bull = 80 mg

- 1 ounce milk chocolate = 6 mg

- 1 ounce dark chocolate = 20 mg

- 1 cup chocolate milk = 5 mg

- ½ cup coffee ice cream = 20 to 40 mg

no need to. Just make your morning joe regular and your afternoons decaf. Or order your latte with mostly decaf shots instead of regular—or with less espresso and more milk (you'll get a bigger calcium bonus anyway).

If it's the lift you crave—and that your body has become accustomed to—cutting back will be a taller order (make that a venti order). As any coffee lover is well aware, it's one thing to be motivated to cut back on or kick caffeine altogether and another thing to

do it. Caffeine is addictive (that's where the craving comes in), and quitting—or even cutting way back on—a heavy habit comes with its own set of withdrawal symptoms, including headache, irritability, fatigue, and lethargy. That's why it's a good idea to ease off heavy consumption gradually. Try cutting back a cup at a time, and give yourself a few days to adjust to the lower dose before cutting back by another cup. Another way to cut back: Take each cup half-caf, gradually going full decaf in more and more cups—until your total caffeine consumption is down to that two-a-day-or-less goal.

No matter what's been driving you to the coffee bar, cutting back on or kicking caffeine will be less of a drag if you follow these energizing solutions:

- Boost your blood sugar to boost your energy. You'll get a longer-lasting boost from snacking on healthy foods often, especially complex carbs and protein (a combo that will give you the lift that keeps on lifting).

- Get some pregnancy-appropriate exercise each day. Working out will help you work out those caffeine cravings, but it'll also raise the energy roof while releasing those feel-good endorphins. Adding fresh air to the exercise mix will give you an extra energy boost.

- Get your buzz from z's. Clocking in the sleep your body needs at night (which will probably be easier to do without all that caffeine keeping you wired) will help you feel more refreshed in the morning, even before you've filled your first mug.

- Keep an eye on the prize—and on your savings. Do the math: Cutting back on visits to the coffee bar means you'll be able to stash cash to use on gearing up for your baby-to-be.

Drinking

"I had a few drinks before I knew I was pregnant. Could that have hurt the baby?"

Wouldn't it be nice to get a text from your body the moment sperm and egg meet up? ("Just wanted to let you know we have a baby on board—time to trade that wine in for water.") But since there's no app for that (at least not yet), many moms-to-be are clueless that baby making has begun until several weeks into pregnancy—especially if they weren't keeping track of their fertility. And in the meantime, they're apt to have done a thing or two they wouldn't have done if they'd only known. Like having a few, a few times too many. Which is why your concern is shared by so many other new moms-to-be.

Fortunately, it's a concern that you can cross off the list. There's no evidence that a couple of drinks on a couple of occasions very early in pregnancy, when you didn't even know you were pregnant, can harm a developing embryo. So you—and all the other moms who didn't get the message right away—can relax.

That said, it's definitely time to change your drink order now. Keep reading to find out more.

"I've heard that it's okay to have an occasional glass of wine with dinner when you're pregnant. Is that true?"

It's been passed around the pregnancy grapevine a lot lately, but there's no research to support that an occasional glass of wine (or beer, or cocktail) is a safe bet when you're expecting. In fact, the Surgeon General, the CDC, ACOG, AAP, and many other experts advise that no amount of alcohol is safe for pregnant women.

You can check in with your practitioner for a recommendation—some practitioners are more lenient when it comes to alcohol in pregnancy (especially that occasional glass of wine, sipped with food), taking a page from medical texts in the U.K. and many European countries, where light drinking for two is considered acceptable.

But here's why the medical consensus in the U.S comes down so definitively against drinking during pregnancy. First, it's to be on the safe side—which, when you think about it, is always the best side to be on when you have a baby on board. Though nobody knows for sure whether there is a safe limit when it comes to alcohol consumption during pregnancy (or whether that limit would be different in different women and for different babies), it is known that an expectant mom never drinks alone—she shares each glass of wine, each beer, each cocktail equally with her baby. The alcohol enters the fetal bloodstream in about the same concentrations present in the mom-to-be's blood, but it takes the fetus twice as long to eliminate the alcohol from its system. Second, for some moms-to-be, having an occasional drink during pregnancy can be a slippery slope—one mom's sip of wine may be another mom's 12 ounces—making it wiser to just stay away from alcohol altogether. Glass sizes and pours (whether at home or in a restaurant) vary widely, too—another good reason to toe the teetotaling line. Certainly more than occasional, light drinking is associated with proven, serious risks to a developing baby; see box, page 66.

Passing up a drink during pregnancy is as easily done as said for some women, especially those who develop an aversion to alcohol in early pregnancy that sometimes lingers through delivery. For others, particularly those who are accustomed to unwinding with a beer at the end of the day or to sipping

Drinking That Can Devastate

At what point does a drink become one drink too many for a developing fetus? It's hard to put a number on that, since every woman and every fetus is different (and the amount of alcohol in different drinks and pours varies). However, drinking heavily throughout pregnancy or binge drinking (having 4 or more drinks at a time, even occasionally) can result not only in serious obstetrical complications, but in fetal alcohol syndrome. This condition produces babies who are born small for gestational age, with facial deformities, and with brain damage (which later shows up as tremors, motor development problems, attention deficits, learning disabilities, lower IQ, and possibly other mental deficiencies). But even drinking moderately throughout pregnancy can increase the risk of miscarriage and stillbirth, as well as the risk of developmental and behavioral problems in a child.

The effects of drinking during pregnancy are devastating, permanent, and completely preventable by completely avoiding alcohol. The sooner a drinker stops drinking during pregnancy, the less risk there is to her baby and her pregnancy. If you can't stop drinking, talk to your practitioner and get help right away.

a glass of red with dinner, abstinence may require a concerted effort and include a lifestyle change. If you drink to relax, for example, try substituting other methods of relaxation: music, a bath, prenatal yoga, or meditation or visualization. If drinking is part of a daily ritual that you don't want to give up, try a Virgin Mary (a Bloody Mary without the vodka) at brunch, sparkling juice or nonalcoholic beer at dinner, or a half-juice, half-sparkling water spritzer—served at the usual time, in the usual glasses (unless, of course, these look-alike beverages trigger a yen for the real stuff). If your spouse joins you on the wagon (at least while in your company), the ride will be considerably smoother.

If you're having trouble giving up alcohol, ask your practitioner for help and for a referral to a program that can help you quit.

Smoking

"I've been smoking cigarettes for 10 years. Will this hurt my baby?"

Happily, there's no clear evidence that any smoking you've done before pregnancy—even if it's been for 10 or more years—will harm the baby you're now busy making. But it's well documented (as well as plastered on cigarette packs) that smoking during pregnancy, particularly beyond the 3rd month, isn't hazardous to just your health but to your baby's as well.

In effect, when a mom smokes, her fetus is confined in a smoke-filled womb. Its heartbeat speeds up and, worst of all, because of insufficient oxygen, it can't grow and thrive as it should.

The results can be devastating. Smoking around the time of conception increases the risk of ectopic pregnancy and continued smoking can increase the risk of a wide variety of pregnancy complications, including abnormal implantation or premature detachment of the placenta, premature rupture of the membranes, and early delivery.

There is also strong evidence that a baby's development in utero is adversely and directly affected by a mom's smoking. The most widespread risks for babies of smokers are low birthweight, shorter length, and smaller head circumference, as well as cleft palate or cleft lip, and heart defects. And being born too small is the major cause of newborn illness and death.

There are other potential risks as well. Babies of smokers are more likely to die from SIDS (sudden infant death syndrome). They are also more prone to apnea (breathing lapses), and in general, aren't as healthy at birth as babies of nonsmokers. And evidence indicates that, on average, these children will suffer long-term physical and intellectual deficits, especially if parents continue to smoke around them. Children of mothers who smoked while pregnant are hospitalized more often in their first year of life, and are particularly prone to a lowered immune system, respiratory diseases, ear infections, colic, tuberculosis, food allergies, asthma, short stature, obesity, and problems in school, including attention deficit hyperactivity disorder (ADHD). They're also more likely to be abnormally aggressive as toddlers and to have behavioral and psychological problems into adulthood. Other research suggests that daughters born to mothers who smoked during pregnancy are at higher risk of developing gestational diabetes when they become pregnant later in life. Finally, children of moms who smoked during pregnancy are also more likely to grow up to be smokers themselves.

The effects of tobacco use, like those of alcohol use, are dose related: Tobacco use reduces the birthweight of babies in direct proportion to the number of cigarettes smoked, with a pack-a-day smoker 30 percent more likely to give birth to a low-birthweight child than a nonsmoker. So cutting down on the number of cigarettes you smoke

FOR FATHERS

Your Secondhand Smoke

Moms-to-be definitely carry a heavy load—and most of the baby-nurturing responsibilities, at least until baby's born. The exception: When it comes to providing a smoke-free environment, mom can't do it alone. If there is smoke in her environment, there's smoke (and harmful tobacco by-products) in baby's. Even if she doesn't light up herself, but you (or others around her) do, baby's body is going to pick up nearly as much contamination as it would if she smoked. Doing your smoking away from your pregnant partner is better than smoking around her, but you'll still be exposing her (and baby) to the toxins that stick to your clothes and skin.

A very big (yet very little and vulnerable) reason to quit: to give your baby-to-be the very best chances possible of being born healthy. But the benefits to your baby of having a smoke-free dad don't end at delivery. Smoking by either parent increases the risk of SIDS in infancy and of respiratory problems, lung damage, and other illnesses at all ages. And it ups the chances that your little one will become a smoker one day. Quitting now will give your baby a healthier home to be born into— and a healthier life to live. Not to mention, a chance to grow up with a healthier dad who's likely to live longer. For help quitting, see box, page 68.

Your baby will thank you, also, for not smoking cigars and pipes. Because they aren't inhaled, they release even more smoke into the air than cigarettes, making them more potentially harmful to your baby. So pass the chocolate cigars, instead.

Help Quitting

Congratulations—you've decided to give your baby a smoke-free environment, in utero and out, and you're mega-motivated to quit. Luckily, there is plenty of help for smokers who want to kick butt. Among the strategies that have made quitters out of smokers: hypnosis, acupuncture, and relaxation techniques. If you're comfortable with a group approach to quitting—which builds in support—consider programs run by Nicotine Anonymous, the American Lung Association, the American Cancer Society, and SmokEnders. Or seek support online from other pregnant women who are trying to call it quits. Check out smokefree.gov or cdc.gov/tobacco/ quit_smoking for more information and help.

Wondering about the safety of nicotine replacement therapy (nicotine patches, lozenges, or gums) or Chantix (a prescription drug used to curb cravings) when you're expecting? Ask your practitioner. Most experts don't recommend these as first-line treatment for smoking cessation during pregnancy.

---

may help some. But cutting down can be misleading, because a smoker often compensates by taking more frequent and deeper puffs and smoking more of each cigarette. This can also happen when a smoker switches to low-tar or low-nicotine cigarettes.

What about e-cigarettes? Despite little research on electronic cigarettes during pregnancy, most experts say it's best not to puff on those, either. Electronic cigarettes, which claim to have significantly fewer toxins and less nicotine than traditional cigarettes, still contain enough to potentially affect your baby. Plus, until FDA regulation is implemented across the board, it'll be hard to know just how much nicotine you're exposing yourself (and your baby) to—even from e-cigarettes that are marketed as "nicotine-free." Additives and flavorings used in many e-cigarettes may also be questionable when you're growing a baby. Bottom line: Until more is known—and until more regulation is in place—you're better off staying away from e-cigarettes.

Same goes for a hookah, in which the smoke from specially made tobacco passes through water and is then drawn through a rubber hose to a mouthpiece. Smoking a hookah is as toxic as smoking a cigarette. Despite what you may have heard, the water in the hookah does not filter out the toxic ingredients (like tar, carbon monoxide, and heavy metals) in the tobacco smoke. And what's worse, hookah smokers may actually breathe in more nicotine than cigarette smokers do because of the large volume of smoke they inhale during a session.

Eager to kick the smoking habit? You should be, because some studies show that women who quit smoking early in pregnancy—no later than the 3rd month—can eliminate all of the associated risks. For some smoking women, quitting will never be easier than in early pregnancy, when they might develop a sudden distaste for cigarettes—probably the warning of an intuitive body. Sooner is better, but quitting even in the last month can help preserve oxygen flow to the baby during delivery. See the box above for more on quitting.

Marijuana Use

"I have smoked pot socially for years. Could this be harmful to the baby I'm now pregnant with? And is smoking pot during pregnancy dangerous?"

You can safely put past pot behind you. Although it's usually recommended that couples trying to conceive pass on pot because it can interfere with conception, you're already pregnant—so that won't be a problem for you. And there's no present evidence that the marijuana you've smoked before you conceived will harm your fetus.

What about the risks of weed now that you're pregnant? All the research isn't in yet, and the research that's been done so far hasn't been very helpful. That's because, on average, women who smoke pot regularly during pregnancy are more likely to make other pregnancy-unfriendly choices (smoking cigarettes, drinking, not getting regular prenatal care)—making it hard to identify which choice is to blame when the baby of a pot smoker doesn't thrive or isn't born healthy. Some studies show a relationship between regular pot smoking and a baby being born too small for gestational age, others studies don't. And still other research has pointed to attention, learning, and behavioral disorders later in childhood for babies of moms who used marijuana throughout pregnancy.

What is known definitively so far is that marijuana passes through the placenta, so a smoking mom shares the drug with her baby. And with no sure proof that it's safe to use weed during pregnancy—and some evidence that suggests it may be quite harmful—it's smart to pass on pot during pregnancy. Pass, too, on edibles (the same potential risks apply to weed you eat in treats).

If you've already smoked or indulged in edibles early in your pregnancy, don't

---

Prescription for a Healthy Pregnancy

Coming into pregnancy with a squeaky clean lifestyle—no drinking, no smoking, and definitely no drugs? That's great news for you and your baby. But what about prescription medications? Depending on the meds you take, it may be time for some changes now that you're expecting. For the lowdown on Rx med safety during pregnancy, see page 538.

---

worry. But do quit now. Try to find ways to unwind and net that natural high (endorphin-releasing exercise, yoga, meditation, hypnosis, acupuncture). If your use of marijuana has been for medical reasons, say, to relieve chronic pain, ask your practitioner about pregnancy safe therapies.

If you can't seem to stop smoking weed, speak to your practitioner and seek professional help as soon as possible.

Cocaine and Other Drug Use

"I did some cocaine a week before I found out I was pregnant. Now I'm worried about what that could have done to my baby."

Don't worry about past cocaine use—just make sure it was your last. On the upside: Using cocaine once or twice before you found out you were pregnant isn't likely to have had any effect. On the downside: Continuing to use it during pregnancy could be dangerous. How dangerous isn't quite clear. Since many cocaine users are also

Domestic Violence

Protecting her baby from harm is every expectant mother's most basic instinct. But sadly, some women can't even protect themselves during pregnancy. That's because they're victims of domestic violence.

Domestic violence can strike at any time, but it's especially common during pregnancy. While having a baby brings out a new (or renewed) tenderness in many relationships, it rocks others, sometimes triggering unexpectedly negative emotions in a woman's partner (from anger to jealousy to a feeling of being trapped), particularly if the pregnancy wasn't planned. In some cases, unfortunately, those emotions play out in the form of violence against both the mother and her unborn baby. Sometimes, cultural or financial factors, or a family history of domestic violence against women can contribute to a partner's aggression, too.

The statistics are alarming. Nearly 20 percent of all pregnant women experience violence at the hands of their partners, which means that an expectant mother is twice as likely to be the victim of domestic violence as she is to develop preeclampsia or deliver prematurely. More shockingly and tragically still, domestic violence is the single leading cause of death among pregnant women.

Domestic abuse (emotional, sexual, and physical) against pregnant women carries more than just the immediate risk of injury to the mother-to-be and her baby (such as uterine rupture or hemorrhaging). Being battered during pregnancy can lead to numerous negative health consequences, including poor nutrition, poor prenatal care, substance abuse, and so on. Its effects on the pregnancy can also include miscarriage or stillbirth, preterm labor, premature rupture of the membranes, and low birthweight. And once a baby is born into a physically abusive household, he or she can easily become a victim of direct violence—as well as emotional abuse.

Abuse doesn't discriminate—it crosses every socioeconomic profile, every religion, every age, every race and ethnicity, and every educational level. If you're the victim of domestic violence, remember that it's not your fault. You've done nothing wrong. If you are in an abusive relationship, don't wait for things to get better—get help now. Without intervention, the abuse is likely not only to continue but to get worse. Keep in mind that if you're not safe in your relationship, your baby won't be safe, either.

Talk to your practitioner, tell your trusted friends and family, and call a local domestic violence hotline. Many states have programs that can help you with shelter, clothing, and prenatal care. Check out the National Coalition Against Domestic Violence at ncadv.org and the CDC's domestic violence resource page at cdc.gov/violenceprevention or call the National Domestic Violence Hotline at 800-799-7233 (thehotline.org). If you are in immediate danger, call 911.

cigarette smokers, it's hard to separate the probably negative effects of cocaine use from the documented negative effects of smoking. What many studies have shown is that cocaine not only crosses the placenta, but can damage it, reducing fetal growth, particularly of a baby's head. It's also believed to lead to preterm birth, low birthweight, withdrawal symptoms in the newborn, and long-term neurological, behavioral, and developmental problems for the child, along with possibly lower IQ. Certainly, the more a mom-to-be uses cocaine, the greater the risk to her baby.

Tell your practitioner about any cocaine use since you've conceived. As with every aspect of your medical history, the more he or she knows, the better care you will receive. If you have any difficulty giving up cocaine entirely, seek professional help immediately.

Not surprisingly, there are serious risks to babies exposed prenatally to other illicit drugs (including heroin, meth, crack, ecstasy, "ice," and PCP). But also potentially dangerous are some prescription drugs that are often abused and that can, with continued use, cause serious harm to a developing fetus and/or to pregnancy. Then, if you are still using drugs, get professional support to help you quit now. Enrolling in a drug-free pregnancy program now can make a tremendous difference in the outcome of your pregnancy.

Mobile Devices

"I spend hours a day on my smartphone, both for work and for fun . . . and all things baby. Is that safe during pregnancy?"

A re you obsessed with your cell? A message board maniac? Just plain app happy? If so, this should make you extra happy: Evidence suggests it's unlikely mobile devices and the radiation they emit pose any risk to your baby-to-be.

Eager to play it safe but still keep playing on your phone? Experts suggest that you avoid carrying your mobile on your waist (or where your waist once was) and keep it on silent when it's near your bump. Research shows that fetuses startle when they hear that beeping or buzzing or ringing so close by, possibly rattling their sleep-wake cycle.

One well-documented danger of

Wild Rides

S o pregnancy isn't enough of a roller coaster for you? Thinking of something even more daring? There's no need to skip your day at the amusement park (or county fair), but consider keeping it more chill, less thrill—sitting out high-speed or jerky rides now that you're expecting. There's a reason why the signs on those extreme rides warn moms-to-be to steer clear: Rapid starts and stops and jarring forces could possibly lead to placental abruption or other complications. Don't worry about rides you've already taken— just take a pass from now on.

mobile devices whether you're pregnant or not comes from using a handheld mobile phone (for texting or talking) while driving. In fact, in many areas it's illegal. Even hands-free devices can be distracting when you're driving, and you're better off putting your phone on silent (so you don't hear any rings or text dings or social media notification zings) or turning it off altogether when you're in the car. Play it safe by pulling over to a safe area before making a call or texting.

Walking while distracted (using your cell while walking) can also land you in trouble. You're already a little more prone to falls as pregnancy progresses (your center of gravity is off, you can't see your feet), and there's no reason to add another risk factor to the mix. Park yourself on a park bench, stand against a wall in the mall, or stop in your tracks on the track before you text or check how many likes the photo you posted last night has gotten.

Something else to keep in mind: Using a phone or tablet before bed can keep you busy (and productive, when there's so much to do on your to-do list), but it can also keep you from sleeping once you turn in. Light from the screen alters sleepiness and alertness, and also suppresses levels of melatonin, the hormone that regulates your internal clock and plays a role in your sleep cycle. So power down your devices at least an hour before turning in.

Microwaves

"I use my microwave practically every day to heat up food or even cook. Is microwave exposure safe during pregnancy?"

Microwave away, mom. All the research indicates that microwaves are completely safe to use during pregnancy (and at all other times). Just a couple of sensible precautions: Use only cookware that is specifically manufactured for use in the microwave (look for a microwave-safe BPA-free container), and don't let plastic wrap touch foods during microwaving, covering food with an appropriate microwave-safe top or with a paper towel instead. Definitely continue

to practice these protocols after baby arrives—they're not just for pregnancy.

Hot Tubs and Saunas

"We have a hot tub. Is it safe for me to use it while I'm pregnant?"

You won't have to switch to cold showers, but it's probably a good idea to stay out of the hot tub. Anything that raises body temperature over 102°F and keeps it there for a while—whether it's a soak in a hot tub or an extremely hot bath—is potentially hazardous to a developing embryo or fetus, particularly in the early months. Some studies have shown that a hot tub doesn't raise a woman's temperature to dangerous levels immediately—it takes at least 10 minutes (longer if the shoulders and arms are not submerged or if the water is 102°F or less). But because individual responses and circumstances vary, play it safe by keeping your bump out of the hot tub. Feel free, however, to soak your aching feet.

If you've already had some brief dips in the hot tub, there's probably no

---

Is Hot Stuff Not So Hot?

Considering cuddling up with an electric blanket when the winter chill sets in? Or easing that achy-breaky back with a heating pad? Too much heat isn't so hot when you're pregnant, because it may raise your body temperature excessively. So cuddle up to your sweetie instead of that electric blanket (or if his tootsies are as icy as yours, invest in a down comforter, push up the thermostat, or heat the bed with an electric blanket and then turn it off before you turn in). Still feeling the chill? Keep in mind that as the months pass, you'll probably be keeping

yourself so warm—thanks to a pregnancy-boosted metabolism—that you'll be kicking off all your covers anyway.

As for that heating pad, wrap it in a towel before you apply it to your back, belly, or shoulders to reduce the heat it passes along (an ankle or knee can take the heat), keep it at the lowest setting, limit applications to 15 minutes, and avoid sleeping with it. You've already spent some time under that electric blanket or heating pad? Not to worry—there's no proven risk.

What about heat patches? See page 254.

cause for concern. Most women spontaneously get out of a hot tub before their body temperatures reach 102°F because they become uncomfortable. It's likely you did, too.

Take a pass, too, on the sauna and steam room when you're expecting, since they can also raise body temperature excessively—as well as lead to dehydration, dizziness, and low blood pressure.

For more information on the safety of other types of spa treatments, see page 149.

The Family Cat

"I have cats at home. I've heard that cats carry a disease that can harm babies. Do I have to get rid of my pets?"

Before you throw the kitties out with the kitty litter, keep in mind that the risk of infection with toxoplasmosis (a parasite that cats and other animals can carry and excrete in their feces and that can be harmful to a baby) is very remote if you have indoor cats. What's more, if you've had cats for a while, you're likely to already be immune to toxoplasmosis (because you've probably already been infected with it—most cat owners have been). A simple blood test is available that will confirm your immunity, but it won't be useful unless you were tested before you conceived (that's because the tests are not sensitive enough to show whether you have a new infection or simply have antibodies from an old infection). Talk to your practitioner to see if you were tested before you became pregnant.

If you were tested before you conceived and were not immune, or if you're not sure whether you are immune or not, take the following precautions to avoid infection:

■ Have your cats tested by the vet to see if they have an active infection. If they

> ## No Cat, No Toxoplasmosis?
>
> Cats aren't the only culprits when it comes to spreading toxoplasmosis. It's also possible to catch this infection through handling or eating contaminated raw meat or fruits and veggies that have been grown in soil that may have toxoplasmosis parasites in it. Fortunately, the risk of becoming infected is low. Still, to stay on the safe side, follow these smart food-prep tips (which just happen to be best practices for food safety anyway):
>
> ■ Wash fruits and vegetables, especially those grown in home gardens, rinsing very thoroughly, and/or peel or cook them.
>
> ■ Don't eat raw or undercooked meat or unpasteurized milk or dairy products.
>
> ■ Wash your hands thoroughly after handling raw meat.

do, board them at a kennel or ask a friend to care for them for at least 6 weeks, when the infection is transmissible. If they are free of infection, keep them that way by not allowing them to eat raw meat, roam outdoors, hunt mice or birds (which can transmit toxoplasmosis to cats), or hang out with other cats.

■ Have someone else handle the litter box. If you must do it yourself, use disposable gloves and wash your hands when you're finished, as well as after you touch your cats. The litter should be scooped at least daily.

■ Wear gloves when gardening. Don't garden in areas where your cats (or other cats) may have deposited feces.

Though universal screening for toxoplasmosis is not currently recommended by ACOG, some practitioners are urging routine testing before conception or in very early pregnancy for all women, so that those who test positive can relax, knowing they are immune, and those who test negative can take the necessary precautions to prevent infection. Check with your practitioner to see what he or she recommends.

Household Hazards

"How much do I really have to worry about household hazards like cleaning products and BPA? And what about tap water—is it safe to drink it while I'm pregnant?"

A little perspective goes a long way when you're expecting. The reality is that your home is probably a very safe place for you and your baby to hang out—especially if you couple a little caution with a lot of common sense. Here's what you need to know about so-called household hazards:

Household cleaning products. Mopping your kitchen floor or polishing your dining room table may be tough on your pregnant back, but it's not typically tough on your pregnancy. Still, it makes sense to clean with care when you're expecting. Let your nose and the following common sense tips be your guide:

- Go green. As much as you can, prefer products that clean the green way, with nontoxic ingredients (many are surprisingly effective). Going green when you clean is a good habit to get into now, before baby starts crawling around your home (and trying to put everything into that cute little mouth).

- If the product has a strong odor or fumes, don't breathe it in directly. Use it in an area with plenty of ventilation, or don't use it at all.

- Never (even when you're not pregnant) mix ammonia with chlorine-based products. The combination produces deadly fumes.

- Try to avoid using products such as oven cleaners that are plastered with warnings about toxicity levels.

- Wear rubber gloves when you must use a really strong product. Not only will this spare your hands a lot of wear and tear, but it'll prevent the absorption of chemicals through the skin.

Lead. Exposure to lead isn't potentially harmful just to small children but to pregnant women and their fetuses as well. Fortunately, there are steps you can take to reduce lead exposure around your house, allowing you to bring baby home to a safer environment. Here's how to steer clear of some common sources of lead:

- Check your tap. Since tap water is a common source of lead, be sure yours is lead-free (see facing page).

- Check your paint. Old paint is a major source of lead. If your home dates back to 1955 or earlier and layers of paint are to be removed for any reason, stay away from the house while the work is being done. If you find paint is flaking in an older home, or if you have a piece of old painted furniture that's flaking, see about having the walls or furniture repainted to contain the flaking lead paints, or have the old paint removed—again, stay away while the job is being done.

- Check your china. Flea market fan? Lead can also be leached from antique, handmade, and imported ceramicware and pottery. If you're unsure whether your ceramic, clay, or other china dishes, bowls, or pitchers are lead-free (look for a label), don't use them for food or drinks. Using them for decoration is fine.

- Check your unusual cravings. Pica, a craving for nonfood items, can lead some expectant moms to consume soil, clay, or paint chips, any of which may contain lead.

Tap water. It's still the best drink in the house—and in most houses, water is completely safe and drinkable straight from the tap. To be sure that when you fill a glass of water you'll be drinking to your good health—and your baby's—do the following:

- Contact your local water supplier or health department, the EPA (epa.gov), or a consumer advocacy group. If there is a possibility that your home's or your community's water supply is unsafe (because of pipe deterioration, a contaminated water source, or proximity to a waste disposal area, or because of odd taste or color), arrange to have it tested. Your local EPA or health department can tell you how.

- If testing reveals your water is contaminated with unsafe contaminants, invest in a filter (the kind depends on what turns up in your water) or use bottled water for drinking and cooking. Be aware, however, that bottled waters are not automatically free of impurities. Some contain more than tap water, and some are actually bottled directly from a tap. Many bottled waters also don't contain fluoride, an important mineral, especially for growing teeth (your baby's). To check the purity of a particular brand, search for it at NSF International (nsf.org) or check the bottle's label for NSF certification. Also look for bottles that don't contain BPA (see page 76) by checking for

the recycling code "1" on the bottom. Avoid distilled waters (from which beneficial minerals have been removed).

- If testing shows lead in your water, switch to bottled water or water that comes from a filtration system certified to reduce or eliminate lead for cooking, drinking, and brushing your teeth. Bathing and showering using water that has tested positive for lead is not a problem since lead from water can't be absorbed through the skin.

- If your water smells and/or tastes like chlorine, boiling it or letting it stand, uncovered, for 24 hours will allow much of the chemical to evaporate.

Pesticides. Can't live with roaches, ants, and other yucky insects? Fortunately, pest control and pregnancy can be completely compatible, with a few precautions. If your neighborhood is being sprayed, avoid hanging around outside for long periods until the chemical odors have dissipated, usually about 2 to 3 days. When indoors, keep the windows closed. If spraying for roaches or other insects is necessary in your apartment or house, be sure all closets and kitchen cabinets are tightly closed and all food-preparation surfaces are covered. Ventilate with open windows until the fumes have dissipated. Once the spray has settled, make sure food-preparation surfaces in or near the sprayed area have been thoroughly cleaned.

Inside the house, use "motel" or other types of traps, strategically placed in heavy bug traffic areas, to get rid of roaches and ants. Use cedar blocks instead of mothballs in clothes closets, and use the least toxic or most environmentally friendly (aka green) pesticides possible. Also, whenever possible, try to take a natural approach to pest control. For example, invest in an infantry of ladybugs or other beneficial predators (available from some garden supply houses) that like to feed on the bugs that are bugging you.

Most important, keep in mind that brief, indirect exposure to insecticides or herbicides isn't likely to be harmful (though best to avoid, if possible). What does increase the risk is frequent, long-term exposure, the kind that working daily around such chemicals (as in a factory or heavily sprayed fields or gardens) would involve.

Paint. Is baby's room getting a makeover that includes painting? Happily, today's paints don't contain lead or mercury, so they're safe to use when you're pregnant. And there are plenty of eco-friendly paints—ones made without volatile organic compounds (VOCs), toxic fungicides, and chemical pigments—on the market that you can use for your baby's nursery.

Still, even if the paint you're using isn't potentially harmful, the actual painting may be, so there are plenty of good reasons why you should pass the paintbrush to someone else—even if you're trying desperately to keep busy in those last weeks of waiting. The repetitive motion of painting can be a strain on back muscles already under pressure from the extra weight of pregnancy—and balancing on a ladder is precarious for the pregnant, to say the least. What's more, paint odors (though most are not harmful) can offend the pregnant nose and bring on a bout of nausea—a good reason to try to arrange to be out of the house while the painting is being done. Whether you're there or not, keep windows open for ventilation.

Avoid exposure to paint removers entirely, because they are highly toxic, and steer clear of the paint-removing process (whether chemicals or sanders are used), particularly if the paint that's

being removed is older and might contain mercury or lead.

BPA. Excessive exposure to BPA (bisphenol-A)—a chemical found in some plastic containers, cans, and even some store receipts—may pose a pregnancy risk. That's because BPA is believed to mimic hormones and disrupt the endocrine system that's responsible for assuring proper fetal development. BPA is everywhere (according to the CDC, 93 percent of all Americans have BPA in their bloodstreams), but the good news is that it's becoming easier to avoid excessive exposure. You can do this by:

- Opting for canned foods that are labeled "BPA-free" or choosing food packaged in glass jars instead
- Selecting storage containers, cutting boards, and utensils made from BPA-free plastic or from glass, wood, or ceramic
- Using stainless steel or "BPA-free" water bottles (those with recycle codes "3" and "7" are more likely to contain BPA)

Phthalates. Phthalates, sometimes known as plasticizers, come from compounds that enhance the flexibility of plastics. They're found in IV tubing, flexible PVC pipes used for plumbing, some flexible plastic bags (like single-use shopping bags), and some food and drink containers, among a variety of other products. Phthalates are also found in many personal care products, from fragrances to lipstick, shampoo to nail polish—and there's a growing case against them. Research has found that excessive exposure to phthalates during pregnancy can damage cells and DNA in the body, possibly leading to pregnancy complications including preeclampsia, preterm birth, and miscarriage. Too much exposure to phthalates in utero has also been linked to lower IQ and higher risk of learning disabilities in children.

The good news is that more products are being manufactured without phthalates. You can reduce exposure not only by choosing products labeled "phthalate-free" but also by watching out for the word "fragrance" (a blanket term that can hide phthalates) on the ingredient list of a product not labeled "phthalate-free." Also cut back on the use of plastic (use cloth bags instead of plastic, and use glass food and drink containers instead of plastic). Not ready to give up on plastic storage containers altogether? Choose ones from the growing number that are labeled BPA- and phthalate-free, or at least be sure not to heat up foods or drinks in regular plastic containers, since heating plastics allows the chemicals to break down and leach into the food.

Air Pollution

"Can city air pollution hurt my baby?"

Take a deep breath. Ordinary breathing in the big city is a lot safer than you'd think. After all, millions of women live and breathe in major cities across the nation and give birth to millions of healthy babies. Still, it's always sensible to avoid high doses of most air pollutants, since studies have shown that extremely high exposure to air pollution can put a baby at risk of being born at a low birthweight, having a higher risk of autism, or developing asthma later in life. Here's how to breathe easier for two:

- Pay attention to outdoor air quality. Try to limit time spent outdoors when the air quality is poor and keep windows closed. Check the air quality near you with the American Lung Association's State of the Air app (lung.org/healthy-air).

- Fuel up at night. Filling your gas tank after dusk, especially during warmer months, releases less harmful pollution than fueling up by day.

- Have the exhaust system on your car checked to be sure there is no rusting or leakage of noxious fumes. Never start your car in the garage with the garage door closed, and keep the tailgate on an SUV or minivan closed when the engine is running.

- Idle wisely. Keep your car windows and outdoor air vents closed in heavy traffic, and avoid standing near idling cars.

- Don't run, walk, or bike along congested roads, since you breathe in more air—and pollution—when you're active. Instead, choose a route with little traffic and a lot of trees. Trees, like indoor greenery, help to keep the air clean.

- Keep indoor air clean. The EPA recommends changing the air filters on HVAC units regularly. Another tip: Place potted plants around your home, since research shows they can actually suck up irritating chemicals like formaldehyde, leaving your air cleaner. In making your selections, however, be sure to avoid plants that are toxic when ingested, such as philodendron or English ivy. You won't likely be munching on shrubbery, but the same can't necessarily be said for your baby once he or she begins crawling around the house.

- Make sure fireplaces, gas stoves, and wood-burning stoves in your home are vented properly. Also, make sure the fireplace flue is open before lighting a fire.

ALL ABOUT:
Complementary and Alternative Medicine

Maybe you're already a reflexology regular. Or your chiropractor has had your (once aching) back for years. Maybe you've tried acupuncture a few times for headaches, or dabbled in hypnotherapy when you were trying to quit smoking. Maybe a monthly therapeutic massage is your drug-free answer to a chill pill (and speaking of drug-free, maybe you're a regular in the herbal supplement aisle, too). Or maybe you've always been curious about these and other complementary and alternative medicine (CAM) therapies—but couldn't help thinking that CAM might just be a scam.

And maybe, now that you're expecting, you're wondering whether CAM has a place in your pregnancy. After all, pregnancy isn't an illness, it's a normal part of the life cycle—making the holistic view of health and well-being that CAM encompasses (which integrates not only physical influences, but nutritional, emotional, and spiritual ones, too) seem like a pregnancy natural.

And for more and more pregnant women—and the traditional medicine doctors and midwives who care for them—it is. A variety of CAM practices are currently being used in pregnancy, with varying degrees of success, including the following:

Acupuncture. Acupuncture is based on correcting imbalances and blockages of what Chinese medicine refers to as qi, or chi (pronounced CHEE), the flow of vital energy along internal energy pathways (known as meridians) in your body. It might sound a little on the fringe—or even off the wall—but acupuncture has been working its medical magic for thousands of years to relieve any number of pregnancy woes and conditions.

How is it done? An acupuncturist inserts dozens of thin needles at prescribed points (there are more than 1,000 acupuncture points) along invisible meridians on the body. Lost you at "needles"? Most people say acupuncture doesn't hurt at all, or only for a moment (just don't watch if the needles unnerve you—close your eyes and get some much-needed relaxation). Researchers have found that the points correspond to deep-seated nerves, so that when the needles are twirled (or electrically stimulated, in a procedure known as electropuncture), the nerves are activated, leading to the release of endorphins—and relief from stress, depression, back pain, fatigue, headaches, sciatica, carpal tunnel pain, and possibly other pregnancy symptoms like heartburn and constipation. Acupuncture has also been shown to be particularly good at easing morning sickness even in its most severe form, hyperemesis gravidarum, and it may also be used during labor to relieve pain, as well as to help speed progress along. Acupuncturists say just a single treatment per month during pregnancy can help you de-stress and enjoy this amazing (if sometimes uncomfortable) time in your life more fully. Be sure to choose an acupuncturist who is experienced and uses clean and sanitary procedures (meticulously sterilized or single-use disposable needles, for example). And your acupuncturist should avoid having you lie flat on your back after your 4th month.

Acupressure. Acupressure—or shiatsu—works on the same principle as acupuncture, except that instead of poking you with needles, your practitioner will use thumb or finger pressure, or will apply firm pressure with small beads, to stimulate the points. Pressure on a certain point just above your inner wrist can ease nausea (which is why acupressure wristbands can also work; see page 137). Acupressure on the center of the ball of the foot is said to help back labor. In fact, acupressure is said to relieve the same aches, pains, and symptoms of pregnancy that acupuncture does. There are several acupressure points (such as those in the ankle) that are said to induce contractions—which is why these particular pressure points should be avoided until term (at which point, impatient moms-to-be might want to give them a try).

Moxibustion. This CAM therapy combines acupuncture with the burning of mugwort, an herb. In addition to—or instead of—inserting needles into your skin, the practitioner will burn long sticks of mugwort near certain acupuncture points. Though most scientific research shows a low success rate, many in the CAM community say that moxibustion performed on the outside of the little toe can turn a breech baby. If you're thinking of trying moxibustion—or your practitioner has suggested giving it a go—look for an acupuncturist who is experienced in the technique. It generally requires multiple sessions, starting sometime between the end of the 7th month and the middle of the 8th month.

Chiropractic medicine. This therapy uses physical manipulation of the spine and other joints to enable nerve impulses to move freely through an aligned body, encouraging the body's natural ability to heal. During pregnancy your body produces ligament-relaxing hormones—a good thing, since your baby's head would never be able to fit through your pelvis otherwise. But those hormones, combined with your spectacularly swollen belly, can leave you loose-limbed, swaybacked, and unusually clumsy because of a rapidly lowering center of gravity (look out below!). All of this can do quite a number on your spine. Chiropractic care may be able to undo much of this damage and get your lower body in proper alignment for an easier birth. Some chiropractors also claim that chiropractic adjustments can reduce the likelihood of miscarriage, control morning sickness, and lower your risk of preterm delivery. The chiropractor's ability to realign and, in many cases, relax the ligaments and muscles in your pelvis has led to what is known as the Webster Technique, a method that is said to help breech babies turn themselves, naturally.

It's very important that any chiropractic practitioner you see has experience treating expectant women. You should be placed on a special table made to keep pressure off your belly during treatments, and your chiropractor should avoid having you lie flat on your back, especially during your last trimester. Finally, as with any type of CAM treatment, make sure you clear it first with your ob, who may have a very specific reason you should avoid spinal realignment.

Massage. Ahhhh . . . massage. Anyone who's ever had a professional massage knows that both body and mind feel better after a good rubdown. And studies back up the feel-good message about massage, showing that it can reduce stress hormones in your body and relax and loosen tense muscles—all welcome benefits when you're expecting. It can also increase blood flow and circulation—good for you and baby—and keep your lymphatic system working at peak efficiency, flushing out toxins from your body. But massage is more than just a day in the spa (which you can read more about on page 153). Massage in the hands of a trained physical therapist can help relieve joint pain, neck and back pain, hip pain, leg cramps, and sciatica. It can also reduce swelling in your hands and feet (as long as that swelling isn't a result of preeclampsia), relieve carpal tunnel pain, and alleviate headaches and sinus congestion—all common side effects of baby making. Because physical therapists create individualized treatment plans for pain relief, yours can teach you stretches and exercises that you can do at home to help relieve any aches and pains you're experiencing. Many of these stretches are also designed to improve the strength, flexibility, and stability in your muscles. And in most cases, practitioner-prescribed physical therapy is covered by insurance.

Reflexology. Similar to acupressure, reflexology is a therapy based on the notion that areas on the feet and hands are linked to other areas and organs of the body. Reflexology is used to treat symptoms in many parts of your body by using fingertip pressure on specific areas on your feet primarily, and sometimes on your hands as well. The idea is that this pressure allows blocked energy to flow freely, which increases blood flow to the corresponding part of your body and an uptick in the removal of toxic wastes. During pregnancy, reflexology can be used to soothe the aches and pains in your back and joints that are taking a beating from your growing girth. But that's not all. Reflexologists say their fancy footwork can give you relief from some of your most persistent and wide-ranging woes. These may include morning sickness, heartburn, mild swelling, constipation, high blood pressure (but not preeclampsia), insomnia, bladder problems, and even hemorrhoids. In addition, reflexology seems to reduce emotional stress and ease mild depression and anxiety. It may even be helpful after you give birth—some studies show it stimulates milk production.

It's important to know that reflexologists often work on the area between your ankle and heel to stimulate labor and contractions. Unless you've reached full term, make sure the therapy avoids stimulating this area for any length of time.

As with almost any alternative therapy, check with your practitioner before you begin reflexology treatments, and be sure that your reflexologist has been properly trained and has experience working with pregnant women. Keep in mind, too, that some reflexologists prefer to wait until an expectant mom is out of her first trimester before working on her, and that there are certain complications for which reflexology is specifically not recommended.

Hydrotherapy. The therapeutic use of warm water is particularly effective during pregnancy because the body's physiological response to water helps improve your circulation, ease your aching back (and feet, knees, you name it), ease the pain of labor and delivery, and generally make you a happier mama. There are a variety of ways to harness the power of water. Soaking in a warm tub is one of them. During labor, spraying your face with cold water may help you concentrate and stay calm. A cold compress on your neck may help you breathe more steadily and deeply, and increase energy while decreasing exhaustion. A warm compress placed on the lower back can help your pelvic muscles relax between contractions.

Some women believe so deeply in the power of hydrotherapy that they choose to spend much of their labor immersed in water, and some even deliver their babies there. One reason water works so well is that floating eases pressure on your spine, helping the pelvis to open. Once you're in the tub (or a special birthing pool), you no longer need to concentrate on your posture—your body is decompressed, which helps minimize the pain of contractions.

Since it's important to keep your body temperature in a safe range during pregnancy, think soothingly warm, not blisteringly hot, when it comes to your tub water. And while hydrotherapy is fine (actually, amazing) for almost any pregnant woman and an awesome option for pain management during labor, delivering underwater is usually reserved for low-risk births.

Meditation, visualization, and relaxation techniques. Deep relaxation techniques, meditation, and visualization can help you cope with a variety of physical and emotional stresses during pregnancy (from the miseries of morning sickness to the pain of labor and delivery), enabling you to relax and focus your concentration, reduce stress, lower your blood pressure, and enhance your peace of mind. They can work wonders on an expectant mom's anxiety, too. See page 148 for a relaxation exercise you can try, or try a meditation app that can transport you to your happy place as needed.

Hypnotherapy. Hypnosis—when your conscious (rational) mind takes a backseat and your subconscious mind (feelings, memories, emotions) drives the car for a while—usually involves music, soothing images, and guided visualization. Natal hypnotherapy (the kind that's used during pregnancy) uses deep relaxation and the power of suggestion to tap into the part of your mind that's responsible for bodily functions (your heart rate, hormone production, and digestive system, as well as your emotions) and helps you cope with the anxiety that's sometimes part of the pregnancy package. Many women use hypnosis to ease (or even eliminate) the pain of childbirth (see page 335), but proponents say hypnosis can also be effective in relieving pregnancy symptoms (from nausea to headaches), helping to hold off premature labor, ease stress, or help turn a breech baby.

Keep in mind that hypnosis isn't for everyone. About 25 percent of the population is highly resistant to hypnotic suggestion, and many more aren't suggestive enough to use it for effective pain relief (though even then, there can be relaxing benefits). Hypnosis is also not a last-minute option—you've got to learn (and practice) hypnosis techniques in advance of labor for it to be effective. And of course, make sure any hypnotherapist you use or train with is certified and experienced in pregnancy therapies.

Biofeedback. Biofeedback is a method that helps patients learn how to recognize and control their biological responses to physical pain or emotional stress. How does it work? Your therapist applies sensors to your body that provide feedback on factors such as muscle tension, brain-wave activity, respiration, heart rate, blood pressure, and temperature. As the practitioner monitors the feedback these sensors provide, he or she uses relaxation techniques to calm you, reducing muscle tension and easing your pain or stress. Over time, you should be able to control your body's responses by yourself through self-guided relaxation, without needing the therapist or the biofeedback machine.

CAM Caveats

Clearly, CAM is making an impact in pregnancy care. Even the most traditional obs are realizing that it's a holistic force to be reckoned with, and one to begin incorporating into ob business as usual. But in making CAM a part of your pregnancy, it's wise to proceed with sensible caution and with these caveats in mind:

- The "C" stands for complementary. So check in with your traditional practitioner before you book an appointment with a CAM therapist. Even better, ask for therapist recommendations first.

- The "M" stands for medicine. CAM medications can be strong medicine, just as traditional prescriptions or over-the-counter medication can be, but with an important distinction: Because they are not FDA regulated or approved, their safety hasn't been clinically established. Which is not to say there aren't CAM medications that are safe to use during pregnancy, just that there is no official system in place to determine those that are and those that aren't (or those that are effective and those that aren't). All the more reason to avoid any herbal or homeopathic remedy, as well as any dietary supplement or aromatherapy treatment, unless it has been prescribed or recommended by your ob or midwife—same as you would do with any other medication during pregnancy.

- CAM rules change during pregnancy. You've been seeing the same chiropractor for the same adjustments for years? Or getting a massage from the same therapist every time your back acts up? Just remember: What's safe for the nonpregnant may not be safe when you're expecting. That's why you should choose a therapist who is trained and experienced in the special precautions needed for pregnant patients.

Biofeedback can be used safely to lower blood pressure and combat depression, anxiety, and stress, as well as to relieve a variety of pregnancy symptoms, including headache, backache, and other pains, plus insomnia and possibly morning sickness. It can also be an effective treatment for urinary incontinence, both during and after pregnancy.

Herbal remedies. "Botanicals" have been used since humankind first began looking for relief from ailments. Now more often manufactured than foraged for, herbal remedies are touted by some as a natural treatment for many of pregnancy's peskiest symptoms, from leg cramps to hemorrhoids. And while some are probably harmless and possibly effective (say a cup of chamomile tea when you get up in the morning to calm a queasy tummy, or a cup of raspberry leaf tea to jump start contractions when your due date has come and gone), most experts don't recommend herbal remedies for pregnant women because adequate studies on safety haven't been done.

Also important to keep in mind: Just because a product is natural doesn't mean it's safe. In fact, there are certain herbs that are known to be dangerous during pregnancy (and that might be lurking in herbal remedies without you even knowing). For instance, aloe, barberry, black cohosh, blue cohosh, dong quai, feverfew, goldenseal, juniper, and wild yam are uterine stimulants and could potentially lead to miscarriage or premature contractions. Autumn crocus, mugwort (used for moxibustion, but not safe for ingestion), pokeroot, and sassafras have been linked to birth defects. Comfrey and mistletoe can have a toxic effect.

Another reason to proceed with care down the herbal aisles of your health food market: Herbal supplements are not regulated by the FDA the way prescription and over-the-counter medications are. Though herbal remedies manufactured in Germany, Poland, Austria, and the U.K. are regulated, which means they undergo careful scrutiny, those produced in other countries (including the U.S.) are not. This means their strength, quality, and even ingredients may vary from brand to brand and package to package. They may contain contaminants (possibly including lead, depending on the country of origin), ingredients not listed on the label, higher levels of active ingredients than listed, or no active ingredients at all.

So treat herbal remedies (including herbal teas) as you would treat any medication during pregnancy: Don't use them unless they've been cleared by your practitioner.

CHAPTER 4

Nine Months of Eating Well

There's a tiny new being developing inside of you—a baby in the making. Adorable little fingers and toes are sprouting, eyes and ears are forming, brain cells are rapidly growing. And before you know it, the speck of a fetus inside you will come to resemble the baby of your dreams: fully equipped and suitable for cuddling.

Not surprisingly, a lot goes into making a baby. Happily for babies and the parents who love them, nature's incredibly good at what it does. Which means that the chances that your baby will be born not only perfectly cuddly, but perfectly healthy, are already excellent. What's more, there's something you can do to help make those excellent chances even better—while helping yourself to a healthier and more comfortable pregnancy. It's something that's relatively easy to do (except maybe when you're feeling queasy)—and something that you probably already do at least 3 times a day. Yes, you guessed it: eat. But the challenge during pregnancy isn't just to eat (though that may be challenge enough during those early months)—it's to eat as well as you can. Think of it this way: Eating well when you're expecting is one of the first and best gifts you can give your soon-to-arrive bundle of joy—and it's a gift that

can keep on giving, handing out not just a healthier start in life but a healthier lifetime.

The Pregnancy Diet is an eating plan dedicated to baby's good health—and yours. What's in it for your baby? Among many other impressive benefits, a better chance for a healthy birthweight, improved brain development, reduced risk for certain birth defects—and as a bonus, believe it or not, better and potentially less picky eating habits as baby grows (a perk you'll really appreciate when broccoli's on the dinner menu). It may even make it more likely that your yet-to-be-born baby will grow to be a healthier adult.

And your baby's not the only one who's likely to benefit. The Pregnancy Diet can also increase the chances that you'll have a safe pregnancy (some complications, such as anemia, gestational diabetes, and preeclampsia, are less common among women who eat well and avoid excess weight gain), a comfortable pregnancy (the right foods can minimize morning sickness, fatigue, heartburn, constipation, and a host of other pregnancy symptoms), better balanced emotions (good nutrition may help moderate those wild mood swings), a full-term pregnancy (in general, moms-to-be who eat regularly and well are less likely to deliver too early), and a speedier postpartum recovery (a well-nourished body can bounce back faster and more easily, and weight that's been gained at a sensible rate can be shed more quickly). For more on the many benefits of a healthy diet during pregnancy, see *What to Expect: Eating Well When You're Expecting.*

Luckily, scoring those benefits is a piece of (carrot) cake, especially if you're already eating pretty well, and even if you're not (you'll just have to be a little more selective before bringing fork to mouth). That's because the Pregnancy Diet isn't all that different from the average healthy diet. While a few modifications have been made for the pregnant set (not surprisingly, baby making requires more calories and more of certain nutrients), the foundation is the same: a good, balanced mix of lean protein and calcium, whole grains, a rainbow of fruits and vegetables, and healthy fats. Sound familiar? It should—after all, it's what good nutrition is all about.

And here's some more good news. Even if you're coming to your pregnancy (and bellying up to the table) with less than ideal eating habits, changing them to follow the Pregnancy Diet won't be that tough, especially if you're committed to making the changes. There are healthy alternatives for almost every less healthy food and beverage you've ever brought to your lips (see box, page 87), which means there are nourishing

Have It Your Way

Have your doubts about diets? Not a fan of eating plans? Just don't like being told what to eat—or how much? No problem. The Pregnancy Diet is one way to feed yourself and your baby well, but it definitely isn't the only way. A balanced, healthy diet—one that includes plenty of lean protein, calcium-rich foods, whole grains, a rainbow of fruits and vegetables, healthy fats, plus about 300 extra calories a day—will get the job done, too. So if you'd rather not keep track—don't. Eat well, your way!

ways to have your cake (and cookies and chips and even fast food) and eat it, too. Plus, there are countless ways to sneak crucial vitamins and minerals into recipes and favorite dishes—so you can pump up your pregnancy nutrition without shortchanging your taste buds.

And now for the reality check. What's presented in this chapter is the ideal, the best possible plan for eating well when you're expecting. Something you should strive for, absolutely—but nothing you should stress over. Maybe you'll choose to follow the diet closely, at least most of the time. Or you'll follow it loosely, all of the time. Or you'll do the best you can, which won't always be that great—especially when you're crazy queasy . . . or when food cravings send you careening into the candy aisle . . . or when reflux keeps coming up. But even if you keep your allegiance to burgers and fries, you'll pick up at least a few pointers in the pages that follow that will help nourish you and your baby better during the next 9 months (salad with that burger?).

Nine Basic Principles for Nine Months of Healthy Eating

Bites count. Chew on this: You've got 9 months of meals, snacks, nibbles, and noshes ahead of you. Each one of them is an opportunity to feed your baby well before he or she is even born—a chance to make a down payment on a healthier future for your little one. So open wide, but think first. Try to make your pregnancy bites count by choosing them (at least most of the time) with baby in mind.

All calories are not created equal. Choose your calories with care, selecting quality over quantity when you can. It may seem obvious—and inherently unfair—but those 200 calories in a donut are not equal to the 200 calories in a whole grain muffin. Also not equal: the 100 calories in a handful of potato chips and the 100 calories in a handful of almonds. Your baby will benefit a lot more from 2,000 nutrient-rich calories daily than from 2,000 mostly empty ones. And your body will show the benefits postpartum as well.

Starve yourself, starve your baby. Your baby needs regular nourishment at regular intervals—and as the sole caterer of your uterine cafe, only you can provide it. Even if you're not hungry, your baby is. So try not to skip meals. In fact, eating frequently may be the best route to a well-nourished fetus. Research shows that moms-to-be who eat at least 5 times a day (3 meals plus 2 snacks or 6 mini-meals, for instance) are more likely to carry to term. Of course, that's easier said than done, especially if even the thought of eating has you hugging the toilet. And what if your heartburn has made eating a pain—literally? You'll find plenty of tips on how to eat around these appetite-cramping pregnancy symptoms on pages 132 and 159.

Efficiency is effective. Think it's impossible to meet every Daily Dozen (see page 90) each and every day (let's see, 6 whole grains means 1 every 4 hours . . .)? Worried that even if you do manage to eat it all, you'll end up looking like a pregnant blimp? Think again, and worry no more. Instead, become an efficiency expert. Get more nutritional bang for your buck by choosing foods that are lightweights when it comes to calories, heavy hitters

1,000 Days to a Healthier Future

Want to know how to unlock a healthier future for your yet-to-be-born baby? Scientists have found one of the most important keys: good nutrition for the first 1,000 days of baby's life, counting from pregnancy to the second birthday. These first 1,000 days can lay the foundation for a lifetime of good health—lowering a baby's risk of becoming obese and a host of preventable chronic diseases (from Type 2 diabetes to heart disease). They can also boost brain development and improve the chance of success in school and beyond. Think of these next 9 months of eating well as the first installment of your baby's vital first 1,000 days. To learn more, go to thousanddays.org.

Try These Instead

Looking for healthy alternatives to your not-so-healthy favorite foods? Here are some ideas to get you started:

INSTEAD OF	TRY
Potato chips	Lentil, soy, kale, or whole grain corn chips
A bag of M&M's	Trail mix (with a few M&M's)
Skittles	Frozen grapes
Before-dinner pretzels	Before-dinner edamame
Hot fudge sundae	Frozen yogurt with fruit and nuts
Taco chips and cheese sauce	Veggies and cheese sauce
French fries	Baked sweet potato fries
Anything on white bread	Anything on whole wheat bread
Soda	Sparkling water with a splash of juice
A slice of apple pie	A baked apple

when it comes to nutrients. Need an example? A crispy (read: fried) chicken sandwich, at about 700 calories, is a considerably less efficient way of netting a protein serving than a turkey burger (about 300 calories). A cup and a half of ice cream (about 500 calories, way more if you're choosing the premium stuff) is a fun but less efficient way of scoring a calcium serving than a cup of nonfat frozen yogurt (still fun, but with 200 fewer calories). Using the same model of efficiency, choose lean meats over fatty ones, fat-free or low-fat milk and dairy products over full-fat versions, grilled or broiled foods over fried, and sauté using a tablespoon of olive oil, not a quarter of a cup. Another trick of the efficient-eating trade: Select foods that are overachievers in more than 1 Daily Dozen category, so you can fill 2 or more requirements at once.

Efficiency is important, too, if you're having trouble gaining weight. To start tipping the scale toward a healthier weight gain, choose foods that are dense in nutrients and calories—avocados, nuts, and dried fruits, for instance—that can fill you and your baby out without filling you up too much.

Carbohydrates are a complex issue. What do you think of when you think of carbs? If it's "extra pounds," you're not alone. Carbs have long been dissed and dismissed out of hand—and off the table—by the weight conscious. And that's too bad, especially when it comes to weight conscious expecting moms—who could stand to gain a lot of nutrients (without gaining a lot of weight) by eating the right kind of carbs: the complex kind. Sure, refined carbs (white rice, white bread and pastries, white potatoes) are nutritional slackers, adding calories but little else. Another downer: They can send blood sugar soaring . . . and then crashing.

Skip That Side of Guilt

Willpower has its place, particularly while you're trying to eat well for two. Still, everyone needs to give in to temptation now and then, without feeling guilty about it. So treat yourself to a treat when you really want one, and without a side of eater's remorse.

But even as you venture down the path of least nutritious, try to pump it up—add fresh strawberries and walnuts to your sundae, choose a dark chocolate bar that's filled with almonds.

Share that serving of onion rings, or take a slender slice of pecan pie instead of a slab. And remember to stop before you get too carried away—otherwise, you might just begin to feel that guilt coming your way after all.

But complex carbohydrates (whole grain breads and cereal, brown rice, fruits and veggies, and beans) supply a bundle of B vitamins, trace minerals, protein, and fiber, contributing way more than calories. They're good not only for baby, but also for you (they'll help keep nausea and constipation in check). And because they are filling and fiber-rich, they'll help keep your weight gain in check, too. Research suggests yet another bonus for complex carb consumers: Eating plenty of fiber may reduce the risk of developing gestational diabetes.

Sweet nothings are exactly that. There's no gentle way to put this: Sugar calories, sadly, are empty calories. And empty calories aren't sugar's only shortfall. A heavy consumption has been linked to a variety of health concerns, from obesity to colon cancer. In pregnancy, too much sugar can turn into too many pounds, but it can also increase the risk of developing gestational diabetes, as well as tooth decay (you're already extra susceptible when you're expecting). Another strike against sugar: Large amounts are likely to show up in nutritionally underachieving foods and drinks you're probably better off skipping anyway (say, candy and soda).

Refined sugar goes by many names on the supermarket shelves, including corn syrup and dehydrated cane juice. Honey, an unrefined sugar, has a nutritional edge because it contains disease-fighting antioxidants. Plus, it is more likely to find its way into more nutritious foods. Still, it's smart to try limiting your intake of sugar in all its forms.

Satisfy your sweet tooth the wholesome way by substituting fruit (fresh, dried, or freeze-dried), fruit juice concentrate, and fruit purees for sugar whenever you can. You can also find sweet revenge in the calorie-free or low-calorie sugar substitutes that seem to be safe for pregnancy use (see page 111).

Good foods remember where they came from. Nature knows a thing or two about nutrition. So it's not surprising that the most nutritious foods are often the ones that haven't strayed far from their original, nature-formulated recipe. Choose fresh vegetables and fruits when they're in season, or nothing-added frozen when fresh are unavailable or you don't have time to prepare them. Freeze-dried is another nutritious (and convenient) way to go—you'll find the flavor of freeze-dried fruits and veggies is more intense, the texture crunchy and satisfying, and the calorie counts low compared with traditionally dried. And when it comes to

Eating Well with WIC

Worried you won't be able to afford to eat well when you're expecting? If your income qualifies you, you could be eligible for the Women, Infants, and Children's program (WIC), a supplemental food and nutrition program for pregnant women, new moms, and children under 5. Through the WIC program, moms-to-be and their little ones receive checks or vouchers that can be used in the local grocery store to buy healthy food such as eggs, milk, cheese, beans, whole grain bread, and fruits and vegetables. WIC also provides nutrition education and counseling at their clinics, as well as screening and referrals to other health, welfare, and social services. For more information and to see if you're eligible, go to fns.usda.gov/wic.

prep, less is more—more nutrients, that is. Try to eat some raw vegetables and fruit every day, and when you're cooking, opt for steaming or a light stir-fry, so more vitamins and minerals will be retained.

It's no secret that processed foods don't grow on trees—they're produced on an assembly line, where they not only pick up plenty of chemicals, fat, sugar, and salt, but lose a lot of nutritional value, too. So stick with nature's model when you can, and choose fresh roasted turkey breast over processed turkey, mac and cheese made with whole grain macaroni and natural cheese over that bright orange variety, fresh oatmeal made from rolled oats over the lower-fiber and super-sugary instant varieties.

Healthy eating begins at home. Let's face it. It isn't easy to nibble on fresh fruit when your darling dearest is diving headfirst into a vat of ice cream—right next to you on the sofa. Or to reach for a cheese stick when he's filled the cabinets with Cheez Doodles. So enlist him—and other family members—in making your home a healthy food zone. Make whole grain your house bread, stock your freezer with frozen yogurt, and ban the unhealthy snacks you can't help attacking when they're within reach. And don't stop after delivery. Healthy eating is linked not only with a better pregnancy outcome but with a lower risk of many diseases, including Type 2 diabetes and heart disease.

Bad habits can sabotage a good diet. Eating well is only part of the healthy prenatal picture. If you haven't already, change your other lifestyle habits for the better.

The 6-Meal Solution

Too bloated, queasy, heartburned, or constipated (or all of the above) to contemplate a full meal? No matter what tummy troubles are getting you down (or keeping food from staying down), you'll find it easier to spread your Daily Dozen (see page 90) into 5 or 6 mini-meals instead of those standard 3 squares. A grazing approach keeps your blood sugar level, so you'll get an energy boost, too (and who couldn't use that?). And you'll have fewer headaches—and fewer wild mood swings.

The Pregnancy Daily Dozen

Calories. Technically, a pregnant woman is eating for two (rejoice, food lovers). But it's important to remember that one of the two is a tiny developing fetus whose caloric needs are significantly lower than mom's—a mere 300 on average a day, more or less (sorry, food lovers). So, on average, you now need only about 300 calories more a day than you used to eat prepregnancy—the equivalent of 2 glasses of skim milk and a bowl of oatmeal (not exactly the all-you-can-eat sundae bar you might have been envisioning). Pretty easy to spend (or overspend), given the extra nutritional requirements of pregnancy. What's more, during the first trimester you probably don't need any extra calories at all (that baby you're growing is only pea size), unless you're trying to compensate for starting out underweight. By the time your metabolism speeds up during the second trimester, you can aim for 300 to 350 extra calories. Later in pregnancy (when your baby is much bigger) you may even need more, or upward of about 500 extra calories a day.

Eating more calories than you and your baby need isn't only unnecessary, but it can lead to excessive weight gain. Eating too few calories, on the other hand, is also unhealthy as pregnancy progresses. Moms-to-be who don't take in enough calories during the second and third trimesters can slow the growth of their babies.

There are 4 exceptions to this basic formula—and if any apply to you, it'll be important to ask your practitioner for input on your calorie input. If you're overweight, you can possibly do with fewer calories, as long as you have the right nutritional guidance (you'll have to focus even more on quality). If you're seriously underweight, you'll need more calories so you can catch up weight-wise. If you're a teen, you're still growing yourself, which means you have unique nutritional needs (though calories, again, may depend on whether you're underweight, overweight, or just about the right weight). And if you're carrying multiples, you'll have to add about 300 calories for each baby.

But while calories count during pregnancy, they don't have to be literally counted. No need to add them up at every meal or keep a running log of what you ate when. How will you know if you're getting the right number of calories then? Simple—just watch your weight gain. If your weight gain is right on target, you're eating the right number of calories. If you're gaining too little or too slowly, you're eating too few calories—and if you're gaining too much too fast, you're eating too many. Just maintain or adjust your food intake as necessary, but be careful not to cut out nutrients you need along with calories—just be extra efficient in your eating. See page 177 for more on weight gain.

Protein foods: 3 servings daily. How does your baby grow? Using, among other nutrients, the amino acids (the building blocks of human cells) from the protein you eat each day. Because your baby's cells are multiplying rapidly, protein is an extremely vital component of your pregnancy diet. If the recommended 75 grams per day sounds like a lot, keep in mind that most Americans (including you, most likely) consume at least that much daily without even trying, and those on high-protein diets pack away a lot more. When tallying

Animal-Free Protein

Early pregnancy queasiness and aversions are pushing meat and other animal proteins off the menu? Or are you a vegetarian or vegan? Here's some good news. There are plenty of ways to net your Protein requirements without dipping into the animal kingdom. Even better news? Many of these foods fulfill the requirements for Whole Grains as well as Protein, and some add a little calcium to the equation.

LEGUMES
(half Protein servings)

¾ cup cooked beans, lentils, split peas, or chickpeas (garbanzos)

½ cup cooked edamame

¾ cup green garden peas

1½ ounces peanuts

3 tablespoons peanut or nut butter

¼ cup miso

4 ounces tofu (bean curd)

3 ounces tempeh

1½ cups soy milk*

3 ounces soy cheese*

½ cup vegetarian "ground beef"*

1 large veggie "hot dog" or "burger"*

1 ounce (before cooking) soy or high-protein pasta**

GRAINS
(half Protein servings)

3 ounces (before cooking) whole wheat pasta

⅓ cup wheat germ

¾ cup oat bran

1 cup uncooked (2 cups cooked) oats

2 cups (approximately) whole grain ready-to-eat cereal*

½ cup uncooked (1½ cups cooked) bulgur, buckwheat, or whole wheat couscous

½ cup uncooked quinoa

4 slices whole grain bread**

2 whole grain pitas or English muffins**

NUTS AND SEEDS
(half Protein servings)

3 ounces nuts, such as walnuts, pecans, or almonds

2 ounces sesame, sunflower, or pumpkin seeds

*Protein content varies widely, so check labels for 12 to 15 grams protein per half serving.

**High-protein pastas or breads may contain far more protein, so check labels.

your Protein servings, don't forget to count the protein found in many high-calcium foods, like cheese and yogurt (especially Greek), as well as in whole grains and legumes.

Every day aim to have 3 of the following (each is 1 Protein serving, or about 25 grams of protein), or a combination equivalent to 3 servings. Keep in mind that most of the dairy options also fill your Calcium requirement, which make them especially efficient choices (see box, this page, for a list of plant proteins):

24 ounces (three 8-ounce glasses) of milk or buttermilk

1 cup cottage cheese

Whey to Go?

With whey protein bars, powders, and shake mixes way popular these days, you might be wondering whether they're, well, the way to go when you're trying to get your share of pregnancy protein. While there's a lack of scientific evidence on the use of whey protein during pregnancy or breastfeeding, most experts say it's probably okay to turn to in moderation as long as you follow these caveats.

First, since whey protein is made from cow's milk, you'll have to avoid it if you're allergic to milk or are lactose intolerant. Second, check out all the ingredients in whey products, since some contain added sweeteners (artificial and natural), herbs, enzymes, and other components that may not be pregnancy-appropriate. Third, be sure to check the vitamin and mineral content of the whey products you're eating—some are so heavily fortified, they could put you way over the limits for certain nutrients. And finally, remember that whey protein shouldn't be the only way you score protein—try to balance it with other sources.

---

2 cups yogurt or 1¼ cups Greek yogurt

3 ounces (¾ cup grated) cheese

4 large whole eggs

7 large egg whites

3½ ounces (drained) canned tuna or sardines

4 ounces (drained) canned salmon

4 ounces cooked shellfish

4 ounces (before cooking) fresh fish

4 ounces (before cooking) skinless chicken, turkey, duck, or other poultry

4 ounces (before cooking) lean beef, lamb, veal, pork, or buffalo

Calcium foods: 4 servings daily. Back in elementary school, you probably learned that growing children need plenty of calcium for strong bones and teeth. Well, so do growing fetuses on their way to becoming growing children. Calcium is also vital for muscle, heart, and nerve development, blood clotting, and enzyme activity. But it's not only your baby who stands to lose when you don't get enough calcium. If incoming supplies aren't keeping up, your baby-making factory will tap into the calcium in your own bones to help meet its quota, setting you up for osteoporosis later in life—another good reason to bone up on calcium now.

Can't stomach the taste of milk by the glassful? Luckily, calcium doesn't have to be served in glasses at all. It can be served up as a cup of yogurt or a piece of cheese. It can be enjoyed in smoothies, soups, casseroles, cereals, dips, sauces, desserts, and more.

The lactose-intolerant can easily substitute lactose-free dairy products (milk, cottage cheese, and even ice cream come lactose-free). For those who don't eat dairy products at all, calcium also comes in nondairy form. A glass of calcium-fortified orange juice, for instance, efficiently provides a serving of Calcium (along with a serving of Vitamin C). A glass of calcium-fortified almond milk also provides a serving of Calcium (and tastes great in smoothies). You'll find more non-dairy sources of calcium listed below.

For vegans or others who can't be sure they're getting enough calcium in their diets, a supplement (one that includes vitamin D) may be recommended.

Aim for 4 servings of calcium-rich foods each day, or any combination of them that is equivalent to 4 servings (so don't forget to count that half cup of yogurt, that sprinkle of cheese). Each serving listed below contains about 300 mg of calcium (you need a total of about 1,200 mg a day), and many also fill your Protein requirements:

¼ cup grated cheese

1 ounce hard cheese

½ cup pasteurized ricotta cheese

1 cup milk or buttermilk

5 ounces calcium-added milk

1 cup yogurt or Greek yogurt

1½ cups frozen yogurt

1 cup calcium-fortified juice or almond milk

4 ounces canned salmon with bones

3 ounces canned sardines with bones

3 tablespoons ground sesame seeds

1 cup cooked greens, such as kale or collards

1½ cups cooked Chinese cabbage (bok choy)

1½ cups cooked edamame

You'll also score a calcium bonus by eating cottage cheese, tofu, dried figs, almonds, broccoli, spinach, and dried beans.

Vitamin C foods: 3 servings daily. You and baby both need vitamin C for tissue repair, wound healing, and various other metabolic (nutrient-using) processes. Your baby also needs it for proper growth and for the development of strong bones and teeth. Since vitamin

Count 'Em Once, Count 'Em Twice

Many of your favorite foods fill more than one Daily Dozen requirement in each serving, giving you two for the calorie price of one. Case in point: A slice of cantaloupe nets a serving in the Green Leafy and Yellow category and one in the Vitamin C category—both in one delicious package. One cup of yogurt yields 1 Calcium serving and ½ a Protein serving (nearly a whole serving if you're reaching for Greek yogurt). Use such overlappers as often as you can to save yourself calories and stomach space.

C is a nutrient the body can't store, a fresh supply is needed every day. Lucky for you, vitamin C usually comes from foods that naturally taste good—even when you're feeling green. As you can see from the list of Vitamin C foods below, the old standby orange juice (reliable as it is) is far from the only, or even the best, source of this essential vitamin.

Aim for at least 3 Vitamin C servings every day—again, your body needs a daily dose since it can't be stashed. (Fruit fanatic? Help yourself to more.) Keep in mind that many Vitamin C foods also fill the requirement for Green Leafy and Yellow Vegetables and Yellow Fruit:

½ medium grapefruit

½ cup grapefruit juice

½ medium orange

½ cup orange juice

2 tablespoons juice concentrate

¼ cup lemon juice

½ medium mango

¼ medium papaya

⅛ small cantaloupe or honeydew
(½ cup cubed)

⅓ cup strawberries

⅔ cup blackberries or raspberries

½ medium kiwi

½ cup diced fresh pineapple

2 cups diced watermelon

¼ cup freeze-dried mango, strawberries,
or other vitamin C–rich fruit

¼ medium red, yellow, or orange bell
pepper

½ medium green bell pepper

½ cup raw or cooked broccoli

1 medium tomato

¾ cup tomato juice

½ cup vegetable juice

½ cup raw or cooked cauliflower

½ cup cooked kale

¾ cup kale chips

1 packed cup raw spinach, or
½ cup cooked

¾ cup cooked collard, mustard, or
turnip greens

2 cups romaine lettuce

¾ cup shredded raw red cabbage

1 sweet potato or baking potato,
baked in skin

1 cup cooked edamame

**Green Leafy and Yellow Vegetables
and Yellow Fruits: 3 to 4 servings
daily.** These bunny favorites supply the
vitamin A, in the form of beta-carotene, that is vital for cell growth (your
little bunny's cells are multiplying at a
fantastic rate), and healthy skin, bones,
and eyes. This brightly-colored family of vegetables and fruits also deliver
doses of other essential carotenoids and
vitamins (vitamin E, riboflavin, folic
acid, and other B vitamins), numerous
minerals (many green leafy vegetables
provide a good deal of calcium as well
as trace minerals), disease-fighting
phytochemicals, and constipation-
fighting fiber. A bountiful selection of
Green Leafy and Yellow Vegetables
and Yellow Fruit can be found in the
list that follows. Have a long-standing
anti-vegetable agenda (or a brand new
one, thanks to pregnancy aversions)?
You may be pleasantly surprised to discover that broccoli and spinach are far
from the only sources of vitamin A. In
fact, orange is the new green when it
comes to vitamin A: This vitamin comes
packaged in some of nature's sweetest
orange-fleshed offerings—including
apricots, mangoes, yellow peaches, and
cantaloupe, as well as butternut squash,
pumpkin, and sweet potato. And those
who like to drink their vegetables can
count a glass of vegetable juice, a bowl
of carrot soup, or a mango smoothie
toward their daily Green Leafy and
Yellow goal.

Try to eat at least 3 to 4 servings a
day—aim to have some raw and some
cooked, some green and some yellow
each day (but don't force the green if
it turns you green—stick with the mel-
low yellows). Remember, many of these
foods also fill a Vitamin C serving:

⅛ cantaloupe (½ cup cubed)

2 large fresh apricots or 6 dried apricot
halves

½ medium mango

¼ medium papaya

1 large nectarine or yellow peach

1 small persimmon

You Can't Tell a Fruit by Its Cover

When it comes to nutrition, the more vibrant the color of most fruits and vegetables, the more antioxidants, vitamins (especially vitamin A), and minerals you'll be able to harvest from them. Explore the color purple (cabbage, potatoes, even cauliflower come in purple), a rainbow assortment of berries, orange carrots and mangoes, bright red, orange, and yellow bell peppers and tomatoes, and all the greens you can think of, from broccoli to kale to Swiss chard. But keep in mind that it's the color inside—not outside—that usually signals exceptionally good nutrition. So while cucumber (pale inside) is a lightweight, cantaloupe and kiwi (dark inside) are standouts.

¼ cup freeze-dried mango or other vitamin A–rich fruit

¾ cup pink grapefruit juice

1 pink or ruby red grapefruit

1 clementine

½ carrot (¼ cup grated)

½ cup raw or cooked broccoli pieces

1 cup coleslaw mix

¼ cup cooked collard greens, Swiss chard, or kale

1 packed cup green leafy lettuce, such as romaine, arugula, or red or green leaf

1 packed cup raw spinach, or ½ cup cooked

¼ cup cooked winter squash

½ small sweet potato or yam

2 medium tomatoes

½ medium red bell pepper

¼ cup chopped parsley

Other Fruits and Vegetables: 1 to 2 servings daily. While Others were once considered the produce department's nutritional B-listers, they're now getting a second look. Turns out they're rich not only in minerals, such as potassium and magnesium, that are vital to good pregnancy health, but also in a host of other trace minerals. Many also have phytochemicals and antioxidants in abundance (particularly those that sport the colors of the rainbow, so pick produce that's brightly hued for the biggest nutritional return). From that apple a day to those headline-making blueberries and pomegranates, Other Fruits and Vegetables are definitely worthy of a spot in your daily diet.

Round out your produce picks with 1 to 2 from this list daily:

1 medium apple

½ cup apple juice or applesauce

2 tablespoons apple juice concentrate

1 medium banana

½ cup blueberries

½ cup pitted fresh cherries

1 cup grapes

1 medium peach

1 medium pear or 2 dried halves

½ cup unsweetened pineapple juice

2 small plums

½ cup pomegranate juice

¼ cup freeze-dried fruit of the Other variety

½ medium avocado

½ cup cooked green beans

White Whole Wheat

Not a wholehearted fan of whole wheat? Craving the comfort of white during your queasy days? There's a new bread in town that might be just the ticket. White whole wheat breads are made with whole white wheat, a grain that has a milder, sweeter taste than the red wheat that regular whole wheat's made from. Is white whole wheat the best thing since sliced bread? It may well be if you're a white bread fan, since it offers the same nutritional benefits of regular whole wheat—including the bran—with that just-like-white taste and texture. Just be sure to read labels, since white wheat bread isn't whole grain unless it says so. You can also find white whole wheat in flour form—use it instead of regular whole wheat flour for lighter, less dense baked goods, pancakes, and more.

½ cup fresh raw mushrooms

½ cup cooked okra

½ cup sliced onion

½ cup cooked parsnips

½ cup cooked zucchini

1 small ear cooked sweet corn

1 cup shredded iceberg lettuce

½ cup green garden peas or snow peas

Whole Grains: 6 or more servings a day. There are plenty of reasons to go with the grain. Whole grains are packed with nutrients, particularly the B vitamins (except for vitamin B_{12}, found only in animal products) that are needed for just about every part of your baby's body. These concentrated complex carbohydrates are also rich in iron and trace minerals, such as zinc, selenium, and magnesium, all very important in pregnancy. An added plus: Carbs can calm a queasy tummy and combat constipation. Though these selections have many nutrients in common, each has its own strengths. To net the best benefits, include a variety of whole grains and legumes in your diet. Be adventurous: Coat your fish or chicken with whole wheat bread crumbs seasoned with herbs and Parmesan cheese. Try quinoa (a tasty high-protein grain) or whole wheat couscous as a side dish, or add bulgur or wheat berries to a wild rice pilaf. Use oats in your favorite cookie recipe. Substitute navy beans for limas in your soup. And though you'll likely sometimes eat them, remember that refined grains just don't stack up nutritionally. Even if they're "enriched," they are still lacking in fiber, protein, and more than a dozen vitamins and trace minerals that are found in the original whole grain.

Aim for about 6 from this list every day. Don't forget that many also contribute to your protein intake, often significantly:

1 slice whole wheat, whole oat, brown rice, whole rye, or other whole grain bread (or white whole wheat)

½ whole grain pita, roll, bagel, 12-inch wrap, tortilla, or English muffin

1 ounce whole grain, crackers, soy crisps, or lentil chips

1 cup cooked whole grain cereal, such as oatmeal

1 cup whole grain ready-to-eat cereal (serving sizes vary, so check labels)

½ cup granola

2 tablespoons wheat germ

½ cup cooked brown, black, or wild rice

½ cup cooked millet, bulgur, couscous, buckwheat, barley, farro, or quinoa

1 ounce (before cooking) whole grain or soy pasta

½ cup cooked beans, lentils, split peas, or edamame

2 cups popcorn

¼ cup whole grain or soy flour

Iron-rich foods: some daily. Since large amounts of iron are essential for the developing blood supply of your baby and for your own expanding blood supply, you'll need to pump up your iron intake during these 9 months.

Because it's often difficult to fill the pregnancy iron requirement through diet alone, your practitioner may recommend that you take a daily iron supplement in addition to your prenatal vitamins from the 20th week on, or whenever routine testing shows an iron shortfall. To enhance the absorption of the iron, take it between meals with a fruit juice rich in vitamin C (caffeinated beverages, antacids, high-fiber foods, and high-calcium foods can interfere with iron absorption). Eat your Iron-rich foods with a side of C, too.

Small amounts of iron are found in most of the fruits, vegetables, grains, and meats you eat every day. But try to have some of the following Iron-rich foods daily. Again, many Iron-rich foods also fill other requirements at the same time:

Beef, buffalo, duck, turkey

Cooked clams, oysters, mussels, and shrimp

Sardines

Spinach, collard, kale, and turnip greens

Seaweed

Pumpkin seeds

Oat bran

Barley, bulgur, quinoa

Beans and peas

Edamame and soy products

Dried fruit

Fats and high-fat foods: about 4 servings daily. Now, here's a requirement that's not only easy to fill, but easy to overfill. And though there's no harm—and probably some benefit—in having a couple of extra Green Leafies or Vitamin C foods, excess Fat servings could spell excess pounds. Still, though sensibly moderating your fat intake during pregnancy is a good idea, eliminating all fat from your expectant diet isn't. Fat is vital to your developing baby. The essential fatty acids in them are just that—essential. Especially beneficial in the third trimester are omega-3 fatty acids (see page 98).

Keep track of your fat intake—fill your daily quota but try not to overfill it. And in keeping track, don't forget that the fat used in cooking and preparing

Fat Matters

Trying to keep those calories down by skipping the dressing on your salad or the oil in your stir-fry? You'd be getting an A for willpower—but less vitamin A in your veggies. Research shows that many of the nutrients found in vegetables aren't well absorbed by the body if not accompanied by a side of fat. So make a point of including a little fat with your veggies: Enjoy oil with your stir-fry, a sprinkle of nuts on your broccoli, and dressing with your salad.

foods counts, too: the butter you scrambled your eggs in, the mayo you tossed your coleslaw with. The good news is, adding some fat to the preparation of your veggies boosts your body's absorption of their nutrients (see box, page 97).

If you're not gaining enough weight, and increasing your intake of other nutritious foods hasn't done the trick, try adding an extra Fat serving each day—the concentrated calories it provides may help you hit your optimum weight-gain stride. If you're gaining too quickly, you can cut back by 1 or 2 servings—but again, don't cut fat out altogether.

The foods on this list are made up completely (or mostly) of fat. They certainly won't be the only source of fat in your diet (full-fat cheeses and yogurts, some meats, and nuts and seeds are all high in fat), but these "added fats" are the only ones you'll want to keep track of. If your weight gain is on target, aim for about 4 full (about 14 grams each) or 8 half (about 7 grams each) Fat servings each day. If it's not, consider adjusting your fat intake up or down:

1 tablespoon oil, such as vegetable, olive, canola, grapeseed, or sesame

1 tablespoon regular butter or margarine

1 tablespoon regular mayonnaise

2 tablespoons regular salad dressing

2 tablespoons heavy or whipping cream

¼ cup half-and-half

¼ cup whipped cream

¼ cup regular sour cream

2 tablespoons regular cream cheese

2 tablespoons peanut, almond, or other nut butter

Omega-3 fatty acids. Are you fat phobic (especially since pregnancy put you on the weight-gain fast track)? Fear not your fat—just choose the right ones. After all, not all fats are created equal. Some fats are good ones—and they're especially good (make that great) when you're expecting. Omega-3 fatty acids, most notably DHA, are the best addition you can make to your diet when you're eating for two. That's because DHA is essential for proper brain growth and eye development in fetuses and young babies. In fact, researchers have found that toddlers whose moms consumed plenty of DHA during pregnancy had better hand-eye coordination than their peers, though it's unclear if this translates to boosted brainpower later in childhood. Getting enough of this vital baby brain fuel in your diet is especially important during the last trimester (when your baby's brain grows at a phenomenal pace) and while you're nursing (the DHA content of a baby's brain triples during the first 3 months of life).

And what's good for the expected is also good for the expecting. For you, getting enough DHA may mean moderated mood swings and a lowered risk of postpartum depression. Another potential postpartum perk? Getting enough DHA when you're expecting could mean your baby will have better sleep habits later on. Luckily, DHA is found in plenty of foods you probably already eat—and like to eat:

Salmon (choose wild when you can) and other higher-fat fish, such as sardines

Canned light tuna

Walnuts

Arugula

DHA-rich eggs (often called omega-3 eggs)

A Grain of Salt

Trying to shake the salt habit because you're afraid it'll lead to water retention and swelling? Well, it may—but that's not such a bad thing when you're pregnant. In fact, some increase in body fluids in pregnancy (aka that swelling you're figuring isn't so swell) is necessary and normal, and a moderate amount of salt (sodium) is needed to maintain that extra fluid. Seriously skimping on sodium can actually be harmful during pregnancy.

Still, most Americans (including pregnant Americans) consume far too much sodium. Consuming very large quantities of salt and very salty foods frequently (such as those pickles you can't stop eating, extra soy sauce on your already-salty stir-fry, and super-salty potato chips by the bagful) isn't good for anyone, pregnant or not. High sodium intake is closely linked to high blood pressure, a condition that can cause complications in pregnancy, labor, and delivery. As a general rule, salt only lightly—or don't salt at all—during cooking. Salt your food to taste at the table instead. Have a pickle when you crave it, but try to stop at 1 or 2 instead of eating half the jar. And unless your practitioner recommends otherwise (because you are hyperthyroid, for example), use iodized salt to be sure you meet the increased need for iodine in pregnancy. In fact, be sure to check the label of the salt you're using to make sure it's got iodine in it (most sea salts, for example, don't contain iodine). About one-third of moms-to-be are iodine deficient—a problem when you're growing a baby, since iodine is needed for healthy brain development of the fetus.

Grass-fed beef and buffalo

Crab and shrimp

Chicken (free-range—or pasture-raised—chickens usually have more DHA)

You can also ask your practitioner about pregnancy-safe mercury-free DHA supplements (many prenatal supplements contain up to 200 to 300 mg of DHA already). Not a fan of the fishy aftertaste some DHA supplements leave behind (and that often repeat)? There are vegetarian and vegan alternatives that are fish-free.

Fluids: as much as you need. You're not only eating for two, but drinking for two. Your baby's body, like yours, is composed mostly of fluids. As that little body grows, so does its demand for fluids. Your body needs fluids more than ever, too, since pregnancy pumps up fluid volume significantly. Water also eases constipation, rids your body of toxins and waste products (and baby's, too), and reduces excessive swelling and the risk of UTIs and preterm labor. So it's important you get enough fluids when you're expecting.

But just how much is "enough"? You've probably heard that everyone should get at least 8 glasses (or 64 ounces) a day, but there's really no scientific basis for that one-size-fits-all formula for fluid intake. How much fluid a person needs varies a lot—it depends on her activity level, where she lives, what she eats, her BMI, and a whole host of other variables (including whether or not she's pregnant). It can even vary from day to day (if

What's in a Supplement?

What's in a prenatal pill, powder, or gummy? That depends on which one you're taking. Since there aren't any standards set for prenatal supplements, formulas vary. Chances are your practitioner will prescribe or recommend a supplement, which will take the guesswork (and homework) out of choosing a formula yourself. If you're facing the pharmacy shelves without a recommendation, look for a formula that contains:

- No more than 4,000 IU (800 mcg) of vitamin A (amounts over 10,000 IU could be toxic). Many manufacturers have reduced the amount of vitamin A in their vitamin supplements or have replaced it with beta-carotene, a much safer source of vitamin A.

- At least 400 to 600 mcg of folic acid (folate)

- 250 mg of calcium—though if you're not getting enough calcium in your diet, you will need to take an extra calcium supplement to reach the daily pregnancy quota for calcium of 1,200 mg. Do not take more than 250 mg of calcium at the same time as supplementary iron, because calcium interferes with iron absorption.

- 30 mg iron

- 50 to 80 mg vitamin C

- 15 mg zinc

- 2 mg copper

- 2 mg vitamin B_6

- At least 400 IU of vitamin D

- Approximately the DRI for vitamin E (15 mg), thiamin (1.4 mg), riboflavin (1.4 mg), niacin (18 mg), and vitamin B_{12} (2.6 mg). Most prenatal supplements contain 2 to 3 times the DRI of these. There are no known harmful effects from such doses.

- 150 mcg of iodine (not all prenatals contain iodine or this amount of it)

- Some formulas may also contain magnesium, selenium, fluoride, biotin, choline, phosphorus, pantothenic acid, extra B_6 (to combat queasiness), ginger (ditto), and/or baby brain–boosting DHA.

Also important: Scan for ingredients that shouldn't be in your prenatal supplement, such as herbs. When in doubt, ask your practitioner.

one day is spent at a sunny beach and the next at an air-conditioned mall, or one day is active and one is sedentary). Fortunately, your body is likely to tell you how much fluid it needs—so listen. Drink up whenever you're starting to feel thirsty, or preferably, before. Reach for the water bottle, too, when you're sweating more than usual (such as when you're exercising or when it's hot outside), when you've been vomiting, or if you're retaining a lot of fluid

(paradoxically, extra fluids can flush out excess fluids). And the best gauge of your fluid intake: your fluid output. If your urine is pale straw colored and there's plenty of it, you're getting enough to drink. If it's dark yellow and scant, you need to drink more.

Of course, not all your fluids have to come from water. You get a good share of fluids from milk (which is two-thirds water), almond milk, coconut water, fruit and vegetable juices, and soups.

Fruit and vegetables count, too—especially juicy ones, like watermelon.

Prenatal vitamin supplements: a pregnancy formula taken daily. With all the nutrients already packed into the Daily Dozen (or any healthy diet), why would you need to add a prenatal vitamin to the mix? Couldn't you fill all of your requirements by filling yourself with the right foods? Well, you probably could—that is, if you lived in a laboratory where your food was precisely prepared and measured to calculate an adequate daily intake, and if you never ate on the run, had to work through lunch, or felt too sick to eat. In the real world—the one you most likely live in—a prenatal supplement provides extra health insurance for you and your baby, covering those nutritional bases when your diet doesn't. And that's why taking one daily is recommended.

Still, a supplement is just a supplement. No pill (or powder), no matter how complete, can replace a good diet. It's best if most of your vitamins and minerals come from foods, because that's the way nutrients can be most effectively used. Fresh foods contain not only nutrients that we know about and can be synthesized in a pill, but probably lots of others that are as yet undiscovered. Food also supplies fiber and water (fruits and vegetables are loaded with both) and important calories and protein, none of which comes efficiently packaged in a pill.

But don't think that because a little is good, a lot is better. Any vitamin or mineral supplementation beyond what's found in your prenatal should be taken only if your practitioner has recommended it—and the same goes for herbal supplements, too. As for vitamins and minerals you can get from your diet, you can't overdo the nutrients by piling up your plate at the salad bar—so no need to hold back when the carrots call or the broccoli beckons.

What You May Be Wondering About

Milk-Free Diet

"I'm lactose intolerant, and drinking 4 glasses of milk a day would make me feel really sick. But don't babies need milk?"

It's not milk your baby needs, it's calcium. Since milk is one of nature's finest and most convenient sources of calcium in the American diet, it's the one most often recommended for filling the greatly increased requirement during pregnancy. But if milk leaves you with more than a sour taste in your mouth and a white mustache above your lips (got gas?), you probably think twice before reaching for that glass of the white stuff. Fortunately, you don't have to suffer so your baby can grow healthy teeth and bones. If you're lactose intolerant or just don't have a taste for milk, plenty of substitutes are available that fill the nutritional bill just as well.

Even if regular milk turns your tummy, you can easily turn to lactose-free varieties (ditto other lactose-free dairy). You may find that your tummy tolerates hard cheeses and fully processed yogurts (the active cultures in them actually help your digestion), as well as dairy products made from pasteurized goat's or sheep's milk. Another

Pasteurized, Please

When it was invented by French scientist Louis Pasteur in the mid-1800s, pasteurization was the greatest thing to happen to dairy products since cows. And it still is, particularly as far as pregnant women are concerned. To protect yourself and your baby from harmful bacteria, make sure all the milk you drink is pasteurized and all the dairy products you eat are made from pasteurized milk ("raw" dairy is not pasteurized). Be especially careful when it comes to soft cheeses (fresh mozzarella, feta, Brie, blue cheese, soft Mexican-style cheese) made from raw milk, since these can be contaminated with listeria, a particularly dangerous bacteria (see page 118). Choose pasteurized varieties of these cheeses (domestic is more likely to be pasteurized than imported, but always check the label) or heat until bubbly before eating. Keep in mind that the raw rage has expanded the number of non-pasteurized products on the market, so pregnant buyer be wary.

And dairy doesn't corner the market when it comes to pasteurization. Eggs come pasteurized, too (eliminating the risk of salmonella)—a good choice if you're whipping up a homemade Caesar dressing or prefer your yolks runny or your scrambles soft. Juices you drink should also be pasteurized (to eliminate E. Coli and other harmful bacteria). Most (but not all) commercially packaged juice is pasteurized, so always check the label before you buy. Not sure if a juice is pasteurized or pretty sure it isn't (say, freshly squeezed at the juice bar)? Don't drink it. Ditto for smoothies made with juice, unless you're sure it's pasteurized. Fresh coconuts cut open right in front of you and served with a straw are fine to drink since the coconut water is sterile and well protected inside the hard coconut shell.

Wondering about "flash-pasteurized"? It's a faster but just as effective pasteurization process, which kills bacteria while preserving flavor. And how about juicing you do at home? That's all good (and yummy, and nutritious)—as long as you've thoroughly washed the produce first.

---

advantage of using lactose-free milk products: Some are fortified with extra calcium (check labels and choose one that is). Taking a lactase tablet before ingesting regular milk or milk products, or adding lactase drops to regular milk, can also minimize or eliminate dairy-induced tummy troubles.

Even if you've been lactose intolerant for years, you may be pleasantly surprised to discover that your tummy no longer puts up a fuss in the second and third trimester, conveniently when baby's needs for calcium are greatest. If so, go ahead and indulge in dairy—just keep in mind that your tummy may have its limits, so keep those lactose-free

options open, too. Also remember, your free pass to the dairy case will probably expire once baby arrives.

If you can't handle any dairy products or are allergic to them, you can still get all the calcium your baby requires by drinking calcium-fortified juices or almond milk and eating the nondairy foods listed under calcium foods on page 93.

If your problem with milk isn't physiological but just a matter of taste, try some of the dairy or nondairy calcium-rich alternatives. There are bound to be plenty that your taste buds can embrace. Or disguise your milk in cereal, soups, and smoothies.

If you can't seem to get enough calcium into your diet, ask your practitioner to recommend a calcium supplement (there are plenty of chewable varieties that are sweet revenge for those who find a pill hard to swallow). You'll also need to be sure that you're getting enough vitamin D (which is added to cow's milk). Many calcium supplements include vitamin D (which actually boosts absorption of calcium), and you'll also be getting some in your prenatal supplement.

Red-Meat-Free Diet

"I eat chicken and fish but no red meat. Will my baby get all the necessary nutrients without it?"

Your baby won't have a beef with your red-meat-free diet. Fish and lean poultry, in fact, give you more baby-building protein and less fat for your calories than most beef, pork, and lamb—making them more efficient pregnancy choices. And like red meat, they're also rich sources of many of the B vitamins your baby needs. The only nutrient poultry and fish can't always compete with meat for is iron (duck, turkey, and shellfish are iron-rich exceptions), but there are plenty of other sources of this essential mineral, which is also easy to take in supplement form.

Vegetarian Diet

"As a vegetarian I'm wondering if I have to change anything in my diet now that I'm expecting a baby."

Vegetarians of every variety can have healthy babies without compromising their dietary principles—they just have to be a little more careful in planning their diets than meat-eating moms-to-be. When choosing your meat-free menus, make sure you get all of the following:

Enough protein. For the ovo-lacto vegetarian, who eats eggs and dairy products, getting enough protein is as easy as getting enough of these dairy-case favorites (particularly if you seek Greek yogurt, an especially potent protein source). If you're a vegan (a vegetarian who doesn't eat any animal products, including eggs and dairy), you may find you'll need to work a little harder in the protein department, turning to ample quantities of dried beans, peas, lentils, tofu, and other soy products (see page 91 for more vegetarian proteins).

Enough calcium. This is no tall order for the vegetarian who eats dairy products, but it can be trickier for those who don't. Luckily, dairy products are the most obvious but not the only sources of calcium. Calcium-fortified almond milk and juices offer as much calcium as milk, ounce for ounce (just make sure you shake them before using). Other nondairy dietary sources of calcium include dark leafy green vegetables, sesame seeds, almonds, and many soy products (such as soy milk, soy cheese, tofu, and tempeh). For added insurance, vegans should probably also take a calcium supplement in addition to their prenatal vitamin, so check with your practitioner for a recommendation (preferably one with vitamin D added; see page 104).

Vitamin B_{12}. Though B_{12} deficiencies are rare, vegetarians, particularly vegans, often don't get enough of this vitamin because it is found only in animal foods. So be certain to take supplemental B_{12}, as well as folic acid and iron (ask your practitioner if you need more B_{12} than what's provided in your prenatal vitamin). Other dietary sources include B_{12}-fortified soy milk, fortified cereals, nutritional yeast, and fortified meat substitutes.

Don't Be D-eficient

While the body produces vitamin D when exposed to sunlight, making enough can be challenging—especially for those who have darker skin, live in less-sunny climates, don't get outdoors enough, or wear sunscreen. Can you eat (or drink) your D? Not easily, since it isn't found in large amounts in any food. Fortified milk and juices contain some, as do sardines and egg yolks, but not nearly enough to prevent a D deficit. Your best bet: Ask your practitioner about testing your vitamin D levels and prescribing a supplement as needed.

Vitamin D. Everyone needs vitamin D in their diet, but vegans who aren't drinking milk or eating fish need to be especially mindful about finding ways to get their D (see the box above).

Low-Carb Diet

"I've been on a low-carb/high-protein diet to lose weight. Now that I'm pregnant, can I continue eating this way to keep from gaining too much weight?"

Here's the low-down on low-carb: When you're expecting, low isn't the way to go. Going low on any essential nutrient, in fact, isn't smart when you're growing a baby. Your highest pregnancy priority: getting a balance of all the best baby-making ingredients, including the right kind of carbs (those complex ones). As popular as they are, diets that limit all carbohydrates (including fruits, vegetables, and whole grains) limit the nutrients—especially folic acid—that growing fetuses need. And what's bad for baby can also be bad for mom: Skimp on complex carbohydrates and you'll be skimping on constipation-fighting fiber, plus all the B vitamins known to battle morning sickness and pregnancy-unsettled skin.

Thinking about being a pregnant Paleo? The Paleo diet, which mimics the menu of our cave-dwelling ancestors, doesn't quite measure up for modern moms-to-be. Though it includes plenty of animal protein, vegetables, and some fruit and nuts, it excludes dairy, whole grains, and beans, all good sources of essential pregnancy-friendly nutrients. Queasy moms-to-be may also find that having crackers (and bread, and other often stomach-settling carb options) off the table may be challenging.

Raw Diet

"I've been eating an all-raw diet, which makes me feel amazing—full of energy. Do I have to stop now that I'm expecting?"

Eating a completely raw diet may be a raw deal for you and your baby, for a couple of reasons. Most important: There's always the possibility that raw foods may be contaminated with bacteria that cooking or pasteurizing would otherwise kill. That holds true not only for the obvious suspects (raw

Diet Don'ts

Pregnancy is a time for healthy eating, not for dieting. So shelve those weight-loss books, power down those diet apps, skip the juice cleanses, free yourself of that gluten-free diet (unless you have celiac disease or gluten intolerance), be sensible when going raw, and stay well balanced for a well-fed baby.

A Walk Down the Health Food Aisle

Maybe you're a regular at the health food store (or aisle)—or maybe you're wondering if you should visit it for the first time now that you're trying to be healthy for two. But are health foods always a healthy choice for mamas-to-be? For the most part, yes . . . with a side of caution. Take flaxseed products, for example—touted for their health benefits, of which they have many. Some practitioners recommend limiting how much flax expectant moms consume (in oil, seed, or supplement form), citing animal studies that show that very large amounts may affect a baby's development—though there's no clear evidence that the same would hold true for human moms and babies. Other practitioners say moderate amounts of flax are fine during pregnancy—especially because it's a good source of baby-friendly omega-3 fatty acids. Unsure whether to reach for the flax? Ask your practitioner for his or her recommendation.

What about other health food favorites? Hemp seed, hemp food products, and hemp seed oil in moderation (1 to 2 servings a day) are probably safe for expectant moms—and a good source of protein, fiber, and fatty acids. But since hemp's use during pregnancy has not been well studied, it makes sense to avoid it in large concentrations (as it would be in supplement form). Chia seeds are an excellent source of fiber, omega-3 fatty acids, protein, calcium, and iron—but while a sprinkle on a salad, yogurt, or cereal, or in a smoothie is likely a safe and nutritious bet, check in with your practitioner before you chow down on chia because (surprise!) its safety hasn't been studied in pregnancy. The pregnancy safety of spirulina (a natural algae powder that is high in protein and calcium and is a good source of antioxidants, B vitamins, and other nutrients) also hasn't been established, leading some practitioners to suggest that moms-to-be limit or even avoid using this nutrient-packed powder. Another reason to consider pausing when pregnant before using spirulina: It's sometimes contaminated with toxins, including heavy metals, as well as harmful bacteria. Same goes for popular "green food" powders, some of which also contain herbs and supplements that might not be pregnancy safe. Wheat grass doesn't get a pass, either— not only because there's no proof that it's safe during pregnancy, but also because it, too, can be contaminated with bacteria.

Thinking about shaking things up with a protein shake mix? Think about running the label by your practitioner first, since many contain suspect supplements and too-high levels of vitamins and minerals.

Had a couple of shots of wheat grass or a few green powder smoothies before you got the go-ahead from your practitioner? No worries— just remember that going forward it's always a good idea to get clearance from your practitioner before you clear off the shelves of your health food market.

dairy products, raw meat and fish), but also for "raw" ready-to-eat foods sold in health food markets that aren't prepared or stored safely. Another consideration: It's hard to get all the nutrients you need during pregnancy when you're eating only raw—some vitamins are better absorbed when they're cooked. The most notable nutrients you'll miss: vitamins B_{12} (which is impossible to get from raw, plant-based foods) and D, selenium, zinc, iron, and DHA. Plus,

Shortcuts to Healthy Eating

Healthy food can be fast food, too. Here's how:

- If you're always on the run, remember that it takes no more time to slap together a roast turkey, cheese, lettuce, and tomato sandwich to take to work (or to order one at the deli) than it does to stand in line for fast food.

- If the prospect of preparing a real dinner every night seems overwhelming, cook enough for 2 or 3 dinners at one time and give yourself alternate nights off.

- Keep it simple when you're cooking healthy. For a quick meal, bake or broil a fish fillet and top it with your favorite jarred salsa, a little chopped avocado, and a squeeze of fresh lime juice. Layer tomato sauce and mozzarella cheese on a cooked boneless chicken breast, and then run it under the broiler. Or scramble some eggs and wrap them in a corn tortilla along with shredded cheddar and some microwave-steamed vegetables.

- When you don't have time to start from scratch (when do you ever?), turn to canned beans, soups, frozen or packaged ready-to-prepare healthy entrees, frozen vegetables, or the fresh prewashed veggies sold in supermarket produce sections.

---

if you're going all raw, you'll have a hard time getting your protein quota safely (which vegetarians and vegans can net from cooked beans and quinoa, for instance—something a raw foodie can't).

A good compromise when you're expecting? Dig into those raw veggies, serve those salads, and by all means eat that apple (and fresh peach, and fresh mango) a day—but also remember that some foods were made to be cooked (or heat-pasteurized), at least when you're baking a baby bun.

Junk Food Junkie

"I'm addicted to junk foods like cookies, chips, and fast food. I know I should be eating healthier—and I really want to—but I'm not sure I can change my habits."

Ready to junk the junk food? Getting motivated to change your eating habits is the first and most important step—so congratulate yourself on taking it. Actually making the changes will involve some serious effort—but the effort will be seriously worth it, for baby and for you. Here are several ways to make your withdrawal from your junk food habit almost as painless as it is worthwhile:

Move your meals. If the coffee cake calls when you breakfast at your desk, fill up on a better breakfast at home (foods that are packed with the blood-sugar-stabilizing, stick-with-you combo of complex carbs and protein, like oatmeal, will actually help you fight those junk food cravings when they strike later on). If you know you can't resist the golden fries once you pass through the Golden Arches, don't go there—literally. Order in a healthy sandwich from the local deli—or head to that wrap place that doesn't fry anything.

Plan, plan, and plan some more. Planning for meals and snacks ahead of time (instead of grabbing what's easiest or nearest, like that package of bright orange cheese crackers from the vending machine) will keep you eating well throughout your pregnancy. So pack those brown bags and bento boxes. Keep a supply of takeout menus from restaurants that offer healthy options or opt for a delivery app, so a nourishing meal is always just an order away (and place your order before hunger strikes). Stock up with wholesome but satisfying snacks: fresh, dried, or freeze-dried fruit (try freezing grapes at home for a cold, sweet snack), nuts, healthy chips (baked soy, lentil, whole corn, kale, or other veggie varieties), whole grain granola or cereal bars and crackers, individual-size yogurts or smoothies, string cheese or wedges (or crunchy Moon Cheese). So that the soda won't speak to you next time you get thirsty, keep water at the ready.

Don't test temptation. Keep candy, chips, cookies, and sugar-sweetened soft drinks out of the house so they'll be out of reach (if not out of mind). Step away from the pastry case before that cupcake makes eye contact with you. Drive the long way home from the office if it means you won't drive by the drive-through.

Make substitutions. Crave a Krispy Kreme with your morning coffee? Dunk a whole grain bran muffin instead. The midnight munchies have you digging for Doritos? Settle for the baked whole grain corn chips (dipped in salsa for more flavor and a healthy helping of vitamin C). Is your sweet tooth aching for ice cream (with Oreos mixed in)? Stop for a thick, creamy, sweet fruit smoothie instead.

Keep baby on your mind. Your baby eats what you eat, but that's sometimes hard to remember (especially when the smell of a cinnamon bun tries to seduce you at the mall). If you find it helps keep baby feeding front of brain, put pictures of cute, healthy babies wherever you might need a little inspiration (and a lot of willpower). Keep one on your desk, in your wallet, in your car (so when you're tempted to veer into the drive-through, you'll drive by instead). Or let that ultrasound photo of your own little cutie talk you off the junk food ledge.

Know your limits. Some junk food junkies can handle a once-in-a-while approach to indulging their cravings, others can't (and you know who you are). If enough junk food is never enough for you—if a snack-size leads to king-size, if a single donut leads to a box of 6, if you know you'll polish off the whole bag of chips once you tear it open—you might have an easier time quitting your habit cold turkey than trying to moderate it.

Remember that good habits can last a lifetime, too. Once you've put the effort into developing healthier eating habits, you might want to consider keeping them. Continuing to eat well after delivery will give you more of the energy you'll need to fuel your new-mom lifestyle. Plus, since your little one will learn future eating habits (the good, the bad, and the junky) from you, it'll make it more likely that he or she will grow up with a taste for the healthier things in life.

Eating Out

"I try hard to stay on a healthy diet, but I eat out so often, it seems impossible."

For many moms-to-be, it isn't substituting mineral water for martinis that poses a challenge at the restaurant table—it's trying to put together a meal that's baby-friendly and doesn't break

Cholesterol Concerns

Here's a happy fat fact: Cholesterol doesn't have to be off the table when you're expecting. Pregnant women are protected against the artery-clogging effects of cholesterol. In fact, cholesterol is a must-have for healthy fetal development, so much so that the mom's body automatically steps up its production, raising blood cholesterol levels by anywhere from 25 to 40 percent. Though you don't have to eat a high-cholesterol diet to help your body rev up production, you don't have to be cholesterol-phobic, either (unless your practitioner advises you otherwise). So go ahead—say cheese, scramble some eggs, and bite into that burger, all without cholesterol concerns. Just remember to make healthy food choices as much as possible for the nutritional benefits they come with (clearly, a typical fast-food burger doesn't stack up to a grass-fed burger on a whole-wheat bun).

the calorie bank. With those goals in mind, and the following suggestions, it's easy to take the Pregnancy Diet out to eat:

- Look for whole grains before you leap into the bread basket. If there aren't any in the basket, ask if there are any in the kitchen. If not, try not to fill up too much on the white stuff. Go easy, too, on the butter you spread on your bread and rolls as well as the olive oil you dip them into. There will probably be plenty of other sources of fat in your restaurant meal—dressing on the salad, butter or olive oil on the vegetables—and, as always, fat adds up quickly.

- Select a salad. Other good first-course choices include shrimp cocktail, steamed seafood, grilled vegetables, or soup.

- If soup's on, look to ones with a vegetable base (such as sweet potato, carrot, winter squash, or tomato). Lentil or bean soups pack a protein punch, too. In fact, a large bowl may eat like a meal, especially if you toss some grated cheese on top. Generally steer clear of creamy soups (unless they get their creamy goodness from yogurt or buttermilk), and take Manhattan-style when it comes to clam chowder.

- Make the most of your main. Get your protein—fish, seafood, chicken breast, or beef—the lean way (good words to look for: "grilled," "broiled," "steamed," and "poached"). If everything comes heavily sauced, ask for yours on the side. And don't shy away from special requests (chefs are used to them—plus, it's hard to say no to a pregnant woman). Ask if that chicken breast can be grilled plain instead of breaded and pan-seared or if the snapper can be broiled or baked instead of fried.

- Be selective on the side, scouting for sweet potatoes, brown or wild rice, quinoa, beans, and fresh vegetables.

- Consider a fruity finish. Fruit alone doesn't cut it (at least not all the time)? Add whipped cream, sorbet, or ice cream to those fresh berries.

Reading Labels

"I'm trying to eat well, but it's hard to figure out what's in the products I buy. The labels are so confusing."

Labels aren't designed to help you as much as to sell you. Keep this in mind when filling your shopping cart, and learn to read the small print, especially the ingredients list and the nutrition label (which is designed to help you).

The ingredients listing will tell you, in order of predominance (with the first ingredient the most plentiful and the last the least), exactly what's in a product. A quick look will tell you whether the major ingredient in a cereal is a whole grain (like "whole grain oats") or a refined one (like "milled corn"). It will also tell you when a product is high in sugar, salt, fat, or additives. For example, when sugar is listed near the top of the ingredients list, or when it appears in several different forms on a list (corn syrup, honey, and sugar), you can suspect that the product is chock-full of it.

Checking the grams of sugar on the label won't be useful until the FDA requires that the grams of "added sugar" be separated from the grams of "naturally occurring sugar" (those found in the raisin part of the raisin bran, or in the milk part of the yogurt). Though the number of grams of sugar on the present label may be the same on a container of orange juice and a container of fruit drink, they aren't equivalent. It's like comparing oranges and corn syrup: The real OJ gets its naturally occurring sugar from fruit, while the fruit drink relies on added sugar.

Nutrition labels, which appear on most packaged products on your grocer's shelves, can be particularly helpful if you're tracking your protein or fat intake (listed in grams per serving) or keeping an eye on calories (listed in number per serving). Just be aware that serving sizes may be much smaller than you'd think, another reason to read the fine print (that candy bar might seem like a bargain at 100 calories, until you realize the bar contains 2½ servings, 100 calories each). The listing of percentages of the DRI really isn't all that useful, because the DRI for pregnant women is different from the one for average adults. Still, a food that scores high in a wide variety of nutrients is a good product to drop into your cart.

While it's important to pay attention to the small print, it's sometimes just as important to ignore the large print. When a box of English muffins boasts, "Made with whole wheat, bran, and honey," reading the small print may reveal that the major ingredient (first on the list) is wheat flour, not whole wheat flour, that the muffins contain barely any bran (it's near the bottom of the ingredients list), and that there's a lot more white sugar (it's high on the list) than honey (it's low). Remember that "wheat," like "oats" or "corn," refers to the variety of grain, not to whether it's whole or not (if it is, it'll say so).

"Enriched" and "fortified" are also buzz words to be wary of. Adding a few vitamins to a not-so-good food doesn't make it a good food. You'd be much better off with a bowl of oatmeal, which comes by its nutrients naturally, than with a refined cereal that contains 12 grams of added sugar and tossed-in vitamins and minerals.

Sushi Safety

"Sushi is my favorite food, but I heard you're not supposed to eat it while you're pregnant. Is that true?"

Sorry to say, but sashimi and sushi made with raw fish don't make the cut when you're expecting, at least according to most experts. Same holds true for the rest of the raw bar, including raw oysters and clams, ceviche, fish tartares or carpaccios, and other raw or barely cooked fish and shellfish. That's because when seafood isn't cooked, there's a slight chance that it can cause food poisoning (something you definitely don't want when you're pregnant). But that doesn't mean you can't belly up to the sushi bar. Rolls that are made with cooked fish or seafood and/or vegetables are, in fact, healthy options—especially if your local sushi bar offers brown-rice sushi.

Worried about the raw fish you've downed before you read this? Don't be (after all, you didn't get sick)—just skip it from now on.

Fish Safety

"Should I eat fish while I'm pregnant, or should I stay away from it? I keep on hearing conflicting information."

Fish is an excellent source of lean protein, as well as baby brain–building omega-3 fatty acids, good reasons to keep it on your pregnancy menu—or even to consider adding it if you've never been a fish fan before. In fact, research has shown brain benefits for babies whose moms eat fish when they're expecting. So go fish, by all means, aiming for at least 8 and up to 12 ounces of fish each week (about 2 or 3 servings weekly).

But when you're casting your fishing net, be sure to fish selectively, sticking to those varieties that are lower in mercury—a chemical that in large, accumulated doses can possibly be harmful to a fetus's developing nervous system. Luckily, many of the most commonly consumed fish are low in mercury: Choose from salmon (wild caught is best), sole, flounder, haddock, trout, halibut, ocean perch, pollack, cod, light canned tuna, catfish, and other smaller ocean fish (anchovies, sardines, and herring are not only safe, but also loaded with omega-3s).

It's smart to avoid shark, swordfish, king mackerel, and tilefish (especially from the Gulf of Mexico), since these types of fish contain high levels of mercury. Don't worry if you've already enjoyed a serving or two—any risks would apply to regular consumption—just skip these fish from now on.

Also limit your consumption of freshwater fish recreationally caught to an average of 6 ounces (cooked weight) per week—commercially-caught fish usually has lower levels of contaminants, so you can safely eat more. Steer clear of fish from waters that are contaminated (with sewage or industrial runoff, for example) and tropical fish, such as grouper, amberjack, and mahimahi (which sometimes contain toxins).

What about tuna, America's favorite fish in a can? The EPA, the FDA, and ACOG all agree that canned light tuna is safe to eat because it's not high in mercury. Solid or chunk white tuna (usually albacore) contains 3 times the mercury of light varieties, and experts recommend limiting white tuna to no more than 6 ounces per week (the same limit applies to tuna steaks). Since some experts feel that's still too much for expectant moms, check in with your practitioner before opening that can . . . of white tuna. Or switch to canned salmon or sardines (or light tuna).

For the latest information on fish safety, go to fda.gov (search for "fish").

Spicy Food

"I love spicy food—the hotter, the better. Is it safe to eat it while I'm pregnant?"

Hot mamas-to-be can continue testing their taste buds with 4-alarm chilis, salsas, stir-fries, and curries. The only risk of eating spicy food during pregnancy is that you'll be following it up with indigestion, especially later in pregnancy (chili today, heartburn tomorrow . . . or, let's face it, tonight).

If that's a risk worth taking for you, go ahead and spice things up—just don't forget to have some Tums (or a glass of almond milk, known for its heartburn-cooling benefits) ready for dessert.

An unexpected hot pepper perk? Hot peppers, like all peppers, are packed with vitamin C.

Spoiled Food

"I ate a container of yogurt this morning without realizing that it had expired a week ago. It didn't taste spoiled, but should I worry?"

No need to cry over spoiled milk . . . or yogurt. Though eating dairy products that have expired is never a good idea, it's rarely a dangerous one. If you haven't gotten sick from your postdate snack (symptoms of food poisoning usually occur within 8 hours), there's obviously no harm done. Besides, food poisoning is an unlikely possibility if the yogurt was refrigerated continuously. In the future, however, check dates more carefully before you buy or eat perishables, and, of course, don't eat foods that smell or taste off, or appear to have developed mold. For more on food safety, see on page 117.

"I think I got food poisoning from something I ate last night, and I've been throwing up and having diarrhea. Will that hurt my baby?"

You're much more likely to suffer from the food poisoning than your baby is. The major risk—for you and your baby—is that you'll become dehydrated from vomiting and/or diarrhea. So make sure you get plenty of fluids (which are more important in the short term than solids) to replace those that you're losing. And contact your practitioner if your diarrhea is severe and/ or your stools contain blood or mucus. See page 530 for more on stomach bugs.

Sugar Substitutes

"I use Splenda in my coffee, drink a lot of diet soda, and eat sugar-free yogurt. Are sugar substitutes safe during pregnancy?"

They sound like a sweet deal, but the truth is that sugar substitutes are a somewhat mixed bag for expectant moms. Though most are generally considered safe for use during pregnancy, some research suggests that the artificial ones on this list may increase baby's later risk of being overweight or obese. Here's the lowdown on sugar substitutes:

Sucralose (Splenda). It's sugar, sort of. At least it starts out life that way, before being chemically processed into a form that your body won't be able to absorb, making it essentially calorie free. Sucralose, which has less of that aftertaste that gives sweeteners a bad name, appears to be safe during pregnancy and has been approved by the FDA for pregnant women to consume—so sweeten your day (and your coffee, tea, yogurt, and smoothies) with it if you want, or with foods and drinks pre-sweetened with it. It's also stable for cooking and baking (unlike aspartame), making that sugar-free chocolate cake less pipe dream, more possibility. Just make moderation your motto.

Aspartame (Equal, NutraSweet). Many experts believe it's harmless, and others think it's an unsafe artificial sweetener, whether you're pregnant or not. While the FDA has approved aspartame for pregnant women, they do recommend that moms-to-be limit consumption. A packet or two of the blue stuff now and then, a can of diet Coke every once in a while—no problem. Just avoid consuming aspartame during pregnancy in large

A Gut Check About Fermented Foods

Are you sweet on sauerkraut, crazy for kimchi, and nutty for natto? Old favorites in many cultures, fermented foods like these (and many others, including yogurt, kefir, tempeh, and miso, to name a few) are new again—and they're hitting the shelves with lots of health claims, too. For one, they're packed with friendly bacteria that help to ensure good gut health (and what pregnant woman couldn't use better gut health?).

But are all fermented foods your friend during pregnancy? Probably not. Some have high amounts of added sugars or sodium, some don't contain any healthy probiotic bacteria at all, and others can cause minor headaches, stomachaches, and bloating. Play it safe and ask your practitioner about the fermented foods you favor.

Kombucha have you curious? This fermented drink, made with tea, sugar, bacteria, and yeast, comes with many purported benefits (from improved digestion and liver function to a stimulated immune system), but none of these have actually been substantiated by science yet. If you crave kombucha, check with your practitioner before you chug, since it's unclear whether it's safe during pregnancy. It can also cause stomach upset in some new drinkers. Keep in mind, too, that unpasteurized kombucha (particularly home-brewed varieties) can be contaminated with harmful bacteria and that some kombuchas contain alcohol (clearly a no-go when you're expecting).

amounts, and steer clear of it altogether if you have PKU. Some diet sodas are sweetened with sucralose instead of aspartame, so they might be a better choice for expectant moms.

Saccharin (Sweet'N Low). The FDA has deemed saccharin safe, but some studies suggest that saccharin gets to your baby through the placenta, and when it does, it's slow to leave. For that reason, you might want to stay away from the pink packets—or pick them up only occasionally (say, when there's no yellow in sight).

Acesulfame-K (Sunett). This sweetener, 200 times sweeter than sugar, is approved for use in baked goods, gelatin desserts, chewing gum, and soft drinks. The FDA says it's okay to use in moderation during pregnancy, but since few studies have been done to prove its safety, ask your practitioner what he or she thinks before gobbling the stuff up.

Sorbitol. Sorbitol is actually a nutritive sweetener, which is fine during pregnancy. But while it can't hurt your baby, it can have unpleasant effects on your tummy: In large doses, it can cause bloating, gas pains, and diarrhea— a digestive trio no pregnant woman needs. Sorbitol is safe in moderate amounts, but keep in mind that it has more calories than other substitutes and less sweetness than regular sugar (so its calories can add up).

Mannitol. Less sweet than sugar, mannitol is poorly absorbed by the body and thus provides fewer calories than sugar (but more than other sugar substitutes). Like sorbitol, it is safe in modest amounts, but large quantities can cause gastrointestinal unrest (and pregnancy already comes with plenty of that).

Xylitol. A sugar alcohol derived from plants (it's naturally occurring in many fruits and veggies), xylitol can be found in chewing gum, toothpaste, candies, and some foods. Considered safe during pregnancy in moderate amounts, it has 40 percent fewer calories than sugar and has been shown to prevent tooth decay—a good reason to grab a stick of xylitol-sweetened gum after meals and snacks when you can't brush.

Stevia (Sweetleaf, Truvia). Derived from a South American shrub, stevia appears to be safe during pregnancy, but since it's relatively new to the sweetening scene, check with your practitioner before you dip deeply.

Agave. Because it's low in glucose, agave doesn't spike your blood sugar like regular sugar does. But it contains more fructose than any other common sweetener, including high-fructose corn syrup, and experts believe that fructose is converted into fat more rapidly than glucose—which means using agave as a sugar substitute won't help in the weight department (or in blood sugar regulation). Agave syrup is also highly processed. It's probably safe for use during pregnancy, but use it in moderation.

Lactose. This milk sugar is one-sixth as sweet as table sugar and adds light sweetening to foods. For those who are lactose intolerant, it can cause uncomfortable symptoms—otherwise it's safe.

Whey Low. Fructose (the sugar in fruit), sucrose (regular sugar), and lactose (milk sugar) are blended to create this low-glycemic sweetener that the makers say doesn't get completely absorbed into the body, giving you only one-quarter of the calories of sugar. It's probably safe for use during pregnancy, but run it by your practitioner.

Honey. Everyone's all abuzz about honey because of its high levels of antioxidants (darker varieties, such as buckwheat honey, are the richest in antioxidants). But it's not all sweet news. Though it's a good substitute for sugar, honey is definitely not low-cal. It's got 19 more calories per tablespoon than sugar does. How's that for sticky?

Fruit juice concentrates. Fruit juice concentrates, such as white grape and apple, are a safe (if not low-calorie) sweetener to turn to during pregnancy. You can substitute them for the sugar in many recipes, and they're readily available in frozen form at the supermarket. Look for them in commercial products, too, from jams and jellies to whole grain cookies, muffins, cereals, and granola bars, to pop-up toaster pastries, yogurt, and sparkling sodas. Unlike most products sweetened with sugar or other sugar substitutes, many fruit-juice-sweetened products are made with nutritious ingredients, such as whole grain flour and healthy fats.

Herbal Tea

"I drink a lot of herbal tea. Is it safe to drink it while I'm pregnant?"

Should you take (herbal) tea for two? Unfortunately, since the effect of herbs in pregnancy has not been well researched, there's no definitive answer to that question yet. Some herbal teas are probably safe in small amounts (chamomile, for instance), some probably not—and some, such as red raspberry leaf, taken in very large amounts (more than four 8-ounce cups a day), are thought to trigger contractions (good if you're 40 weeks and impatient, not good if you haven't reached term). Until more is known, the FDA has urged caution on the use of most herbal teas in pregnancy and when you're breastfeeding. And though many women have drunk lots of herbal teas throughout pregnancy without a problem, it is probably safest to stay away from, or at least limit, most herbal teas while you're expecting—unless they've been specifically recommended or cleared by your practitioner. Check with your practitioner for a list of which herbs he or she believes are safe and which are pregnancy no-no's.

To make sure you're not brewing up trouble (and an herb your practitioner hasn't cleared) with your next cup of tea, read labels carefully—some brews that seem from their names to be fruit based also contain a variety of herbs. Stick to regular (black) tea that comes flavored, or mix up your own by adding any of the following to boiling water or regular tea: orange, apple, pineapple, or other fruit juice; slices of lemon, lime, orange, apple, pear, or other fruit; mint leaves, cinnamon, nutmeg, cloves, or ginger (believed to be an effective calmer of the queasies). Chamomile is also considered safe in small amounts during pregnancy and can be soothing to a pregnancy-unsettled tummy. The jury's still out on green tea, which can decrease the effectiveness of folic acid, that vital pregnancy vitamin—so if you're a green tea drinker, drink in moderation. And never brew a homemade tea from a plant growing in your backyard, unless you are absolutely certain what it is and that it's safe for use during pregnancy.

Chemicals in Foods

"With pesticides on vegetables, PCBs and mercury in fish, antibiotics in meat, and nitrates in hot dogs, is there anything I can safely eat during pregnancy?"

Eating for two may sound twice as risky, but the truth is you don't have to go crazy (or hungry . . . or even broke) to protect your baby from the chemicals in (and on) food. That's because few chemicals have been proved absolutely harmful during pregnancy—especially in the context of a mostly healthy diet.

Still, it's smart to reduce risk whenever you can—particularly when you're reducing risk for two. And it's not that difficult to do, especially these days. To feed yourself and your baby as safely as you can, use the following as a guide to help you decide what to drop into your shopping cart and what to pass up:

■ Choose your foods from the Pregnancy Diet. Because it steers away from processed foods, this eating plan steers you clear of many questionable and unsafe substances. It also supplies green leafies and yellows, rich in protective beta-carotene, as well as other fruits and vegetables rich in phytochemicals, which may counteract the effects of toxins in food.

■ Whenever possible, cook from scratch with fresh ingredients or use frozen or packaged organic ready-to-eat foods. You'll avoid many questionable additives found in processed foods, and your meals will be more nutritious, too.

■ Go as natural as you can, when you can. Whenever you have a choice (and you won't always), choose foods that are free of artificial additives (colorings, flavorings, and preservatives). Read labels to screen for foods that are either additive-free or use natural additives (a cheddar cheese cracker that gets its orange hue from annatto instead of red dye #40, and its flavor from real cheese instead of artificial cheese flavoring). Keep in mind that although some artificial additives are considered safe, others are of questionable safety, and many are used to enhance foods that aren't very nutritious to start with. (For a listing of

What to Know About GMOs

How do those tomatoes and plums stay so pristine from farm to supermarket—especially when the drive is clear cross-country? In some cases it could be because growers are tapping into GMOs. Genetically engineered foods and plants (known in the food business as GMOs, for genetically modified organisms) have their DNA modified so that they acquire more desirable traits—like staying fresher longer or being able to thrive on a steady diet of weed killer and pesticides. These days anything from corn to papayas, plums to potatoes, rice to soybeans, and squash to tomatoes is allowed to be genetically engineered in the U.S. Problem is, the FDA doesn't require GMO foods to be labeled as such, which makes it hard to know whether the food you're buying is made with genetically modified ingredients or not.

Are GMOs unsafe during pregnancy? Safety of GMOs in general is a growing controversy, with organizations and industries on both sides of the argument firmly planted in their position. Not willing to take a chance with your baby-to-be's health while you wait out the debate? Look for foods that are labeled "USDA organic"—they'll be free of GMOs, as well as questionable additives or chemicals. Or check for certification by the Non-GMO Project. And stay tuned, because many states are passing legislation that requires labeling of GMO foods, which means it may soon be easier to shop for non-GMO foods.

questionable and safe additives, go to cspinet.org).

- Generally avoid foods preserved with nitrates and nitrites (or sodium nitrates), including many varieties of hot dogs, salami, bologna, and smoked fish and meats. Look for those brands (you'll find plenty on the market these days) that do not include these preservatives. Any ready-cooked meats or smoked fish should be heated to steaming before eating (not to avoid chemicals, but to avoid listeria; see page 118).

- Choose lean cuts of meat and remove visible fat before cooking, since chemicals that livestock ingest tend to concentrate in the fat of the animal. With poultry, remove both the fat and the skin to minimize chemical intake. And for the same reason, don't eat organ meats (such as liver and kidneys) very often, unless your meat or poultry is organic.

- When it's available and your budget permits, buy meat and poultry that has been raised organically (or grass-fed), without hormones or antibiotics (remember, you eat what your dinner ate). Choose organic dairy products and eggs, when possible, for the same reason. Free-range chickens (and eggs) are not only less likely to be contaminated with chemicals, but are also less likely to carry such infections as salmonella because the birds are not kept in cramped, disease-breeding quarters. And here's a plus when it comes to grass-fed beef: It's likely to be lower in calories and fat, higher in protein, and a better source of those baby-friendly omega-3 fatty acids.

- Buy organic produce when possible and practical. Produce that is certified

Pick and Choose Organic

Though prices on organic foods are going down as demand goes up (a good reason to demand it at your local market), it can be budget-busting to fill your shopping cart with organic-only produce and products. Here's the lowdown on when to spring for the organic and when it's safe to stick with conventional:

Best to buy organic (because even after washing, these foods still carry higher levels of pesticide residue than others): apples, cherries, grapes, peaches, nectarines, pears, raspberries, strawberries, bell peppers, celery, potatoes, and spinach.

No need to go organic on these foods (because these products generally don't contain pesticide residue on them): bananas, kiwi, mango, papaya, pineapples, avocado, asparagus, broccoli, cauliflower, corn, onions, and peas.

Consider organic for milk, beef, and poultry because they won't contain antibiotics or hormones, though they will cost more. Grass-fed beef usually is considered organic, but check labels. Don't bother with so-called organic fish. There are no USDA organic certification standards for seafood (which means producers are making their own claims about why it's organic). Instead, fish selectively using the guide on page 110.

organic usually is as close as possible to being free of all chemical residues. "Transitional" produce (from farms that aren't yet completely organic but are moving in that direction) may still contain some residues from soil contamination but should be safer than conventionally grown produce. If organic produce is available locally and you can afford the premium price, make it your choice—just keep in mind as you load up your shopping cart that organic produce will have a much shorter shelf life (same goes for organic poultry and meats). If price is an object, pick organic selectively (see box, this page).

Want to take your conscientious produce shopping to the next level? While not necessarily more nutritious, "biodynamic" produce (you'll notice the labels in some health food stores) is certified to be grown, processed, and brought to market in a way that is healthy for the planet. And that's a win-win-win—healthy for you, healthy for your baby, and healthy for the world your baby is about to be born into. The catch: the price, which can be hefty (consumer demand for both organic and biodynamic products will help bring those prices down).

- Give all vegetables and fruits a bath. Washing produce thoroughly is important no matter what (even organic produce can wear a coating of bacteria), but it's key to removing chemical pesticides your fruits and veggies may have picked up in the field. Water will wash off some, but a dip in or a spray with produce wash will take off much more (rinse thoroughly afterward). Scrub skins when possible and practical to remove surface chemical residues, especially when a vegetable has a waxy coating (as cucumbers and sometimes tomatoes, apples, peppers, and eggplant do). Peel skins that still seem "coated" after washing.

- Favor domestic produce. Imported (and foods made from such produce) sometimes contain higher levels of pesticides than U.S.-grown equivalents, because pesticide regulation in some countries is lax or nonexistent.

- Go local. Locally grown produce is likely to contain more nutrients (it's fresh from the field) and possibly sport less pesticide residue. Many of the growers at your local farmers market may grow without pesticides (or with very little), even if their products aren't marked "organic." That's because certification is too expensive for some small growers to afford.

- Vary your diet. Variety ensures not only a more interesting eating experience and better nutrition but also better chances of avoiding too much exposure to any one chemical if you're eating conventionally grown produce.

> ## Something's Cooking
>
> You can find recipes that put it all together in *What to Expect: Eating Well When You're Expecting.*

- Drive yourself to the health food market, but don't drive yourself nuts (or let a lack of access to organic drive you away from nutritious foods, like fruits and veggies). Though it's smart to try to avoid theoretical hazards in food, making your life stressful (or budget-busting) in the pursuit of a purely natural meal isn't necessary. Do the best you can manage and afford—and then sit back, eat well, and relax.

ALL ABOUT:
Eating Safely for Two

Worried about the pesticides your peach picked up in South America? That's sensible, especially because you're trying to eat safely for two. But what about the sponge you're about to use to wipe that peach down (the one that's been hanging around your sink for the last 3 weeks)? Have you thought about what that might have picked up lately? And the cutting board you were planning to slice your peach on—isn't that the same one you diced that raw chicken on last night when you were prepping the stir-fry? Here's a food-safety reality check: A more immediate—and proven—threat than the chemicals in your food are the little organisms, bacteria, and parasites that can contaminate it. It's not a pretty picture (or one that's visible without a microscope), but these nasty bugs can cause anything from mild stomach upset to severe illness. To make sure that the worst thing you'll pick up from your next meal is a little heartburn, shop, prepare, and eat with care:

- When in doubt, throw it out. Make this your mantra of safe eating. It applies to any food you even suspect might be spoiled. Always check freshness dates on food packages.

- When food shopping, avoid fish, meat, and eggs that are not well refrigerated or kept on ice. Toss jars that are leaky or don't "pop" when you open them and cans that are rusty or seem swollen or otherwise misshapen

The Lowdown on Listeria

So what's this you hear about eating your cold cuts warm now that you're pregnant? And skipping the feta on your Greek salad? These pregnancy diet restrictions may seem random—and unfair—but they're actually designed to protect you and your unborn baby from listeria. This bacteria can cause a serious illness (listeriosis) in high-risk individuals, including young children, the elderly, those with compromised immune systems, and pregnant women, whose immune systems are also somewhat suppressed. Though the overall risk of contracting listeriosis is extremely low—even in pregnancy—the potential of it causing problems in pregnancy is higher. Listeria, unlike many other germs, enters the bloodstream directly and therefore can get to the baby quickly through the placenta (other food contaminants generally stay in the digestive tract and may pose a threat only if they get into the amniotic fluid).

So, clearly, it's important to prevent infection in the first place by staying away from the risky foods that might possibly carry listeria. These include cold cuts (deli meats), hot dogs, cold smoked fish (unless heated until steaming), unpasteurized milk and cheeses made from unpasteurized milk (including some mozzarella, blue cheese, Mexican cheese, brie, camembert, and feta—unless cooked until bubbly), unpasteurized juice, raw or undercooked meat, fish, shellfish, poultry, or eggs, and unwashed raw vegetables and salad.

(beyond a dent). Wash can tops before opening (and wash your can opener frequently in hot soapy water or in the dishwasher).

■ Wash your hands before handling food and after touching raw meat, fish, or eggs. If you use gloves, remember that unless they're disposable, they need to be washed as often as your bare hands.

■ Keep kitchen counters and sinks clean. Same goes for cutting boards (wash with soap and hot water or in the dishwasher). Wash dishcloths frequently and keep sponges clean (replace them often, wash them in the dishwasher each night, or periodically pop dampened ones into the microwave for a couple of minutes), since they can harbor bacteria. Or look for sponges that can be machine washed in hot water.

■ Use separate cutting boards for produce, fish, and meat.

■ Serve hot foods hot, cold foods cold. Leftovers should be refrigerated quickly and heated until steaming before reusing. (Toss perishable foods that have been left out for more than 2 hours.) Don't eat frozen foods that have been thawed and then refrozen.

■ Keep an eye on the fridge interior temperature with a refrigerator thermometer and be sure it stays at 41°F or less. Keep your freezer at 0°F or below to maintain the quality of frozen foods.

■ Thaw foods in the fridge, time permitting. If you're in a rush, thaw food in a watertight plastic bag submerged in cold water (and change it every 30 minutes). Never thaw foods at room temperature. When thawing food in a microwave, select the defrost feature. If your microwave doesn't automatically rotate food, turn it yourself about halfway through the thawing process. Plan to cook the food immediately after thawing, because some areas of the food may become unsafely warm (allowing bacteria to grow and spread).

- Marinate meat, fish, or poultry in the refrigerator, not on the counter. Don't reuse the marinade.

- Don't eat raw or undercooked meats poultry, fish, or shellfish while you're expecting. Always cook meat and fish to medium (to 160°F) and poultry thoroughly (to 165°F). Fish should be cooked until it easily flakes with a fork, and poultry until the juices run clear (and the proper temperatures are reached).

- Eat eggs cooked through, not runny, and if you're mixing a batter that contains raw eggs, resist the urge to lick the spoon (or your fingers). The exception to this rule: if you're using pasteurized eggs.

- Wash raw fruits and vegetables thoroughly (especially if they won't be cooked before eating or juicing). Even the freshest organic produce can wear a coating of bacteria.

- Avoid alfalfa and other sprouts, which can be contaminated with bacteria.

For the latest information on food safety, visit cdc.gov/foodsafety.

PART 2

Nine Months & Counting

From Conception to Delivery

CHAPTER 5

The First Month

Approximately 1 to 4 Weeks

Congratulations, and welcome to your pregnancy! Though you almost certainly don't look pregnant this early on, you may already be starting to feel it. Maybe it's just tender breasts or a little fatigue you're experiencing, maybe it's every pregnancy symptom in the book. But even if there's not a single pregnancy sign in sight yet (at least as far as you've noticed), your body is gearing up for the months of baby making to come. As the weeks and months pass, you'll notice more and more changes in parts of your body you'd expect (like your belly), as well as places you wouldn't expect (your feet and your eyes). You'll also notice changes in the way you live—and look at—your life. The information you'll find in this chapter may apply to you already, or may be just around the bend (or may never apply at all, since every woman and every pregnancy is different). Just try not to think (or read) too far ahead. For now, sit back, relax, and enjoy the beginning of one of the most amazing adventures of your life.

Your Baby This Month

Week 1 The countdown to baby begins this week. Only thing is, there's no baby in sight—or inside. So why call this week 1 of pregnancy if you're not even pregnant? Here's why. It's extremely hard to pinpoint the precise moment when sperm meets egg (sperm from your partner can hang out in your body for several days before your egg comes out to greet it, and your egg can wait for up to 24 hours for sperm to make their appearance).

What isn't hard to pinpoint, however, is the first day of your last menstrual period (LMP—so mark the calendar), allowing your practitioner to use that as the standard starting line for your 40-week pregnancy. The upshot of this dating system (besides a lot of potential for confusion)? You get to clock in 2 weeks of your 40 weeks of pregnancy before you even get pregnant.

Week 2 Nope, still no baby yet. But your body isn't taking a break this week. In fact, it's working hard gearing up for the big O—ovulation. The lining of your uterus is thickening (feathering its nest for the arrival of the fertilized egg), and your ovarian follicles are maturing—some faster than others—until one becomes dominant, destined for ovulation. And waiting in that dominant follicle is an eager egg with your baby's name on it (or, if you're about to conceive fraternal twins, 2 eager eggs will be waiting in 2 follicles)—ready to burst out and begin its journey from single cell to bouncing boy or girl. But first it will have to make a journey down your fallopian tube in search of Mr. Right—the lucky sperm that will seal the deal.

Week 3 Congratulations—you've conceived! Which means your baby-to-be has started its miraculous transformation from single cell to fully formed baby boy or girl. Within hours after sperm meets egg, the fertilized cell (aka zygote) divides, and then continues to divide (and divide). Within days, your baby-to-be has turned into a microscopic ball of cells, around one-fifth the size of the period at the end of this sentence. The blastocyst—as it is now known (though you'll almost certainly come up with a cuter name soon)—begins its journey from your fallopian tube to your waiting uterus. Only 8½ more months—give or take—to go!

Week 4 It's implantation time! That ball of cells that you'll soon call baby—though it's now called embryo—has

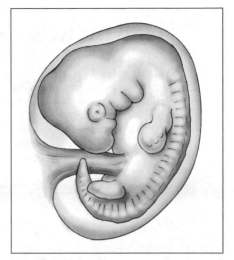

Your Baby, Month 1

reached your uterus and is snuggling into the uterine lining, where it'll stay connected to you until delivery. Once firmly in place, the ball of cells undergoes the great divide—splitting into 2 groups. Half will become your son or daughter, while the other half will become the placenta, your baby's lifeline during his or her uterine stay. And even though it's just a ball of cells right now (no bigger than a poppy seed, actually), don't underestimate your little embryo—he or she has already come a long way since those blastocyst days. The amniotic sac—otherwise known as the bag of waters—is forming, as is the yolk sac, which will later be incorporated into your baby's developing digestive tract. Each layer of the embryo—it has 3 now—is beginning to grow into specialized parts of the body. The inner layer, known as the endoderm, will develop into your baby's digestive system, liver, and lungs. The middle layer, called the mesoderm, will soon be your baby's heart, sex organs, bones, kidneys, and muscles. The outer layer, or ectoderm, will eventually form your baby's nervous system, hair, skin, and eyes.

What Week Am I In, Anyway?

Though this book is organized month-by-month, corresponding weeks are also provided. Weeks 1 to 13 (approximately) make up the first trimester and are months 1 to 3; weeks 14 to 27 (approximately) are the second trimester and are months 4 to 6; and weeks 28 to 40 (approximately) are the third trimester and are months 7 to 9. Just remember, you're counting from the beginning of a week or month. So, for example, you start your 3rd month when you've finished 2 months. You begin your 24th week when you complete your 23rd.

Your Body This Month

While it's true that pregnancy has its share of wonderful moments and experiences to cherish, it also has a boatload (make that a bloatload) of less than fabulous symptoms. Some you're probably expecting to have (like that queasy feeling that might already be settling in). Others you'd probably never expect (like drooling—who knew?). Many you'll probably not discuss in public (and will try your best not to do in public, like passing gas), and many you'll probably try to forget (which you might, by the way, since forgetfulness is another pregnancy symptom).

Here are a couple of things to keep in mind about these and other pregnancy symptoms. First, every woman and every pregnancy is different, which means different women experience different pregnancy symptoms. Second, the symptoms that follow are a good sampling of what you might expect to experience (though, thankfully, you probably won't experience them all—at least not all at once), but there are plenty more where these came from. Chances are just about every weird and wacky sensation you feel during the next 9 months (both the physical ones and the emotional ones) will be normal for pregnancy. But if a symptom ever leaves you with a nagging doubt (can this really be normal?), always check it out with your practitioner, just to be sure.

Though you most likely won't have confirmation that you're expecting until you're nearing the end of the month, you might begin noticing that

Symptoms? Starting Soon

Most early pregnancy symptoms begin making their appearance around week 6, but every woman—and every pregnancy—is different, so many may begin earlier or later for you (or not at all, if you're lucky). If you're experiencing something that's not on this list or in this chapter, look ahead to the next chapters or check out the index.

something's up—even this early on. Or, you might not. Here's what you might experience this month:

Physically

- Possible staining or spotting when the fertilized egg implants in your uterus, around 6 to 12 days after conception (see page 142)

- Breast changes, such as fullness, heaviness, tenderness, tingling, darkening of the areolas

- Bloating, gas

- Fatigue, lack of energy, sleepiness

- More frequent urination than usual

- Beginnings of nausea, with or without vomiting (though this doesn't typically kick in until week 6 or even later)

- Excess saliva

- Increased sensitivity to smells

Emotionally

- Emotional ups and downs (like amped-up PMS), which may include mood swings, irritability, irrationality, inexplicable weepiness

- Anxiety/anticipation while waiting for the right time to take a home pregnancy test

Your Body This Month

There's definitely no way to tell this book by its cover yet. Though you may recognize a few physical changes in yourself—your breasts may be a little fuller, your tummy a tad rounder (though that's from bloat, not baby)—no one else is likely to have noticed. Make sure you take a good look at your waist: It may be the last time you'll see it for many months to come.

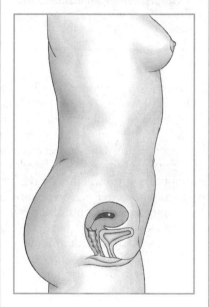

What You Can Expect at Your First Prenatal Visit

Your first prenatal visit probably will be the longest you'll have during your pregnancy—and definitely will be the most comprehensive. Not only will there be more tests, procedures (including several that will be performed only at this visit), and information gathering (in the form of a complete medical history), but there will be more time spent on questions (questions you

Make the Pregnancy Connection

Log on to WhatToExpect.com or the What To Expect app—your interactive pregnancy companion—for week-by-week info on your baby's growth and development, plus a whole lot more. Connect on the message boards with other moms who are going through the same experience (and the same queasiness) at the same time. After all, nobody gets pregnancy like another pregnant woman!

have for your practitioner, questions he or she will have for you) and answers. There will also be plenty of advice to take in—on everything from what you should be eating (and not eating) to what supplements you should be taking (and not taking) to whether (and how) you should be exercising. So be sure to come equipped with a list of the questions and concerns that have already come up, as well as with a notebook, the *What to Expect Pregnancy Journal and Organizer,* your smartphone, or the What To Expect app to jot down those answers.

Keep in mind that your first official prenatal visit will probably be scheduled sometime in your 2nd month (see page 8), not the 1st month—though some offices offer earlier pre-ob visits.

One practitioner's routine may vary slightly from another's. In general, the exam will include:

Confirmation of your pregnancy. Even if you've already passed your pregnancy test at home, your practitioner will most likely repeat a urine test and also do a blood test. The following will also be checked: pregnancy symptoms you're experiencing, the date of your LMP to determine your estimated date of delivery (EDD, aka due date; see page 8), and your cervix and uterus for signs and approximate gestational age of the pregnancy. Most practitioners also do an early ultrasound, which is the most accurate way of dating a pregnancy (see page 170).

A complete history. To give you the best care possible, your practitioner will want to know a lot about you. Come prepared by checking records at home or calling your primary care doctor to refresh your memory on the following: your personal medical history (immunizations you've had, chronic illness, previous major illnesses or surgeries, known allergies, including drug allergies), supplements (vitamins, minerals, herbal, homeopathic) or medications (over-the-counter or prescription) you take or have taken since conception, your mental health history (any history of depression, anxiety disorder, or other mental health conditions), your gynecological history (age at first period, details about your cycle, whether you have problems with PMS or PMDD, prior gynecological surgeries, history of abnormal Pap smears or of STDs), and your obstetrical history if any (including any pregnancy complications or losses, details about previous deliveries). Your practitioner will also ask questions about your lifestyle habits (what you typically eat, whether you exercise, drink, smoke, or use recreational drugs) and other factors that might affect your pregnancy (information about the baby's father, information on your ethnicities).

A complete physical exam. This may include a general health exam (checking your heart, lungs, breasts, abdomen), measurement of your blood pressure to serve as a baseline reading at future visits, notation of your height and your weight, a look at your arms and legs for varicose veins and swelling to serve as a baseline at future visits, an exam of your external genitals and an internal check of your vagina and cervix (with a speculum in place, as when you get a Pap smear), examination of your pelvic organs bimanually (with one hand in the vagina and one on the abdomen and also possibly through the rectum and vagina), and an assessment of the size of your uterus and the size and shape of the pelvis (through which your baby will eventually try to exit).

A battery of tests. Some tests are routine for every pregnant woman, some are routine in some areas of the country (or in some practices), and some are performed only when necessary. The most common prenatal tests given at the first visit include:

■ Urine test to screen for glucose (sugar), protein, white blood cells, blood, and bacteria

■ Blood test to determine blood type and Rh status (see page 35), to check for anemia, and to measure hCG levels. Your blood will also be screened for antibody titers (levels) and immunity to certain diseases (like rubella and chicken pox), and possibly for vitamin D deficiency.

■ Tests to screen for syphilis, gonorrhea, hepatitis B, chlamydia, and HIV

■ A Pap smear (just like the one you get at your annuals) to screen for abnormal cervical cells

What's a Rubella Titer?

One lab result your practitioner will look for in your first blood test is a rubella titer, a measurement of the level of antibodies you have for rubella, aka German measles. Low titers means you're due for a booster vaccine (or to be vaccinated if you've never been), but you won't roll up your sleeve for that until after you deliver. Happily, the CDC considers rubella to be eradicated in the U.S., which means that it's next to impossible to catch it here now—even if your titers are low. See page 535 for more.

Depending on your particular situation, and if appropriate, you may also receive:

■ Genetic tests for cystic fibrosis (all moms-to-be are offered this test), sickle cell anemia, thalassemia, Tay-Sachs, or other genetic diseases if you weren't screened before conception (see page 48 for more on genetic screening)

■ Possibly, a blood sugar test if you're obese, had gestational diabetes (and/or a very large baby) in a previous pregnancy, have a family history of diabetes, or have other risk factors for gestational diabetes (see page 294 for more on screening for gestational diabetes).

An opportunity for discussion. Here's the time to bring out that list of questions and concerns.

What You May Be Wondering About

Breaking the News

"I just found out I'm pregnant, and I can't wait to break the news to everyone. But is it too early to tell my family and friends?"

Bursting with the news—almost as much as your bladder is bursting with urinary frequency? It's not surprising that you're eager to alert the social media (and your family and other friends), especially if this is your first pregnancy. But how long should you wait to share? When should you let this still very tiny kitten out of the bag?

That's actually your call (or text, or email, or post). Some couples opt to hold off on any announcements until the first trimester has passed, and some keep the secret as long as they can—say, until the baby bump (or the sudden passing up of wine, or the ever-green look on her face)—starts making it obvious. Others have rushed off to tell the world (or at least, everyone on their contact list) before the pee has even dried on the pregnancy test. Still others tell selectively, starting with those nearest and dearest (or those who can be trusted not to blab until you've given the go-ahead). Since there's no right or wrong time to tell or way to tell, do whatever works for you. Tell now, tell later, tell some, tell all. Keep them in the loop, or keep them guessing.

Just remember, once you share your happy news (or it becomes oh-so-obvious), people you know (and, yes, even those you don't) will be more than happy to share unsolicited advice, comments about your weight, nightmare labor stories, and finger-wagging critiques of your morning latte—not to mention those belly rubs you didn't ask for. A reason to hold off? You decide.

So talk it over with your partner, and do what feels most comfortable. Just remember: In spreading the good news, don't forget to take the time to savor it as a twosome.

For tips on when to break the news at work, see page 199.

Prenatal Supplements

"I hate swallowing pills. Do I really have to take a prenatal, even though I eat pretty well?"

Virtually no one gets a nutritionally perfect diet every day—especially early in pregnancy, when round-the-clock morning sickness is a common appetite suppressant, or when the little nutrition you do manage to get down often doesn't stay down, or when aversions kill your taste for anything remotely healthy. Though a daily prenatal supplement can't take the place of a good prenatal diet, it can serve as some dietary insurance, guaranteeing that your baby won't be cheated if you don't always hit the nutritional mark you're aiming for—especially during the early months, when so much of your baby's most crucial construction occurs.

And there are other good reasons to take your prenatals. For one thing, studies show that taking a supplement containing folic acid and vitamin B_{12} during the first months of pregnancy (especially if it's started in the months before pregnancy) significantly reduces the risk of neural tube defects (such as spina bifida), congenital heart defects, and autism in a baby, and helps prevent preterm birth. For another, research

The Downside (and Flip Side) to Telling Early

Even as they celebrate a positive pregnancy test—and think about sharing the happy news with friends, family, and maybe the world—just about every couple worries about the "what-if." What if the happy news turns to sad news—what if pregnancy ends soon after it has started, with a miscarriage? More than any other reason, that's why many couples hold off on announcing pregnancy until the first trimester is safely behind them.

And that's understandable—especially if you've had previous pregnancy losses. But here's the flip side to keeping pregnancy completely to yourselves early on. Should the unthinkable—and unlikely—actually happen, whether that's a miscarriage or a devastating result on prenatal testing, will going it alone make the sad news harder to handle? Will you be relieved you haven't told anyone—after all, then there's no need to tell them what happened—or will you be craving support from friends and family when you need it the most?

Something to think about—but something only you and your partner can decide, together.

has shown that taking a supplement containing at least 10 mg of vitamin B_6 before and during early pregnancy can minimize morning sickness. And yet another: Many women are deficient in vitamin D (you can ask your practitioner about testing for D deficiency)—and taking a prenatal can help bump up your D levels to where they should be.

Which prenatal should you take? Since there are an overwhelming number of formulations on the market (available both over-the-counter and by prescription), it's always a good idea to ask your practitioner to recommend or prescribe one. If size matters to you (say, you find that the typical horse-size prenatal supplement is hard to gag down) ask for one that's smaller, coated, or a gel cap. Or look into ditching the pill entirely—formulas come in powder, gummy, or chewable form, too (just ask first, since not all prenatals are equivalent). A slow-release formula may prove less upsetting to your pregnancy-sensitive tummy, especially if you've been hit hard by morning sickness, and added B_6 and/or ginger may help ease quease,

too. Taking the supplement with food or at the time of the day when you're least likely to upchuck it (maybe after dinner, before bed) may also help you get it (and keep it) down.

If you decide to switch prenatals from one that your practitioner recommended or prescribed to one that's easier for you to take, run the formula by your practitioner first. Any prenatal you choose should approximate the requirements for prenatal supplements (see page 100 for details).

Some moms-to-be find the iron in a prenatal vitamin causes constipation or diarrhea. Again, switching formulas may bring relief. Taking a prenatal without iron and adding an iron supplement as prescribed (you probably won't require extra iron until midway through pregnancy) may also help. Your practitioner can suggest an iron supplement that's easier on the tummy.

"I eat a lot of cereals and breads that are enriched. If I'm also taking a prenatal supplement, will I be taking in too many vitamins and minerals?"

You can get too much of a good thing, but not usually this way. Taking a prenatal vitamin along with eating the average diet, which typically includes plenty of enriched and fortified products, isn't likely to lead to excessive intake of vitamins and minerals. To take in that many nutrients, you'd have to be adding other supplements beyond the prenatal—something an expectant mama should never do without her practitioner's advice. It's wise, however, to be wary of any foods, drinks, or other dietary supplements that are fortified with more than the recommended daily allowance of vitamins A, E, and K, because these can be toxic in large amounts. Most other vitamins and minerals are water soluble, meaning any excesses that the body can't use are simply excreted in the urine. Which is why—fun fact—supplement-crazy Americans are said to have the most expensive urine in the world (if pee could be sold, that is).

Fatigue

"Now that I'm pregnant, I'm tired all the time. Sometimes I feel as if I won't even be able to get through the day."

Can't lift your head off the pillow each morning? Dragging your feet all day? Can't wait to crawl into bed as soon as you arrive home at night? If it seems like your get-up-and-go has left the building—and doesn't seem to have plans to return anytime soon—it's not surprising. After all, you're pregnant. And even though there might not be any evidence on the outside that you're busily building a baby, plenty of exhausting work is going on inside. In some ways, your pregnant body is working harder when you're resting (even when you're sleeping!) than a nonpregnant body is when running a marathon—only you're not aware of the exertion.

So what exactly is your body up to? For one very significant thing, it's manufacturing your baby's life-support system, the placenta—a massive project that won't be completed until the end of the first trimester. For another, your body's hormone levels have increased significantly, you're producing more blood, your heart rate is up, your blood sugar is down, your metabolism is burning energy overtime (even when you're lying down), and you're using up more nutrients and water. And if that's not enough to wear you out, just toss into the draining equation all the other physical and emotional demands of pregnancy that your body is adjusting to. Add it all up, and it's no wonder you feel as if you're competing in a triathlon each day—and coming in dead last (or at least, dead tired).

Happily, there is some relief headed your way—eventually. Once the herculean task of manufacturing the placenta is complete (around the 4th month) and your body has adjusted to the hormonal and emotional changes pregnancy brings, you'll feel a little peppier.

In the meantime, keep in mind that fatigue is a sensible signal from your body that you need to take it easier these days. So listen up, and get the rest your body needs. You may also be able to recapture some of that get-up-and-go with some of the following tips:

Baby yourself. If you're a first-time mom-to-be, enjoy what will probably be your last chance for a long while to focus on taking care of yourself without feeling guilty. If you already have children at home, you'll definitely have to divide your focus. But either way, this is not a time to strive for super-mom-to-be status. Getting enough rest is more important than keeping your house spotless or cooking 4-star dinners (or cooking dinner at all—that's what takeout was created for). Let the dishes wait until later, and turn the other way as the dust bunnies breed under your dining table. Order your groceries (and anything else you can think of) online instead of dragging yourself to the store. If it's affordable for you, become a regular on the GrubHub or Seamless (or other food delivery services) circuit, and tap into TaskRabbit (or others like it) to outsource errands. Don't book activities—or take care of chores—that aren't must-do's. Never been a slacker? There's never been a better time to try it on for size.

Let others baby you. You'll be doing plenty of heavy lifting in the months to come, so your partner will need to be doing his fair share (how does more than half sound?) of household chores, including laundry and grocery shopping. Accept your mother-in-law's offer to cook dinner when she's visiting. Have a pal pick up some essentials for you while she's going on a shopping run anyway. That way, you might actually have enough energy left to drag yourself out for a walk . . . before you drag yourself into bed.

Chill out more. Exhausted once the day's over? Spend evenings chilling out (preferably with your feet up) instead of stepping out. And don't wait until nightfall to take it easy. If you can squeeze in a nap, by all means go for it. If you can't sleep, lie down and rest. If you're a working mom-to-be, a nap at the office may not be an option, of course, unless you have a flexible schedule and access to a comfortable sofa, but putting your feet up at your desk or on the sofa in the break room during downtimes and lunch hours may be possible. (If you choose to rest at lunch hour, make sure you make time to eat, too.)

Be a slacker mom. Have other kids? You may be extra tired, for obvious reasons (you have less time to rest, more demands on your body). Or fatigue may be less noticeable, since you're already accustomed to exhaustion—or too busy to pay attention to it. Either way, it's not easy babying yourself when you have other babies (and older children) clamoring for your attention. But try. Explain to them that growing a baby is hard work and it's leaving you beat. Ask for their help around the house and their help in letting you get more rest. Spend more time at quiet pursuits with your kids—reading, doing puzzles, being the patient in a game of "doctor" (you'll get to lie down), watching movies. Napping when you're mothering full-time may also be difficult, but if you can time your rest with naptime (if they still nap), you may be able to swing it.

Push up your bedtime. It may be stating the obvious, but just in case: Getting even an hour more sleep at night can pick you up come morning. Just don't overdo the dozing—too many z's can actually leave you feeling even more tired.

Eat well. To keep your energy up, you need a steady supply of premium fuel. Make sure you're getting enough calories each day and focus on the long-lasting energy boosting combo of protein and complex carbs. Caffeine or sugar (or both, taken together) may seem like the perfect quick fix for an energy slump, but they're not. Though a candy bar or a jolt-in-a-can energy drink might pick you up briefly, that blood sugar high will be followed by a free-falling crash, leaving you dragging more than ever. (Plus, many canned energy drinks may contain dietary supplements that aren't safe for pregnancy use.)

Eat often. Like so many other pregnancy symptoms, fatigue responds well to the 6-Meal Solution (see page 89). Keeping your blood sugar on an even keel will help keep your energy steady, too—so resist meal skipping, and opt for frequent mini-meals and snacks.

Take a hike. Or a slow jog. Or a stroll to the grocery store. Or do a pregnancy exercise or yoga routine. Sure, the couch has never looked more inviting—but paradoxically, too much rest and not enough activity can be a drag on your energy reserves. Even a little exercise (a 10-minute walk, or even 5 minutes of *What to Expect When You're Expecting: The Workout* DVD) can be more rejuvenating than a sofa break. Just don't overdo it—you want to finish up your workout feeling energized, not drained—and be sure to follow the guidelines starting on page 231.

Though your growing fatigue will probably ease up by month 4, you can expect it to return in the last trimester. (Could it be nature's way of preparing you for the long sleepless nights you'll encounter once baby has arrived?)

Morning Sickness

"I haven't had any morning sickness. Can I still be pregnant?"

Morning sickness, like a craving for pickles and ice cream, is one of those truisms about pregnancy that isn't necessarily true. Studies show that nearly three-quarters of all expectant women experience the nausea and/or vomiting associated with morning sickness, which means that a little more than 25 percent of moms-to-be don't. If you're among those who never have a nauseous moment, or who feel only occasionally or mildly queasy, you can consider yourself not only pregnant but also lucky. Consider, too, that this luck may soon run out, since morning sickness often doesn't kick in until 6 weeks or even later.

"My morning sickness lasts all day. I'm afraid that I'm not keeping down enough food to nourish my baby."

Welcome to the queasy club—a club that up to 75 percent of pregnant women belong to. Happily, though you and all the other miserable members are definitely feeling the effects of morning sickness—a misnamed malady, as you've already noticed, since it can strike at morning, noon, night, or, more likely, all the above—your baby almost definitely isn't. That's because your baby's nutritional needs are tiny right now, just like your baby (who's not even the size of a pea yet). Even women who have such a hard time keeping food down that they actually lose weight during the first trimester aren't hurting their babies or their pregnancies as long as they make up for the lost weight, as needed, in later months. Which is usually pretty easy to do, because that trademark nausea and vomiting don't generally linger much beyond the 12th to 14th week.

What causes morning sickness (technically known as the nausea and vomiting of pregnancy, or NVP)? No one knows for sure, but there's no shortage of theories, among them the high level of the pregnancy hormone hCG in the blood in the first trimester, elevated estrogen levels, gastroesophageal reflux (GER), the hormonally relaxed muscle tissue in the digestive tract (which makes digestion less efficient), and the super keen sense of smell that moms-to-be develop.

Not all pregnant women experience morning sickness the same way. Some have only occasional queasy moments, others feel queasy round the clock but never vomit (though they probably sometimes wish they could), others vomit once in a while, and still others vomit frequently. There are probably several reasons for these variations on the morning sickness (or 24/7 sickness) theme:

Hormone levels. Higher-than-average levels (as when a woman is carrying multiple fetuses) can increase morning sickness, while levels on the lower side of normal may minimize or eliminate it (though women with normal hormone levels may also experience little or no morning sickness).

Sensitivity. Some brains have a nausea command post that's more sensitive than others, which means they're more likely to respond to hormones and other triggers of pregnancy queasiness. If you have a sensitive command center (you always get carsick or seasick, for instance), you're more likely to have more severe nausea and vomiting in pregnancy. Never have a queasy day ordinarily? You're less likely to have lots of them when you're expecting.

Stress. It's well known that emotional stress can trigger tummy troubles, so it's not surprising that symptoms of morning sickness tend to get way worse when stress strikes. That's not to say that morning sickness is "in your head" (it's actually in your hormones)—but where your head is at (as in super-stressed-out) can intensify it.

Fatigue. Physical or mental fatigue can also aggravate the symptoms of morning sickness (conversely, severe morning sickness can definitely aggravate physical or mental fatigue).

First-timer status. Morning sickness is more common and tends to be more severe in first pregnancies, which supports the idea that both physical and emotional factors may be involved. Physically, the novice pregnant body is less prepared for the onslaught of hormones and other changes it's experiencing than one that's been there, done that. Emotionally, first-timers are more likely to be subject to the kinds of anxieties and fears that can turn a stomach—while women in subsequent pregnancies may be distracted from their nausea by the demands of caring for older children. (Generalities never hold true for every expectant mom, though, and some women are queasier in subsequent pregnancies than they were in their first.)

One thing that's likely not a contributing factor to whether or not you'll have the pregnancy queasies: the sex of your baby. Sure, some moms swear that morning sickness is worse when they're expecting a girl than when they're carrying a boy. But there are just as many moms who swear the opposite and say they never had a queasy day when they were pregnant with their girls. There is some evidence that moms-to-be who have severe vomiting during pregnancy may be a bit more likely to have a baby girl on board, but experts say these findings don't apply to average morning sickness.

No matter the cause (and does it really matter, when you're upchucking for the third time in one day?), there is no sure cure for the queasies but the passing of time. Luckily there are ways to minimize the misery while you're waiting for a less nauseous day to dawn:

- Eat early. Morning sickness doesn't wait for you to get up in the morning. In fact, nausea's most likely to strike when you're running on empty, as you are after a long night's sleep. That's because when you haven't eaten in a while, the acids churning around inside your empty tummy have nothing to digest but your

Helping Ease Her Quease

Morning sickness is one pregnancy symptom that definitely doesn't live up to its name. It's a 24/7 experience that can send your spouse running to the bathroom morning, noon, and night—and hugging the toilet far more than she'll be hugging you. So take steps to help her feel better—or at least not worse. Lose the aftershave that she suddenly finds repulsive, and get your onion ring fix out of her sniffing range (thanks to her hormones, her sense of smell is supersized). Fill her gas tank so she doesn't have to come nose-to-nozzle with the fumes at the pump. Fetch her foods that quell her queasies and don't provoke another run to the toilet. Good choices include ginger ale, soothing smoothies, and crackers (but ask first—what spells r-e-l-i-e-f for one queasy woman spells v-o-m-i-t for another). Encourage her to eat small meals throughout the day instead of 3 large ones (spreading out the load and keeping her tummy filled may ease her nausea), but don't chide her for her food choices (now's not the time to nag her about eating her broccoli). Be there for support when she's throwing up— hold back her hair, bring her some ice water, rub her back. And remember, no jokes. If you were throwing up for weeks, you wouldn't find it amusing. Not surprisingly, neither does she.

stomach lining—which, not surprisingly, increases queasiness. To head off heaving, don't even consider getting out of bed in the morning without reaching for a nibble (crackers or rice cakes, dry cereal, a handful of trail mix) that you stashed on your nightstand the night before. Keeping nibbles next to the bed also means you don't have to get up for them if you wake up hungry in the middle of the night. It's a good idea to have a bite when you rise for those midnight bathroom runs, too, just so your stomach stays a little bit full all night long.

- Eat late. Eating a light snack high in protein and complex carbs (a muffin and a glass of milk, string cheese and a handful of freeze-dried mango) just before you go to sleep will help ensure a happier tummy when you wake up.

- Eat light. A stuffed tummy is just as prone to puking as an empty one.

Overloading—even when you feel hungry—can lead to upchucking.

- Eat often. One of the best ways to keep nausea at bay is to keep your blood sugar on an even keel—and your stomach a little filled—all the time. To head off an attack of the queasies, join the graze craze. Eat small, frequent meals—6 mini-meals a day is ideal— instead of 3 large ones. Don't leave home without a stash of snacks that your tummy can handle (dried fruit and nuts, freeze-dried fruit, granola bars, dry cereal, crackers, pretzels, Moon Cheese).

- Eat well. A diet high in protein and complex carbohydrates can help combat queasiness. General good nutrition may help, too, so eat as well as you can (given the circumstances, that might not always be so easy).

- Eat what you can. So the eating well thing isn't working out so well for you?

Right now, getting anything in your tummy—and keeping it there—should be your priority. There will be plenty of time later on in your pregnancy for eating well. For the queasy moment, eat whatever gets you through the day (and night), even if it's nothing but ice pops and gingersnaps. If you can manage to make them real fruit ice pops and whole grain gingersnaps, great. If you can't, that's fine, too.

- Drink up. In the short term, getting enough fluids is more important than getting enough solids—particularly if you're losing lots of liquids through vomiting. If you're finding that liquids are easier to get down when you're feeling green, use them to get your nutrients. Drink your vitamins and minerals in soothing smoothies, soups, and juices. If you find fluids make you queasier, eat solids with a high water content, such as fresh fruits and vegetables—particularly melons (watermelon's a winner) and citrus fruits. Some queasy moms-to-be find that drinking and eating at the same meal puts too much strain on their digestive tract—if this is true for you, try taking your fluids between meals. Both electrolyte water and coconut water may be especially helpful if you're vomiting a lot.

- Get chilly. Experiment with temperature, too. Many women find that icy-cold fluids and foods (frozen grapes, for instance) are easier to get down. Others favor warm ones (melted cheese sandwiches instead of cold ones).

- Switch off. Often, what starts out as a comfort food (it's the only thing you can keep down, so you eat it 24/7) becomes associated with nausea—and actually starts to trigger it. If you're so sick of crackers that they're actually beginning to make you sick, switch off to another comforting carb (maybe it'll be Cheerios next).

- If it makes you queasy, don't go there. Period. Don't force yourself to eat any foods that don't appeal or, worse, make you sick. Instead, let your taste buds (and cravings, and aversions) be your guide. Choose only sweet foods if they're all you can tolerate (get your vitamin A and protein from peaches and yogurt at dinner instead of from broccoli and chicken). Or select only savories if they're your ticket to a less tumultuous tummy (have pizza for breakfast instead of cereal).

- Smell (and see) no evil. Thanks to a much more sensitive sense of smell, pregnant women often find once-appetizing aromas suddenly offensive—and offensive ones downright sickening. So stay away from smells that trigger nausea—whether it's the sausage and eggs your partner likes to make on the weekends or his after-shave that used to make you head over heels (but now makes you head for the toilet). Steer clear, too, of foods that you can't stand the sight of (raw chicken is a common culprit).

- Supplement. Take a prenatal supplement to compensate for nutrients you may not be getting. Afraid you'll have trouble choking the pill down—or keeping it down? Actually, that one-a-day can decrease nausea symptoms (especially if you take a slow-releasing vitamin that's higher in quease-combating vitamin B_6). But take it at a time of day when you are least likely to heave it back up, possibly with a substantial bedtime snack. You can also ask your practitioner about taking extra vitamin B_6 (with or without Unisom SleepTabs, or another OTC version of the antihistamine doxylamine), and/or supplementing with

Your Nose Knows

Have you noticed, now that you're expecting, that you can smell what's on the menu before you even set foot in the restaurant? That heightened sense of smell you're experiencing is actually a very real side effect of pregnancy, caused by hormones (in this case, estrogen) that magnify every little scent that wafts your way. What's worse, this bloodhound syndrome can also ramp up morning sickness symptoms. Smell trouble? Give your nose a break. Here are some strategies to try:

- If you can't stand the smell, get out of the kitchen. Or the restaurant. Or the perfume aisle at Sephora. Or anywhere odors that sicken you hang out.

- Make friends with your microwave. Microwave cooking generally makes less of a stink.

- Too late—there's already a stink? Open your windows whenever possible to banish cooking or musty odors. Or run the exhaust fan on the stove.

- Wash your clothes more often than usual, since fibers tend to hold on to odors. Use unscented detergent and softener, though, if the scented ones bother you (same goes for all your cleaning supplies).

- Switch to unscented or lightly scented toiletries (or scents that don't make you sick).

- Ask those who are regularly within sniffing distance of you (and who you know well enough to ask) to be extra-considerate of your sensitive smell status. Get your spouse to wash up, change his clothes, and brush his teeth after stopping for a chili cheeseburger. Suggest that pals go easy on the perfume when they're with you.

- Try to surround yourself with those scents (if there are any) that actually make you feel better. Mint, lemon, ginger, and cinnamon are more likely to be soothing, especially if you're queasy, though some expectant moms suddenly embrace smells that invoke infants, such as baby powder.

---

magnesium (or using a magnesium spray), which some say can help ease pregnancy nausea.

- Tread gingerly. It's true what the old wives (and midwives) have been saying for centuries: Ginger can be good for what ails a queasy pregnant woman. Use ginger in cooking (carrot-ginger soup, ginger muffins), steep it in tea, nibble on some ginger biscuits, nosh on some crystallized ginger, or suck on some ginger candy or lollipops. A drink made from real ginger (regular ginger ale isn't always, so check the label) may also

be soothing. Even the smell of fresh ginger (cut open a knob and take a whiff) may quell the queasies. Or try another trick of the queasy trade: lemons. Many women find both the smell and taste of oranges or lemons comforting (when life gives you morning sickness, make lemonade?). Sour or peppermint flavored sucking candies spell relief for others. Or try sipping on icy-cold almond milk, also touted for its tummy-settling benefits (it works on heartburn, too).

- Rest up. Get some extra sleep, since fatigue can step up that sick feeling.

- Go slow-mo. Don't jump out of bed and dash out the door—rushing tends to aggravate nausea. Instead, linger in bed for a few minutes, nibbling on that bedside snack, then rise slowly to a leisurely breakfast. This may seem impossible if you have other children, but try to wake up before they do so you can sneak in some quiet time, or let daddy do the dawn shift.

- Minimize stress. Easing the stress can ease the quease. See page 145 for tips on dealing with stress.

- Treat your mouth well. Brush your teeth (with a toothpaste that doesn't increase queasiness) or rinse your mouth after each bout of vomiting, as well as after each meal (ask your dentist to recommend a good rinse). This will not only help keep your mouth fresh and reduce nausea, but decrease the risk of damage to teeth or gums that can occur when bacteria feast on regurgitated residue in your mouth.

- Try Sea-Bands. These 1-inch-wide elastic bands, worn on both wrists, put pressure on acupressure points on the inner wrists and often relieve nausea. They cause no side effects and are widely available at drug and health food stores. Or your practitioner may recommend a more sophisticated form of acupressure: a battery-operated wristband that uses electronic stimulation, like Relief Bands or Psi Bands.

- Consider CAM. A wide variety of complementary medical approaches, such as acupuncture, acupressure, biofeedback, meditation, or hypnosis, can help minimize the symptoms of morning sickness—and they're all worth a try (see page 78).

- Ask about medication. If the do-it-yourself tips don't do the trick, check with your practitioner about whether you might need to step up to a prescription approach. Diclegis (Diclectin in Canada) is a very safe and effective combination of the antihistamine doxylamine and vitamin B_6 (the same combo often recommended in OTC form) in a delayed-release formula that can ease symptoms of morning sickness throughout the day and night with less daytime drowsiness. If morning sickness is really severe, antinausea medication may be added (such as Phenergan, Reglan, or Scopolamine). But don't take any medication (traditional or herbal) for morning sickness unless it is prescribed by your practitioner.

In fewer than 5 percent of pregnancies, nausea and vomiting become so severe that medical intervention may be needed. If this seems to be the case with you, check in with your practitioner and see page 547.

Excess Saliva

"My mouth seems to fill up with saliva all the time—and swallowing it makes me gag. What's going on?"

It may not be cool to drool (especially in public), but for many women in the first trimester, it's an icky fact of life. Overproduction of saliva is a common—and unpleasant—symptom of pregnancy, especially among morning sickness sufferers. And though all that extra saliva pooling in your mouth may add to your queasiness—and lead to a gaggy feeling when you eat—it's completely harmless, and thankfully short-lived, usually disappearing after the first few months.

Tired of being the Spit Girl? Spitting mad about all that spit? Brushing your teeth frequently with a minty toothpaste, rinsing with a minty mouthwash, or chewing sugarless gum can help dry things up a bit.

Metallic Taste

"I have a metallic taste in my mouth all the time. Is this pregnancy related—or is it something I ate?"

So your mouth tastes like loose change? Believe it or not, that metal mouth taste is a fairly common—though not often talked about—side effect of pregnancy and one more you can chalk up to hormones. Your hormones always play a role in controlling your sense of taste. When they go wild (as they do when you have your period—and as they do with a vengeance when you're pregnant), so do your taste buds. Like morning sickness, that yucky taste should ease up—or, if you're lucky, disappear altogether—in your second trimester, when those hormones begin to settle down.

Until then, you can try fighting metal with acid. Focus on citrus juices, lemonade, sour sucking candy, and—assuming your tummy can handle them—foods marinated in vinegar (some pickles with that ice cream?). Not only will such assertive acidics have the power to melt through that metallic taste, but they'll also increase saliva production, which will help wash it away (though that could be a bad thing, if your mouth's already flooded with the stuff). Other tricks to try: Brush your tongue each time you brush your teeth, or rinse your mouth with a salt solution (a teaspoon of salt in 8 ounces of water) or a baking soda solution (¼ teaspoon baking soda in 8 ounces of water) a few times a day to neutralize pH levels in your mouth and keep away that flinty flavor. You might also ask your practitioner about changing your prenatal vitamin, since some seem to lead to metal mouth more than others.

Frequent Urination

"I'm in the bathroom every half hour. Is it normal to be peeing this often?"

It may not be the best seat in the house, but for most pregnant women, it's the most frequented one. Let's face it, when you gotta go, you gotta go—and these days (and nights) you gotta go all the time. And while nonstop peeing might not always be convenient, it's absolutely normal, particularly in early pregnancy.

What causes this frequent urination? First, hormones trigger an increase not only in blood flow but in urine flow, too. Second, during pregnancy the efficiency of the kidneys improves, helping

---

FOR FATHERS

When She's Gotta Go . . . All the Time

There she goes—again. Urinary frequency will be your spouse's constant companion in her first trimester, and it'll come back with a vengeance in the last trimester, too. To make the going (and going) easier, try to practice your best bathroom etiquette. Try not to hog the bathroom, and always leave it ready for her use. Remember to put the seat down after every use (especially at night), and keep the hallway free of obstacles (your gym backpack, your sneakers) and lit by a nightlight so she won't trip on her way to the toilet. And be as understanding as you can (read: no eye rolling) when she has to get up 3 times during the movie or stop 6 times on the way to your parents' house. Keep in mind that urinary frequency is not in her control (sometimes literally) and that frequently trying to hold in her pee can lead to a urinary tract infection.

your body rid itself of waste products more quickly (including baby's, which means you'll be peeing for two). Finally, your growing uterus is pressing on your bladder now, leaving less storage space in the holding tank for urine and triggering that "gotta go" feeling. This pressure is often relieved once the uterus rises into the abdominal cavity during the second trimester and doesn't usually return until the third trimester or when the baby's head "drops" back down into the pelvis in the 9th month (bringing you Urinary Frequency: The Sequel). But because the arrangement of internal organs varies slightly from woman to woman, the degree of urinary frequency in pregnancy may also vary. Some women barely notice it, and others are bothered by it for most of the 9 months.

Leaning forward when you urinate will help ensure that you empty your bladder completely, as will double voiding (pee, then when you're finished, squeeze out some more). Both tactics may reduce the number of trips to the bathroom, though realistically, not by much.

Don't cut back on liquids, thinking it'll keep you out of the bathroom. Your body and your baby need a steady supply of fluids—plus, dehydration can lead to a UTI. But do cut back on caffeine, since large quantities can increase the need to pee (and that fierce urgency of "now!"). If you find that you go frequently during the night, try limiting fluids right before bedtime.

If you're always feeling the urge to urinate (even after you've just peed), talk to your practitioner. He or she might want to run a test to see if you've got a UTI.

"How come I'm not urinating frequently?"

Maybe you're not noticing an increase in urination because you're already a frequent pee-er—or because you're just not keeping track.

But do make sure you're getting enough fluids. Too little fluid intake cannot only cause infrequent urination, but lead to dehydration and urinary tract infection. Keep an eye not only on pee frequency, but on the color of your urine (it should be clear and pale yellow, not dark).

Breast Changes

"I hardly recognize my breasts anymore—they're so huge. And they're tender, too. Will they stay that way, and will they sag after I give birth?"

Looks like you've discovered the first big thing in pregnancy: your breasts. While bellies don't usually do much growing until the second trimester, breasts often begin their expansion within weeks of conception, gradually working their way through the bra cup alphabet, sometimes into double- and triple-letter territory (you may ultimately end up 3 cup sizes bigger than you started out). Fueling this growth are those surging hormones—the same ones that boost your bust premenstrually but at much greater levels. Fat is building up in your breasts, too, and blood flow to the area is increasing. And there's a swell reason for all this swelling—your breasts are gearing up to feed your baby when he or she arrives.

In addition to their expanding size, you will probably notice other changes to your breasts. The areola (the pigmented area around the nipple) will darken and spread, and may be spotted with even darker areas. This darkening may fade but not disappear entirely after birth. The little bumps you may notice on the areola are lubrication glands, which become more prominent during pregnancy and return to normal afterward. The complex road map of blue veins that spreads over the breasts—often vivid on a fair-skinned

When to Call Your Practitioner

What should you call your practitioner about and when? What's possibly an emergency and what probably isn't? Use the following list of symptoms as a general guideline, but keep in mind that your practitioner may want you to call for different reasons or within different parameters. That's why it's a good idea to discuss a protocol (or the following list) with your practitioner before a worrisome symptom strikes or an emergency comes up (some practitioners include a when-to-call and emergency protocol in their first-visit information packet).

If you haven't discussed a protocol with your practitioner and you're experiencing a symptom listed here (or another one that may require immediate medical attention), try the following: First, call the practitioner's office. If he or she isn't available, leave a message detailing your symptoms. If you don't get a call back within a few minutes, call again or call the nearest ER and tell the triage nurse what's going on. If he or she tells you to come in,

head to the ER and leave word with your practitioner. Call 911 if no one can take you to the ER.

When you report any of the following to your practitioner or to the triage nurse, be sure to mention any other symptoms you may be experiencing, no matter how unrelated they may seem. Also be specific, mentioning when you first noticed each symptom, how frequently it recurs, what seems to relieve or exacerbate it, and how severe it is:

CALL IMMEDIATELY IF YOU EXPERIENCE:

- Heavy bleeding or bleeding with cramps or severe pain in the lower abdomen

- Severe lower abdominal pain, in the center or on one or both sides, that doesn't subside, even if it isn't accompanied by bleeding

- A sudden increase in thirst, accompanied by reduced urination, or no urination at all for an entire day

---

woman and sometimes not even noticeable on darker women—represents a mom-to-baby delivery system for nutrients and fluids. After delivery—or, if you're breastfeeding, sometime after baby's weaned—the skin's appearance will return to normal.

Fortunately, that cup-size gain won't continue to come with pain (or uncomfortable sensitivity). Though your breasts will probably keep growing throughout your 9 months, they're not likely to stay super tender to the touch past the 3rd or 4th month. Some women find that most tenderness eases

well before that. In the achy meantime, find relief in cool or warm compresses (whichever is more soothing).

As for whether or not your breasts will end up sagging, a lot of that is up to genetics (if your mom drooped, you may, too), but some of it's up to you. Sagging results not just from pregnancy itself but from a lack of support during pregnancy. No matter how perky your breasts are now, protect them from a floppy future by wearing a supportive bra (though in that tender first trimester, you may want to avoid restrictive underwires). If your breasts are particularly

- Painful or burning urination accompanied by chills and fever over 101.5°F and/or backache

- Bloody diarrhea

- Fever over 101°F

- Very sudden and severe swelling or puffiness of hands, face, and eyes, accompanied by headache or vision difficulties

- Vision disturbances (blurring, dimming, double vision) that persist for more than a few minutes

- A severe headache or a headache that persists for more than 2 or 3 hours

CALL THE SAME DAY (OR THE NEXT MORNING, IF IT'S THE MIDDLE OF THE NIGHT) IF YOU EXPERIENCE:

- Blood in your urine

- Sudden swelling or puffiness of your hands, face, or eyes

- Painful or burning urination

- Fainting or dizziness that's more than momentary

- Chills and fever over 100°F in the absence of cold or flu symptoms (start bringing down any fever over 100°F promptly by taking acetaminophen, such as Tylenol)

- Severe nausea and vomiting; vomiting more often than 2 or 3 times a day in the first trimester; vomiting later in pregnancy when you didn't earlier

- Itching all over, with or without dark urine, pale stools, or jaundice (yellowing of skin and whites of the eye)

- Frequent (more than 3 times a day) diarrhea, especially if it's mucousy

Keep in mind as you look over this list: There might be times when you have none of the symptoms here, but you don't feel "quite right." Or you have different symptoms not listed here or not explained in this book. Chances are what you're feeling is normal and that all you'll need is a good night's sleep to get you back on track. But when in doubt, check it out and call your practitioner.

large or have a tendency to sag, it's a good idea to wear a bra even at night. You'll probably find a cotton sports bra most comfortable for sleeping.

Not all women notice pronounced breast changes early in pregnancy, and some find the expansion takes place so gradually that it's not perceptible. As with all things pregnancy, what's normal is what's normal for your breasts. And don't worry: Though slower growth—or less substantial growth—means you won't have to replace bras so often, it won't have any impact on your ability to breastfeed.

"My breasts became very large in my first pregnancy, but they haven't seemed to change at all in my second. Is that normal?"

Last time your breasts were newbies—this time, they entered pregnancy with previous experience. As a result, they may not need as much preparation—or react as dramatically to those surging hormones—as they did in your first round of baby making. You may find that your breasts will enlarge gradually as your pregnancy progresses—or you may find that their expansion holds off until after delivery, when milk production begins. Either way, this slow growing is completely normal—and an early indication of how very different pregnancies can be.

Lower Abdominal Pressure

"I've been having a nagging feeling of pressure in my lower abdomen. Should I be worried?"

It sounds like you're very tuned in to your body—which can be a good thing (as when it helps you recognize ovulation) or a not-so-good thing (when it makes you worry about the many innocuous aches and pains of pregnancy).

Don't worry. A feeling of pressure or even mild crampiness without bleeding is very common, especially in first pregnancies—and is usually a sign that everything's going right, not that something's going wrong. Chances are, that sensitive body radar of yours is just picking up some of the many dramatic changes that are taking place in your lower abdomen, where your uterus is currently located. What you're feeling may be the sensation of implantation, increased blood flow, the buildup of the uterine lining, or simply your uterus beginning to grow—in other words, your first growing pains. It could also be gas pains or bowel spasms that come with constipation (another common pregnancy side effect).

For further reassurance, ask your practitioner about the feeling (if you're still having it) at your next office visit.

Spotting

"I was in the bathroom and noticed a spot of blood when I wiped. Am I having a miscarriage?"

It's definitely scary to see blood down below when you're pregnant. But what's not definite is that bleeding is a sign that something's wrong with your pregnancy. Many women—about 1 in 5, in fact—experience some bleeding during pregnancy, and most go on to have a perfectly healthy pregnancy and baby. So if you're noticing only light spotting—similar to what you see at the beginning or end of your period—you can take a deep breath and read on for a probable (and probably reassuring) explanation. Such light spotting is usually caused by one of the following:

Implantation of the embryo. Affecting 20 to 30 percent of women, such spotting (called "implantation bleeding" in the ob business) will usually occur before (or in some cases around the time) you expected your period, about 6 to 12 days after conception. Lighter than a period (and lasting anywhere from a few hours to a few days), implantation bleeding is usually spotty and light to medium pink or light brown in color. It occurs when the little ball of cells you'll one day call your baby burrows its way into the uterine wall. Implantation bleeding is not a sign that something is wrong.

Recent sex, an internal exam, or Pap smear. During pregnancy, your cervix becomes tender and engorged with blood vessels and can occasionally become irritated during intercourse or an internal exam, resulting in some light bleeding. This type of bleeding is common, can occur at any time during your pregnancy, and usually doesn't indicate a problem, but do tell your practitioner about any post-sex or post-exam spotting for extra reassurance.

Infection of the vagina or cervix. An inflamed, irritated, or infected cervix or vagina might cause some spotting (though the spotting should disappear once you're treated for the infection).

No Worries

Some expectant moms (make that, most expectant moms) will always find something to worry about—especially in the first trimester and particularly in first pregnancies. Topping the list of most common concerns, understandably, is a fear of miscarriage.

Fortunately, most expectant worriers end up worrying unnecessarily. Most pregnancies continue uneventfully, and happily, to term. Just about every normal pregnancy includes some cramps, some abdominal aches, or some spotting—and many include all three. While any of these symptoms can be understandably unnerving (and when it comes to a stain on your underwear, downright scary), more often than not, they're completely innocuous—and not a sign that your pregnancy is in trouble. Though you should report them to your practitioner at your next visit (or sooner if you need some professional reassurance), the following are no cause for concern. So don't worry if you have:

Mild cramps, achiness, or a pulling sensation in the lower abdomen on one or both sides. Early on, this is probably related to implantation, the increased blood flow to the region, the buildup of your uterine lining, or just all the growing that's going on as your uterus and the ligaments that support it begin stretching. Unless cramping is severe, constant, or accompanied by significant bleeding, there's no need to worry.

Slight spotting that isn't accompanied by cramps or lower abdominal pain. There are plenty of reasons why pregnant women spot, and it often has nothing to do with a miscarriage. See facing page for more on spotting.

Of course, it's not just symptoms that pregnant women worry about in early pregnancy—it's a lack of symptoms, too. In fact, not "feeling pregnant" is one of the most commonly reported first-trimester concerns. And that's not surprising. It's hard to feel pregnant this early on, even if you're experiencing every early pregnancy symptom in the book—and it's far harder still to feel pregnant if you're relatively symptom-free. Without tangible proof yet of that baby-to-be growing inside you (a swelling belly, those first flutters of movement), it's pretty easy to start wondering whether the pregnancy is going well—or whether you're even still pregnant.

Once again, not to worry. A lack of symptoms—such as morning sickness or breast tenderness—is not usually a sign that something's wrong. Consider yourself lucky if you're spared these and other unpleasant early-pregnancy symptoms—and also consider that you might be a late bloomer. After all, since every pregnant woman experiences pregnancy symptoms differently and at different times, these and other symptoms may be just around the corner for you.

Subchorionic bleed. Subchorionic bleeding occurs when there is an accumulation of blood under the chorion (the outer fetal membrane, next to the placenta) or between the uterus and the placenta itself. It can cause light to heavy spotting but doesn't always (sometimes it is detected only during a routine ultrasound). Most subchorionic bleeds resolve on their own and do not end up being a problem for the pregnancy (see page 544 for more).

Spotting is as variable in a normal pregnancy as it is common. Some women spot on and off for their entire pregnancies. Other women spot for just a day or two—and still others for several weeks. Some women notice mucousy brown or pink spotting, others see small amounts of bright red blood. But happily, most women who experience any kind of spotting continue to have completely normal and healthy pregnancies and end up delivering perfectly healthy babies. Which means that there's probably nothing for you to worry about (though, realistically, that doesn't mean you'll stop worrying).

For extra reassurance, put in a call to your practitioner (no need to call immediately or outside of office hours unless your spotting is accompanied by cramping or bright red, soak-through-a-pad bleeding). He or she will likely either order a blood test to check hCG levels (see next question) or perform an ultrasound (or do both). If you're past the 6th week, you'll probably be able to see your baby's heartbeat during the ultrasound, which will reassure you that your pregnancy is progressing along just fine, even with the spotting.

What if the spotting progresses to heavier bleeding similar to a period? Though such a scenario is more cause for concern (especially if it's accompanied by cramps or pain in your lower abdomen) and does warrant an immediate call to your practitioner, it's not a sign that you're inevitably miscarrying. Some women bleed—even heavily—for unknown reasons throughout their pregnancies and still deliver healthy babies.

If it does end up that you're having a miscarriage, see page 582.

hCG Levels

"My doctor gave me the results of my blood test and it says that my hCG level is at 412 mIU/L. What does that number mean?"

It means that you're pregnant. Human chorionic gonadotropin (hCG) is the

---

hCG By the Numbers

Really want to play the hCG numbers game? The following are ranges of "normal" hCG levels based on week of pregnancy. Keep in mind that anywhere in that wide range is normal—your baby doesn't have to be scoring off the charts for your pregnancy to be progressing perfectly—and that a slight miscalculation in your dates can throw the numbers off completely.

WEEKS OF PREGNANCY	AMOUNT OF hCG IN mIU/L
3 weeks	5 to 50
4 weeks	5 to 426
5 weeks	19 to 7,340
6 weeks	1,080 to 56,500
7 to 8 weeks	7,650 to 229,000
9 to 12 weeks	25,700 to 288,000

just-for-pregnancy hormone manufactured by the cells of the newly developing placenta within days after the fertilized egg implants in your uterine lining. HCG is found in your urine (you came face-to-stick with hCG the day that positive readout showed up on your HPT) and in your blood, which explains why your practitioner ran a blood test to find out your expectant status for sure. When you're very early in the pregnancy game (as you are), the level of hCG in your blood will be quite low (it's just starting to show up in your system, after all). But within days, it'll begin to soar, doubling every 48 hours (give or take). The rapid increase peaks somewhere between 7 and 12 weeks of pregnancy and then starts to decline.

But don't start swapping your numbers with mama-to-be buddies. Just as no two women's pregnancies are alike, no two pregnant women's hCG levels are alike, either. They vary from day to day, mom to mom, even as early as the first missed day of a period and continuing throughout pregnancy.

What's more important and relevant to you is that your hCG level falls within the very wide normal range (see box, facing page) and continues to increase over the coming weeks (in other words, look for a pattern of increasing levels instead of focusing on specific numbers). Even if your readings fall outside these ranges, don't worry. It's still quite likely that everything's fine. Your due date might just be off—a very common cause of hCG number confusion—or, less probably, you might be carrying twins. As long as your pregnancy is progressing normally and your hCG levels are increasing during the first trimester, there's no need to obsess about these numbers or even try to find them out (plus, if your practitioner is happy with your numbers, then you can be, too). Ultrasound findings after 5 or 6 weeks

of pregnancy are much more predictive of pregnancy outcome than hCG levels are. Of course, as always, if you have a question or concern, talk with your practitioner about your results.

Stress

"I'm a high-stress person with a high-stress job—and now that I'm pregnant, I'm stressing about stressing too much. Can too much stress be bad for a baby?"

Most mommies-to-be are stressed out sometimes (or even often) during their 9 months. But here's some news that should calm you down: Research shows that pregnancy isn't affected by typical stress levels. If you're able to cope well with your everyday stress (even if it's more than most people could take on), then your baby will be able to cope just fine, too. In fact, a certain amount of stress—if you're good at handling it—can be a pregnancy plus. It can keep you on your toes, keeping you motivated to take the best possible care of yourself, your baby, and your pregnancy.

That said, too much stress—or stress that isn't well managed—can take its toll, particularly if it continues into the second and third trimesters. Which means that learning how to handle stress constructively, or cutting back on it as needed, should become a priority now. The following should help:

Unload it. Allowing your anxieties to surface is the best way of ensuring that they don't get you down. Make sure you have somewhere to vent—and someone to vent to. Maintain open lines of communication with your spouse, spending some time at the end of each day (preferably not too close to bedtime, which should be as stress-free as possible) sharing concerns and frustrations. Together you may be able to find some

Anxiety Over Life Changes

Worried about how different your life will be once you're a dad? Little babies do bring some large life changes, no doubt about it—and all expectant parents worry about them. Thinking about them—and even stressing about them a little—now is actually a really good thing, since it gives you a chance to prepare realistically for the impact parenthood will have on your life. The most common dad-to-be worries include:

Will our relationship change? Let's get real: Yes, your relationship will change. From the moment baby comes into your life, spontaneous intimacy and complete privacy will be precious, and often unattainable, commodities. Romance may have to be planned (during baby's nap) rather than spur of the moment, and interruptions may be the rule. But as long as you both make the effort to make time for each other—whether that means catching up over a late dinner once baby's in bed, or giving up a game with the guys so you can play games of an entirely different kind with your partner, or starting a weekly date night—your relationship will weather the changes well. Many couples, in fact, find that becoming a threesome deepens, strengthens, and improves their twosome—bringing them closer together than they've ever been before.

How will work be affected? That depends on your work schedule. If you currently work long hours with little time off, you may need (and want) to make some changes so that fatherhood can become the priority in your life that you'll want it to be. And don't wait until you officially graduate to dad status. Think about taking time off now for prenatal checkups, as well as to help your exhausted spouse with baby preparations. Start weaning yourself off those 12-hour days, and resist the temptation to continue your day at the office at home. Avoid trips and a heavy workload during the 2 months before and after your baby's arrival, if you can. And if it's at all possible, consider taking paternity leave in the early weeks of baby's life.

Will we have to give up our lifestyle? You probably won't have to say goodbye to activities-as-usual or your social life as you knew it, but you should expect to make some adjustments, at least up front. A new baby does, and should, take center stage, pushing some old lifestyle habits temporarily aside. Parties, movies, and sports may be tricky to fit in between feedings, and cozy dinners for two at your favorite bistro may become noisy meals for three at family restaurants that tolerate squirming infants. Your circle of friends may change somewhat, too—you may suddenly find yourself gravitating

relief, some solutions—and ideally a good laugh or two. Is he too stressed to absorb enough of your stress? Find others who can lend an ear—a friend, another family member, coworkers (who will understand your workplace stress better?), your online buddies, or your practitioner (especially if you're concerned about the physical effects of your stress). If you need more than a friendly ear, consider counseling to help you develop strategies to better deal with your stress.

Do something about it. Identify sources of stress in your life and determine how toward fellow baby-wearers or stroller-pushers for empathetic companionship. Not to say that there won't be a place in your new life with baby for old friends who aren't fathers—and pastimes from your pre-parent past—just that your priorities will likely do some necessary shifting.

Can we afford a larger family? With the cost of having and raising a baby going through the roof, many expectant parents lose sleep over this very legitimate question. But there are plenty of ways to cut those costs, including opting for breastfeeding (no bottles or formula to buy) and accepting all the hand-me-downs that are offered (new clothes start to look like hand-me-downs after a few spitting-up episodes anyway). If either of you plan to take extra time off from work (or to put career plans on hold for a while) and this concerns you from a financial standpoint, weigh it against the costs of high-quality child care and commuting. The income lost may not be such a budget buster after all.

Most important: Instead of thinking of what you won't have in your life anymore (or won't have as much opportunity for), try to start thinking of what you will have in your life: a very special little person to share it with. Will your life be different? Definitely. Will it be better? No doubt about it.

they can be modified. If you're clearly trying to do too much, cut back in areas that are not high priority (this is something you're going to have to do big time anyway, once you have a bigger priority—a new baby—on the agenda). If you've taken on too many responsibilities at home or at work, decide which

can be postponed or delegated. Learn to say no to new projects or activities before you're overloaded (another skill you're wise to cultivate pre-baby).

Sometimes, making lists of the hundreds of things you need to get done (at home or at work), and the order in which you're planning to do them, can help you feel more in control of the chaos in your life. For a satisfying sense of accomplishment, check items off your list as they're taken care of.

Sleep it off. Sleep is the ticket to regeneration—for mind and body. Often, feelings of tension and anxiety are prompted by not getting enough shut-eye—and, of course, having too much tension and anxiety can also prevent you from getting enough shut-eye. So try to break the sleepless-stressed-sleepless cycle. If you're having trouble sleeping, see the tips on page 264.

Nourish it. Hectic lifestyles can lead to hectic eating styles. Inadequate nutrition during pregnancy can be a double whammy: It can hamper your ability to handle stress, and it can eventually affect your baby's wellbeing. So be sure to eat well and regularly (6 mini-meals will best keep you going when the going gets stressful). Focus on complex carbs and protein, and steer clear of excessive caffeine and sugar, two staples of the stressed life that can actually leave you less able to cope.

Wash it away. A warm bath is an excellent way to relieve tension. Try it after a stressful day—it will also help you sleep better.

Run it off. Or swim it off. Or prenatal yoga it off. You might think that the last thing you need in your life is more activity, but exercise is one of the best stress relievers—and mood boosters. Build some into your busy day.

Expect the Best

It's long been speculated that optimistic people live longer, healthier lives. Now it's been suggested that an expectant mom's optimistic outlook can actually improve the outlook for her unborn baby, too. Researchers have found that seeing the bright side reduces the chance of a high-risk woman delivering a preterm or low-birthweight baby.

A lower level of stress in optimistic women definitely plays a part in the lowered risk—high levels of stress, after all, have been implicated in a variety of health problems in and out of pregnancy. But stress itself apparently doesn't tell the whole story. Women who are optimistic, not surprisingly, are more likely to take better care of themselves—eating well, exercising right, getting regular prenatal care, and making good lifestyle choices. And these positive behaviors—fueled by the power of positive thinking—can, of course, have a very positive effect on pregnancy and fetal wellbeing.

Researchers point out that it's never too late to start seeing the bright side when you're expecting. Learning how to expect the best—instead of the worst—can actually help make those expectations come true: a good reason to start seeing that glass of milk as half full instead of half empty.

CAM it. Explore the many complementary and alternative therapies that can promise inner calm, among them biofeedback, acupuncture, hypnotherapy, massage (or even a shoulder rub from your partner). Meditation and visualization can melt the stress away (see box below). See page 78 for more on CAM techniques.

Relaxation Made Easy

Is your growing bundle of joy making you a quivering bundle of nerves? Now's a great time to learn some soothing relaxation techniques—not just because they can help you cope with pregnancy concerns, but because they'll come in handy in your hectic life as a new mom. Yoga's a fabulous de-stresser, if you have time to take a prenatal class or practice with a DVD or online video. If you don't, you can try this simple relaxation technique, which is easy to learn and to do anywhere, anytime. If you find it helpful, you can do it when anxiety strikes and/or regularly several times a day to try to ward it off:

Sit with your eyes closed and imagine your ideal happy place (a sunset over your favorite beach with waves gently lapping the shore, or a serene mountain vista complete with babbling brook), or envision your baby-to-be wrapped in your arms on a sunny day in the park. Then, working your way up from your toes to your face, concentrate on relaxing every muscle. Breathe slowly, deeply, silently noting each inhale or exhale or choosing a simple word (such as "yes" or "one") to repeat aloud every time you exhale. Ten to 20 minutes should do the trick, though even a minute or two is better than nothing.

Get away from it. Combat stress with any activity you find relaxing. Lose it in reading, a good movie or music, knitting (you can relax while you get a head start on those booties), browsing online for baby clothes, lunching with a fun friend, keeping a journal (another good way to vent your feelings), scrapbooking. Or walk away from it (even a quick stroll can be relaxing and rejuvenating).

Cut it back. Maybe what's causing the stress just isn't worth it. If it's your job that's got you too wired, consider taking early maternity leave or cutting back to part-time (if either of these options is financially feasible), or delegating some of your workload to reduce stress to a level that doesn't weigh you down. A change of jobs or careers might be impractical to pull off now, but it might be something to consider once your baby arrives.

If your stress is the kind that causes anxiety, sleeplessness, or depression, triggers physical symptoms (such as chronic headaches or loss of appetite), or even leads to unhealthy behaviors (smoking, for instance), talk to your practitioner.

ALL ABOUT:
Your Pampered Pregnancy

Talk about extreme makeovers. Pregnancy is a radical full-body transformation that may have you feeling your most beautiful (you glow, girl!), your least attractive (those zits! those chin hairs!)—or both in the same day. But it's also a time when your usual beauty regimen might need a makeover. Before you reach into your medicine cabinet for the acne cream you've been using since middle school or head to your favorite spa for a bikini wax and a facial, you'll need to know what's a beauty do—and what's a beauty don't—when you're expecting. Here's the lowdown from tip (highlights) to toes (pedicure) on how you can pamper your pregnant self beautifully—and safely.

Your Hair

When you're expecting, your hair can take a turn for the better (when lackluster hair suddenly sports a brilliant shine) or for the worse (when once-bouncy hair goes limp). One thing's probably for sure: Thanks to hormones, you'll have more of it than ever before (and sadly, probably not just on your head). Here's the heads-up on hair treatments:

Coloring. Here's the root of the problem when it comes to hiding your roots during pregnancy. Even though no evidence suggests the small amount of chemicals absorbed through the skin during hair coloring is harmful when you're expecting, some experts still advise waiting out the first trimester before heading back to the salon (or reaching for your favorite drugstore formula) for retouching. Others maintain that it's safe to dye throughout pregnancy. Check with your practitioner—you'll likely get the green light on color. If you're uncomfortable with a full dye job, consider highlights instead of single-process color. That way the chemicals won't touch your scalp at all, plus highlights tend to last longer than all-over color, which means you'll

A Day at the Spa

Ahhhh, the spa. No one deserves —and needs—a day of pampering more than a mom-to-be. And happily, more and more spas are offering treatments specifically catering to the expectant set. But before you head off for your day of pregnant pampering, ask your practitioner for any specific caveats for your situation. Then, when you call to make your appointment, tell the scheduler that you're expecting. Discuss any restrictions you may have so the spa can tailor treatments to fit your needs. Also be sure to inform any esthetician or therapist who will be working on you that you're pregnant, even if you already mentioned it when making the appointment.

need fewer retouches during your pregnancy. You can also ask your colorist (or beauty supply store) about less harsh processing—an ammonia-free base or an all-vegetable dye, for instance. Just keep in mind that hormonal changes can make your hair react strangely—so you might not get what you expect, even from your regular formula. Try a small test area first so you don't wind up with a headful of punk purple instead of that ravishing red you were hoping for.

Straightening treatments or relaxers. Thinking about a straightening treatment to calm those curls? Though there's no evidence that hair relaxers are dangerous during pregnancy (the amount of chemicals that seep through the scalp and into the blood system is probably minimal), there's no proof they're completely safe, either. Ditto for Brazilian keratin treatments (many contain formaldehyde, which is probably not safe during pregnancy, plus the fumes can be intense). So check with your practitioner—you may hear that it's safest to let your hair do what comes naturally, especially during the first trimester. If you do decide to go straight, keep in mind that there's a possibility that your hormone-infused locks may respond oddly to the chemicals (you might end up with a helmet of frizz instead of ramrod-straight tresses). Plus, your hair will grow faster during pregnancy, making those curls reappear at your roots sooner than you might like. Thermal reconditioning processes that involve different—often gentler—chemicals to tame your frizz may be a safer option (again, ask first). Or just buy a flat iron of your own, and coax your hair into smooth submission.

Permanents or body waves. So your hair's not as full as your figure's becoming? Ordinarily, a permanent or a body wave might be the answer for hair that's limping, but it probably isn't during pregnancy. Not because it isn't safe (it probably is, though check with your practitioner), but because hair responds unpredictably under the influence of pregnancy hormones. A permanent might not take at all—or might result in frizz instead of waves.

Hair removal. If pregnancy has you looking like an extra from *Planet of the Apes,* stay calm—this hairy situation is only temporary. Your armpits, bikini line, upper lip, even your belly may be fuzzier than usual because of those raging hormones (though some lucky moms-to-be find hair growth on their legs slows down). Rather not wear fur? No need to. You can safely turn to all of those hair removal old reliables: shaving, plucking, threading, and waxing. Even a full-on Brazilian wax is fine—just proceed with care, since pregnancy skin can be super-sensitive and easily irritated. If you're heading to the salon, let the esthetician know you're expecting so she can be extra gentle. Wondering about other hair removal options? Like many cosmetic procedures and products, lasers (including at-home varieties), electrolysis, depilatories, and bleaching haven't been studied enough in pregnancy to prove their safety, so ask your practitioner for a deciding vote before opting in. Some practitioners give certain ones the all-clear after month 3, while others will advise holding off on all for the full 9 months.

Eyelash treatments. As for the hair that no one can get enough of—you'll have to make do with the eyelashes you've got for now. The prescription eyelash-growing treatment Latisse, as well as many of the over-the-counter products touted to lengthen lashes, aren't recommended for expectant and breastfeeding moms because (you guessed it) they haven't been studied in pregnancy. It's probably also smart to avoid dying your eyelashes or brows. On the plus side, your lashes may be thicker than ever now that you're expecting.

Your Face

Your pregnancy may not be showing in your belly yet, but it's almost certainly showing on your face. Here's the good, the bad, and the blotchy about face care when you're expecting.

Facials. Face fact: Not every mom-to-be is blessed with that expectant radiance you've always read about. If your glow decides not to show, a facial might be just the ticket, working wonders when it comes to clearing pores clogged by extra oil (thanks to extra hormones). Most facials are safe during pregnancy, as long as they don't incorporate any ingredients that might get the red light (such as retinoids or salicylic acid; see

below). Some of the more aggressively exfoliating treatments (like microdermabrasion or peels) might be especially irritating to skin made super-sensitive by pregnancy hormones—leaving you less glowy, more red and blotchy. Facials that use an electrical microcurrent or lasers are off-limits during pregnancy (ditto for at-home laser facials—better to postpone those treatments until after pregnancy). Discuss with the esthetician which preparations might be most soothing and least likely to provoke a reaction. If you're unsure about a particular treatment's safety, check with your practitioner before signing up.

Antiwrinkle treatments. A wrinkly baby is cute . . . a wrinkly mommy, not so much. But before you stop by your dermatologist's office to treat those fine lines (or fill those lips), consider this: The safety of injectable fillers (such as collagen, Restylane, or Juvederm) during pregnancy hasn't been established through studies yet. The same goes for Botox, which means you're better off staying unfilled (and uninjected) for now. As for antiwrinkle creams, it's best to read the fine print (and check with your practitioner). You'll likely be advised to bid a temporary farewell to products that contain vitamin A (in any of its many retinoid forms), vitamin K, or salicylic acid (also called BHA, or beta-hydroxy acid). Check with your practitioner about other ingredients you're unsure about, too. Most practitioners will green-light products containing AHA (alpha-hydroxy acid) or fruit acids, but get the all clear first. On the bright side, you may find that normal pregnancy fluid retention plumps up your face nicely, leaving your wrinkles less noticeable—and your lips fuller—without the help of cosmetic procedures.

Acne treatments. Got more pimples than a high school marching band? You

Making Up for Pregnancy

Between breakouts, funky skin discolorations, and normal pregnancy swelling, your face will be facing some challenges over the next 9 months. Luckily, you'll be able to make up for them with the right makeup:

- Go under cover. Corrective concealer and foundation can cover a multitude of pregnancy skin issues, including chloasma and other discolorations (see page 258). For those dark spots, look for brands that are designed to cover hyperpigmentation, but make sure all makeup is hypoallergenic. Match both to your skin tone, but select a concealer that's a shade lighter than your natural complexion. Apply the concealer only to the dark spots, stippling the edges to blend. Then lightly blend the foundation over the area. Less is definitely more when it comes to heavy coverage products, so use the least you can get away with—you can always top it off. Set with powder.

  Keep coverage lighter when it comes to pregnancy pimples to avoid calling attention to them (they'll likely call enough attention to themselves). Start with foundation, then apply a concealer—one that matches your skin—directly to the zit, blending with your finger. If you're going to pre-spot before you cover up, use a pregnancy-approved topical that's clear.

- Play with shadows. Chip away at those chipmunk cheeks you'll likely be growing: After you've applied your all-over foundation, apply a highlighting shade (one shade lighter) to the center of your forehead, under your eyes, on the tops of your cheekbones, and on the tip of your chin. Then brush a contouring shade (one shade darker) down the sides of your face, starting at the temples, and under your cheekbones. Blend, and presto—instant contours!

- Stop the spread. Sure, you expect your belly to plump up, and maybe even your hips—but your nose? Don't worry—any widening is temporary, the result of pregnancy swelling. Slim a swollen sniffer by applying a highlighting shade (one shade lighter than your overall foundation) down the center of your nose, then contour the vertical edges of the sides of your nose with a darker shade. Make sure you blend well.

---

can blame pregnancy hormones for that. But before you march to the medicine cabinet for your usual zit zappers, check them out with your practitioner. Exfoliating scrubs and products containing glycolic acid and fruit acids are probably safe to use (though watch out for irritation). Ditto some prescription products (azelaic and topical antibiotics, such as erythromycin), which may be especially helpful when you've got bacne to boot. Two active ingredients commonly found in topical acne medications, beta-hydroxy acid (BHA) and salicylic acid, are typically shelved during pregnancy. Ask your practitioner about the safety of products that contain these ingredients and those that contain benzoyl peroxide (the active ingredient in many pimple preparations and one that also often gets the red light during pregnancy). Accutane (which causes serious birth defects) is definitely off-limits. So is Retin-A (ask your practitioner about over-the-counter products that contain retinol). Laser treatments and chemical peels for acne should also probably wait until after the baby is born. You can absolutely try to tame eruptions naturally by eating well (some women find keeping sugar and refined grains to a minimum helps a lot), and keeping your face clean but not overscrubbed (and don't forget the oil-free moisturizer, since skin that's too dry can actually be more pimple prone). And no popping or picking. See page 166 for more.

Your Teeth

You've got plenty to smile about now that you're expecting, but will your teeth be up for the exposure? Cosmetic dentistry's popular, but not always pregnancy approved.

Whitening products. Eager to flash your pearly whites? While there are no proven risks to tooth whitening during pregnancy, it's a procedure that probably falls into the better-safe-than-sorry category (so you'll be wise to wait a few months to debut that new million-dollar smile). Be sure to keep your teeth clean and well flossed, though. Your pregnancy-sensitive gums will thank you for the attention (and for not exposing them to those irritating whitening products).

Veneers. Here's one more for the better-safe-than-sorry side, even though there are no proven risks to adding veneers to your teeth during pregnancy. There's another reason why you might consider waiting until you're postpartum before you veneer your teeth: Your gums might be extra sensitive when you've got a baby on board, making any dental procedure—including veneers and whitening—more uncomfortable than usual.

Your Body

Your body definitely pays for the privilege of pregnancy—in ways you probably never imagined. So more than any body, it deserves some pampering. Here's how to give it what it needs—safely.

Massage. Aching for some relief from that nagging backache—or from that nagging anxiety that's keeping you up at night? There's nothing like a massage to rub away the aches and pains of pregnancy, as well as the stress and strain. But though a massage may be just what the feel-good doctor ordered, you'll need to follow some guidelines to ensure your pregnancy massages are not only relaxing but also safe:

- Get rubbed by the right hands. Make sure your massage therapist is licensed and well versed in the do's and don'ts of prenatal massage.

- Wait for your rub. Massage during the first 3 months of pregnancy may trigger dizziness and add to morning sickness, so it's best to hold off until the second trimester. But don't worry if you've already had a massage during your first trimester.

- Relax in the right position. It's best to avoid spending a lot of time on your back after the 4th month, so ask your massage therapist to use a table that's equipped with a cutout for your belly, special pillows designed for pregnancy use, or cushioned foam padding that conforms to your body, or to position you on your side.

- Try some non-scents. Ask for an unscented lotion or oil, not only because your pregnancy-sharpened sniffer might be offended by strong fragrances, but also because some aromatherapy oils can stimulate contractions (see next page).

- Rub the right spots (and stay away from the wrong ones). Direct pressure on the area between the anklebone and heel can trigger contractions, so be sure your therapist stays away from there (another good reason to choose a massage therapist with prenatal training). Another spot to steer clear of: the abdomen, for both comfort's and safety's sake (there is a very slight risk that deep abdominal massage could trigger contractions or lead to other complications). And if your therapist is working too deeply or if the massage is too intense, speak up. This is about you feeling good, after all.

Aromatherapy. When it comes to scents during pregnancy, it's good to use some common sense. Because the effects of many plant oils in pregnancy are unknown and some may be harmful, approach any kind of aromatherapy with caution. The following essential oils are considered safe for prenatal massage, though experts recommend that they be mixed at a concentration that's half the standard usage: rose, lavender, chamomile, jasmine, tangerine, neroli, and ylang-ylang. Pregnant women should particularly avoid the following oils, because some of them can trigger uterine contractions: basil, juniper, rosemary, sage, peppermint, pennyroyal, oregano, and thyme. (Midwives often use these oils during labor precisely because they may trigger contractions.) If you've had an aromatherapy massage with these oils (or used them in home baths or treatments), don't worry. The absorption of the oil is very low, especially because the skin on your back is pretty thick. Just steer clear of them in future treatments. Scented lotions or beauty products sold at bath and beauty shops (like peppermint foot lotion, for instance) are fine since the scents aren't concentrated.

Body treatments, scrubs, wraps, hydrotherapy. Body scrubs are generally safe, as long as they're gentle (some scrubs can be too rough on sensitive pregnant skin). Some wraps can be safe, but most are off-limits because they might raise your body temperature excessively. A short warm bath (no hotter than 100°F) as part of hydrotherapy is safe and relaxing, but stay out of the sauna, steam room, and hot tub.

Tanning beds, sprays, lotions. Looking for a way to go beyond the pale (pale skin, that is) during your pregnancy? Sorry, but tanning beds are out. Not only are they bad for your health (they increase your risk of skin cancer), but they speed up the aging process and up your chances of getting chloasma (the skin discoloration called the "mask of pregnancy"). Worse, tanning beds can raise your body temperature to a level that could be harmful to your developing baby. Still a fan of the tan? Before you fake it with sunless tanning lotions and sprays, talk to your practitioner. And even if you get the go-ahead, consider that your hormones can cause your skin to play games with the color (and take a turn for the terra cotta). Plus, as your belly expands, applying a sunless tanner evenly might get tricky (especially once you can no longer see your legs, and even if you're getting a professional spray or airbrush tan).

For information on the safety of tattoos, henna, and piercings during pregnancy, check out pages 169 and 191.

Your Hands and Feet

Yes, even your hands and feet will show the effects of pregnancy (though you won't be able to see the effects on your feet as easily once you reach the third trimester). But even when you're feeling swell—as in fingers and ankles that are puffy with fluids—your hands and feet can still look their best.

Manicure and pedicure. It's perfectly safe to polish while pregnant (and take advantage now, because it's likely that your nails are growing faster and stronger than ever). If you get your nails done in a salon, make sure it's a well-ventilated one. Inhaling those strong chemical smells is never a good idea but especially not when you're breathing for two (and at the very least, the fumes might make you queasy). Do be sure the manicurist doesn't massage the area between your anklebone and heel when you're getting your pedi (it could theoretically trigger contractions). And if you want your calluses removed, have the manicurist do so only with a pumice stone, not a blade (even if it's from a sterile pack and is the disposable kind), since that can lead to infection (never mind the fact that the more you cut calluses, the more they grow back).

If you're worried about the fumes from regular nail polishes, check out the growing number of nontoxic polishes—as well as nontoxic polish removers.

When it comes to long-lasting gel or Shellac polish, there's no proven risk to pregnancy, but there definitely could be to your skin if you're not careful. That's because the lights sometimes used to cure the gel polish emit UV light—the kind used in tanning booths and that has been implicated in premature aging and skin cancer (plus it could lead to blotchy hands during pregnancy). If you do gels, ask for specially made gloves that cover your hands, exposing only your nails to the UV light (or frequent a nail salon that uses LED light that cures far faster). Also wise: getting the green light on gels from your practitioner, especially if you're thinking of getting them regularly during pregnancy.

As for acrylics, there's no proof that the chemicals are harmful, but you might want to err on the cautious side and forgo those tips until post-baby—not only because the application smell can be extremely strong, but because they can become a nail bed for infection, something you might be more prone to while you're pregnant. And remember, you may not need the extra length or strength of acrylics anyway, because your nails will be growing at warp speed and may be stronger than ever.

CHAPTER 6

The Second Month

Approximately 5 to 8 Weeks

E ven if you're not telling anyone you're expecting yet (and even though you're definitely not showing it), your baby's probably starting to spill the beans to you. Not in so many words, but in so many symptoms. Like that nagging nausea that follows you wherever you go, or all that excess saliva pooling in your mouth (am I drooling?). Like the gotta-go feeling you're getting all day (and all night), those oh-so-tender nipples, or that 24/7 bloat you just can't seem to deflate. Even with the ever-growing evidence that you're pregnant, you're probably still getting used to the idea that a new life is growing inside of you. You're also probably just getting used to the demands of pregnancy, from the physical (so that's why I'm tired!) to the logistical (the shortest route to the bathroom is . . .) to the lifestyle (make my Sea Breeze a virgin). It's a wild ride, and it's only just beginning. Hold on tight!

Your Baby This Month

Week 5 Your little embryo, which at this point resembles a tadpole more than a baby (complete with teeny tail), is growing fast and furiously and is now about the size of an orange seed—still small, but exponentially larger than before. This week, the heart is starting to take shape. In fact, the circulatory system, along with the heart, is the first system to be operational. Your baby's heart (about the size of a poppy seed) is made up of 2 tiny channels called heart tubes, and though it's still far from fully functional, it's already beating—something you might be able to see on an early ultrasound. Also in the works is the neural tube, which will eventually become your baby's brain and spinal cord. Right now the neural tube is open, but it will close by next week.

Week 6 Crown (head) to rump (bottom) measurements are used for babies in the first half of pregnancy because their tiny, newly forming legs are bent, making it difficult to estimate the full length of the body. How's baby measuring up this week? That crown to rump measurement has reached somewhere between ⅕- to ¼-inch (no bigger than a nail head). This week also sees the beginning of the development of your baby's jaws, cheeks, and chin. Little indentations on both sides of the head will form into ear canals. Small black dots on the face will form the eyes, and a small bump on the front of the head will turn into a button nose in a few weeks' time. Also taking shape this week: your baby's kidneys, liver, and lungs. Your baby's tiny heart is beating 110 times per minute and getting faster each day—a stat that's probably got your heart racing.

Week 7 Here's an amazing fact about your baby right now: He or she is 10,000 times bigger now than at conception—about the size of a blueberry. A lot of that growth is concentrated on the head (new brain cells are being generated at the rate of 100 cells per minute). Your baby's mouth and tongue are forming this week and so are arm and leg buds, which are beginning to sprout into paddle-like

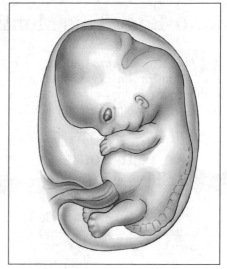

Your Baby, Month 2

appendages and to divide into hand, arm, and shoulder segments—and leg, knee, and foot segments. Also in place now are your baby's kidneys, and they're poised to begin their important work of waste management (urine production and excretion). At least you don't have to worry about dirty diapers yet!

Week 8 Your baby is growing up a storm, this week measuring about ½- to ⅔-inch, or about the size of a large raspberry. And that sweet little raspberry of yours is looking less reptilian and more human (happily), as his or her lips, nose, eyelids, legs, and back continue to take shape. And though it's still too early to hear from the outside, your baby's heart is beating at the incredible rate of 150 to 170 times per minute (that's about twice as fast as your heart beats). Something else new this week: Your baby is making spontaneous movements—twitches of the trunk and limb buds way too tiny for you to feel.

Your Body This Month

What symptoms can you expect this month? Since every pregnancy is different, you may experience all of the following symptoms, or maybe just a few. Don't be surprised if you don't feel pregnant yet, no matter what your symptoms (or lack of symptoms):

Your Body This Month

Even though you still won't look like you're pregnant to those around you, you might notice your clothes are getting a little tighter around the waist. You might also need a bigger bra now. By the end of this month, your uterus, usually the size of a fist, has grown to the size of a large grapefruit.

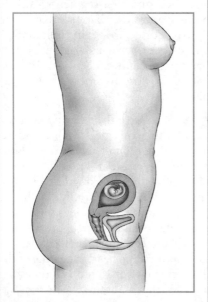

Physically

- Fatigue, lack of energy, sleepiness

- Frequent urination

- Nausea, with or without vomiting

- Excess saliva

- Constipation

- Heartburn, indigestion, flatulence, bloating

- Food aversions and cravings

- Lots of breast changes(see page 139)

- Slight whitish vaginal discharge

- Occasional headaches

- Occasional lightheadedness or dizziness

- A little rounding of your belly, your clothes feeling a little snugger

Emotionally

- Emotional ups and downs (like amped-up PMS), which may include mood swings, irritability, irrationality, crying for no apparent reason

- Joy, excitement, apprehension, doubts—any or all of these

- A sense of unreality about the pregnancy ("Is there really a baby in there?")

What You Can Expect at This Month's Checkup

If this is your first prenatal visit, see page 125. If this is your second visit, it's likely to be a much shorter one—unless you're getting a first-trimester ultrasound to date your pregnancy (see page 170). And if those initial tests have already been taken care of, you probably won't be subjected to much poking and prodding this time. You can expect your practitioner to check the following, though there may be variations, depending on your particular needs and your practitioner's style of practice:

- Weight and blood pressure
- Urine, for sugar and protein
- Hands and feet for swelling, and legs for varicose veins
- Symptoms you've been experiencing, especially unusual ones
- Questions or problems you want to discuss—have a list ready

What You May Be Wondering About

Heartburn (and Other Indigestion)

"I have heartburn all the time. Why, and what can I do about it?"

No one does heartburn like a pregnant woman does heartburn. Not only that, but you're likely to keep doing it—and doing it at least as well—throughout your whole pregnancy (unlike many early pregnancy symptoms, this one's a keeper).

So why does it feel like you have a flamethrower stationed in your chest? Early in pregnancy, your body produces large amounts of the hormones progesterone and relaxin, which tend to relax smooth muscle tissue everywhere in the body, including the gastrointestinal (GI) tract. As a result, food sometimes moves more slowly through your system, resulting in indigestion issues of all kinds, from that bloated, gassy, full feeling to heartburn. This may be uncomfortable for you, but it's actually beneficial for your baby. The digestive slowdown allows for better absorption of nutrients into your bloodstream and subsequently through the placenta and into your baby.

Heartburn occurs when the ring of muscle that separates the esophagus

Bringing Up Reflux

If you have GERD (gastroesophageal reflux disease), heartburn's nothing new, but treating it during pregnancy might be. Now that you're expecting, ask your practitioner about whether the prescription meds you're taking are still okay to take. Some are not recommended for use during pregnancy, but most are safe. Many of the tips for fighting heartburn can also help with your reflux.

Heartburn Today, Hair Tomorrow?

Feeling the burn bad? You may want to stock up on baby shampoo. Research has actually backed up what old wives have maintained for generations: On average, the more heartburn you have during pregnancy, the more likely your baby will be born with a full head of hair. Implausible as it sounds, seems that the hormones responsible for heartburn are the same ones that cause fetal hair to sprout. So pass the Tums, and the detangler.

from the stomach relaxes (like all the other smooth muscle in the GI tract), allowing food and harsh digestive juices to back up from the stomach to the esophagus. These stomach acids irritate the sensitive esophageal lining, causing a burning sensation right around where the heart is located—thus the term heartburn, though the problem has nothing to do with your heart. During the last 2 trimesters, heartburn can be compounded by your expanding uterus as it presses up on your stomach and crowds out the digestive system.

It's nearly impossible to have an indigestion-free 9 months—tummy troubles come with the pregnant territory. There are, however, some effective ways of avoiding heartburn and other indigestion most of the time, and of minimizing the misery when it strikes:

- Don't pull the triggers. If a food or drink brings on the burn (or other tummy troubles), take it off the menu for now. The most common offenders (and you're sure to know those that offend you) are spicy and highly seasoned foods, fried or fatty foods, processed meats, chocolate, coffee, carbonated beverages, and mint.

- Take it small. To avoid digestive system overload (and backup of gastric juices), opt for frequent mini-meals over 3 large squares. The 6-Meal Solution is ideal for heartburn and indigestion sufferers (see page 89).

- Take it slow. When you eat too quickly, you tend to swallow air, which can form gas pockets in your belly. And rushing through meals means you're not chewing thoroughly, which makes your stomach work harder digesting your food—and makes indigestion more likely to happen. So even when you're super hungry or in a super hurry, make an effort to eat slowly, taking small bites and chewing well (your mother would be proud).

- Don't drink and eat at the same time. Too much fluid mixed with your food distends the stomach, aggravating indigestion. So try to drink most of your fluids in between meals.

- Keep it up. It's harder for gastric juices to back up when you're vertical than when you're horizontal. To keep them where they belong (down in your stomach), avoid eating while lying down. Or lying down after eating—or eating a big meal before bed. Sleeping with your head and shoulders elevated about 6 inches can also fight the gastric backup with gravity. Another way: When picking something up, bend at the knees, not at the waist. Anytime your head dips, you're more likely to experience burn.

■ Keep it down. Your weight gain, that is. A gradual and moderate gain will minimize the amount of pressure on your digestive tract.

■ Keep it loose. Don't wear clothing that's tight around your belly or waist. A constricted tummy can add to the pressure, and the burn.

■ Pop some relief. Always keep a supply of Tums or Rolaids at popping distance (they'll also give you a healthy dose of calcium while they ease the burn), but avoid other heartburn medicines unless they've been cleared by your practitioner.

■ Chew on it. Chewing sugarless gum for a half hour after meals can reduce excess acid (increased saliva can neutralize the acid in your esophagus). Some people find that mint-flavored gum exacerbates heartburn—if so, choose a non-minty gum.

■ Add almonds. Eat a few almonds after each meal, since these tasty nuts neutralize the juices in the stomach, which may relieve or even prevent heartburn. Or soothe with a small glass of almond milk—after every meal or whenever heartburn hits (you'll get a calcium bonus). Some moms-to-be find cooling comfort in warm milk mixed with a tablespoon of honey, others find sweet relief by eating fresh, dried, or freeze-dried papaya (which scores vitamin A and C, too).

■ Relax for relief. Stress compounds all gastric upset, so learning to chill can ease that burn (see page 148). Also try some CAM approaches, such as meditation, visualization, acupuncture, biofeedback, or hypnosis (see page 78).

Food Aversions and Cravings

"Certain foods that I've always loved taste strange now. Instead, I'm having cravings for foods that I never liked. What's going on?"

The pregnancy cliché of a harried hubby running out in the middle of the night, parka over his pajamas, for a pint of ice cream and a jar of pickles to satisfy his wife's cravings has definitely played out more often in the heads of old-school sitcom writers than in real life. Cravings don't always carry pregnant women—or their spouses—that far.

Still, the majority of expectant moms find their tastes in food change somewhat in pregnancy—and some

---

FOR FATHERS

Those Crazy Cravings

Have you noticed your spouse is gagging over foods she used to love—or going gaga over foods she's never eaten before (or eaten in such peculiar combinations)? Try not to tease her about these cravings and aversions—she's as powerless to control them as you are to understand them. Instead, indulge her by keeping the offending foods out of smelling distance. (Love chicken wings? Love them somewhere else.) Surprise her with the pickle-melon-and-Swiss sandwich she suddenly can't live without. Go the extra mile—or two miles—for that pineapple pizza, and you'll both feel better.

Sympathy Symptoms

Feeling curiously . . . pregnant? Women may have a corner on the pregnancy market, but they don't have one on pregnancy symptoms. As many as half, or even more, of expectant fathers experience some degree of couvade syndrome, or "sympathetic pregnancy," while their partners are pregnant. The symptoms of couvade can mimic virtually all the normal symptoms of pregnancy, including nausea and vomiting, abdominal pain, appetite changes, bloating, weight gain, food cravings, constipation, leg cramps, dizziness, fatigue, back pain, and mood swings. Which means your partner might not be the only one in your home growing a little belly, heaving at the sight of a burger, or running to the fridge for a midnight olive orgy (or all of the above).

Any number of completely normal (if unexpected) emotions that have settled down in your psyche these days could trigger these symptoms, from sympathy (you wish you could feel her pain, and so you do), to anxiety (you're stressed about the pregnancy or about becoming a father), to jealousy (she's getting center stage and you'd like to share it). But there's more to sympathy symptoms than just sympathy (and other normal father-to-be feelings). Believe it or not, pregnancy gets a dad-to-be's hormones talking, too—stepping up his supply of estrogen (see page 222 for more).

What can you do about those sympathy symptoms (besides stop bringing home Cookies 'n Cream in the economy tubs)? Try channeling your sometimes uncomfortable feelings into productive pursuits (like cleaning out the garage or hitting the gym), applying your sympathy to cooking dinner and scrubbing the toilet, and working through those anxieties by talking them out with your spouse . . . and with friends who are already dads (or connect with dads on social media). You'll also feel less left out by becoming more involved in the pregnancy and baby prep.

Rest assured, all symptoms that don't go away during pregnancy will disappear soon after delivery, though you may find that others crop up postpartum. And don't stress out if you don't have a single sick—or queasy or achy—day during your partner's pregnancy. Not suffering from morning sickness or putting on weight doesn't mean you don't empathize and identify with your spouse or that you're not destined for nurturing—just that you've found other ways to express your feelings. Every expectant dad, like every expectant mom, is different.

find that they change a lot. Most experience a craving for at least one food (most often ice cream, though usually without the pickles), and more than half will have at least one food aversion (poultry ranks right up there, along with vegetables of all varieties). To a certain extent, these suddenly eccentric (and sometimes borderline bizarre) eating habits can be blamed on hormonal havoc, which probably explains why they're most common in the first trimester of first pregnancies, when that havoc is at its height.

Hormones, however, may not tell the whole story. The long-held theory that cravings and aversions are sensible signals from our bodies—that when we develop a distaste for something, it's usually bad for us, and when we lust after something, it's usually something we need—often does seem to stand up. Like when you suddenly can't face the morning coffee you once couldn't face your morning without. Or when a glass of your favorite wine sips like vinegar. Or when you can't gobble up enough grapefruit. On the other hand, when you call foul at the sight of chicken, or your beloved broccoli becomes bitter, or your cravings launch you into a full-fledged fudge frenzy—well, it's hard to credit your body with sending the smartest signals.

The problem is that body signals relating to food are always hard to read when hormones are involved—and may be especially tough to call now that humans have departed so far from the food chain (and now that most food chains sell junk food). Before candy was invented, for instance, a craving for something sweet might have sent a pregnant woman foraging for berries. Now it's more likely to send her foraging for M&M's.

Do you have to ignore your cravings and aversions in the name of healthy pregnancy eating? Even if that were possible (hormone-induced food quirks are a powerful force), it wouldn't be fair. Still, it's possible to respond to them while also paying attention to your baby's nutritional needs. If you crave something healthy—cottage cheese by the carton or peaches by the pound—don't feel like you have to hold back. Go for the nutritious gusto, even if it means your diet's a little unbalanced for a while (you'll make up for the variety later on in pregnancy when the cravings calm down).

If you crave something that you know you'd probably be better off without, then try to seek a substitute that speaks to the craving without throwing nutrition under the bus—or filling you up with too many empty calories (say, baked natural cheese puffs instead of the kind that turn your fingers orange). If substitutes don't fully satisfy, adding sublimation to the mix may be helpful.

When MoonPies howl your name at night, try doing something that takes your mind off them: taking a brisk walk, chatting with message board buddies, checking out maternity jeans online. And of course, completely giving in to less nutritious cravings is fine (as is enjoying them), as long as your indulgences don't regularly take the place of nutritious foods in your diet.

Most cravings and aversions disappear or weaken by the 4th month. Cravings that hang in there longer may be triggered by emotional needs—the need for a little extra attention, for example. If both you and your spouse are aware of this need, it should be easy to satisfy. Instead of requesting a middle-of-the-night pint of Chunky Monkey (with or without the sour dills), you might settle for an oatmeal cookie or two and some quiet cuddling or a romantic bath.

Some women find themselves craving, even eating, such peculiar non-food substances as clay, ashes, and paper. Because this habit, known as pica, can be dangerous and may be a sign of nutritional deficiency (particularly of iron), report it to your practitioner. Craving ice may also mean you're iron deficient, so also report any compulsion to chew ice.

Visible Veins

"I have unsightly blue lines all over my breasts and belly. Is that normal?"

Not only are these veins (which can make your chest and belly look like a road map) normal and nothing to worry about, but they are a sign that your body is doing what it should. They're part of the network of veins that has expanded to carry the increased blood supply of pregnancy, which will be nourishing your baby. They may show up earlier and be more prominent in slim or fair-skinned moms-to-be. In other expectant moms, particularly those who are dark-skinned or overweight, the veins may be less visible or not noticeable at all, or they may not become obvious until later in pregnancy.

Spider Veins

"Since I became pregnant, I've got awful-looking spidery purplish lines on my thighs. Are they varicose veins?"

They aren't pretty, but they aren't varicose veins. They are probably spider nevi, commonly dubbed "spider veins," for obvious reasons. What might prompt spider veins to spin their purplish-red web across your legs during pregnancy? First, the increased volume of blood you're carrying can create significant pressure on blood vessels, causing even tiny veins to swell and become visible. Second, pregnancy hormones can do a number on all your blood vessels, big and small. And third, genetics can predispose you to spider veins at any time in life, but especially during pregnancy (thanks, mom).

If you're destined to have spider veins, there's not much you can do to avoid them altogether, but there are ways to minimize their spread. Since your veins are as healthy as your diet is, try eating enough vitamin C foods (the body uses it to manufacture collagen and elastin, important connective tissues that help repair and maintain blood vessels). Exercising regularly (to improve circulation and leg strength) and getting into the habit of not crossing your legs (which restricts blood flow) will also help keep spider veins at bay.

Prevention didn't do the trick? Some, though far from all, spider veins fade and disappear after delivery. If they don't, they can be treated by a dermatologist—either with the injection of saline (sclerotherapy) or glycerin, or with the use of a laser. These treatments destroy the blood vessels, causing them to collapse and eventually disappear—but they're not cheap and aren't recommended during pregnancy. In the meantime, you can try camouflaging your spider veins with a flesh-toned concealer or an "airbrush" makeup for legs designed to cover all kinds of imperfections.

Varicose Veins

"My mother and grandmother both had varicose veins during pregnancy. Is there anything I can do to prevent them in my own pregnancy?"

Varicose veins run in families—and it definitely sounds like they have legs in yours. But being genetically predisposed to varicose veins doesn't mean you have to be resigned to them, which is why you're wise to be thinking now about bucking this family tradition with prevention.

Varicose veins often surface for the first time during pregnancy, and they tend to get worse in subsequent pregnancies. That's because the extra volume of blood you produce during pregnancy puts extra pressure on your blood vessels, especially the veins in your legs, which have to work against gravity to push all that extra blood back up to your heart. Add to that the pressure your ever-heavier uterus will be putting on your pelvic blood vessels and the vessel-relaxing effects of the extra hormones your body is producing, and you have the perfect recipe for varicose veins.

The symptoms of varicose veins aren't difficult to recognize, but they vary in severity. There may be a mild achiness or severe pain in the legs, or a sensation of heaviness, or swelling, or none of these. A faint outline of bluish veins may be visible, or snakelike veins may bulge from ankle to upper thigh. In severe cases, the skin overlying the veins becomes swollen, dry, and irritated. Occasionally, superficial thrombophlebitis (inflammation of a surface vein, caused by a blood clot) may develop at the site of a varicosity, so always check with your practitioner about varicose vein symptoms.

To give your legs a leg up against varicose veins:

■ Keep the blood flowing. Too much sitting or standing can compromise blood flow, so avoid long periods of either when you can—and when you can't, periodically flex your ankles. When sitting, avoid crossing your legs and elevate them if possible. When lying down, raise your legs by placing a pillow under your feet. When resting or sleeping, try to lie on your left side, the best one for optimum circulation (though either side will do).

■ Watch your weight. Excess poundage increases the demands on your already overworked circulatory system, so keep your weight gain within the recommended guidelines.

■ Avoid heavy lifting, which can make those veins bulge.

■ Push gently during bowel movements. Straining on the toilet can be a strain on the deep leg veins, so take steps to avoid constipation.

■ Wear support panty hose (light support hose seem to work well without being uncomfortable) or elastic stockings. Put them on first thing in the morning (before blood pools in your legs) and take them off at night before getting into bed. While wearing support hose probably won't contribute

to your sexiest pregnancy moment, it may help by counteracting the downward pressure of your belly and giving the veins in your legs a little extra upward push. Plus, support hose have come a long way in style and comfort since grandma's day.

■ Stay away from clothes that might restrict your circulation: tight belts or pants, panty hose and socks with elastic tops, and snug shoes. Also skip high heels, favoring flats (choose ones with good arch support), medium chunky heels, or low wedges instead.

■ Get some exercise every day (see page 229). But if you're experiencing pain, avoid high-impact cardio, jogging, cycling, and weight training.

■ Be sure your diet includes plenty of fruit and vegetables rich in vitamin C, which help keep blood vessels healthy and elastic.

Surgical removal of varicose veins isn't recommended during pregnancy, though it can certainly be considered a few months after delivery. In most cases, however, the problem will improve after delivery, usually by the time prepregnancy weight is reached.

An Achy, Swollen Pelvis

"My whole pelvic area feels achy and swollen, and really uncomfortable—and I think I felt an actual bulge in my vulva. What is that all about?"

Legs may have the market share of varicose veins, but they definitely don't have a monopoly. Varicose veins can also appear in the pelvic area (in the vulva and the vagina), on the buttocks, and in the rectum, for the same reason you might get them in your legs—and it sounds like they've made that appearance in you. Called pelvic congestion syndrome, the symptoms (in addition to bulging in the vulva) include chronic pelvic pain and/or abdominal pain, an achy, swollen, "full" feeling in the pelvic area and the genitals, and sometimes pain with or after intercourse. The tips for minimizing varicose veins in the legs will also help you (see previous question), but do be sure to check with your practitioner, both for the diagnosis and for possible treatment options (usually after delivery).

Breakouts

"My skin is breaking out the way it did when I was in middle school—not cute."

The glow of pregnancy that some women are lucky enough to radiate isn't just a result of joy, but of the stepped-up secretion of oils brought on by hormonal changes. And so, alas, are the less-than-glowing breakouts of pregnancy that some not-so-lucky expectant mamas experience (particularly those who break out like clockwork before their periods). Though such eruptions are hard to eliminate entirely, the following suggestions may help keep them at a minimum—and keep you from resembling your 8th-grade yearbook picture:

- Wash your face 2 or 3 times a day with a gentle cleanser. But don't get overaggressive with scrubs—not only because your skin is extra sensitive during pregnancy, but because over-stripped skin is actually more susceptible to breakouts.

- Get the all clear on any acne medications (topical or oral) before you use them (see page 151).

- Use an oil-free moisturizer to keep skin hydrated. Skin that's dried out by harsh acne cleansers and treatments can become more pimple prone.

- Choose skin care products and cosmetics that are oil-free and labeled "non-comedogenic," which means they won't clog pores.

- Keep everything that touches your face clean, including those blush brushes at the bottom of your makeup bag.

- Pop (and pick) not. Just like your mother always told you, popping or picking at pimples won't make them go away—and can actually make them stick around longer by pushing bacteria back down into the zit. Plus, when you're pregnant, you're more prone to infections. Poked-at pimples can also leave scars.

- Feed your face well. A diet that's low in sugar, loaded with fruits and veggies, and favors whole grains and healthy fats (think the Pregnancy Diet) may help minimize those hormonal breakout performances.

- Got bacne that just won't back off? Besides being faithful to cleanliness and healthy eating habits, ask your practitioner or a dermatologist who knows you're expecting about pregnancy-safe creams that might work (most practitioners give the okay to azelaic acid). The doc might also suggest you wash your back (or chest if that's where the pimples are popping up) with a glycolic or fruit-acid-based cleanser to help clear those angry red bumps.

Dry Skin

"My skin is really dry. Is that pregnancy related, too?"

Feeling a tad reptilian these days? You can blame your hormones for your dry, often itchy, skin. Hormonal changes can sometimes rob your skin of oil and elasticity, giving it that not-so-lovely mama alligator look. To keep your skin as soft as your baby-to-be's bottom:

- Switch to a nonsoap cleanser such as Cetaphil or Aquanil, and use it no more than once a day (at night if you're taking off makeup). Wash with just water the rest of the time.

- Slather on moisturizer while your skin is still damp (after a bath or shower), and use the moisturizer as often as you can—and definitely before you turn in for the night.

- Cut down on bathing and keep your showers short. Too much washing can dry out your skin. Make sure, too, that the water is lukewarm and not hot. Hot water removes natural oil from the skin, making it dry and itchy.

- Add unscented bath oils to your tub, but be careful with the slippery surface you've created. (Remember, as your belly grows, so will your klutz factor.)

- Drink plenty of fluids throughout the day to stay hydrated, and be sure to include good fats in your diet (those omega-3s that are so baby friendly are also skin friendly).

- Keep your home well humidified.

- Wear a sunscreen with an SPF of at least 15 (preferably 30) every day.

Eczema

"I've always been prone to eczema, but now that I'm pregnant, it's gotten much worse. What can I do?"

Unfortunately, pregnancy (or more accurately, its hormones) often exacerbates the symptoms of eczema, and for women who suffer from this skin condition, the itching and scaling can become practically unbearable. (Some lucky eczema sufferers find that pregnancy actually causes the eczema to go into remission.)

Fortunately, low-dose hydrocortisone creams and ointments are safe to use during pregnancy in moderate amounts—ask your practitioner or dermatologist for a recommendation. Antihistamines may also be helpful in coping with the itchiness, but again, be sure to check with your practitioner first. Most other options are off the table now that you're expecting. For instance, cyclosporine, long used on severe cases of eczema that don't respond to other treatment, is generally not prescribed during pregnancy. Nonsteroidals Protopic and Elidel aren't recommended either, because they haven't been studied in pregnancy and can't be ruled safe until more is known. Finally, some topical and systemic antibiotics may be shelved during pregnancy, so get your practitioner's clearance on those, too, before using.

If you're an eczema sufferer, you know that prevention can go a long way in keeping the itch away. Try the following:

- Use a cold compress—not your fingernails—to curb the itch. Scratching makes the condition worse and can puncture the skin, allowing bacteria to enter and cause an infection. Keep nails short and rounded to decrease the chance that you'll puncture your skin when you do scratch.

- Limit contact with potential irritants such as household cleaners, soaps, perfumes, and fruit juices. Wear gloves to protect your hands when cooking and cleaning.

- Moisturize early and often (while skin is still damp, if you're just out of the water) to lock in the skin's own moisture.

- Limit time in the water (especially very warm water).

- Try not to get too hot or sweaty. Of course that's easier said than done when you're pregnant and already one hot, sweaty mama. Stay cool by wearing loose cotton clothes and avoiding synthetic fabrics, wool, or any scratchy material. Avoid overheating by favoring that layered look—and peeling off layers as you start to warm up.

- Try to keep your cool, too, when it comes to stress—a common eczema trigger. When you feel anxiety creeping in, take some relaxation breaths (see page 148).

- Seek alternatives. Acupuncture may work to decrease nerve pain and moderate the itch, and it also helps relieve stress.

- Do a diet check. If you're allergic to a certain food (or suspect you are), cut it out to see if that helps curb your eczema. Though diet seems to have less effect on eczema than internet legend would have you believe, it's worth asking your dermatologist whether a change in what you're eating might help. Ask, too, about adding probiotics to your diet. While studies haven't yet shown that probiotics help ease a

mom's eczema, they may help reduce the chances that your baby-to-be will develop eczema later on. Vitamin D supplementation, though still a bit controversial, has shown some promise as a treatment for eczema, but check with your practitioner first.

Something to keep in mind: Though eczema is hereditary (meaning that your baby has a chance of having it, too), research suggests that breastfeeding may prevent eczema from developing in a child. That's just one more good reason to opt for breastfeeding if you can.

Come-and-Go Belly

"It's the strangest thing—one day it'll look like I'm showing, and the next day my belly will be completely flat again. What's up with that?"

What's up are your bowels, actually. Bowel distension (the result of constipation and excess gas, two of a newly pregnant woman's constant companions) can make a flat belly round in no time flat. And just as quickly as it appeared, your belly can disappear—once you've had a bowel movement,

---

A Pregnant Pose

Maybe you've been dodging the camera lately ("no need to put yet another 10 pounds on me"). Still, you might consider preserving your pregnancy bump for posterity. Sure, you don't have much to show for pregnancy yet (if anything). But taking bump shots right from the start means you'll have plenty to show for it later. Snap them daily, weekly, or monthly—selfie-style in the mirror or with the help of a friend, bump bared or wearing something form-fitting. Then compile your photos in a pregnancy album or custom photo book, post them online for easy viewing by family and friends, or turn them into a video to track your amazing pregnancy story. Lights, camera . . . baby!

Belly Piercings

It's cool, it's stylish, it's sexy—and it's one of the cutest ways to show off a flat, toned tummy. But once your belly starts to bulge, will you have to remove your belly piercing? Nope—not as long as your belly piercing is healed (read: Your trip to the Piercing Pavilion wasn't last month) and healthy (in other words, not red, weeping, or inflamed). Remember, your belly button marks where you connected to your own mom in the womb, not where your baby connects to you—which means a piercing won't provide a path for pathogens to reach your baby. You also don't have to worry about a belly ring interfering with birth, or even a cesarean delivery.

Of course, as your pregnancy progresses and your tummy starts to jut out in earnest, you may find that your belly bar or belly ring becomes too uncomfortable to wear, thanks to your stretched-to-the-limit skin. The belly ring might also start to rub—and even get caught on—your clothing, especially when your belly button "pops" out later in pregnancy. And that rubbing can hurt, big time.

If you do decide to take out the jewelry entirely, just run your belly ring through the hole every few days to keep the piercing from closing up shop (unless you've had it for a number of years, in which case the likelihood that the hole will close is pretty slim). Or consider replacing your bar or ring with a flexible belly bar made of Teflon or PTFE (polytetrafluoroethylene).

As for getting your belly (or anywhere else on your body) pierced during pregnancy: better to hold off until after delivery. It's never a good idea to puncture the skin unnecessarily during pregnancy, because it ups the chances of infection.

Too late—you already commemorated your pregnancy with a fresh piercing, or you pierced just before finding out you were expecting? If the area is not healed yet (it's still red), it's probably best to take the piercing out and repierce after delivery. Not only because of the increased risk of infection, but because the stretching of your belly can stretch a still unhealed hole, leaving it much larger than you'd probably like it to be (as in gaping).

---

that is. A little unnerving, yes ("But I looked pregnant just yesterday!"), but completely normal.

Don't worry. Pretty soon you'll have a belly that doesn't come and go—and that's more baby than bowel. In the meantime, see page 185 for tips on fighting constipation.

Losing Your Shape

"Will I ever get my body back after I have a baby?"

Well, that kind of depends . . . on you. Studies show that 25 percent of all moms of 2- to 3-year-olds are still hanging on to 10-plus pounds of their pregnancy weight. And most new moms find that even if they've gotten close to their prepregnancy weight, their tummy (and hips, and butt) aren't exactly the same after pregnancy. But now's not the time to worry about what'll happen after pregnancy. Focus instead on gaining the right amount of weight, at the right rate, on the right foods. Not only will that enable you to

First-Trimester Ultrasound

You certainly won't be able to make out any adorable baby features yet (or find out whether you're boarding a boy or a girl), but you're still probably pretty excited to know that early ultrasounds (at about 6 to 9 weeks) have become a routine part of prenatal care, allowing eager parents a welcome first glimpse of their still teeny baby bean. In fact, ACOG recommends that all moms-to-be receive an early ultrasound. The top reason why: Combined with the LMP, measurement of the embryo or fetus during early pregnancy is the most accurate way to date a pregnancy (after the first trimester, ultrasound measurements of the fetus are less accurate). An early ultrasound is also used to visualize a heartbeat, as well as to confirm that the pregnancy is taking place where it's supposed to, in the uterus (and to rule out an ectopic, or tubular, pregnancy). And if you're carrying twins (or more), an early ultrasound will issue that double baby bulletin sooner.

How does ultrasound get a picture of life inside your uterus? Through sound waves, emitted by a transducer wand, which bounce off structures (your baby, the gestational sac, and so on) to produce an image that can be viewed on a video screen. If you're getting an ultrasound before week 6 or 7, it's likely you'll have a transvaginal one.

In a transvaginal ultrasound, a long, narrow transducer wand (covered first with a condom-like cover and sterile lubricant) is inserted into the vagina. The practitioner will gently move the wand within the vaginal canal to scan your uterus, allowing for an extra early view of your baby. After week 6 or 7, you'll probably be a candidate for the transabdominal version. For a transabdominal early ultrasound, your bladder must be full (which isn't fun) so the still-small uterus can be seen more easily. Gel (some practitioners warm it up first, otherwise it's chilly) is spread on your abdomen, and then the transducer wand is rubbed over it.

Both procedures can last from 5 to 30 minutes and are painless, except for the discomfort of the full bladder necessary for the first-trimester transabdominal exam, and possibly the discomfort of the vaginal transducer. You'll be able to watch along with your practitioner (though you'll likely need help figuring out what you're seeing), and probably take home a small printout as a souvenir.

While most practitioners will wait until at least 6 weeks to order an early ultrasound, it's possible to see a gestational sac as early as 4½ weeks after a last menstrual period and a heartbeat as early as 5 to 6 weeks (though it isn't always detected that early).

keep your eyes on the real prize—the healthy nourishment of your baby—but it'll also increase your chances of recovering your prepregnancy shape (and even bettering it) once baby is born. Want to up the odds even more? Team your sensible eating efforts with pregnancy-approved exercise, and try as best you can to keep up your regimen after your baby arrives. Mind you, that

recovery won't happen overnight (think 3 months as the best-case scenario, 6 months a more realistic one, and longer than that a real possibility).

Difficulty Urinating

"The last few days it's been really hard to pee, even though my bladder seems very full."

What's a Corpus Luteum Cyst?

If your practitioner said that your ultrasound shows you have a corpus luteum cyst, your first question will probably be—what is it? Well, here's all you need to know. Every month of your reproductive life, a small, yellowish body of cells forms after you ovulate. Called a corpus luteum (literally "yellow body"), it occupies the space in the follicle formerly occupied by the egg. The corpus luteum produces progesterone and some estrogen, and it is programmed by nature to disintegrate in about 14 days. When it does, diminishing hormone levels trigger your period. When you become pregnant, the corpus luteum hangs around instead of disintegrating, continuing to grow and produce enough hormones to nourish and support your baby-to-be until the placenta takes over. In most pregnancies, the corpus luteum starts to shrink around 6 or 7 weeks after the LMP and stops functioning altogether at about 10 weeks, when its work

of providing board for baby is done. But in about 10 percent of pregnancies, the corpus luteum doesn't regress when it's supposed to. Instead, it develops into a corpus luteum cyst.

So now that you know what a corpus luteum cyst is, you're probably wondering—how will it affect my pregnancy? The answer: It probably won't at all. The cyst is usually nothing to worry about—or do anything about. Chances are, it will go away by itself in the second trimester. But just to be sure, your practitioner will keep an eye on its size and condition regularly via ultrasound (which means you get extra peeks at your baby). Some moms-to-be report an ovulation-like pinching sensation on one side of their lower abdomen early in pregnancy that may be related to the corpus luteum or to a corpus luteum cyst. Again, nothing to worry about, but mention it to your practitioner for reassurance.

Sounds like your bladder may be under pressure—from your uterus. About 1 in 5 women have a tilted (aka retroverted) uterus, one that tilts toward the back instead of the front. When it refuses to right itself, a tilted uterus can press on the urethra, the tube leading from the bladder. The pressure of this ever-heavier load can make it feel hard to pee. Urine may also leak when the bladder becomes very overloaded.

In nearly all cases, the uterus shifts itself back into position by the end of the first trimester without any medical intervention. But if you're really uncomfortable now—or if you're finding it especially difficult to urinate—put in a call to your practitioner. He or she might be able to manipulate your uterus by hand to move it off the urethra so

you can pee easily again. Most of the time that works. In the unlikely event that it doesn't, catheterization (removing the urine through a tube) may become necessary.

One other possibility if you're having trouble peeing (and another good reason to put in that call to your practitioner): a UTI (urinary tract infection). See page 528 for more.

Mood Swings

"I know I should feel happy about my pregnancy—and sometimes I am. But other times, I feel so weepy and sad."

They're up—and they're down. The very normal mood swings of pregnancy can take your emotions places

Rolling with Her Mood Swings

Welcome to the wonderful—and sometimes wacky—world of pregnancy hormones. Wonderful because they're working hard to nurture the tiny life that's taken up residence inside your partner's belly (and that you'll soon be cuddling in your arms). Wacky because, in addition to taking control of her body (and often making her miserable), they're also taking control of her mind—making her weepy, over-the-top excited, disproportionately pissed, deliriously happy, and stressed out . . . and that's all before lunch.

Not surprisingly, an expectant mom's mood swings are usually the most pronounced during the first trimester when those pregnancy hormones are in their greatest state of flux (and when she's just getting used to them). But even once the hormones have settled down in the second and third trimesters, you can still expect to be riding the emotional roller coaster with your partner, which will continue to take her to emotional highs and lows (and fuel those occasional outbursts) right up until delivery, and beyond.

So what's an expectant dad to do? Here are some suggestions:

Be patient. Pregnancy won't last forever (though there will be times in the 9th month where you both may wonder if it will). This, too, shall pass, and it'll pass a lot more pleasantly if you're patient. In the meantime, try to keep your perspective—and do whatever you can to channel your inner saint.

Don't take her outbursts personally. And don't hold them against her. They are, after all, completely out of her control. Remember, it's the hormones talking—and crying for no apparent reason. Avoid pointing out her moods, too. Though she's powerless to control them, she's also probably all too aware of them. And chances are, she's no happier about them than you are. It's no picnic being pregnant.

Help slow down the swings. Since low blood sugar can send her mood swinging, offer her a snack when she's starting to droop (a plate of crackers and cheese, a fruit-and-yogurt smoothie). Exercise can release those feel-good endorphins she's in need of now, so suggest a before- or after-dinner walk (also a good time to let her vent fears and anxieties that might be dragging her down).

Go the extra yard. That is, go to the laundry room, to her favorite takeout on the way home from work, to the supermarket on Saturday, to the dishwasher to unload . . . you get the picture. Not only will she appreciate the efforts you make—without being asked—but you'll appreciate her happier mood.

they've never gone before, both to exhilarating highs and depressing lows. Moods that can have you over-the-moon one moment, down-in-the-dumps the next—and weeping inexplicably over insurance commercials in between. Can you blame it on your hormones? You bet. These swings may be more pronounced in the first trimester (when hormonal havoc is at its peak) and, in general, in women who ordinarily experience emotional ups and downs before their periods (it's sort of like PMS pumped up). Feelings of ambivalence about the pregnancy once it's confirmed are common even when a pregnancy is planned, and may exaggerate the swings still more. Not to mention all those changes you're experiencing (the physical ones, the emotional ones, the logistical ones, the relationship ones—all of which can overwhelm your moods).

Mood swings tend to moderate somewhat after the first trimester, once hormone levels calm down a little—and once you've adjusted to some of those pregnancy changes (you'll never adjust to all of them). In the meantime, though there's no sure way to hop off that emotional roller coaster, there are several ways to minimize the mood mayhem:

- Keep your blood sugar up. What does blood sugar have to do with moods? A lot. Dips in blood sugar—caused by long stretches between meals—can lead to mood crashes. Yet another compelling reason to ditch your usual 3-meals-a-day (or fewer) eating routine and switch to the 6-Meal Solution (see page 89). Keep complex carbs and protein in starring roles in your mini-meals so that your blood sugar—and mood—stay stable.

- Keep dietary sugar and caffeine consumption down. That candy bar, that giant cookie, that Coke will give your blood sugar a quick spike—followed soon after by a downward spiral that can take your mood down with it. Caffeine (especially when it's combined with sugar, as in that Mocha Iced Blended) can have the same effect, adding to mood instability. So limit both, for happier results.

- Eat well. In general, eating well will help you feel your best emotionally (as well as physically), so follow the Pregnancy Diet as best you can. Getting plenty of omega-3 fatty acids in your diet (from walnuts, fish, grass-fed beef, and enriched eggs, to name a few foods) may also help with mood

moderating—plus, they're also super-important for your baby's brain development. Studies have shown that a daily dose of dark chocolate can also help boost your mood.

- Get a move on. The more you move, the better your mood. That's because exercise releases feel-good endorphins, which can send your spirits soaring. Build practitioner-approved exercise into your day—every day.

- Get a groove on. If you're in the mood for love (and not too busy puking), sex can turn that frown upside down by releasing happy hormones. It can also bring you closer to your partner at a time when your relationship may be facing new challenges. If sex isn't in the cards—or sexy isn't what you're feeling at the moment—the power of touch in any form (cuddling, hugging, holding hands) can help boost your mood.

- Light up your life. Research has shown that sunlight can actually lighten your moods. When the sun's shining, try catching some daily rays (just don't forget to apply sunscreen first).

- Talk about it. Worried? Anxious? Feeling unsettled? Unsure? Pregnancy is a time of many mixed emotions, which play out in mood swings. Venting some of those feelings—to your spouse (who's probably feeling plenty of the same things), to friends who can relate, to other expectant moms on the WhatToExpect.com message boards—can help you feel better, or at least help you see that what you're feeling is normal. On the other hand, if you're finding that too much message board surfing makes waves with your emotions (you're always worrying about having what she's having—or not having what she's having—symptom-wise), consider taking a board break.

- Rest up. Fatigue can exacerbate normal pregnancy mood swings, so make sure you're getting enough sleep (but not too much, since that can actually increase emotional instability).

- Learn to relax. Stress can definitely take your moods down, so find ways of moderating it or coping with it better. See page 145 for tips.

If there's one person in your life who is more affected—and bewildered—by your mood swings than you are, it's probably your partner. It'll help for him to understand why you're acting the way you are these days (that surges of pregnancy hormones are holding your emotions hostage), but it'll also help for him to know exactly how he can help you. So tell him what you need (more help around the house? a night out at your favorite restaurant?) and what you don't need (hearing that your rear's looking a little wide . . . or seeing a trail of socks and underwear down the hallway) right now, what makes you feel better, and what makes you feel worse. And be specific: Even the most loving spouse isn't a mind reader.

Pregnancy Depression

"I expected some mood swings with pregnancy, but I'm not just a little down—I'm depressed all the time."

Every expectant mom has her ups and downs, and that's normal. But if your lows are consistent or frequent, you may be among the 10 to 15 percent of women who battle mild to moderate depression during pregnancy—and that's not something to write off as part of the pregnancy package.

True depression shows up in a variety of symptoms, both emotional and physical, that go well beyond standard moms-to-be moodiness. These can include feeling sad, empty, hopeless, and emotionally lethargic, having sleep disturbances (you feel like sleeping all the time, or you can't sleep at all), having a change in eating habits (you don't feel like eating at all, or you're eating all the time), feeling fatigued and lacking energy (above what's normal in pregnancy) and/or feeling agitated or restless, losing interest in work, friends, family, and activities you usually enjoy, losing concentration and focus, having exaggerated mood swings (more dramatic than what's normal in pregnancy), and even having self-destructive thoughts. There may also be unexplained aches and pains.

Having had mood disorders in the past or having a family history of mood disorders can increase your chances of depression during pregnancy. Other factors can contribute, too, including stress (financial, relationship, work, or family), lack of emotional support, anxiety over your health or baby's (especially if you've had complications or pregnancy losses in the past), or having pregnancy symptoms that are severe or complications that require lots of extra medical screening, hospitalization, or bed rest.

If you believe that what you're experiencing is depression (or even if you think you might be), start by trying those tips for dealing with mood swings listed in the previous question. If mild to moderate symptoms continue for longer than 2 weeks, speak to your practitioner about treatment options or ask for a referral to a therapist. (Don't wait to call if the symptoms are more serious—for instance, you're unable to function or care for yourself and your baby, or you're having thoughts about harming yourself.) Since thyroid conditions—which are fairly common and can be easily treated—can trigger depression, a thyroid panel may be

Panic Attacks

Pregnancy can be a time of high anxiety, especially for those who are expecting for the first time (and consequently don't know what to expect). And a certain amount of worry is normal, and probably unavoidable. But what about when that worry turns to panic?

If you've had panic attacks in the past, you're probably all too aware of the symptoms (and most women who have panic attacks during pregnancy have had them before). They're characterized by intense fear or discomfort accompanied by an accelerated heart rate, sweating, trembling, shortness of breath, feeling of choking, chest pain, nausea or abdominal distress, dizziness, numbness or tingling, or chills or hot flashes that appear seemingly out of the blue. They can be incredibly unsettling, of course, particularly when they strike for the first time during pregnancy. But happily, though they definitely affect you, there is no reason to believe that panic attacks affect the development of your baby in any way.

Still, if you do experience such an attack, tell your practitioner. Therapy is always the first choice during pregnancy (and other times, too). But if medications are necessary to ensure your wellbeing (and your baby's—if anxiety is keeping you from eating or sleeping or otherwise taking care of your precious cargo), your practitioner, together with a qualified therapist, can work with you to decide which medication offers the most benefits for the fewest risks (and how low a dose you can take and still derive those benefits). If you've been on a medication for panic attacks, anxiety, or depression prepregnancy, a change or an adjustment of dose might be necessary, too.

While medication is one solution to extreme anxiety, it certainly isn't the only one. There are many nondrug alternatives that can be used instead of or in conjunction with traditional therapy. These include eating well and regularly (including plenty of omega-3 fatty acids and some dark chocolate in your diet may be especially helpful), avoiding too much sugar and caffeine (caffeine, in particular, can trigger anxiety), getting regular exercise, and learning meditation and other relaxation techniques (prenatal yoga can be incredibly calming, and can teach you the kind of deep breathing that can alleviate anxiety). Talking your anxieties over with your partner and/or with other expectant moms can also generate relief.

done to rule that out first (ask for one if it's not offered).

Getting the right help, and getting it promptly, is important—not only for your sake, but for your baby's. Depression can keep you from taking optimum care of yourself and your baby, now and after delivery. In fact, depression during pregnancy can increase risks for complications—much as depression can adversely affect your health when you're not pregnant. Continued extreme emotional stress can also negatively impact baby's growth and development.

Happily, there are plenty of effective strategies for treating pregnancy depression. Finding the right treatment (or combination of treatments) can help you feel better, so you can begin enjoying your pregnancy. Options include:

- Supportive therapy. Every treatment plan for depression should include regular visits with an experienced

Your Pregnancy Mood Swings

Dads-to-be share a lot more than an expected bundle of joy with their partners. In fact, long before that bundle arrives, you may share in many of the symptoms, including pregnancy mood slumps—which are surprisingly common in expectant dads. Fluctuations in your hormones can play a role (yes, your hormones are talking, too), but feelings factor in as well. Just about every dad-to-be (like most moms-to-be) experiences a host of conflicted (but completely normal) feelings in the months leading up to one of life's most major changes—from anxiety to fear to ambivalence to a crumbling of confidence. No wonder your moods can take a hit.

But you can help boost your pregnancy mood—and perhaps prevent the postpartum blues, which about 10 percent of new dads find themselves experiencing. Check out the suggestions on page 173 and try:

- Talking. Let your feelings out so they don't bring you down. Share them with your partner (and let her share hers, too), making communication a daily ritual. Talk them over with a friend who recently became a father (no one will get it like he will). Or find an outlet through dad social media.

- Moving. Nothing gets your mood up like getting your pulse up. A workout won't only help you work out your feelings, but those feel-good endorphins can give your mood a long-lasting boost.

- Getting baby-busy. Gear up for the anticipated arrival by pitching in with all the baby gear gathering and other baby prep that's likely going on. You may find that getting in the baby spirit helps give your spirits a boost.

- Cutting out (or cutting down). Drinking a lot can swing your moods even lower. Though alcohol has a reputation for being a mood booster, it's technically a depressant, so there's a reason why the morning after is never as happy as the night before. Plus, it's a coping mechanism that covers up the feelings you're trying to cope with. Ditto with drugs.

- Eating well. Like with the mama-to-be in your life, eating well and keeping your blood sugar on an even keel can help moderate mood swings. Focus on lean protein and complex carbs instead of getting pumped up with sugar and caffeine, which can crash your blood sugar, bringing your mood with it.

Remember, there's a difference between pregnancy mood swings and actual depression during pregnancy—and that goes for both expectant moms and dads. True depression can be physically and emotionally debilitating: It can wear on relationships, impact eating, sleeping, normal functioning, your work and your social life, and keep you from enjoying what should be (and can be!) an exciting, joyful life change. But research shows that a father's depression can ultimately affect his baby's wellbeing, too. So don't wait. If you're having symptoms of depression (especially if you're also have feelings of rage or violent thoughts) seek professional help from your physician or therapist right away.

therapist—and it's always the first-line treatment for mild to moderate pregnancy depression. No matter what's triggering your depression, therapy can help you sort through and deal with the feelings you're having and help you cope with them. Under the ACA, most insurance plans should offer some level of coverage for mental health therapy, though it varies widely, depending on your state and insurance.

- Medication. Deciding whether therapy is enough or whether antidepressant medication will be part of the treatment plan (and which one to use) will require consulting with both your practitioner and your therapist to weigh possible risks against possible benefits (see page 45).

- CAM therapies. Meditation (and other relaxation techniques), yoga, acupuncture, music therapy—these are just some of the CAM therapies that can help relieve symptoms of depression safely. Bright light therapy can also be surprisingly effective in reducing symptoms of pregnancy depression by increasing levels of serotonin, the mood-regulating hormone in the brain, and it's safe and simple: All you do is sit about 2 feet away from a special full-spectrum bright light—one that's 20 times brighter than normal room lighting—for 10 to 45 minutes a day, depending on your response. Don't, however, turn to herbal supplements touted for their mood-boosting properties (such as SAM-e and St. John's wort) without your practitioner's approval—they haven't been studied enough to consider them safe for pregnancy use.

- Exercise. Besides being good for your body and health, exercise has been shown to be a potent mood booster, releasing feel-good endorphins.

- Healthy eating. It probably won't be the first line of treatment for depression, but eating foods rich in omega-3 fatty acids (see page 98 for a list) may help ease pregnancy depression and possibly postpartum depression, too. And since those foods are baby-healthy anyway, it definitely couldn't hurt to try adding them to the mood-boosting mix. You can also ask your practitioner about taking a pregnancy-safe omega-3 supplement. Eating dark chocolate (the higher the cocoa content, the better) may help boost mood and reduce anxiety, too.

Being depressed during pregnancy does somewhat increase the chances of postpartum depression (PPD). But the happy news is that getting the right treatment during pregnancy—and/ or right after delivery—can help prevent PPD. Some doctors prescribe low doses of antidepressants to women with a history of depression as a preventive measure starting during the second trimester, while others recommend that women who are at high risk take antidepressants right after delivery to prevent PPD. Ask your practitioner about this.

ALL ABOUT:
Weight Gain During Pregnancy

Maybe you've been looking forward to putting pounds on after years of dieting to take them off (or at least, keep them from piling on). Maybe you've been dreading watching the numbers on the scale creep up for the same reason. Either way, for most moms-to-be weight gain isn't only a reality during pregnancy, it's a necessity. Gaining the right amount of weight, in fact, is vital when you're growing a baby.

But what is the right amount of weight? How much is too much? How much is too little? How fast should you gain it all? And will you be able to lose it all (or most of it) after delivery? Short answer to that last question: yes—if you gain the right amount of weight at the right rate on the right type of foods.

How Much Should You Gain?

If there were ever a legitimate reason to pile on the pounds, pregnancy is it. After all, when you grow a baby, you've got to do some growing, too. But piling on too many pounds can spell problems for you, your baby, and your pregnancy. Ditto if you accumulate too few.

What's the perfect pregnancy weight gain formula? Actually, since every pregnant woman—and every pregnant body—is different, that formula can vary a lot. Just how many pounds you should aim to add during your 40 weeks of baby growing will depend on how many pounds you were packing before you became pregnant.

Your practitioner will recommend the weight gain target that's right for you and your pregnancy profile—and that's the guideline to follow, no matter what you read here. But in general, weight gain recommendations are based on your prepregnancy BMI, or body mass index. Your BMI (essentially, your body fat level) is calculated by multiplying your weight in pounds by 703, then dividing by your height in inches squared—but it's much easier to skip the math and do the calculations on a BMI app. You can search "adult BMI calculator" at cdc.gov, or use the chart in *What to Expect: Eating Well When You're Expecting*:

- If your BMI is average (between 18.5 and 25), you'll probably be advised to gain between 25 and 35 pounds, the standard recommendation for the average-weight pregnant woman.

- If you start out your pregnancy overweight (BMI between 25 and 30),

---

Why More (or Less) Weight Gain Isn't More

What do you have to lose by gaining too much weight when you're expecting? Packing on too many pounds can present a variety of problems in your pregnancy. More padding can make assessing and measuring your baby more difficult, and added pounds can add to pregnancy discomforts (from backache and varicose veins to fatigue and heartburn). Gaining too much weight can also increase the risk of preterm labor, of developing gestational diabetes or pregnancy-induced hypertension, of ending up with an oversize baby who's difficult or even impossible to deliver vaginally, of complications after a cesarean delivery, of a host of problems for your newborn, and of having more trouble with breastfeeding. Not surprisingly, too, those extra pounds may be extra hard to shed postpartum—and in fact, many women who gain too much weight during pregnancy end up never shedding them all.

Gaining too little weight can also be a losing proposition during pregnancy. Babies whose moms gain less than 20 pounds are more likely to be premature, small for their gestational age, and suffer growth restriction in the uterus. (The exception: obese women, who can safely gain 11 to 20 pounds or less.)

Breaking Down the Weight Gain

Baby	7½ pounds
Placenta	1½ pounds
Amniotic fluid	2 pounds
Uterine enlargement	2 pounds
Mom's breast tissue	2 pounds
Mom's blood volume	4 pounds
Fluids in mom's tissue	4 pounds
Mom's fat stores	7 pounds
Total average	30 pounds overall weight gain

(All weights are approximate)

your goal will be somewhat scaled back—to somewhere between 15 and 25 pounds.

- If you're obese (with a BMI greater than 30), you may be told to hold your total to between 11 and 20 pounds, or perhaps even less than that.

- Are you super skinny (with a BMI of less than 18.5)? Chances are, your target will be higher than average—upward of 28 to 40 pounds.

- Carrying multiples? For moms providing room and board for more than one, extra babies will require extra pounds; see page 446.

It's one thing to set an ideal weight gain goal . . . it's another thing to get there. That's because ideals aren't always completely compatible with reality. Piling on the right number of pounds isn't just about piling the right amount of food on your plate. There are other factors at work, too. Your metabolism, your genes, your level of activity,

your pregnancy symptoms (the heartburn and nausea that make eating too much like hard work, or those cravings for high-calorie foods that make gaining too much too easy)—all play a role in helping you pack on (or in keeping you from packing on) the perfect pregnancy poundage. With that in mind, keep an eye on the scale to ensure that you're reaching your weight gain target.

At What Rate Should You Gain?

Slow and steady doesn't only win the race—it's a winner when it comes to pregnancy weight gain, too. A gradual weight gain is best for your body and your baby's body. In fact, the rate at which weight is gained is as important as the total number of pounds you gain. That's because your baby needs a steady supply of nutrients and calories during his or her stay in your womb—shipments that come in fits and spurts won't cut it once your little one starts

Weight Gain Red Flags

If you experience sudden, rapid weight gain in the second and third trimester, especially if it's accompanied by severe swelling in the legs and feet or puffiness of the face and hands, check with your practitioner. Check, too, if you gain no weight for more than 2 weeks in a row during the 4th to 8th months (unless you're obese and your practitioner has you on a slowed-down weight gain schedule).

doing some significant growing (as will happen during the second and third trimesters). A well-paced weight gain will also do your body good, allowing it to gradually adjust to the increased poundage (and the physical strains that come with it). Gradual gain also allows for gradual skin stretching (think fewer stretch marks). Need more convincing? Pounds put on at a slow and steady rate will come off more easily when the time comes (after you've delivered and you're eager to get back to your prepregnancy shape . . . and into those prepregnancy jeans).

Does steady mean spreading out those 30 pounds or so evenly over 40 weeks? No—even if that were a possible plan, it wouldn't be the best one. Here's how it breaks down trimester by trimester:

- During the first trimester, your baby is tiny, which means that eating for two doesn't require extra eating at all, and only a minimum of weight gain, if any. A good goal for trimester 1 is between 2 and 4 pounds—though many women don't end up gaining any at all or even lose a few (thanks

to nausea and vomiting), and some gain somewhat more (often because their queasiness is comforted only by starchy, high-calorie foods), and that's fine, too. For those who start slowly, it should be easy to play weight gain catch-up during the next 6 months (especially once food starts tasting and smelling good again). For those who begin gangbusters, watching the scale a little more closely in the second and third trimester will keep their total close to target.

- During the second trimester, your baby's getting bigger, which means your weight gain quota will grow, too—picking up to an average rate of about 1 to 1½ pounds per week during months 4 through 6 (totaling 12 to 14 pounds).

- During the third (and last!) trimester, baby's weight gain will pick up steam, but yours may start to taper off to about a pound a week (for a net gain of about 8 to 10 pounds). Some women find their weight holding steady—or even dropping a pound or two—during the 9th month when ever-tighter abdominal quarters can make finding room for food a struggle. A couple of pounds may also be shed once prelabor kicks in.

How closely will you be able to follow this rate-of-gain formula? Realistically, not that closely. There will be weeks when your appetite will rule and your self-control will waver, and it'll be a rocky road (by the half gallon) to your weight gain total. And there will be weeks when eating will seem too much of an effort (especially when tummy troubles send whatever you eat right back up). Not to worry or stress over the scale. As long as your overall gain is on target and your rate averages out to that model formula (a ½ pound one week, 2 pounds the next, 1 the following, and so on), you're right on track.

So for best weight gain results, keep your eye on the scale, since what you don't know can throw your weight gain way off target. Weigh yourself (at the same time of day, wearing the same amount of clothes, on the same scale) once a week—more often and you'll drive yourself crazy with day-to-day fluid fluctuations. If once a week is too much (because you're scale-phobic), twice a month should do the trick. Waiting until your monthly prenatal checkup to check out your weight is fine, too—though keep in mind that a lot can happen in a month (as in 10 pounds) or not happen (as in no pounds), making it harder for you to stay on track.

If you find that your weight gain has crept up higher and faster than you'd planned (for instance, you gained 14 pounds in the first trimester instead of 3 or 4, or you packed on 20 pounds in the second instead of 12), talk it over with your practitioner and discuss a strategy. It'll probably make sense to take action to see that the gain gets back on a sensible track, but not to stop it in its tracks. Dieting to lose weight is never appropriate when you're pregnant, and neither is using appetite-suppressing drinks or pills (these can actually be very dangerous). Instead, with your practitioner's help, readjust your goal to include the excess you've already gained and to accommodate the weight you still have to gain.

CHAPTER 7

The Third Month

Approximately 9 to 13 Weeks

As you enter the last month of your first trimester (that's something to celebrate), many of those early pregnancy symptoms are probably still going strong (and that's nothing to celebrate). Which means it's probably hard to tell whether you're exhausted because of first-trimester fatigue—or because you woke up 3 times last night to go to the bathroom (it's likely a little of both). But chin up, if you have the strength to lift it. There are better days ahead. If morning sickness has had you—and your appetite—down, there's a less queasy day soon to dawn. As energy levels pick up, you'll soon have more get-up-and-go—and as urinary urges ease, you may have to get up and go less often. Even better, you may hear the amazing sound of your baby's heartbeat with a Doppler at this month's checkup, which might make all those uncomfortable symptoms seem much more worthwhile.

Your Baby This Month

Week 9 Your baby has grown to approximately 1 inch in length, about the size of a medium green olive. The head is continuing to develop and take on more babylike proportions. This week, tiny muscles are starting to form. This will allow your fetus to move his or her arms and legs, though it'll be at least another month or two before you'll be able to feel those little punches and kicks. While it's way too early to feel anything, it's not too early to hear something (possibly). The awesome sound of your baby's heartbeat might be audible via a Doppler device at your practitioner's office. Take a listen—that thump-thump is sure to make your heart beat a little faster.

Week 10 At nearly 1½ inches long (about the size of a prune), your baby—who has officially graduated now from embryo to fetus—is growing by leaps and bounds. And in gearing up for those first leaps and bounds (and baby steps), bones and cartilage are forming—and small indentations on the legs are developing into knees and ankles. Even more unbelievably for someone the size of a prune, the elbows on baby's arms are already working. Tiny buds of baby teeth are forming under the gums. Farther down, the stomach is producing digestive juices, the kidneys are producing larger quantities of urine, and, if your baby's a boy, his testes are producing testosterone (boys will be boys—even this early on).

Week 11 Your baby is just over 1½ inches long now and weighs about ¼ of an ounce. Baby's body is straightening out and the torso is lengthening. Hair follicles are forming, and fingernail and toenail beds are beginning to develop (nails will actually start to grow within the next few weeks). Those nails are forming on individual fingers and toes, having separated recently from the webbed hands and feet of just a few weeks ago. And though you can't tell baby's sex by looking yet (even with an ultrasound), ovaries are developing if it's a girl. What you would be able to see, if your womb had a view, is that your fetus has distinct human characteristics by now, with hands and feet in the front of the body, ears nearly in their final shape (if not final location), open nasal passages on the tip of the nose, a tongue and palate in the mouth, and visible nipples.

Week 12 Your baby has more than doubled in size during the past 3 weeks, weighing in now at ½ ounce and measuring about 2 to 2¼ inches. The size of a small plum, your baby's body is hard at work in the development department.

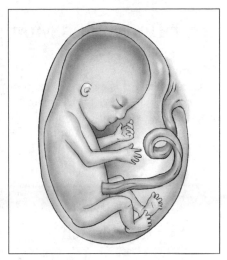

Your Baby, Month 3

Though most systems are fully formed, there's still plenty of maturing to do. The digestive system is beginning to practice contraction movements (so your baby will be able to eat), the bone marrow is making white blood cells (so your baby will be able to fight off all those germs passed around the playgroup), and the pituitary gland at the base of the brain has started producing hormones (so your baby will one day be able to make babies).

Week 13 As your first trimester comes to a close, your fetus (who seems to be working its way through the produce section) has reached the size of a sweet peach, about 3 inches long. Your baby's head is now about half the size of his or her crown-to-rump length, but that cute little body is picking up steam and will continue growing overtime (at birth, your baby will be one-quarter head, three-quarters body). Meanwhile, your baby's intestines, which have been growing inside the umbilical cord, are starting the trek to their permanent position in your baby's abdomen. Also developing this week: your baby's vocal cords (the better to cry with . . . soon!).

Your Body This Month

Here are some symptoms you may experience this month (or may not experience, since every pregnancy is different). Some of these symptoms may be continuing from last month, while others may be brand new:

Your Body This Month

This month, your uterus is a little bigger than a grapefruit and your waist may start to thicken. By the end of the month, your uterus can be felt right above your pubic bone in the lower abdomen.

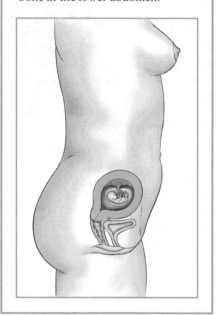

Physically

- Fatigue, lack of energy, sleepiness
- Frequent urination
- Nausea, with or without vomiting
- Excess saliva
- Constipation
- Heartburn, indigestion, flatulence, bloating
- Food aversions and cravings
- Increasing appetite, especially if morning sickness is easing
- Breast changes, continued (see page 139)
- Visible veins on your abdomen, legs, and elsewhere, as your blood supply pumps up
- Slight increase in vaginal discharge
- Occasional headaches
- Occasional lightheadedness or dizziness
- A little more rounding of your belly, your clothes feeling a little snugger

Emotionally

- Continued emotional ups and downs, which may include mood swings, irritability, irrationality, weepiness
- Joy, excitement, apprehension, doubts—any or all
- A new sense of calm
- Still, a sense of unreality about the pregnancy ("Is there really a baby in there?")

What You Can Expect at This Month's Checkup

This month, you can expect your practitioner to check the following, though there may be variations, depending on your particular needs and your practitioner's style of practice:

- Weight and blood pressure
- Urine, for sugar and protein
- Fetal heartbeat

- Size of uterus, by external palpation (feeling from the outside)
- Height of fundus (the top of the uterus)
- Hands and feet for swelling, and legs for varicose veins
- Questions or problems you want to discuss—have a list ready

What You May Be Wondering About

Constipation

"I've been terribly constipated for the past few weeks. Is this common?"

Irregularity—that bloated, gassy, clogged-up feeling—is a very regular pregnancy complaint. And there are good reasons why. For one, the high levels of progesterone circulating in your expectant system cause the smooth muscles of the large bowel to relax, making them sluggish and allowing food to hang around longer in the digestive tract. The upside: There's added time for nutrients to be absorbed into your bloodstream, allowing more of them to reach your baby. The downside: You end up with what amounts to a waste-product traffic jam, with nothing going anywhere anytime soon. Another reason for the clogged-up works: Your growing uterus puts pressure on the bowel, cramping its normal activity. So much for the process of elimination, at least as you once knew it.

But you don't have to accept constipation as inevitable just because you're pregnant. Try these measures to combat your colon congestion (and

head off hemorrhoids, a common companion of constipation, especially during pregnancy):

Fight back with fiber. You—and your colon—need about 25 to 35 grams of fiber daily. No need to actually keep count. Just focus on fiber-rich selections such as fresh fruit (but not bananas, which are constipating) and vegetables (raw or lightly cooked, with skin left on when possible), whole grains, legumes (beans and peas), and dried or freeze-dried fruit. Going for the green can also help get things going—look for it not only in the form of green vegetables, but in the juicy, sweet kiwi, a tiny fruit that packs a potent laxative effect. If you've never been a big fiber fan, add these foods to your diet gradually or you may find your digestive tract protesting loudly. (But since flatulence is a common complaint of pregnancy as well as a frequent, but usually temporary, side effect of a newly fiber-infused diet, you may find your digestive tract protesting for a while anyway.)

Really plugged up? You can try adding some bran or psyllium to your diet,

Another Reason for
Being Tired, Moody, and Constipated

Have you been tired, moody, and constipated lately? Welcome to the pregnancy club. Surging gestational hormones trigger those pesky symptoms in most moms-to-be. But did you know that out-of-whack thyroid hormones can cause (or intensify) those very same symptoms, as well as many others common in pregnancy, including excessive weight gain, skin problems of all kinds (very dry, or pimply), muscle aches and cramps, headaches, a decrease in libido, problems with memory and concentration (that "foggy" feeling), depression, and swelling of the hands and feet? The fact that so many symptoms of a thyroid condition overlap with symptoms of pregnancy make it an easy diagnosis to miss in a mom-to-be. (Another common symptom, an increased sensitivity to cold, is more clear-cut during pregnancy, since expectant moms tend to be warmer rather than chillier.) Yet hypothyroidism (having too little thyroid hormone because of a sluggish thyroid-producing gland), which affects around 2 to 3 percent of expectant moms, can show up for the first time during pregnancy or in the postpartum period. And since it can (if untreated) lead to pregnancy problems (as well as postpartum depression later on; see page 498), proper diagnosis and treatment are vital.

Hyperthyroidism (when too much thyroid hormone is produced by an overactive gland) is seen less often in pregnancy, but it can also cause complications if left untreated. Symptoms of hyperthyroidism—many of which may also be hard to distinguish from pregnancy symptoms—include fatigue, insomnia, irritability, warm skin and sensitivity to heat, rapid heartbeat, and weight loss (or trouble gaining weight).

If you're experiencing some or all of the symptoms of hypo- or hyperthyroidism (and especially if you have a family history of thyroid disease), check with your practitioner. A simple blood test can determine whether you have a thyroid condition that needs treating.

For more on thyroid conditions during pregnancy, see page 43.

starting with a sprinkle and working your way up, as needed. Don't overdo these fiber powerhouses, though—as they move speedily through your system, they can carry away important nutrients before they've had the chance to be absorbed.

Resist the refined. While high-fiber foods can keep things moving, refined foods can clog things up. So steer clear of the refiner things in life, such as white bread and white rice.

Drown your opponent. Constipation doesn't stand a chance against an ample fluid intake. Most fluids—particularly water and juice—are effective in softening stool and keeping food moving along the digestive tract. Another time-honored way to get things moving: Turn to warm liquids, including that spa staple, hot water and lemon. They'll help stimulate peristalsis, those intestinal contractions that help you go. Truly tough cases may benefit from that geriatric favorite, prune juice.

When you gotta go, go. Holding in bowel movements regularly can weaken muscles that control them and lead to constipation. Timing can help avoid this problem. For example, have your high-fiber breakfast a little earlier than usual, so it will have a chance to kick in before you leave the house—instead of when you're in the car stuck in traffic.

Don't max out at mealtime. Big meals can overtax your digestive tract, leading to more congestion. Opt for those 6 minimeals a day over 3 large ones—you'll also experience less gas and bloating.

Check your supplements and medications. Ironically, many of the supplements that do a pregnant body good (prenatal vitamins, calcium, and iron supplements) can also contribute to constipation. Ditto every pregnant woman's best buddy, antacids. So talk to your practitioner about possible alternatives or adjustments in dosages or switching to a slow-release formula. Also ask your practitioner about taking a magnesium supplement to help fight constipation (taking it at night may relax achy muscles and help you sleep better, too).

Go pro. Probiotics (aka "good bacteria") may stimulate the intestinal bacteria to break down food better, aiding the digestive tract in its efforts to keep things moving. Enjoy probiotics in yogurt and yogurt drinks that contain active cultures. You can also ask your practitioner to recommend a good probiotic supplement—in capsules, chewables, or a powder form that can be added to smoothies.

Get a move on. An active body encourages active bowels (even a brisk 10-minute walk can get things moving). So make sure you're getting the recommended amount of practitioner-approved exercise (see page 236). One essential exercise for combating constipation: Kegels. These pelvic floor exercises can keep you regular when practiced regularly (see page 229 for more on Kegels).

If your anti-constipation campaign doesn't get things moving, consult with your practitioner. He or she may prescribe a bulk-forming stool softener for occasional use. Don't use any laxative (including herbal remedies or castor oil) unless your practitioner specifically recommends it.

Lack of Constipation

"All my pregnant friends seem to have problems with constipation. I don't—in fact, I'm going more than ever. Is my system working right?"

From the sound of things, your system couldn't be working better. Chances are, your digestive efficiency is a credit to healthy eating and exercise habits—after all, consuming lots of fiber-rich foods (like fruits, veggies, whole grains, and beans), drinking plenty of water, and staying (or getting) active can all combine to counteract the natural digestive slowdown of pregnancy and keep things moving smoothly.

Sometimes a change for the healthier in eating habits can temporarily cause too much of a good thing, bowel-movement-wise. Chances are, production will slow down as you get used to the rough(age) stuff—as will the extra gas you may pass as a result of it—but you'll still stay "regular."

If your stools are very frequent (more than 3 a day) or watery, bloody, or mucousy, check with your practitioner. This kind of diarrhea could require prompt intervention during pregnancy.

Gas

"I'm very bloated, and I'm passing gas all the time. Will I be this gassy the whole pregnancy?"

Wondering if you'll ever run out of gas—and the overwhelming need to pass it? Probably not, since pregnancy brings out the gas in just about every expectant mom. Happily, while endless flatulence can be endlessly embarrassing for you (especially when there's no dog nearby to blame), it's no problem at all for your baby. Snug and safe in a uterine cocoon that's protected on all sides by impact-absorbing amniotic fluid, your very little one is probably soothed by the bubbling and gurgling of your gastric Muzak.

Baby won't be happy, though, if bloating—which often worsens late in the day and, yes, generally persists throughout pregnancy—keeps you from eating regularly and well. To cut down on the sounds and smells from down under and to make sure your nutritional intake doesn't take a hit, take the following measures:

Stay regular. Constipation is a common cause of gas and bloating. See the tips on page 185.

Graze, don't gorge. Large meals just add to that bloated feeling. They also overload your digestive system, which isn't at its most efficient anyway in pregnancy. Instead of those 2 or 3 supersize squares, nibble on 6 mini-meals.

Don't gulp. When you rush through meals or eat on the fly, you're bound to swallow as much air as food. This captured air forms painful pockets of gas in your gut that will seek release the only way they know how.

Keep calm. Particularly during meals. Stress can cause you to swallow air, which can give you a tank full of gas. Taking a few deep breaths before meals may help relax you.

Steer clear of gas producers. Your tummy will tell you what they are. Common offenders beyond the notorious beans include onions, cabbage, fried foods, sugary sweets, and carbonated beverages.

Don't be quick to pop. Ask your practitioner before popping your usual anti-gas medications (some are safe, others are not recommended) or any remedy, over-the-counter or herbal. Sipping a little chamomile tea, however, may safely soothe all kinds of pregnancy-induced indigestion. Ditto for hot water with lemon, which can cut through gas as well as any medication.

Headaches

"I find that I'm getting a lot more headaches than ever before. Can I take something for them?"

Pregnancy can be a headache—make that, a lot of headaches. Especially once you discover that some of your go-to headache relievers are no-go's when you're expecting (and, ironically, just when you're having more headaches than you've ever had before).

Why the increase in headaches during pregnancy—even in women who haven't previously experienced a lot of everyday headaches? The number one culprit (and you've probably guessed this): those pregnancy hormones. Other headache triggers include fatigue (got plenty of that when you're expecting), tension (and that), blood sugar drops (ditto), physical or emotional stress (double ditto), nasal congestion (expectant moms are stuffy moms), overheating (enough said)—or a combination of any or all of these.

While they're a pain, the vast majority of pregnancy headaches aren't anything to worry about. There are plenty of ways around a headache (and some surprisingly effective ones don't come in capsule form). In many cases you'll be able to fit the probable cause with the possible cure:

For tension headaches and migraines. Try lying in a dark, quiet room with

Heading Off Headaches

Finding that pregnancy headaches are a pain? How about stopping them before they start? Check out these headache-checking tips:

- Relax. Pregnancy can be a time of high anxiety—and lots of tension headaches. Reduce your stress level, and you may reduce your headaches. Try meditation or prenatal yoga to find your inner calm, mom.

- Get enough rest. Pregnancy can also be a time of extreme fatigue, particularly in the first and last trimesters. Making a conscious effort to get more rest can help keep headaches at a minimum. But be careful not to overdo the z's—too much sleep can also give you a headache.

- Seek some peace and quiet. Noise can give you a headache, especially if you're extra sound-sensitive, which many pregnant women are. Make it a point to avoid noisy locales (the mall, loud parties, restaurants with bad acoustics). If your job is extra noisy, talk to your boss about taking steps to reduce the excess noise—or even ask for a transfer to a quieter area, if possible. At home, keep TV and music volumes low (keep it down in your car, too).

- Eat regularly. To avoid hunger headaches triggered by low blood sugar, be sure not to run on empty. Carry high-energy snacks (such as lentil chips, granola bars, nuts, freeze-dried fruit) with you in your bag, stash them in the glove compartment of your car and in your office desk drawer, and always keep a supply on hand at home.

- Don't get stuffy. An overheated room or unventilated space can give anyone a headache—but especially an expectant mom, who's overheated to start with. So try not to get stuffy, but when you can't avoid it (it's 2 days before Christmas and you have to brave that jam-packed mall—or you work there), step out for a stroll and a breath of fresh air when you can. Dress in layers when you know you're going somewhere stuffy, and keep comfortable (and hopefully, headache-free) by removing layers as needed. Stuck inside? Try to crack a window, at least.

- Make a light switch. Take the time to examine your surroundings, particularly the lighting around you, in a whole new, well, light. Some women find that a windowless workspace lit by fluorescent bulbs can trigger headaches. Switching to CFL or LED lighting and/or a room with windows may help—though unless you're the boss (or in charge of office decor), it's probably not going to happen. If you're stuck under that fluorescent glow, take outdoor breaks when you can. Take breaks from your laptop, desktop, or tablet, too, since too much screen time can be a portal to headaches.

- Straighten up. Slouching while at the computer or looking down to swipe on your tablet, scour baby gear sites, or do other close work for long stretches of time can also trigger an aching head, so watch your posture.

your eyes closed. If you're at work, even a few minutes with your feet up and your eyes closed might help (you can say you're brainstorming). Or put an ice pack or cold compress on the back of your neck for 20 minutes while you relax. Some CAM approaches—including acupuncture, acupressure, biofeedback, and massage—can also bring headache relief (see page 78).

For sinus headaches. To unclog the congestion that's triggering the pain, try steam inhalation, running a cool mist humidifier, drinking plenty of fluids, and irrigating your nasal passages regularly with saline spray or rinses. To ease the pain, apply hot and cold compresses to the achy spots (often right above or around the eyes, cheeks, and forehead), alternating 30 seconds of each for a total of 10 minutes, 4 times a day. If you run a fever and/or the pain continues, check with your doctor to see if a sinus infection (common during pregnancy) may be causing your headaches.

For all headaches. First the bad news: Ibuprofen (Advil, Motrin) is pretty much off-limits when you're expecting. Now the good news: You can find relief in acetaminophen (Tylenol), which is considered safe for occasional use during pregnancy (check with your practitioner for recommendations on dosing). Never take any pain medication—over-the-counter, prescription, or herbal—without getting the all clear from your practitioner first.

Often, the best way to treat a headache is by trying to prevent it from happening in the first place (see box, page 189). If an unexplained headache persists for more than a few hours, returns very often, is the result of fever, or is accompanied by visual disturbances or severe puffiness of the hands and face, notify your practitioner right away. Ditto if you get for the first time what you suspect might be a migraine. See below and alert your practitioner about your symptoms.

"I get migraines, and I heard they're more common in pregnancy. Is this true?"

Call it a matter of pregnant providence: Some mamas-to-be find their migraines strike more frequently during their 9 months of pregnancy, others (the lucky ones) find that these mother-of-all headaches come less often. It isn't known why this is true, or even why some people have recurrent migraines and others never have a single one.

Since you've had migraines in the past, discuss with your physician which migraine medications are pregnancy approved so you'll be prepared for dealing with these monster headaches should they strike while you're expecting. Think prevention, too. If you know what brings on an attack, you can try to avoid the culprit. Stress is a common one, as are chocolate, cheese, and coffee. Try to determine what, if anything, can stave off a full-blown attack once the warning signs appear. You may be helped by one or more of the following: splashing your face with cold water or applying a cold cloth or ice pack, lying down in a darkened quiet room for 2 or 3 hours, eyes covered (napping, meditating, or listening to music), or trying CAM techniques such as biofeedback or acupuncture (see page 78).

Stretch Marks

"I'm afraid I'm going to get stretch marks. Can they be prevented?"

Nobody likes stretch marks, especially come skin-baring season. Still, they're not easy to escape when you're expecting. The majority of pregnant women develop these pink or reddish (sometimes purplish), slightly indented, sometimes itchy streaks on their breasts, hips, and/or abdomen sometime during pregnancy.

Stretch marks are caused by tiny tears in the supporting layers of tissue under your skin as it becomes stretched

Body Art for Two?

Heading off to The House of Ink for a "hot mama" tattoo? Think before you ink. While the ink itself won't enter your bloodstream, there is a risk of infection any time you get stuck with a needle, and why take that risk when you've got a baby on board?

Something else to ponder before getting a tattoo for two. What looks symmetrical on your pregnant skin might become lopsided or distorted after you regain your prepregnancy shape. So keep your skin free of any new marks for now, and wait until after you've weaned your baby to express yourself through ink.

If you already have a tattoo, no problem—just sit back and watch it stretch. And don't worry about that lower back tattoo and how it might affect the epidural you were hoping for come labor day. As long as the tattoo ink is fully dried and the wound is healed, sticking that epidural needle through it won't be risky. Something else not to worry about: a healed tattoo on your breast, even near your areola, won't affect your breast milk or your nursing baby.

What about using henna as body art during pregnancy? Since henna is plant based—and temporary—it's probably safe to use. Still, it's wise to follow certain caveats: Make sure the henna artist uses natural henna (it stains the skin reddish brown), not the kind that contains the potentially irritating chemical paraphenylendiamine (which stains black), and check the artist's references (read: no fair doing it at a street fair). To be extra cautious (always the best way to be), ask your practitioner before using henna.

Keep in mind, too, that pregnant skin is often extra sensitive skin, so there's a chance you'll have an allergic reaction to the henna, even if you've had it applied before without incident. To test your reaction to it, place a small amount of henna on a patch of skin and wait 24 hours to make sure no irritation appears.

---

to its limit. Expectant moms who have good elastic skin tone (because they inherited it and/or earned it by eating well, exercising regularly, and avoiding yo-yo dieting) may slip through several pregnancies without a single telltale mark. And actually, your mother may be your best crystal ball when it comes to predicting whether you'll end up with stretch marks: If she sailed through her pregnancies with smooth skin intact, odds are you will, too. If stretch marks struck her, they'll likely strike you, too.

You might be able to minimize, if not prevent, stretch marks by keeping weight gain steady, gradual, and moderate (the faster skin stretches, the more likely the stretching is to leave its mark). Promoting elasticity in your skin by nourishing it with a good diet (especially those vitamin C foods) may also help. And though no topical preparation has been proven to prevent stretch marks from zigzagging their way across your skin, there's no harm in applying pregnancy-safe moisturizers, such as cocoa or shea butter. Even without the scientific proof to back them up, many mamas swear they work—and if nothing else, they'll prevent the dryness and itching associated with pregnancy-stretched skin. An added plus: It may be fun for your spouse to rub them gently on your tummy (and baby will enjoy the massage, too).

If you do develop stretch marks (frequently referred to as the red badge of motherhood, albeit a badge most mothers would prefer not to wear), you can console yourself with the knowledge that they will gradually fade to a silvery sheen some months after delivery. You can also discuss with a dermatologist the possibility of reducing their visibility postpartum with laser therapy or Retin-A. In the meantime, try to wear them with pride—or at least, as a reminder of the reward within.

First-Trimester Weight Gain

"I'm nearing the end of the first trimester, and I'm surprised that I haven't gained any weight yet."

Many moms-to-be have trouble putting on an ounce in the early weeks, and some even lose a few pounds, courtesy of morning sickness and food aversions. Fortunately, nature has your baby's back, offering protection even if you're too queasy or food averse to eat much (or keep much down). Tiny fetuses have tiny nutritional needs, which means that your lack of weight gain now won't have any effect on your baby's growth or development.

Not so, however, once you enter the second trimester. As your baby gets bigger and your baby-making factory picks up steam, calories and nutrients will be more and more in demand— and you'll need to begin playing weight gain catch-up, piling on the pounds at a steady pace (that is, unless your practitioner has prescribed otherwise). Happily, appetite usually picks up just as baby's needs do, which will make gaining weight a piece of cake . . . even if you don't overdo the cake.

Boys Will Be Boys

Hungry, Mom? As you close in on your second trimester, you'll likely notice that your appetite (which you may have lost somewhere around week 6 or so) is starting to make a comeback. But if you're bellying up to the refrigerator with the regularity of a teenage boy, you may be expecting one (or, at least, a male fetus on his way to becoming a teenage boy). Research shows that moms-to-be carrying boys tend to eat more than moms expecting girls—which could explain why boys tend to be heavier at birth than girls. Food (and more food) for thought!

So don't worry—chances are the wait for weight gain will soon be over, and in the meantime, your lightweight baby doesn't mind a bit. From the 4th month forward, though, do start watching your weight to make sure it begins to move upward at the appropriate rate (see page 179). If you continue to have trouble gaining weight, try packing in more calories (preferably nutrient-dense ones) through efficient eating (see page 86). Try, too, to eat a little more food each day, by adding more frequent snacks. If you can't eat a lot at one sitting (which isn't so good for pregnancy digestion anyway), graze on 6 small meals daily instead of 3 big squares. Save fill-you-up beverages for after meals to avoid putting a damper on your appetite. Enjoy foods high in baby-friendly fats (nuts, seeds, avocados, olive oil). But don't try to add pounds by adding lots of junk food to your diet. Ultimately, weight gained on empty calories may add to your bottom line, but not necessarily to baby's.

"I'm 11 weeks pregnant and I was shocked to find out that I'd already gained 12 pounds. What should I do now?"

First of all, don't panic. Lots of women have that "oops" moment—when they step on the scale at the end of their first trimester and discover they've gained 8, 10, a dozen pounds, or more. Sometimes it's because they've taken "eating for two" just a tad too literally (you are eating for two, but one of you is really, really small), relishing sweet release from a lifetime of dieting. Sometimes it's because they've found that comfort from queasiness can come in high-calorie packages (ice cream, pasta, or just bread by the loaf).

Either way, all is not lost if you've gained a little too much in the first trimester. True, you can't turn back the scales—or apply the first 3 months of gain neatly to the next 6. Your baby needs a steady supply of nutrients (especially in the second and third trimester, when he or she will be growing overtime), so cutting way back on calories now isn't a smart plan. But you can aim to keep your gain on target for the rest of your pregnancy—slowing it down, without putting the brakes on it altogether—by watching the scale (and what you eat) more carefully.

Check with your practitioner and work out a safe and sensible weight gain goal for the next 2 trimesters. Even if you stay in the pound-a-week club through month 8 (most women find their weight gain slows or stops in the 9th month), you won't end up more than a few pounds over the outside limit for recommended weight gain (35 pounds). Check out the Pregnancy Diet (Chapter 4) to find out how to eat healthily for two without ending up looking like two (of you). Gaining efficiently, on the highest-quality foods possible, will not only accomplish that goal but make the weight you do gain easier to shed postpartum.

Showing Early

"Why am I already showing if I'm only in my first trimester?"

Have lots more to show for your first trimester than you expected? Because every belly is different, some stay flat well into the second trimester, while others seem to pop by week 6. An early bump can be disconcerting ("If I'm this big now, what will I look like in a few months?"), but it can also be welcome, tangible proof that there's actually a baby in there.

Several possibilities might explain why you're showing so early:

- Bloating. Excess gas and bloating are often behind a prematurely protruding tummy. Bowel distension can contribute, too, if you've been very constipated.

- Extra pounds. Not surprisingly, if you've been packing away extra calories, you may be piling on extra pounds—and extra inches around your middle.

- Small build. If you begin thin, your growing uterus may have nowhere to hide, creating a bulge even when it's still relatively little.

- Less muscle tone. An expectant mom with loose abdominal muscles may produce a pronounced pooch faster than a mom-to-be with a taut and toned torso. That's why second timers tend to show earlier—their abs have already been stretched.

Could your early baby bump be caused by multiple babies? Not likely. Twins usually show up on early ultrasound, not early bellies.

Baby's Heartbeat

"My friend heard her baby's heartbeat with a Doppler at 10 weeks. I'm a week ahead of her, and my doctor hasn't picked up my baby's yet."

The lub-dub of a baby's heartbeat is definitely music to every parent-to-be's ears—that is, once they finally get to hear it. Even if you've already had a listen to that beautiful sound on an early ultrasound (it may be audible as soon as 6 to 8 weeks that way), there's nothing like hearing it on a regular basis—as you likely will at your monthly checkups via Doppler (a handheld ultrasound device that amplifies the sound with the help of a special jelly on the belly).

Some lucky expectant moms and dads get that monthly chance to feast their ears on that sweet beat starting as early as 10 to 12 weeks—others have to wait a little longer. Your baby's position may be the cause of the inaudible heartbeat, or maybe the location of the placenta is muffling the sound (sometimes extra fat padding can do the same). A slightly miscalculated due date may also explain why the Doppler isn't yet picking up your baby's heartbeat.

By your 14th week, the miraculous sound of your baby's heartbeat is certain to be available for your listening pleasure via Doppler. If it isn't, or if you are very anxious, your practitioner will likely do an ultrasound (or a repeat one) to see and hear what the Doppler hasn't yet.

When you do get to hear the heartbeat, listen carefully. Your normal heart rate is usually under 100 beats per minute, but your baby's will be around 110 to 160 beats per minute during early pregnancy and average between 120 and 160 beats per minute by midpregnancy. Don't compare fetal heartbeats with your pregnant pals, though—every baby beats to his or her own drummer, and normal fetal heart rates vary a lot.

Starting at about 18 to 20 weeks, the heartbeat can be heard without Doppler amplification, using a regular stethoscope.

I Heart Girls (or Boys)

Is it a boy or a girl, and can your baby's heart rate give you a clue? While old wives—and some practitioners—have been telling tales for ages (a heart rate of above 140 promises a girl, one under 140 delivers a boy), studies show no correlation between fetal heart rate and the baby's gender. It may be fun to make predictions based on your baby's heart rate (you'll be right 50 percent of the time, after all), but you might not want to make nursery color choices based on it.

Sexual Desire

"Ever since I became pregnant, I'm turned on all the time and I can't get enough of sex. Is this normal?"

Feeling a little hot under the collar (and under those very snug jeans)? Is your turn-on switch always on? Lucky you. While some women find their sex lives coming to a screeching halt in the first trimester (what with all those early pregnancy symptoms kicking their libidos out of bed), others—like you—find they just can't get enough of a good thing. You can thank those extra hormones surging through your body these days, as well as the increase in blood flow to your pelvic region (which can make your genitals feel fabulously engorged and ever-tingly), for turning

At-Home Dopplers

Tempted to buy one of those inexpensive prenatal "heart listeners" so you can stay tuned in to your baby's heartbeat between practitioner visits? Being able to monitor your baby's heart rate can be loads of fun and may even help you have a better night's sleep if you're a stresser by nature. But listen to this: Though these devices (and apps) are considered safe to use, they're not as sophisticated as the one your practitioner uses—and most aren't nearly sensitive enough to pick up fetal heart tones until after the 5th month of pregnancy. Use one before then, and you'll likely be met with silence—or other clicks, swishes, and wooshes (from air moving through your GI tract or blood flowing in your arteries) instead of a steady beat, which can increase worry unnecessarily instead of putting it to rest.

Even later on in pregnancy, at-home Dopplers can't always pick up what you're looking for (baby's position or a bad angle on the device can easily throw off an at-home Doppler, or you may pick up the sound of blood flowing through the placenta and mistake it for a heartbeat). That's especially true about the stand-alone apps (where you use your phone's microphone to hear the in-utero sounds)—they're notoriously unreliable even during the third trimester. And if you do manage to find your baby's heartbeat, the way you interpret the readings might not be accurate (you might not be able to recognize changes in the rate or rhythm that may indicate a problem, for instance) or the readings might be different enough from the ones you're used to getting at your checkups to prompt undue concern.

Still can't resist having a heart listener of your own? You should get your practitioner's okay before placing your order, especially because the FDA considers them "prescription devices" that should be used only under the supervision of a medical professional. And keep in mind that you get what you pay for, and you might get somewhat less than you bargained for.

---

up the sexual thermostat. On top (so to speak) of that are the new curves you're sprouting and the larger-than-life breasts you're likely sporting, all of which can make you feel like one sexy mama. Plus, it might be the first time in your sexual life that you're able to make love when the mood moves you—without having to spoil the moment while you run to the bathroom for your diaphragm or calculate your fertility with an ovulation predictor. This happy state of sensual affairs may be most pronounced during the first trimester, when hormonal havoc is at its height, or it can continue right up until delivery day.

Since your increased sexual appetite is perfectly normal (as is a lack of sexual desire), don't worry or feel guilty about it. And don't be surprised or concerned if your orgasms are more frequent or more intense than ever (and if you're having orgasms for the first time, that's even more reason to celebrate). As long as your practitioner has green-lighted sex in all its forms (and that's usually the case), seize the moment and your partner. Explore different positions before that belly of yours makes many of them a physical impossibility. And most of all, enjoy that cozy twosome while you can (and before your libido takes its very likely postpartum nosedive). In other words, get it while you can. For more on sex during pregnancy, see page 273.

Libido Now

Sexual desire—yours and your partner's—will be up and down during pregnancy. Here are some of the unexpected things you may expect when you're expecting . . . sex:

She's turned on all the time. The rumors are true: Some women really can't get enough sex when they're expecting. And for good reason. Her genitals are swollen with hormones and blood, leaving the nerves down below set on tingle mode. Other parts are swollen, too (you might have noticed), including places like those breasts and hips that can make a woman feel more womanly than ever—and more sensually charged. So be there for the taking whenever she's in the mood to grab you. Feel lucky that you're getting lucky so often. But always take your cues from her, especially now. Proceed with seduction if she's up for it and into it, but don't go without the green light.

Though some women are in the mood throughout their 9 months, others find that the party doesn't get started until the second trimester . . . or that desire dips in the third. Be ready to roll with her changing sexual agenda when she goes from turned on to turned off in 60 seconds. Keep in mind, too, that there'll be some logistical challenges in mid to late pregnancy as her body goes from two-seater to semi.

She's never in the mood. So many factors, both physical and emotional, can affect sexual desire. It could be that pregnancy symptoms have leveled her libido (it's not so easy to lose yourself in the moment when you're busy losing your lunch, or to get hot when you're bothered by backache and swollen ankles and super painful nipples, or to get it on when you barely have the energy to get up), particularly in this uncomfortable first trimester. Or that she's as turned off by her new roundness as you are turned on by it (what you see as a sexy round bottom, she may see as a big fat ass). Or that she's preoccupied with all things baby and/or having a hard time blending the roles of mom and lover. Or that—and this happens to many expectant moms, even the normally libidinous ones—she just doesn't want to be touched. At all. Period.

When she's not in the mood (even if she's never in the mood), don't take it personally. Try, try again another time, but always be a good sport while you're waiting for your ship to come in. Accept those "not now"s and those "don't touch there"s with an understanding smile and a hug (if she's open to touching) that lets her know you love her even when you can't show it the way you'd like to. Remember, she's got a lot going on in her mind (and in her body) right now, and it's a safe bet that your sexual needs aren't front and center on her plate. So don't push the sexual agenda, but do step up the romance, communication, and cuddling. Not only will these bring you closer together, but because they're powerful aphrodisiacs for many women, they may just bring you what you're craving. And don't forget to tell your partner—often—how sexy and attractive you find the pregnant her. Women may be intuitive, but they're not mind readers.

You're not interested in getting it on anymore. There are plenty of good reasons why your sex drive may be in a slump now. Perhaps you and your spouse worked so conscientiously at conception that sex suddenly feels too much like hard work. Maybe you're so focused on the baby and on becoming a dad that your sexual side is taking a backseat. Or the changes in your spouse's body are taking some getting used to. Or fear that you'll hurt her or your baby during sex (you won't) has sent your mojo into hiding. Or it could be a hang-up thing—the hang-up being that you've never made love to a mother before (even though that mother happens to be a woman you've always loved making love to). Or it could be the weirdness factor that's keeping you down: Getting close to your pregnant partner might mean getting too close for comfort to your baby during a decidedly adult activity (even though baby's completely oblivious). The normal hormonal changes that expectant fathers experience can also slow them sexually.

Confusing these conflicted feelings even more could be miscommunication: You think she's not interested, so you subconsciously put your urges on ice. She thinks you're not interested, so she gives desire a cold shower.

Try to focus less on the quantity of sex in your relationship and more on the quality of the intimacy you're sharing. Less may not be more, but it can still be fulfilling. You might even find that stepping up the other kinds of intimacy—the hand-holding, the unexpected hugs, the confiding of your feelings—might put you both more in the mood for lovemaking. Don't be surprised, too, if your libido gets a boost once both of you have adjusted to the emotional and physical changes of pregnancy.

It's also possible that your sexual slowdown will continue throughout the 9 months—and beyond, too. After all, even couples who can't get enough while they're expecting find that their sex lives can come to a screeching halt once there's a baby in the house, at least for the first couple of months. All of this is fine—and all of it is temporary.

Meanwhile, make sure the nurturing of your baby doesn't interfere with the care and feeding of your relationship. Put romance on the table regularly (and while you're at it, put some candles there, too, plus a dinner you cooked up while she was napping). Surprise her with flowers or a sexy negligee (they make them for expectant moms, too). Suggest a moonlit stroll or hot cocoa and cuddles on the couch. Share your feelings and encourage her to share hers. Keep the hugs and kisses coming (and coming . . . and coming). You'll both stay warm while you're waiting for things to heat up again.

Most important, be sure that your partner knows that your lack of libido has nothing to do with her physically or emotionally. Expectant moms can suffer a crumbling of confidence when it comes to their pregnant body image, particularly as those pounds start piling on. Letting her know (often, through words and touch) that she's more attractive to you than ever will help keep her from taking your drop in sexual interest personally.

For more tips on sex during pregnancy, see page 273.

"All of my friends say that they had an increased sex drive early in pregnancy. How come I feel so unsexy?"

Pregnancy is a time of change in many aspects of your life, not the least of them sexual. Hormones, which, as you've undoubtedly noticed, play a role in every physical and emotional high and low, also play an important role in sexuality. But those hormones hit every woman differently, turning up the heat for some and spraying a cold shower on others. Some women who have never had either an orgasm or much of an appetite for sex suddenly experience both for the first time when they're expecting. Other women, accustomed to being sexually insatiable and easily orgasmic, suddenly find that they're completely lacking in libido and are difficult to arouse—or don't even want to be touched. And even if your hormones have pushed your passion turn-on button, pregnancy symptoms (that nausea, that fatigue, those painfully tender breasts) can stand between you and a good time when things get real. These changes in sexuality can be thrilling, disconcerting, guilt provoking, or a confusing combination of all three. And they are all perfectly normal.

Most important is recognizing that your sexual feelings during pregnancy—and your partner's as well—may be more erratic than erotic: You may feel sexy one day and not the next. Mutual understanding and open communication will see you through, as will a sense of humor. And remember (and remind your partner) that many women who've lost that loving feeling in the first trimester get it back in the second, in spades, so don't be surprised if a very warm front moves into your bedroom soon. Until then, you might want to try the tips on page 279 to help heat things up.

Cramp After Orgasm

"I get crampy after orgasm. Is that normal, or does it mean something's wrong?"

Not to worry—and not to stop enjoying sex, either. Cramping (sometimes accompanied by lower backache)—both during and after orgasm—is common and harmless during a low-risk pregnancy. Its cause can be physical: a combination of the normal increased blood flow to the pelvic area during pregnancy, the equally normal congestion of the sexual organs during arousal and orgasm, and the normal contractions of the uterus after orgasm. Or it can be psychological: a result of the common, but unfounded, fear of hurting the baby during sex. Or it can be a combination of physical and psychological factors, since the mind-body connection is so strong when it comes to sex.

In other words, that cramping isn't a sign that you're hurting your baby while you're enjoying yourself. In fact, unless your practitioner has advised you otherwise, it's perfectly safe to mix the pleasure of sex and the business of making a baby. If the cramps bother you, ask your partner for a gentle low back rub. It may relieve not only the cramps but any tension that might be triggering them. Some women also experience leg cramps after they have sex; see page 291 for tips on relieving those.

ALL ABOUT:
Pregnant on the Job

If you're pregnant, you've already got your work cut out for you. Add a full-time job to the full-time job of baby making, and your workload doubles. Juggling it all—practitioner visits with client meetings, trips to the bathroom with trips to the conference room, morning sickness with business lunches, telling your best friend in accounting (who'll be excited for you) with telling your boss (who might not be), staying healthy and comfortable with staying motivated and successful, preparing for baby's arrival with preparing for maternity leave—can be a 9-to-5 challenge that keeps you working overtime. This section can help the employed mama-to-be navigate what's to come.

When to Tell the Boss

Wondering when to belly up to your boss's desk to spill the pregnancy beans? There's no universally perfect time (though it's a sure bet you should do it before that bump gets too big to miss). A lot will depend on how family friendly (or unfriendly) your workplace is. Still more will depend on your feelings (the physical and emotional). Here are some factors to consider:

How you're feeling and whether you're showing. If morning sickness has you spending more time hovering over the toilet than sitting at your desk, if first-trimester fatigue has you barely able to lift your head off your pillow in the morning, or if you're already packing a pooch that's too big to blame on your breakfast, you probably won't be able to keep your secret long. In that case, telling sooner makes more sense than waiting until your boss (and everyone else in the office) has come to his or her own conclusions. If, on the other hand, you're feeling fine and still zipping your pants up with ease, you may be able to hold off on the announcement until later.

What kind of work you do. If you work under conditions or with substances that could be harmful to your pregnancy or your baby, you'll need to make your announcement—and ask for a transfer or change of duties, if at all feasible—as soon as possible.

How work is going. A woman announcing her pregnancy at work may unfortunately—and unfairly—raise many red flags, including, "Will she still have the energy to produce while pregnant?" and "Will her mind be on work or on her baby?" and "Will she leave us in the lurch?" You may head off some of those concerns by making your announcement just after finishing a report, scoring a deal, ringing up record sales, coming up with a great idea, or otherwise proving that you can be both pregnant and productive.

Whether reviews are coming up. If you're afraid your announcement might influence the results of an upcoming performance or salary review, try to wait until the results are in before sharing your news. Keep in mind that proving you've been passed up for a promotion or raise based solely on the fact that you're expecting (and that you'll soon be a worker and a mother, not necessarily in that order) may be difficult.

Whether you work in a gossip mill. If gossip is one of your company's chief

The Pregnant Worker's Rights

There is much room for improvement in the U.S. workplace when it comes to families and their needs—in fact, the U.S. is one of only a tiny handful of countries in the world that don't mandate paid leave for moms. Though individual policies on what's due a pregnant or new mom worker vary from company to company, here's what federal law recognizes:

■ The Pregnancy Discrimination Act of 1978. This act prohibits discrimination based on pregnancy, childbirth, or related medical conditions. Under this law, employers must treat you as they would treat any employee with a medical disability. However, it does not protect you if you end up not being able to do the job you were hired to do—or require that you be offered a transfer to a position with less physical stress while you're expecting.

It is considered discriminatory—and illegal—to pass up a woman for a promotion or a job or fire her solely on the basis of her pregnancy. But this kind of discrimination, like all kinds of discrimination, can be difficult to prove. Complaints of pregnancy discrimination can be reported to the U.S. Equal Employment Opportunity Commission (EEOC) at eeoc.gov.

■ The Family and Medical Leave Act (FMLA) of 1993. All public agencies and private-sector companies that employ at least 50 workers within a 75-mile radius of each other are subject to regulation under this act. If you have been employed by such a company for at least a year (working at least 1,250 hours during the year), you are entitled to take a total of up to 12 weeks of unpaid maternity

---

products, be especially wary. Should word of mouth of your pregnancy reach your boss's ears before your announcement does, you'll have trust issues to deal with in addition to the pregnancy-related ones. Make sure that your boss is the first to know—or, at least, that those you tell first can be trusted not to squeal.

What the family-friendliness quotient is. Try to gauge your employer's attitude toward pregnancy and family if you're not sure what it is. Ask coworkers who have walked in your soon-to-be-swollen footsteps before, if there are any (but keep inquiries discreet). Check the policies on maternity leave in the employee handbook. Or set up a confidential meeting with someone in human resources or the person in charge of

benefits. If the company has had a history of being supportive of moms and moms-to-be, you may be inclined to make the announcement sooner. Either way, you'll have a better sense of what you'll be facing.

Making the Announcement

Once you've decided when to make your announcement, you can take some steps to ensure that it's well received:

Prepare yourself. Before you break the news, do your research. Learn everything you need to know about your employer's maternity-leave policy (or lack of). Some companies offer paid leave, others unpaid. Still others allow leave (the leave can also be used to care for a sick child or another family member) each year that you are employed. Barring unforeseen complications or early delivery, you must notify your employer of your leave 30 days in advance. During your leave, you must continue to collect all benefits (including health insurance), and when you return, you must be restored to an equivalent position with equal pay and benefits. Keep in mind, too, that you're entitled to use some of your leave during your pregnancy if you're not feeling well. In some cases, companies may be able to exclude from FMLA women who are considered key employees—those the company can't do without for 12 weeks and who are in the top 10 percent compensation bracket. The Wage and Hour Division of the U.S. Department of Labor can offer information on FMLA. For more help, contact them at dol.gov.

- State and local laws. Some state and local laws offer additional protection against pregnancy discrimination. A few states and some larger companies also offer "temporary disability insurance," which allows for partial wages during time off for medical disabilities, including pregnancy. Three states (California, New Jersey, and Rhode Island) offer 4 to 6 weeks of paid leave—though not at full salary—to bond with a new baby or care for a seriously ill family member.

Don't like what you're reading about your rights as a pregnant worker who's about to become a new mom worker? Use social media and your vote to mom-mobilize around the issue. And consider supporting companies that voluntarily offer a substantial amount of paid leave to their employees, sometimes for both moms and dads.

you to use sick days or vacation days as part of your leave.

Know your rights. Pregnant women—and parents in general—have fewer rights in the U.S. than almost anywhere in the world. Still, some baby steps have been made on behalf of expectant workers (see box, above). Many other big steps—including paid leave for new moms and dads—have been taken voluntarily by some forward-thinking, family-friendly companies.

Put together a plan. Efficiency is always appreciated on the job, and being prepared invariably impresses. So before you go in to make your announcement, prepare a detailed plan that includes how long you plan to stay on the job (barring any unforeseen complications),

how long your maternity leave will be, how you plan to finish up business before you leave, and how you propose that any unfinished business be handled by others. If you would like to return part-time at first, propose that now. Writing up your plan will ensure you won't forget the details, plus it may score you extra efficiency points.

Set aside the time. Don't try to tell your boss the news when you're on the way to a meeting or when he or she's got one foot out the door Friday night. Make an appointment to meet, so no one will be rushed or distracted. Try to make it on a day and at a time that is usually less stressful at your workplace. Postpone the meeting if things suddenly take a turn for the tense.

The Juggling Act

Even if you don't have any kids at home yet, staying on the job while you're expecting will require that you practice the fine art of juggling work and family (or, at least, a family-to-be). Especially during the first trimester and the last, when the symptoms of pregnancy may be dragging you down and the distractions of pregnancy may be competing for your attention, this juggling act may be exhausting, and sometimes overwhelming—in other words, good preparation for the years of working and parenting you may have ahead of you. These tips won't make working simultaneously at those dual jobs easier, but they may help make your working life work more smoothly with your making-a-baby life:

- Schedule smart. Make appointments for checkups, ultrasounds, blood tests, that glucose tolerance test, and other procedures before your workday begins (you may be too tired afterward) or during your lunch break. If you need to leave work in the middle of the day, explain to your boss that you have a doctor's appointment, and keep a log of the visits (just in case anyone accuses you of slacking off). If necessary, request a note from your practitioner verifying your appointment, and give it to your employer or someone in your human resources department.

- Remember not to forget. If your brain cells seem to be dropping like flies, you can blame your hormones—and start taking precautions so your pregnancy-impaired memory doesn't get you into workplace hot water. To ensure that you don't forget that meeting, that lunch date, those calls that had to be made by noon: Make lists, set reminders, load up on post-its, and keep your smartphone or tablet handy (if you can remember where you put it).

- Know your limits and stop before you reach them. This isn't the time to volunteer to take on extra projects or extra hours unless it's absolutely necessary. Focus on what needs to be done—and realistically can be done—without wearing yourself out. To avoid feeling overwhelmed, complete one task at a time.

- Just say yes. If coworkers offer to help out when you're not feeling well, don't hesitate to take them up on their kindness (maybe you can return the favor someday). And for all of you expectant micromanagers: If there were ever a time to learn how to delegate, this would be it.

- Recharge as needed. When you find yourself emotionally overwhelmed, and you will (a stuck stapler can start the tears flowing when you're pregnant), take a brief walk, a bathroom break, or some relaxation breaths to clear your head. Keep a stress ball handy, to knead as needed, too.

- Speak up. Not only are you only human, but you're human and pregnant. Which means you can't do it all and do it all well—especially if you feel crappy, as you will sometimes feel. If you can barely lift your head off your pillow (or leave the bathroom for more than 5 minutes) and you've got a pile of stuff on your desk or a major deadline looming, don't panic. Tell your boss you need extra time or extra help. And don't beat yourself up—or let anyone else beat you up. You're not lazy or incompetent, you're making a baby—and that's the hardest job of all.

Accentuate the positive. Don't start your announcement with apologies or misgivings. Instead, let your boss know that you are not only happy about your pregnancy but confident in your ability and committed in your plan to mix work and family.

Be flexible (but not spineless). Have your plan in place, and open it up to discussion. Then be ready to compromise (make sure there is room for negotiation built into your plan) but not to back down completely. Come up with a realistic bottom line and stick with it.

Set it in writing. Once you've worked out the details of your pregnancy protocol and your maternity leave, confirm it in writing so there won't be any confusion or misunderstanding later (as in, "I never said that . . .").

Never underestimate the power of parents. If your company is not as family friendly as you'd like, consider joining forces to petition for better parental perks. Making sure that similar allowances are made for employees who must take time off to care for sick spouses or parents may help unite, rather than divide, the company around the cause.

Staying Comfortable on the Job

Between nausea and fatigue, backaches and headaches, puffy ankles and a leaky bladder, it's hard for any expectant mom to have a completely comfortable day. Put her at a desk or on her swollen feet or at a job that requires standing, and you've got a recipe for even more pregnancy discomfort. To stay as comfortable as possible on the job when you're expecting, try these tips:

- Dress for success and comfort. Avoid tight, restrictive clothing, socks or knee-highs that cut off circulation, and heels that are too high or too spiky (2-inch chunky heels, low wedges, or flats with arch support work best). Wearing support hose designed for pregnancy will help ward off or minimize a variety of symptoms, from swelling to varicose veins, and may be especially important if you're spending a lot of the day on your feet. As you get bigger and achier, you may find that a belly sling or band is your favorite workday accessory.

- Watch the weather—inside you. No matter the climate in your city (or your office), when you're pregnant, the forecast is for wildly swinging body temperatures. Sweating one minute and chilly the next, you'll want to favor the layered look—and have a layer ready for every possible condition. Thinking of bundling up in a wool turtleneck to brave a subfreezing day? Don't do it unless you've got a lightweight layer underneath that you can strip down to when a hormone-driven heat wave starts burning inside. And even if you're usually toasty in just a tee, stash a sweater in your drawer or locker. Your body temp goes both ways fast these days.

- Stay off your feet—at least as much as possible. If your job demands that you stand for long stretches, take sitting or walking breaks. If possible, keep one foot on a low stool, knee bent, while you stand, to take some of the pressure off your back. Switch feet regularly. Flex them periodically, too.

- Put your feet up. Find a box, low stool, or other tip-proof object on which to discreetly rest your weary feet under your desk (see illustration, page 253).

- Take a break. Often. Stand up and walk around if you've been sitting,

Working with Carpal Tunnel

If you spend your day (and maybe your nights, too) tap-tap-tapping on a keyboard, you may already be familiar with the symptoms of carpal tunnel syndrome (CTS). A well-known worker's malady, CTS causes pain, tingling, and numbness in the hands and most often strikes those who spend a lot of time doing repetitive tasks (typing, punching numbers, working a smartphone). What you might not know, however, is that CTS affects the majority of pregnant women. Even moms-to-be who rarely touch a keyboard are prone to it, thanks to swollen tissue in the body that presses on nerves. The good news is that carpal tunnel syndrome is not dangerous—just uncomfortable, especially on the job. Even better, you can try a number of remedies until you see the light at the end of the carpal tunnel:

- Raise your office chair so your wrists are straight and your hands are lower than your elbows as you type.

- Switch to a wrist-friendly ergonomic keyboard (one that has a wrist rest) as well as a mouse that offers wrist support.

- Wear a wrist brace while typing.

- Take frequent breaks from the computer.

- Go hands-free if you're on the phone a lot.

- In the evenings, soak your hands in cool water to reduce any swelling.

- Ask your practitioner about other possible remedies, including vitamin B_6 supplements, acupuncture, or pain relievers.

For more tips, see page 291.

sit down with your feet up if you've been standing. If there's a spare sofa and a slot in your schedule, lie down for a few minutes. Do some stretching exercises, especially for your back, legs, and neck. At least once (or even twice) every hour, do this 30-second stretch: Stand up, raise your arms above your head, clasp your fingers, palms up, and reach up. Next, place your hands on a desk or table, step back a bit, and stretch out your back. Sit down and rotate your feet in both directions. If you can bend over and touch your toes—even from a seated position—go for it to release the tension in your neck and shoulders. (Looking for more desk-side exercises? The *What to Expect When You're Expecting: The Workout* DVD has plenty.)

- Adjust your chair. Back hurt? Add a lumbar cushion for extra support. Bottom sore? Slide a soft pillow onto your seat. Hips bothering you? Be sure to get up and walk around at least once an hour, if not more. If your chair reclines, consider setting it back a few notches to create more (and more!) space between your belly and your desk. And if you need more belly support, try a belly band.

- Hang out by the water cooler. Not just for the latest office dish but for frequent refills of your cup. Or keep a refillable water bottle at your desk. Drinking plenty of water can keep many troublesome pregnancy symptoms at bay, including excessive swelling, and may help prevent a UTI.

- Don't hold it in. Emptying your bladder as needed (but at least every 2 hours) also helps prevent UTIs. A good strategy: Plan to pee every hour or so, whether you need to or not. You'll feel better overall if you avoid getting to the bursting point.

- Take time for your tummy. Every expectant mom's job description includes feeding her baby regularly, no matter what else is on her workday agenda. So plan accordingly—making room in even your busiest days for 3 meals, plus at least 2 snacks (or 6 mini-meals). Scheduling meetings as working meals may help. So will keeping a supply of nutritious snacks in your desk, as well as in the office fridge, if there is one. Rediscover brown bags, or pack your lunch or mini-meals in some easy-to-tote food storage containers—that way you'll be able to keep baby fed even when time's not on your side.

- Keep an eye on the scale. Make sure job stress—or erratic eating—isn't keeping you from gaining enough weight, or is contributing to too many pounds (as it can for stress eaters, especially if they work near a vending machine).

- Pack a toothbrush. If you're suffering from morning sickness, brushing your teeth can protect them between bouts of vomiting—plus it helps freshen up your breath when it most needs freshening. Mouthwash will also be a welcome addition to the breath-freshening team, and it can help dry out a mouth that's full of excess saliva (drooling and gagging are common in the first trimester and can be extra embarrassing at work).

- Lift with care. Do any necessary lifting properly, to avoid strain on the back (see page 253).

- Watch what you breathe. Stay out of smoke-filled areas, even outdoor areas where smokers take their breaks. Not only is secondhand smoke bad for you and your baby, but it can also increase fatigue.

- Chill mama, chill. Too much stress isn't good for you or your baby. So try to use breaks to relax as fully as you can: Listen to music or a nature sounds app, close your eyes and meditate, do some soothing stretches, or take a 5-minute stroll around the building.

- Listen to your body. Try to slow down your pace if you're feeling tired.

Staying Safe on the Job

Most jobs are completely compatible with the job of making a baby, which is very good news to the millions of expectant moms who must manage to work full time at both occupations. Still, some jobs are obviously safer and better suited to pregnant women than others. Most on-the-job problems can be avoided with the right precautions or a modification of duties (check with your practitioner for other workplace recommendations in your case):

Office work. Anyone with a desk job knows the pain of stiff necks, aching backs, and headaches, all of which can make a pregnant woman feel more uncomfortable than she already is. No harm done to baby—but a lot of wear and tear on your achy expectant body. If you spend a lot of time sitting, be sure to stand up, stretch, and walk away from your desk frequently. Stretch your arms, neck, and shoulders while sitting in your chair, discreetly put your feet up on a low box or stool to reduce swelling, and support your back with a cushion.

Quiet, Please

By about 24 weeks, your baby's outer, middle, and inner ear are well developed. By 27 to 30 weeks, your baby's ears are mature enough to start responding to the sounds that filter into the womb. The sounds, of course, are muffled—and not just by the physical barrier of amniotic fluid and your own body. In his or her fluid-filled home, a baby's eardrum and middle ear can't do their normal job of amplifying sounds. So even sounds that are quite loud to you won't be for your baby.

Still, since noise is one of the most prevalent of all occupational hazards and has long been known to cause hearing loss in those exposed to it regularly, you might want to play it safe when it comes to excessive noise during pregnancy. That's because studies suggest that prolonged and repeated exposure to very loud noise raises the odds of a baby suffering some hearing loss, especially at lower frequencies. Such prolonged noise exposure—say, daily 8-hour shifts in an industrial workplace where the sound level is more than 90 or 100 decibels (about the same as standing next to a loud lawn mower or a chain saw)—can also increase the risk of premature delivery and low-birth-weight babies. Repeated brief exposure to extremely intense sound of 150 or 155 decibels (like standing next to a screaming jet engine) can cause similar problems. Generally, it's safest to avoid more than 8 hours of continuous exposure to noises louder than 85 or 90 decibels (such as a lawn mower or truck traffic) or more than 2 hours a day of exposure to noise louder than 100 decibels (such as that from a chain saw, pneumatic drill, or snowmobile).

More research needs to be done, but in the meantime, expectant mothers who work in an extremely noisy environment—such as a club where loud music is played, in a subway, or in a factory where protective hearing devices are required (you can't put these devices on your fetus)—or who are exposed to heavy vibrations on the job should play it safe and seek a temporary transfer or a new job. And try to avoid prolonged exposure to very loud noises in your everyday life: Don't take front seats at a concert, turn down the volume in your car, and wear headphones instead of blasting the music while you're vacuuming.

What about computer safety? Luckily, computer monitors are not a hazard to pregnant women, and neither are laptops. More worrisome is the multitude of physical discomforts, including wrist and arm strain, dizziness, and headaches, that can result from too much time spent in front of the computer. For fewer aches and pains, use a height-adjustable chair with a backrest that supports your lower back. Adjust the monitor to a comfortable height; the top should be level with your eyes and about an arm's length away from you. Use an ergonomic keyboard, designed to reduce the risk of carpal tunnel syndrome (see box, page 204), if possible, and/or a wrist rest. When you put your hands on the keyboard, they should be lower than your elbows and your forearms should be parallel to the floor.

Health care work. Staying healthy is every health care professional's top on-the-job priority, but it ranks even higher when you're staying healthy for two. Among the potential risks you'll need to protect yourself and your baby from are exposure to chemicals (such as ethylene oxide and formaldehyde) used for sterilization of equipment, to some anticancer drugs, to infections (such as hepatitis B and HIV), and to ionizing radiation. Most technicians working with low-dose diagnostic x-rays are not exposed to dangerous levels of radiation. It is recommended, however, that women of childbearing age working with higher-dose radiation wear a special device that keeps track of daily exposure, to ensure that cumulative annual exposure does not exceed safe levels (most health care professionals wear these exposure trackers anyway).

Depending on the particular risk you are exposed to, you might want to either take safety precautions as recommended by NIOSH (see box, page 208) or switch to safer work for now, if possible.

Manufacturing work. If you have a factory or manufacturing job that has you operating heavy or dangerous machinery, talk to your boss about a change of duties while you're pregnant, if possible. You can also contact the machinery's manufacturer (ask for the corporate medical director) for more information about the product's safety. How safe conditions are in a factory depends on what's being made in it and, to a certain extent, on how responsible and responsive the people who run it are. OSHA lists a number of substances that a pregnant woman should avoid on the job. Where proper safety protocols are implemented, exposure to such toxins can be avoided. Your union or other labor organization may be able to help you determine if you are properly protected. You can also get useful information from NIOSH or OSHA.

Physically strenuous work. Work that involves heavy lifting, physical exertion, long hours, rotating shifts, or continuous standing may somewhat raise an

expectant mom's risk for preterm delivery. If you have such a job, you should request a transfer to a less strenuous position by 20 to 28 weeks until after delivery and postpartum recovery. (See page 208 for recommendations on how long it is safe for you to stay at various strenuous jobs during your pregnancy.)

Emotionally stressful work. The extreme stress in some workplaces seems to take its toll on workers in general and on pregnant women in particular. So it makes sense to cut down on the stress as much as possible, especially now. An obvious (but not often feasible) way to do that is to switch to a job that is less stressful or take early maternity leave. Understandably, if the job is critical financially or professionally, you may find yourself even more stressed if you leave it.

You might, instead, consider ways of reducing stress, including meditation and deep breathing, regular exercise (to release those feel-good endorphins), and taking breaks when you can. If you're self-employed, cutting back may be even tougher (you're probably your own most demanding boss), but wise to consider.

Other work. Teachers and social workers who deal with young children may come into contact with infections that can potentially affect pregnancy, such as chicken pox, fifth disease, and CMV. Animal handlers, meat cutters, and meat inspectors may be exposed to toxoplasmosis (though if they've developed immunity already, their babies would not be at risk). If you work where infection is a risk, be sure you're immunized as needed and take appropriate precautions, such as washing hands frequently and thoroughly, wearing protective gloves and a mask, and so on.

Flight attendants or pilots may be at a slightly higher risk for miscarriage

Getting All the Facts

By law, you have the right to know what chemicals you are exposed to on the job, and your employer is obliged to tell you. The Occupational Safety and Health Administration (OSHA) is the regulatory body that monitors those laws. Contact them for more information on your rights regarding workplace safety at osha.gov. Further information on workplace hazards can also be obtained by contacting the National Institute for Occupational Safety and Health (NIOSH), Clearinghouse for Occupational Safety and Health Information, cdc.gov/niosh/topics/repro.

If your job does expose you to hazards, either ask to be transferred temporarily to a safer post or, finances and company policy permitting, begin your maternity leave early.

---

or preterm labor (though studies are inconclusive) because of exposure to radiation from the sun during high-altitude flights, and they might want to consider switching to shorter routes (they're usually flown at lower altitudes) or to ground work during pregnancy.

Artists, photographers, hairstylists, cosmeticians, dry cleaners, those in the leather industry, agricultural and horticultural workers, and others may be exposed to a variety of possibly hazardous chemicals in the course of work, so be sure to wear gloves and other protective gear. If you work with any suspect substances, take appropriate precautions, which in some cases may mean avoiding the part of the job that involves the use of chemicals.

Staying on the Job

Planning to work until that first contraction hits? Many women successfully mix business with baby making right through the 9th month, without compromising the wellbeing of either occupation. Still, some jobs are better suited to pregnant women during the long haul (so to speak) than other jobs. And chances are, the decision of whether you'll continue to work until delivery will be impacted by the kind of work you do. If you have a desk job, you can probably plan on going straight from the office to the birthing room. A sedentary job that isn't particularly stressful may actually be less of a strain on both you and baby than staying at home nesting. And some walking—an hour or two daily, on the job or off—is not only harmless but beneficial (assuming you aren't carrying heavy loads as you go).

Jobs that are strenuous, very stressful, and/or involve a great deal of standing, however, may be another, somewhat controversial, matter. Some research has found that women who were on their feet 65 hours a week didn't seem to have any more pregnancy complications than women who worked many fewer and usually less stressful hours. Other research, however, suggests that steady strenuous or stressful activity or long hours of standing after the 28th week—particularly if an expectant mother also has other children to care for at home—may increase the risk of certain complications, including premature labor, high blood pressure, and a low birthweight baby.

Should women who stand on the job work past the 28th week? Most practitioners give the green light to work longer if a mom-to-be feels fine and her pregnancy is progressing normally. Standing on the job all the way to term, however, may not be a good idea, less because of the theoretical risk to the pregnancy than the real risk that such pregnancy discomforts as backache, varicose veins, and hemorrhoids will be aggravated.

It's probably a good idea to take early leave, if possible, from a job that requires frequent shift changes (which can upset appetite and sleep routines, and worsen fatigue); one that seems to exacerbate any pregnancy problems, such as headache, backache, or fatigue; or one that increases the risk of falls or other accidental injuries. But the bottom line: Every pregnancy, every woman, and every job is different. Together with your practitioner, you can make the decision that's right for your workplace situation.

Changing Jobs

With all the changes going on in your life (like your growing belly and the ever-expanding responsibilities that come with it), it may seem counterintuitive to want to add another to your list. But there are dozens of valid reasons why an expectant mom might consider a job change. Maybe your employer isn't family friendly and you're concerned about balancing career and motherhood when you return from maternity leave. Maybe the commute is too long, the hours are inflexible, or the grind is all-consuming. It could be that you're bored or not fulfilled (and, hey—change is in the air anyway, so why not make the most of it?). Or perhaps you're worried that your current workplace might be hazardous to you and your developing baby. Whatever your reason, here are some things to consider before you make a job move:

- Looking for work takes time, energy, and focus—three things you may be lacking these days as you concentrate on having a healthy pregnancy. Will you be up for all those interviews (especially if morning sickness has you frequently running for the nearest toilet or if pregnancy forgetfulness has you fumbling for your thoughts)? Even if you're confident you can ace the interview process, consider that starting a new job also demands a great deal of concentration (all eyes are on you, so you have to be extra careful not to make mistakes).

- Before you jump ship, you'll need to be sure the new job you're seeking out is really all it's cracked up to be (in

---

Unfair Treatment at Work

Think you're being treated unfairly on the job because of your pregnancy? Don't just sit there, do something. Let someone you trust—your supervisor, someone in human resources—know how you feel. If that doesn't fix the problem, see if there is a procedure for employees to follow in the case of pregnancy discrimination (you can probably find it in your employee handbook, if there is one).

If that still doesn't work, contact the U.S. Equal Employment Opportunity Commission (eeoc.gov) to find your local office. They'll be able to help you determine if you have a legitimate complaint.

Remember to keep records of everything that'll bolster your claim (copies of emails, letters, a journal of events). This trail will also be helpful in case you ever need to contact an attorney.

your mind, at least). Does the company you're smitten with offer twice as much vacation time but charge double for health insurance? Do they allow employees to work from home yet expect them to be on call morning, noon, and night? Are the salaries higher and, likewise, the travel demands? Keep in mind that what looks like a great job now may not be so great when you're juggling it with new-baby care (your home life will be a lot more complicated, so you might not want your workplace life to be). Also consider that companies often offer fewer paid short-term disability days or pay a lower percentage of your salary during leave if you have been employed for less than one year.

- By law, your potential employer has no right to ask whether you're pregnant (if it isn't already obvious)—and can't deny you an offer because you're pregnant, though that kind of discrimination is often hard to prove. Consider that some companies will have a hard time justifying (as justified as it may be by law) bringing you on, training you, and then letting you take maternity leave so quickly. And not all employers appreciate what they consider to be a bait-and-switch strategy (you accept a job, then tell them you'll be out on maternity leave). So though it may be smart in the short run to keep your pregnancy a secret as you interview, it may damage your relationship with the company in the end. On the other hand, sometimes it's better to secure the offer first and then discuss the future once you know the company wants to hire you—but before you accept the position.

- What if you started a new job before you found out you were pregnant? Be up front about the situation, and then get down to the business of doing your job to the best of your expectant ability. Just make sure you know your rights about job security should the situation take a negative turn.

The Fourth Month

Approximately 14 to 17 Weeks

Finally, the beginning of the second trimester—which for most expectant moms is the most comfortable of the three. And with the arrival of this momentous milestone (1 down, 2 to go!) often come some welcome changes. For one, most of the more pesky early pregnancy symptoms may be gradually easing up or even disappearing. That queasy cloud may be lifting (which means that food may actually smell and taste good for the first time in a long time). Your energy level should be picking up (which means you'll finally be able to pick yourself up off the sofa), and your visits to the bathroom should be dropping off. And though your breasts will likely still be supersize, they're less likely to be super tender. Another change for the better: By the end of this month, the bulge in your lower abdomen may be looking less like a large lunch and more like a pregnant belly.

Your Baby This Month

Week 14 Beginning in the second trimester, fetuses (like the children they'll eventually become) start growing at different paces, some faster than others, some more slowly. Despite the differences in growth rates, all babies follow the same developmental path in utero. This week, that path is leading your baby—who is about the size of your clenched fist—toward a straighter position as the neck gets longer and the head more erect. And on top of that

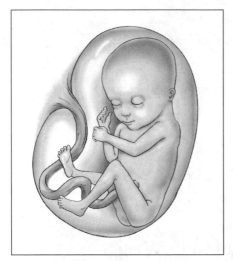

Your Baby, Month 4

cute little head, your baby might actually be sprouting some hair. Eyebrow hair is also filling in about now, as is body hair, called lanugo. Don't worry, it's not permanent. This downy coating of hair is there to keep your baby warm for now—like a furry blanket. As baby fat accumulates later on in your pregnancy, most of that hair will be shed—though some babies, especially those born early, still have a temporary fuzzy coating at delivery.

Week 15 Your baby, who measures approximately 4 inches this week and weighs around 2½ ounces, is about the size of a navel orange and looking more and more like the baby you're picturing in your dreams: His or her ears are positioned properly on the sides of the head (they used to be in the neck), and the eyes are shifting from the sides of the head to the front of the face. By now your baby has the coordination, strength, and smarts to wiggle his or her fingers and toes and even suck a thumb. But that's not all your baby can do now. He or she can make breathing movements, suck, and swallow—all in preparation for that big debut and

life outside the womb. And though it's still unlikely that you'll be feeling any movements from your little one this week, your baby is certainly getting a workout—kicking, flexing, and moving those arms and legs.

Week 16 With a whopping weight of anywhere from 3 to 4 ounces and a length (crown to rump) of 4 to 5 inches, your baby is growing up fast. Muscles are getting stronger (you'll start to feel movement in a few weeks), especially the back muscles, enabling your little one to straighten out even more. Your baby-to-be is looking more baby-like with a face that has eyes (complete with eyebrows and eyelashes) and ears in the right spots. What's more, those eyes are finally working! Yes, it's true: Your baby's eyes are making small side-to-side movements and can even perceive some light, though the eyelids are still sealed. Your baby is also becoming more sensitive to touch. In fact, he or she will squirm if you poke your belly (though you probably won't be able to feel those squirms just yet).

Week 17 Take a look at your open hand. Your baby is about palm-size now, with a crown-to-rump length of 5 inches and an approximate weight of 5 (or more) ounces. Body fat is just beginning to form (baby's fat, that is, though yours is probably forming pretty quickly these days, too), but your little one is still quite skinny, with skin that is practically translucent. This week, your baby is all about practice,

More Baby

For week-by-week videos of your baby's amazing development, download the What To Expect app.

practice, practice in preparation for birth. One important skill your baby is busy sharpening: sucking and swallowing—to get ready for that first (and second . . . and third) suckle at breast or bottle. Your baby's heart rate is regulated by the brain now (no more spontaneous beats) and clocks in at 140 to 150 beats per minute (roughly twice your own heart rate).

Your Body This Month

Here are some symptoms you may experience this month (or may not experience, since every pregnancy is different). Some of these symptoms may be continuing from last month, while others may be brand new. With the start of the second trimester, some symptoms may be tapering off, others intensifying:

Physically

- Fatigue
- Decreasing urinary frequency
- An end to, or a decrease in, nausea and vomiting (for a few women, morning sickness will continue—for a very few, it is just beginning)
- Constipation
- Heartburn, indigestion, flatulence, bloating
- Continued breast enlargement, but usually decreased tenderness
- Occasional headaches
- Occasional lightheadedness or dizziness, particularly with sudden change of position
- Nasal congestion and occasional nosebleeds; ear stuffiness

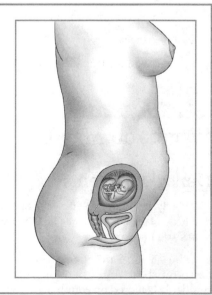

Your Body This Month

Your uterus, now about the size of a small melon, has grown large enough to rise out of the pelvic cavity, and by the end of the month, you'll be able to feel the top of it around 2 inches below your belly button (if you don't know what you're feeling for, ask your practitioner for some pointers at your next visit). You'll probably begin to outgrow your regular clothes, though some moms can zip their way comfortably through 5 months or more without turning to maternity clothes, and that's normal, too.

- Sensitive gums that may bleed when you brush

- Increased appetite

- Mild swelling of ankles and feet, and occasionally of hands and face

- Varicose veins of legs or vulva

- Hemorrhoids

- Slight increase in vaginal discharge

- Fetal movement near the end of the month (but usually not this early, unless this is your second or subsequent pregnancy)

Emotionally

- Mood swings, which may include irritability, irrationality, inexplicable weepiness

- Excitement and/or apprehension— if you have started to feel and look pregnant at last

- Frustration at being "in between"— your regular wardrobe doesn't fit anymore, but you're not looking pregnant enough for maternity clothes

- A feeling you're not quite together— you're scattered, forgetful, drop things, have trouble concentrating

What You Can Expect at This Month's Checkup

This month, you can expect your practitioner to check the following, though there may be variations, depending on your particular needs and on your practitioner's style of practice:

- Weight and blood pressure

- Urine, for sugar and protein

- Fetal heartbeat

- Height of fundus (top of the uterus)

- Size of uterus, by external palpation (feeling from the outside)

- Hands and feet for swelling, and legs for varicose veins

- Symptoms you've been experiencing, especially unusual ones

- Questions or problems you want to discuss—have a list ready

What You May Be Wondering About

Dental Problems

"Suddenly my gums bleed every time I brush, and I think I have a cavity. Is it safe to have dental work done?"

Smile—you're pregnant! But with so much of your attention understandably centered on your belly during pregnancy, it's easy to overlook your mouth—until it starts screaming for equal time. For starters, pregnancy hormones aren't kind to your gums— which, like your other mucous membranes, become swollen and inflamed, and tend to bleed easily. Those same hormones also make the gums more

Expecting X-Rays?

Routine dental x-rays (and other routine x-rays or CT scans) are usually postponed until after delivery, just to be on the extra-safe side. But if putting off x-rays during pregnancy just isn't a good idea (the risk of having one is outweighed by the risk of not having one), most practitioners will green-light the procedure. That's because the risks of x-rays during pregnancy are really very low and can be easily made even lower. Dental x-rays target your mouth, of course, which means the rays are directed far away from your uterus. What's more, a typical diagnostic x-ray of any kind rarely delivers more radiation than you'd get from spending a few days in the sun at the beach. Harm to a fetus occurs only at very high doses, doses you're extremely unlikely to ever be exposed to. Still, if you do need an x-ray during pregnancy, keep the following guidelines in mind:

- Always inform the doctor or dentist ordering the x-ray and the technician performing it that you're pregnant, even if you're pretty sure they know and even if you checked it off on any forms you filled out.

- Have any necessary x-ray done in a licensed facility with well-trained technicians.

- The x-ray equipment should, when possible, be directed so that only the minimum area necessary is exposed to radiation. A lead apron will be used to shield your uterus, and a thyroid collar should protect your neck.

Most important, if you had an x-ray before you found out you were pregnant, don't worry.

susceptible to plaque and bacteria, which can soon make matters worse in some moms-to-be, possibly leading to gingivitis (inflammation of the gums) and tooth decay.

To keep your mouth happy:

- Floss and brush regularly using a soft toothbrush, and use toothpaste with fluoride for cavity protection. Brush up on your technique, too, since brushing too aggressively can injure sensitive gums, leading to bleeding and even recession. Brushing your tongue (with a tongue scraper or a separate toothbrush) will also help combat bacteria while keeping your breath fresher.

- Ask your dentist to recommend a rinse to reduce bacteria and plaque, protecting your gums and your teeth.

- When you can't brush after eating, chew gum. Chewing sugarless gum increases the amount of saliva, which rinses the teeth, and if the gum's sweetened with xylitol, chewing can actually help prevent decay. Or nibble on a chunk of hard cheese (it decreases the acidity in your mouth, and it's the acid that causes tooth decay).

- Watch what you eat, particularly between meals. Save sweets (especially sticky ones, and even dried fruit or fruit leather) for times when you can brush soon after. Chow down on fruits and veggies high in vitamin C, which strengthens gums, reducing the possibility of bleeding. Also be sure to fill your calcium requirements daily. Calcium is needed throughout life to keep teeth strong and healthy—plus

A Gum Bump

If it's not one thing for your poor pregnant gums, it's another. Besides inflammation and sensitivity, canker sores are more common when you're expecting. And your gums might encounter other bumps, as well—literally. If you notice a bump on your gum that bleeds when you brush, get it checked out. It's probably a pyogenic granuloma (also known as a "pregnancy tumor," despite the fact that it's perfectly harmless, if often uncomfortable). These bumps usually regress on their own, but if it becomes really annoying, it can be removed by a dentist or doctor.

you'll be giving baby's growing teeth a boost, too.

- See your dentist. Even if you're not having any noticeable dental discomfort, be sure to make an appointment with your dentist for a checkup and cleaning at least once during your 9 months—preferably earlier than later. The cleaning is important to remove plaque, which can not only increase the risk of cavities but also make your gums more vulnerable. You may also need to schedule an appointment with the periodontist if you've had gum problems in the past. Stay away from any sealants or any cosmetic dental procedures (like whitening; see page 153) until after delivery (though topical fluoride treatment should be safe during pregnancy). Wondering about the safety of routine x-rays? See the box, page 215, for the lowdown.

- Don't keep your pregnancy a secret. From the dentist, that is. Even if you haven't broken the news widely, your dentist and hygienist should both get the heads-up before you open wide. Not only so they can take extra precautions with x-rays and treatment plans, but also because your gums may need to be handled with extra care. Something else you may want to share with them: if pregnancy has revved up your gag reflex.

Seeing your dentist or periodontist is especially important if you suspect a cavity or other tooth or gum trouble. Untreated gingivitis can develop into periodontitis, a more serious gum condition associated with a variety of pregnancy complications such as preeclampsia. Decay that isn't cleaned up or other tooth issues that aren't tended to can also become a source of infection (and infection isn't good for you or your baby).

What happens if major dental work becomes necessary during pregnancy? Luckily, in most dental procedures a local anesthetic will suffice, and that's safe. A low dose of nitrous oxide (laughing gas) is also safe to use after the first trimester, but more serious sedation should be avoided during pregnancy. In some cases, it may be necessary to take an antibiotic before or after major dental work, so check with your practitioner.

Breathlessness

"Sometimes I feel a little breathless. Is this normal?"

Take a deep breath (if you can!) and relax. Mild breathlessness is normal, and many pregnant women experience it beginning in the second trimester. And you can blame—what else?—those pregnancy hormones for taking your breath away. Here's why:

Those hormones stimulate the respiratory center to increase the frequency and depth of your breaths during pregnancy, which can give you that out-of-breath feeling after nothing more strenuous than a trip to the bathroom. They also swell the capillaries in the body—including those of the respiratory tract—and relax the muscles of the lungs and bronchial tubes, making those breaths seem even harder to catch. Your ever-growing uterus will also likely contribute to your breathlessness as pregnancy progresses, pushing up against your diaphragm as it swells, crowding your lungs and making it more difficult for them to expand fully (something else to look forward to!).

Fortunately, though the mild breathlessness you're experiencing may make you feel uncomfortable, it doesn't affect your baby—who isn't breathing at all yet, but (not to worry) is kept well stocked with oxygen through the placenta. If, however, you're feeling constantly breathless, mention it to your practitioner, who may want to test your iron levels (see page 251). And if you're having a very hard time breathing, if your lips or fingertips seem to be turning bluish, or if you have chest pain and a rapid pulse, call your practitioner right away.

Nasal Stuffiness and Nosebleeds

"My nose has been stuffed up a lot, and sometimes it starts bleeding randomly. Is that pregnancy related?"

Your belly's not the only thing that's starting to swell these days. Thanks to the high levels of estrogen and progesterone circulating in your body, which bring with them increased blood flow, the mucous membranes of your nose start to swell, too, and soften (much as the cervix does in preparation for childbirth). Those membranes also produce more mucus than ever, with the intention of keeping infections and germs at bay. What's not so swell is the result—which your nose undoubtedly already knows: congestion, and possibly even nosebleeds. Also not so swell: The stuffiness may only get worse as your pregnancy progresses. You may develop postnasal drip, too, which in turn can occasionally cause coughing or gagging at night (as if you didn't have enough other things keeping you up—or enough gagging going on).

You can safely try saline sprays or rinses, or sleep with a nasal strip (like Breathe Right) to ease nighttime stuffiness. A cool mist humidifier in your room may also help overcome the dryness associated with any congestion. Medications or antihistamine nasal sprays are usually not prescribed during pregnancy, but do ask your practitioner what he or she recommends (some practitioners okay decongestants or steroid nasal sprays after the first trimester; see page 539).

Taking an extra 250 mg of vitamin C (with your practitioner's okay), plus eating plenty of vitamin C–rich fruits and veggies, may help strengthen your capillaries and reduce the chance of bleeding. Sometimes a nosebleed will follow overly energetic nose blowing, so easy does it.

To stem a nosebleed, sit or stand leaning slightly forward, rather than lying down or leaning backward. Using your thumb and forefinger, pinch the area just above your nostrils and below the bridge of your nose, and hold for 5 minutes. Repeat if the bleeding continues. If the bleeding isn't controlled after 3 tries, or if the bleeding is frequent and heavy, call your practitioner.

Snoring

"My husband tells me that I've been snoring lately. Is this another pregnancy symptom, hopefully a temporary one?"

Men get the snoring blame in most households—and for good reason, since they're twice as likely to snore as women. That is, until pregnancy hormones invade the bedroom—then all bets are off on who's disturbing whose sleep.

Yes, that's right—you can add snoring to the list of unexpected (and thankfully temporary) symptoms of expecting. Usually, pregnancy snoring is nothing to lose sleep over (though your bedmate may be losing plenty over it). The noisy nasal soundtrack that plays as you sleep is probably triggered by normal pregnancy stuffiness, which increases when you're lying down. Sleeping with a nasal strip on and a humidifier running can ease the congestion and help everyone sleep better—as can keeping your head well elevated with several pillows (which will also help with any heartburn you're having, so win-win). Extra weight can also contribute to snoring, so make sure you aren't gaining too much.

Rarely, snoring can signal an elevated risk for gestational diabetes or be a sign of sleep apnea, a condition in which breathing stops briefly during sleep. Since you're breathing for two, it's a good idea to mention your snoring to your practitioner at your next visit.

Allergies

"My allergies seem to have gotten worse since I've been pregnant. My nose is runny all the time."

Expectant noses are stuffy noses, so it's possible that you're mistaking the normal (though uncomfortable) congestion of pregnancy for allergies. But it's also possible that pregnancy has aggravated your allergies. Though some lucky expectant allergy sufferers (about a third) find a temporary respite from their symptoms during pregnancy, the less lucky (also about a third) find their symptoms get worse, and the rest (that final third) find their symptoms stay about the same. Since it sounds like you're among the less lucky third, you're probably itching (and tearing and sneezing) for relief. But before you join the rest of the other allergy sufferers in the antihistamine aisle, check with your practitioner to see what you can safely pull off the shelf or have filled at the pharmacy. Some antihistamines and other medications are safe for use in pregnancy, while others (which may or may not include your usual over-the-counter or prescription medication) may not be. Don't worry about any that you took before you knew you were pregnant or before you read this.

Allergy shots are considered safe for pregnant women who were on the receiving end of them before they

---

Snooze or Lose

Are pregnancy hormones—or that growing belly—getting between you and a good night's sleep? Sleep problems are common in pregnancy, and while insomnia may be good preparation for the sleepless nights that lie ahead once your baby arrives, you're likely eager to catch some expectant z's while you can. Before turning to over-the-counter (or prescribed) sleep aids, however, talk to your practitioner. He or she may have other suggestions to help summon the sandman. You can also read the tips on page 284 to help with your insomnia.

Breathing Easier with Asthma

Being pregnant can leave you breathless—literally, once your growing uterus starts crowding out your diaphragm. But what if you're pregnant, breathless, and asthmatic, too? While it's true that poorly controlled severe asthma does put a pregnancy at a somewhat higher risk for complications (such as preterm delivery, low birthweight, or preeclampsia), this risk can be almost completely eliminated. In fact, if you're under close, expert medical supervision by a team that includes your ob, your internist, and/or your asthma doctor, and you keep your asthma well controlled, your chances of having a normal pregnancy and a healthy baby are about as good any mama's (which means you can breathe a little easier now).

You and your doctors may need to take a fresh look at the medications you're taking for your asthma (in general, inhaled medications like budesonide appear to be safer than oral meds). Since you're breathing for two now, getting enough oxygen is doubly important. Treating an asthma attack promptly with prescribed medication—usually albuterol—will help ensure your baby isn't shortchanged on oxygen. Since an asthma attack may trigger early uterine contractions, be sure to call your doctor or head for the nearest emergency room if your rescue inhaler doesn't help. Happily, any contractions that are triggered by an attack will usually stop when the attack does—which is why it's so important to stop it quickly.

When it comes to labor and delivery, yours is likely to be pretty much like other moms', though if your asthma has been serious enough to require oral steroids or cortisone-type medications, you may also require IV steroids to help you handle the added stress of childbirth.

Though well-controlled asthma has only a minimal effect on pregnancy, pregnancy can have an effect on asthma. But the effect varies from expectant mom to expectant mom. For about a third of pregnant asthmatics, the effect is positive: Their asthma improves. For another third, their condition stays about the same. For the remaining third (usually those with the most severe form of the disease), the asthma worsens. Happily, no matter what pregnancy does to your asthma, your chances of having a healthy, safe pregnancy with well-controlled asthma are excellent.

conceived. Most allergists say it's not a good idea to start allergy shots during pregnancy because they may cause unexpected reactions.

In general, however, the best approach to dealing with allergies in pregnancy is prevention—which can be worth a pound of tissues this season. Steering clear of what causes your allergies may also reduce the risk that your baby will develop allergies to those triggers.

To ease the sneeze, try these tips:

- If pollens or other outdoor allergens trouble you, stay indoors in an air-conditioned and air-filtered environment as much as you can during your susceptible season. When you come indoors, wash your hands and face and change clothes to remove pollen. Outdoors, wear large curved sunglasses to keep pollens from floating into your eyes.

Peanuts for Your Little Peanut?

It's as American as the sandwich bread it's spread on—plus it makes a convenient and wholesome snack—but is peanut butter safe for the little peanut you're feeding in utero? Will eating it now cause your peanut to have a peanut allergy later?

Good news: The latest research suggests that eating peanuts while pregnant not only doesn't trigger peanut and other allergies in babies-to-be, but it may actually prevent them. So as long as you're not personally allergic to peanuts, there's no need to skip the Skippy—and maybe more reason than ever to reach for it.

Ditto for dairy products or other highly allergenic foods. If you're not allergic to them yourself (in which case you'd clearly want to steer clear), there's no reason to avoid any allergenic foods during pregnancy. Eating them will not trigger allergies in your little one.

That said, if you yourself have ever suffered from allergies, speak to your practitioner and an allergist about whether you should think about restricting your diet in any way while you're pregnant and/or breastfeeding. The recommendations may be slightly different for you.

- If dust is a culprit, make sure someone else does the dusting and sweeping (how's that for a good excuse to get out of housecleaning?). A vacuum cleaner (especially one with a HEPA filter), or a damp mop or sweeper kicks up less dust than an ordinary broom, and a microfiber cloth will do better than a traditional feather duster. Stay away from attics, basements, and other musty places.

- If animals bring on allergy attacks, keep your distance from cats and dogs. And of course, if your own pet is suddenly triggering an allergic response, try to keep one or more areas in your home (particularly your bedroom) pet-free.

Vaginal Discharge

"I've noticed a slight vaginal discharge that's thin and whitish. Does this mean I have an infection?"

A thin, milky, mild-smelling discharge (known in the ob business as leukorrhea) is normal throughout pregnancy. Its purpose is noble: to protect the birth canal from infection and maintain a healthy balance of bacteria in the vagina. Unfortunately, in achieving its noble purpose, leukorrhea can make a mess of your underwear. Because it increases as pregnancy progresses and may become quite heavy, you may be more comfortable wearing panty liners during the last trimester. Don't use tampons, which could introduce unwanted germs into the vagina.

Though it might make you feel a little icky and sticky (or possibly be a tad of a turn-off during oral sex), this discharge is nothing to worry about. Just keep yourself clean (daily showers or baths) and dry (choose panties with breathable cotton liners). One thing you don't need to do (and shouldn't): douche. Douching upsets the normal balance of microorganisms in the vagina and can lead to bacterial vaginosis (BV; see page 529). You also don't need feminine vaginal wipes, since the vagina does a pretty good job of keeping itself clean. If you really can't live without that "fresh feeling," be sure to choose wipes that are pH safe, and free of alcohol and chemicals (changing the pH of your natural juices could increase the risk of infection). If you notice any unusual vaginal odors (fishy smelling, for instance), gray or green discharge, irritation, burning, or any other signs of infection (see page 529), be sure to tell your practitioner.

Elevated Blood Pressure

"My blood pressure was up a little bit at my last visit. Should I be worried?"

Relax. Worrying about your blood pressure will only send the readings higher. Besides, a slight increase at one visit is probably nothing to worry about at all, and might have been just a temporary blip. Maybe you were stressed because you were caught in traffic on the way to your appointment or because you were having a bad day at work. Maybe you were just nervous—you were afraid you'd gained too much weight or not enough, or you had some strange symptoms to report, or you were eager to hear the baby's heartbeat. Or maybe just being in a medical office set you on edge, elevating your blood pressure in what's commonly dubbed "white coat hypertension." To make sure anxiety doesn't do a number on those numbers again, do some relaxation exercises and some deep breathing (see page 148) while you're waiting for your next appointment—and, especially, while your blood pressure's being taken (think happy baby thoughts).

Even if your blood pressure remains slightly elevated at your next reading, such transient high blood pressure (which about 1 to 2 percent of women develop during pregnancy) is perfectly harmless and disappears after delivery (so you can still relax).

Most expectant mothers will see a slight drop in blood pressure readings during the second trimester as blood volume increases and the body starts working long hours to get that baby-making factory up to speed. But when you hit the third trimester, it usually begins to rise a bit. If it rises too much (if systolic pressure, the upper number, is 140 or more or the diastolic pressure, the lower number, is over 90) and stays up for at least 2 readings, your practitioner will monitor you more closely. That's because elevated readings in pregnancy sometimes increase cardiovascular risk later in life—but more relevant now, if it's also accompanied by protein in the urine, excessive swelling of the hands, ankles, and face, and/or severe headaches, it may turn out to be preeclampsia (see page 550).

Sugar in the Urine

"At my last office visit, the doctor said there was sugar in my urine, but that it wasn't anything to worry about. Isn't it a sign of diabetes?"

Take your doctor's advice—don't stress. Your body is probably doing just what it's supposed to do: making sure that fetus of yours, which depends on you for its fuel supply, is getting enough glucose (sugar).

The hormone insulin regulates the level of glucose in your blood and ensures that enough is taken in by your body cells for nourishment. Pregnancy triggers anti-insulin mechanisms to make sure enough sugar remains circulating in your bloodstream to nourish your fetus. It's a perfect idea that doesn't always work perfectly. Sometimes the anti-insulin effect is so strong that it leaves more than enough sugar in the

It's Your Hormones (Really)

Think just because you're a guy, you're immune to the hormonal swings of pregnancy? Not so much. Research has revealed that expectant and new dads experience a drop in the famously male sex hormone testosterone and a surge in the famously female sex hormone estrogen. And these hormonal fluctuations, which are actually common across the animal kingdom, aren't random or a sign of Mother Nature's twisted sense of humor. It's speculated that they're designed to turn up the tenderness in males—to bring out a soon-to-be dad's nurturing side, and bring out the parent in him. Which doesn't only help prepare you for the diaper changing ahead, but helps you cope with the changes (including the changes in the dynamics of your relationship) that you're both facing now.

These hormonal shifts may also contribute to some pretty strange and surprising pregnancy-like symptoms in dads-to-be (see page 162). What's more (or less), they may keep dad's libido in check (often a good thing, since a raging sex drive can sometimes be inconvenient during pregnancy—and definitely when there's a new baby in the house). Hormone levels typically return to normal within 3 to 6 months of baby's arrival, bringing with them an end to those pseudo pregnancy symptoms—and a return to libido business as usual (though not necessarily to sex life as usual until baby's sleeping through the night).

blood to meet the needs of both mom and baby—more than can be handled by the kidneys. The excess is "spilled" into the urine. So, "sugar in the urine" is not uncommon in pregnancy, especially in the second trimester, when the anti-insulin effect increases. In fact, roughly half of all pregnant women show some sugar in the urine at some point in their pregnancies.

In most women, the body responds to an increase in blood sugar with an increased production of insulin, which usually eliminates the excess sugar by the next office visit. This may well be the case with you. But some moms-to-be, especially those who are diabetic or have tendencies toward diabetes (because of a family history or because of their age or weight), may be unable to produce enough insulin at one time to handle the increase in blood sugar, or they may be unable to use the insulin they do produce efficiently. If that's the case with you, you'll continue to show high levels of sugar in both blood and urine as your pregnancy progresses. If you weren't previously diabetic, this means you have developed gestational diabetes (see page 548).

You—like every pregnant woman—will be given a glucose screening test around the 28th week to check for gestational diabetes (those at higher risk, such as obese women, may be screened earlier). Until then, don't give the sugar in your urine another thought.

Fetal Movement

"I haven't felt the baby moving yet—could something be wrong? Or could I just not be recognizing the kicking when I feel it?"

Forget that positive pregnancy test, the early ultrasound, that expanding belly, or even the lub-dub of a baby's heartbeat. Nothing says you're pregnant like fetal movement.

That is, when you finally feel it. And you're sure you felt it. However, few expectant moms, particularly first timers, feel the first kick—or even the first flutter—in the 4th month. Though an embryo starts making spontaneous movements by the 7th week, these movements, made by very tiny arms and legs, don't become apparent to mom until much later. That first flutter can be felt anytime between the 14th and 26th week, but most moms feel it closer to the average of 18 to 22 weeks. A mom expecting her second baby is likely to feel those early flutters sooner than a mom who's expecting her first, not only because she knows what a kick feels like, but because her looser uterine and abdominal muscles make it easier to feel a kick. A mom who's on the skinny side may notice early flutters, while one who's sporting lots of padding on her belly may not be aware of movements until they start packing more of a punch. The position of the placenta can also play a role: If it's facing front (an anterior placenta), it can muffle the movements and make the wait for those kicks weeks longer. Even then, the movements may feel weaker.

Sometimes, fetal movements aren't noticed when expected because of a miscalculated due date. Other times, mom doesn't recognize the movement when she feels it—she may mistake it for gas or other digestive gurgles.

So what do early movements feel like? They're almost as hard to describe as they are to recognize. Maybe it'll feel like a flutter (sort of like the "butterflies" you can get when you're nervous). Or a twitch. Or a nudge. Or even like the growling of hunger pangs. Maybe it'll feel like a bubble bursting—or that upside-down, inside-out sensation you get on a roller coaster. No matter what it feels like, it's bound to put a smile on your face—at least once you figure out for sure what it is.

Body Image

"I've always watched my weight—and now when I look in the mirror or step on a scale, I get so depressed. I feel so fat."

When you've watched your weight for so many years, watching the numbers on the scale creep up in a matter of weeks can be unnerving—and maybe a little depressing, too. But it shouldn't be. If there's one place where thin is never in, it's in pregnancy. You're supposed to gain weight when you're pregnant. And there's a very important difference between pounds gained from overeating (say, from too many midnight dates with Ben and Jerry) and pounds gained from making a baby.

In the eyes of most beholders, a pregnant woman's rounded silhouette is among the most sensuous of female shapes—beautiful not only on the inside, but on the outside as well. So instead of longing for the thinner old days (they'll be back, eventually), try getting on board with your expectant body. Embrace those new curves (which will become even more fun to embrace as they grow). Celebrate your new shape. Relish being rounder. Enjoy the pounds you pack on, instead of dreading them. As long as you're eating well and not exceeding the recommended guidelines for pregnancy weight gain, there's no reason to feel "fat"—just pregnant. The added inches you're seeing are all legitimate by-products of pregnancy, and they're temporary. The baby will be a keeper, for sure—but the extra inches won't be.

If you are packing on too many pounds too fast, feeling down probably won't keep your weight from climbing ever higher—and if you're a typical estrogen producer, will only send you to the freezer for that vat of vanilla more often. But taking a good look at your eating habits might. Remember, the idea isn't to stop the weight gain (your baby needs that weight to grow)—only to slow it down to the right rate if it's adding up a little too quickly. To do that, become more efficient in your eating—for instance, instead of digging into a pint of ice cream to score some calcium, sip a strawberry smoothie (you'll get far more calcium, far fewer calories, plus a bonus of vitamin C).

Watching your weight gain isn't the only way to give your image an edge. Exercise will definitely help, too, by ensuring that the weight you do gain ends up in all the right places (more belly, less hips and thighs). Another workout plus: It'll give you a mood lift (it's hard to host a pity party when you've got an exercise-induced endorphin high going).

Being maternity fashion-forward can also help you make friends with your mirror. Instead of trying to squeeze into your civilian wardrobe (nothing flattering about the mommy muffin-top look, especially when buttons keep popping), choose from the vast selection of creative maternity styles that accentuate the pregnant shape, rather than trying to hide it. You'll like your mirror image better, too, if you get a hairstyle that's slimming, pamper your complexion, and experiment with new makeup routines (the right techniques can take pounds off your pregnancy-rounded face; see page 152).

Most of all, remember that the body that's reflected in your mirror is working hard making a baby. And what could be more beautiful than that?

Maternity Clothes

"I can't squeeze into my regular clothes anymore, but I dread buying maternity clothes."

There's never been a more styling time to be pregnant. Gone are the days when pregnancy wardrobes were limited to polyester pup tents intended to keep the pregnant shape under cover. Not only are today's maternity clothes a lot more fashion-forward and practical to wear, but they're designed to hug (and highlight) your beautiful baby-filled belly. Visit a nearby maternity store (or shop one online) and you'll likely be filled with excitement instead of dread.

Here are some tips to consider when clothes shopping for two:

- You still have a long way to grow. So don't set off on a spending spree on the first day you can't button your jeans. Maternity clothes can be costly, especially when you consider the relatively short period of time they can be worn. So buy as you grow, and then buy only as much as you need. Though the pregnancy pillows available in maternity store dressing rooms can give a good indication of how things will fit later, they can't predict how you will carry (high, low, big, small) and which outfits will end up being the most comfortable when you crave comfort most.

- You're not limited to maternity clothes. If it fits, wear it. Buying non-maternity clothes for maternity use (or using items you already own) is, of course, the best way to avoid investing a fortune on outfits you'll wear only briefly. And depending on what the stores are showing in a particular season (hopefully the look will be flowy and drapey), anywhere from a few to many of the fashions on the regular racks may be suitable for pregnant shapes—though you may need to size up. Still, be wary of spending a lot on such purchases. Though you may love the clothes now, you may love them considerably less after you've worn them throughout your pregnancy. Plus, if you've bought them on the big side, they may not fit once you've shed your baby fat.

Trimming Tricks

Big is beautiful when you're expecting, but that doesn't mean you can't try some tricks of the trim. With the right fashion choices, you can highlight your baby-licious bump while slimming your overall silhouette. Here's how to show in all the right places:

Make black a basic. And navy blue, chocolate brown, deep purple, dark maroon, or charcoal. You've heard this before, but dark colors are slimming, minimizing body bulk and giving you an overall trimmer appearance, even if you're wearing a t-shirt and yoga pants.

Think monotone. One color fits all—or at least looks slimmer. Sticking to a single hue (or to one color with slight variations) from top to bottom will make you look longer and leaner. A two-tone look, however, will create a break in your figure, causing the eye to stop right at the color change (and possibly right where your hips start spreading).

Be picky with prints. Tired of the monotone and want to add some pattern to your life? Choose a print that's just the right size. Too small and you'll look large, too large and you'll look even larger. Aim for a print that's midsize—about the size of a golf ball—to get it just right. And look for prints that have only 2 or 3 colors. More just makes, well, more.

Go long. It's the oldest trick in the fashion book, but for good reason—it works. As you widen, choose clothes with vertical lines (which create height and give you a leaner look) instead of horizontal lines (which widen you even further). Look for clothes with vertical stripes, vertical zippers, vertical stitching, and vertical rows of buttons. Go vertical with jewelry and accessories, too: a low-hanging necklace, mega-dangling earrings, an extra long scarf.

Focus on the pluses. Like those probably plus-size breasts of yours (there's never been a better time to spotlight your cleavage). And minimize attention to the spots that you might be less inclined to want to show off, such as those swollen ankles (keep them under pants, long flowing skirts, or comfortable boots, or wear slimming black tights or leggings).

Stay fit. With your clothes, that is. While you'll definitely want clothes that have room to grow in the bust and the belly, look for tops—shirts, sweaters, jackets, and dresses—that fit you well in the shoulders (probably the only part of your body that won't be widening). Hanging shoulders will give you a sloppy (and bulky) look. And though clinging can be slimming, watch out for clothes that are so clingy they appear too tight—like you've outgrown them (which you probably have). The overstuffed sausage look is never in style, after all.

- You've got it, so flaunt it. Bellies are out of the closet—and out from under those mama muumuus. Most maternity clothes celebrate the pregnant bump (and the more voluptuous rump) with clingy fabrics and snug-fitting styles (say, in a wrap dress, instead of under wraps). And that's something to celebrate, since belly-accentuating maternity wear actually slims your silhouette down. Not crazy about the cling? Long, flowing maxidresses are comfortable and easy-to-wear options, too, especially as your belly grows. Another great option: low-rise jeans and pants that can be worn under your belly. A low rise is also elongating because it doesn't cut you off in the middle (and what expectant mom couldn't use a little elongating?).

And talking about flaunting what you've got, pick a body part that you feel most comfortable with (let's say your arms or legs . . . or cleavage) and choose clothes that highlight that great asset (or butt) of yours.

- Dip into his dresser. It's all there for the taking (though it's probably a good idea to ask him first): oversize shirts that look great over pants or leggings, sweatpants that accommodate more inches than yours do, running shorts that will keep up with your waistline for at least a couple more months, belts with the few extra notches you need. Keep in mind, though, that by the 6th month (possibly a lot sooner), no matter how big your man is around the middle, you're likely to outgrow him and his clothes.

- Both a borrower and a lender be. Accept all offers of used maternity clothes, as long as they fit. In a pinch, any extra dress, skirt, or pair of jeans may do—you can make any borrowed item your own with accessories. When your term is over, offer to lend those maternity outfits you bought and can't or don't want to wear post-partum to newly pregnant friends. Between you and your friends, you'll be getting your money's worth.

- Be a renter, too. Have a wedding or other formal event to attend and don't feel like shelling out the big bucks for a one-night-only maternity ensemble? Consider renting it from one of the growing number of maternity clothing rental services (some moms even rent their entire maternity wardrobes!)

- Don't overlook those accessories the public never sees. A well-fitting, supportive bra should be your bosom buddy during pregnancy, especially as that bosom expands . . . and expands. Skip the sale racks and put yourself in the hands of an experienced fitter at a well-stocked lingerie department or shop. With any luck, she will be able to tell you approximately how much extra room and support you need and which kind of bra will provide it. But don't stock up. Buy just a couple, and then go back for another fitting when you graduate to the next cup.

Special maternity underwear isn't usually necessary, but if you do decide to go that route, you'll probably be relieved to find that it's a lot sexier than it used to be (goodbye granny panties, hello thongs and bikinis). You can also opt for regular bikini panties—bought in a larger-than-usual size if you need the room—worn under your belly. Buy them in favorite colors and/or sexy fabrics to give your spirits a lift (but make sure the crotches are cotton).

- Cotton is cooler. Hot stuff (fabrics that don't breathe, such as nylon and other synthetics) isn't so hot when you're pregnant. Because your metabolic rate is higher than usual, making you feel warmer than usual, you'll feel more comfortable in cotton. You'll also be less likely to get heat rash (a common complaint among the pregnant set). Knee highs or thigh highs will also be more comfortable than tights or panty hose, but avoid those that have a narrow constrictive band at the top. If you do tights, opt for cotton (yes, even support hose come in cotton). Light colors, mesh weaves, and looser fits will also help you keep your cool in warm weather. When the weather turns cold, dressing in layers is ideal, since you can selectively peel off as you heat up or when you go indoors.

Unwanted Advice

"Now that it's obvious I'm expecting, everyone—from my mother-in-law to strangers on the elevator—has advice for me. It drives me crazy."

There's just something about a bulging bump that brings out the so-called expert in everyone—and breaks down social barriers that usually keep strangers minding their own business. Take your morning jog around the park and someone is sure to chide, "You shouldn't be running in your condition!" Lug home 2 bags of groceries from the supermarket and you're bound to hear, "Do you think you should be carrying that?" Double dip at the ice cream shop, and expect the fingers to start wagging: "That baby fat's not going to be easy to lose, honey."

Between the pregnancy police, the gratuitous advice-givers, and all those inevitable predictions about the sex of the baby, what's an expectant mother to do? First of all, keep in mind that most of what you hear is probably nonsense. Old wives' tales that do have foundation in fact have been, for the most part scientifically substantiated and have become part of standard medical practice. Those that do not might still be tightly woven into pregnancy mythology but can be confidently dismissed. Those recommendations that leave you with a nagging doubt ("What if they're right?") are best checked out with your doctor, midwife, or childbirth educator.

Whether it's possibly plausible or obviously ridiculous, however, don't let unwanted advice get you going—who needs the added stress anyway? Instead, keep your sense of humor handy and try one of these approaches: Politely inform the well-meaning stranger, friend, or relative that you have a trusted practitioner who counsels you on your pregnancy and that, even though you appreciate the thought, you can't accept advice from anyone else. Or, just as politely, smile, say thank you, and go on your way, letting their comments go in one ear and out the other—without making any stops in between.

But no matter how you choose to handle unwanted advice, you might also want to get used to it. If there's anyone who attracts a crowd of advice-givers faster than a woman with a belly, it's a woman with a new baby.

Unwanted Belly Touching

"Now that I'm showing, everyone—even people I barely know—comes up to me and touches my belly, without even asking. I find that kind of creepy."

They're round, they're cute, and they're filled with something even cuter. Let's face it, pregnant bellies just scream out to be touched, and they often are—usually without permission. And that's just fine with some moms-to-be, who don't mind being the center of so much touching attention—or even enjoy it. Still, bottom line: your belly, your business. It may take a village, after all, but bumps aren't the communal property some people view them as—and bellies can (and should) have borders. If the uninvited rubbing is rubbing you the wrong way, you have every right to head off those hands headed toward your bump.

You can do this bluntly (if politely): "I know you find my belly tempting to touch, but I'd really rather you didn't." Or playfully: "No touching, please—the baby's sleeping!" Or, you can try turning the tummy tables, rubbing the rubber right back (patting someone's paunch might make him or her think twice before touching another pregnant belly without permission). Or make your statement without saying a word: Cross your arms protectively over your bump, or take the rubber's hand off your midsection and place it somewhere else (like on his or her own belly).

Forgetfulness

"Last week I left the house without my cell phone. This morning I completely forgot an important appointment. I can't focus on anything, and I'm beginning to think I'm losing my mind."

You're in good (forgetful) company. Many moms-to-be begin to feel that as they're gaining pounds, they're losing brain cells. Even women who usually manage to micromanage to the max, stay focused and organized in the face of chaos, and cope with (no, crush!) whatever a day sends their way, suddenly find themselves forgetting appointments, missing meetings, losing their train of thought (along with their cool . . . and their wallets and cell phones). And this pregnancy forgetfulness isn't in their heads—it's in their brains. Researchers have found that a woman's brain-cell volume actually decreases during pregnancy (which could explain why you won't remember what you just read in that last paragraph). And—for reasons as yet unexplained—moms expecting girls are more forgetful, on average, than those carrying boys. Fortunately, this pregnancy brain fog (similar to what many women experience with PMS, only thicker) is only temporary. Your brain will plump back up a few months after delivery.

Like most pregnancy symptoms, pregnancy forgetfulness (often dubbed "placenta brain" or "pregnancy brain") is hormonally triggered. Sleep deprivation can also play a role (the less you sleep, the less you remember), as can

the fact that you're constantly low on energy—energy your brain needs to stay focused. Also contributing to your scatterbrained self: the mom-to-be mind overload that's keeping all brain circuits busy.

Feeling stressed about this intellectual fogginess will only make it worse (stress also compounds forgetfulness). Recognizing that it is normal (and not imagined), even accepting it with a sense of humor, may help to ease it—or, at least, make you feel better about it. Realistically, it might just not be possible to be as efficient as you were before you took on the added job of baby making. Keeping checklists on your smartphone (along with reminder alarms) can help contain the mental chaos—that is, if you can remember where you put your phone last. Set electronic reminders of important dates and appointments, and tap into the What to Expect app. Strategically placed post-its (one on the front door to remind you to take your keys, for instance) can also help keep you on track.

Although ginkgo biloba has been touted for its memory-boosting properties, it's not considered safe for use during pregnancy, so you'll have to forget about using that and any other herbal preparation in your battle against pregnancy-induced forgetfulness. You may find more focus, though, from regular infusions of protein and complex carbs—in the form of those maxi-sustaining mini-meals. Low blood sugar caused by too-long stretches between eating (and eating well) can definitely contribute to that foggy feeling.

And you might as well get used to working at a little below peak efficiency. The fog may well continue after your baby's arrival (because of fatigue, not hormones) and perhaps may not lift completely until baby (and you) start sleeping through the night.

ALL ABOUT:

Working Out When You're Expecting

You're aching and you can't sleep and your back is killing you and your ankles are swelling and you're constipated and bloated and you're passing more gas than a busload of high school football players who just stopped for fast food. In other words, you're pregnant. Now, if only there were something you could do that might minimize the aches and pains and unpleasant side effects of pregnancy.

Actually, there is, and it'll take just minutes (make that 30 minutes) a day: exercise. Thought pregnancy was a time to take it easy? Not anymore. Lucky for you (or unlucky, if you're a member of the couch potato club), the official advice of ACOG reads like a personal

Your Main Squeeze

Looking for a workout that you can do anytime, anywhere (on the sofa, at your desk, in line at the supermarket, sitting in traffic, eating lunch, browsing baby sites, even while you're having sex)—without heading to the gym or breaking a sweat?

Say hello to the Kegel—an exercise that works out one of the most important sets of muscles in your body: your pelvic floor muscles. Never thought much about your pelvic floor muscles—or maybe never even realized you had them? It's time to start paying attention. They're the muscles that support your uterus, bladder, and bowels, and they're designed to stretch so your baby can come out. They're also the muscles that keep your urine from leaking when you cough or laugh (a skill set you're likely to appreciate only when it's gone, as can happen with postpartum incontinence). These multitalented muscles can also make for a much more satisfying sexual experience.

Luckily, Kegels can easily whip those miracle muscles into shape with minimal time and minimal effort. Just 5 minutes of Kegels, 3 times a day, and you'll tone your way to a long list of both short- and long-term benefits. Toned pelvic floor muscles can ease a host of pregnancy and postpartum symptoms from hemorrhoids to urinary and fecal incontinence. They can help you prevent an episiotomy or even a tear during delivery. Plus, doing your Kegels faithfully during pregnancy will help your vagina snap back more gracefully after your baby's grand exit (and even if you end up having a c-section).

Ready to Kegel? Here's how: Tense the muscles around your vagina and anus and hold (as you would if you were trying to stop the flow of urine), working up to 10 seconds. Slowly release and repeat; shoot for 3 sets of 20 daily. Keep in mind when you Kegel that all your focus should be on those pelvic muscles—and not any others. If you feel your stomach tensing or your thighs or buttocks contracting, your pelvics aren't getting their full workout. Make Kegels your main squeeze during pregnancy, and you'll reap the benefits of stronger pelvic floor muscles for a lifetime. Try doing them during sex, too—both you and your partner will feel the difference (now, that's a workout you can get excited about!).

trainer's pep talk: Women with normal pregnancies should get 30 minutes or more a day of moderate exercise on most (if not all) days.

And barring any activity restrictions from your practitioner, you can, too. It doesn't matter whether you started out as an iron woman in peak physical condition or a sofa slacker who hasn't laced up sneakers since your last gym class (except as a fashion statement). There are plenty of perks to exercising for two.

The Benefits of Exercise

So what's in it for you? Regular exercise can help:

- Your stamina. It seems counterintuitive, but sometimes getting too much rest can actually make you feel more tired. A little exercise can go a long way when it comes to giving your energy level the boost it needs.

- Your sleep. Many pregnant women have a hard time falling asleep (not to mention staying asleep), but those who exercise consistently often sleep better and wake up feeling more rested. Just don't work out right before bed.

- Your health. Exercise, especially when teamed with reasonable weight gain and a healthy diet, may prevent gestational diabetes, a growing problem among pregnant women.

- Your mood. Exercise causes your brain to release endorphins, those feel-good chemicals that give you a natural high—improving your mood, diminishing stress and anxiety.

- Your back. A strong set of abs is the best defense against back pain, which bothers many pregnant women. But even exercise that's not directly targeting the tummy can also relieve back pain and pressure. An example: Swimming or water aerobics can be the perfect prescription for pregnancy back pain (sciatic pain, too).

- Your (tense) muscles. Stretching does your body good—especially a pregnant body, which is more prone to muscle cramps in the legs (and elsewhere). Stretching can help you uncover little pockets of tension, warding off sore muscles. Plus you can do it anywhere, anytime—even if you spend most of your day sitting down—and you don't even have to break a sweat.

- Your bowels. An active body encourages active bowels. Even a 10-minute stroll helps get things going. Kegels can, too (see box, page 229).

- Your labor. Though exercise during pregnancy can't guarantee that you'll race through childbirth, moms who exercise tend to have shorter labors and are less likely to need labor and delivery interventions (including c-sections).

- Your postpartum recovery. The more fit you stay during pregnancy, the faster you'll recover physically after childbirth (and the sooner you'll be zipping up those skinny jeans again).

What's in it for baby? Plenty. Researchers theorize that changes in heart rate and oxygen levels in exercising moms-to-be stimulate their babies. Babies are also stimulated by the sounds and vibrations they experience in the womb during workouts. Exercise regularly during pregnancy, and your baby might end up being:

- More fit. On average, babies of moms who exercise during pregnancy are

Working in Workouts

Your mission when it comes to exercise during pregnancy, should you choose to accept it (and there are lots of reasons why you should), is to work your way up to 30 minutes of some sort of activity a day. And if that sounds daunting, keep in mind that three 10-minute walks or even six 5-minute mini-workouts sprinkled throughout the day are just as beneficial as 30 minutes on the treadmill. (See, it's not as hard as it sounds.)

Still not convinced that you have the time? To make your mission possible, try thinking of exercise as part of your day—like brushing your teeth and going to work—and build it into your routine (that's how it becomes routine, after all).

If there's no place in your schedule to block out gym time, just incorporate exercise into your daily activities: Get off the bus 2 stops from the office, and walk the rest of the way. Park your car in a faraway spot at the mall instead of cruising for the closest (and while you're at the mall, take a few extra laps around—those count, too). Take a brisk walk to the deli instead of ordering in your sandwich. Use the stairs instead of the elevator. Walk up the escalator instead of going along for the ride. Use the restroom that's farther away instead of the one across the hall.

Have the time but lack the motivation? Find it in a pregnancy exercise class (the camaraderie will help cheer you on) or by exercising with a friend (form a lunchtime walking club or hit the hiking trails with your buds on Saturdays before your weekly brunch). Just plain bored with your workouts? Switch it up—try pregnancy yoga if you're tired (literally) of running, or swimming (or water aerobics) if the stationary cycle is getting you nowhere. Find your exercise excitement in a pregnancy workout video.

Sure, there'll be days (especially in those fatigue-prone first and third trimesters), when you're too pooped to lift your legs off the coffee table, never mind actually do leg lifts. But there's never been a better time, or better reasons, to get yourself moving.

born at healthier weights, are better able to weather labor and delivery (they're less stressed by it), and recover from the stresses of birth more quickly. And since a baby's heart rate gets pumped up as his or her mom pumps up, it's as if the baby is also getting a cardio workout, which may result in a healthier heart later in life.

- Smarter. Believe it or not, research shows that babies of moms who exercise throughout pregnancy score higher, on average, on IQ tests by age 5 (meaning that your workout may boost both your muscle power and baby's brain power!).

- Easier. Babies of pregnant exercisers, on average, tend to sleep through the night sooner, are less prone to colic, and are better able to soothe themselves.

Exercising the Right Way

Not only does your pregnant body not fit into your regular workout clothes anymore—it may not fit into your regular workout routine, either. Now that you're exercising for two, you'll need to make doubly sure you're exercising the right way. Here are some

Exercise Smarts

Exercising with a baby on board? Remember to use your exercise smarts:

- **Replenish fluids.** For every half hour of moderate activity, you will need at least a full glass of extra liquid to compensate for fluids lost through perspiration. You will need more in warm weather or whenever you're sweating a lot. Drink before, during, and after exercising—but no more than 16 ounces at a time. It's a good idea to start your fluid intake 30 to 45 minutes before your planned workout.

- **Bring on the snacks.** A light but sustaining before-workout snack will help keep your energy up. Follow up with a light snack, too, especially if you've burned a lot of calories. You'll have to consume about 150 to 200 additional calories for every half hour of moderate exercising.

- **Stay cool.** Any exercise or environment that raises a pregnant woman's temperature more than 1.5 degrees should be avoided (it causes blood to be shunted to the skin and away from the uterus as the body attempts to cool off). So stay out of saunas, steam rooms, or hot tubs, and don't exercise outdoors in very hot or humid weather or indoors in a stuffy, overheated room (no Bikram or hot yoga). If you generally walk outdoors, try an air-conditioned mall instead when the temperature soars.

- **Dress for exercise success.** Play it cool by wearing loose, breathable, stretchable clothes. Choose a sports bra that provides plenty of support for your probably bigger breasts but doesn't pinch once you get moving.

- **Put your feet first.** If your sneakers are showing their age, replace them now to minimize your chances of injury or falls. And make sure you choose workout shoes that are designed for the sport you're pursuing.

- **Select the right surface.** Indoors, a wood floor or a tightly carpeted

pointers, whether you're a gym junkie or a Sunday stroller:

The starting line is the practitioner's office. Before you lace up your sneaks and hit the cardio class, make a pit stop at your practitioner's office for the workout green light. You'll almost certainly get it—most women do. But if you have any medical or pregnancy complications, your practitioner may limit your exercise program, nix it entirely, or—if you have or are at increased risk for gestational diabetes—even encourage you to exercise more. Be sure you're clear about what exercise programs are appropriate for you and whether your normal fitness routine (if you have one) is safe to continue while you're expecting. If you're in good health, your practitioner will likely encourage you to stick with your regular routine as long as you feel up to it, with certain modifications (especially if your regular routine includes pregnancy-taboo sports, like ice hockey).

Respect your body as it changes. Expect your routines to change as your body does. You'll need to modify your workouts as your sense of balance shifts, and you'll probably also have to slow down to avoid taking a spill (especially surface is better than tile or concrete for your workouts. (If the surface is slippery, don't exercise in socks or footed tights.) Better yet, invest in a yoga mat that can do double duty as a surface for your cardio workout as well. Outdoors, soft running tracks and grassy or dirt trails are better than hard-surfaced roads or sidewalk, and level surfaces are better than uneven ones.

- Stay off the slopes. Because your growing bump will affect your sense of balance, ACOG suggests women in the latter part of pregnancy avoid sports that come with a higher risk of falling or abdominal injury. These include gymnastics, downhill skiing or snowboarding, ice skating, vigorous racquet sports (play doubles instead of singles), and horseback riding, as well as cycling and contact sports such as ice hockey, soccer, and basketball (see page 236 for more).

- Stay on the level. Unless you're living at high altitudes, avoid any activity that takes you up more than 6,000 feet. On the flip side, scuba diving, which poses a risk of decompression sickness for your baby, is also off-limits, so you'll have to wait until you're no longer carrying a passenger to take your next dive.

- Stay off your back. After the 4th month, don't exercise flat on your back. The weight of your enlarging uterus could compress major blood vessels, restricting circulation.

- Avoid certain moves. Some moms-to-be find that pointing (or extending) their toes can lead to cramps in their calves. If that's the case with you (and it probably won't be if you're a regular at the barre), flex your feet instead, turning your toes up toward your face. Full sit-ups or double leg lifts pull on the abdomen, so they're probably not a good idea when you've got a baby on board. Also avoid any activity that requires "bridging" (bending over backward) or other contortions, or that involves deep flexion or extension of joints (such as deep knee bends), jumping, bouncing, sudden changes in direction, or jerky motions.

once you can no longer see your feet). Also expect workouts to feel different, even if you've been doing a particular routine for years. If you're a walker, for example, you'll feel more pressure on your hips and knees as your pregnancy progresses and as your joints and ligaments loosen. After the first trimester, you'll also have to accommodate your pregnant body by possibly avoiding any exercise that requires you to lie flat on your back or stand without moving (like some yoga and tai chi poses do). Both can restrict your blood flow.

Start slow. If you're new at this, start slowly. It's tempting to begin with a bang, running 3 miles the first morning or working out twice the first afternoon. But such enthusiastic beginnings usually lead not to fitness but to sore muscles, sagging resolve—and abrupt endings. Start the first day with 10 minutes of warm-ups followed by 5 minutes of a more strenuous workout (but stop sooner if you begin to tire) and a 5-minute cool down. After a few days, if your body has adjusted well, increase the period of strenuous activity by about 5 minutes until you are up to 30 minutes or more, if you feel comfortable.

Already a gym rat? Remember that while pregnancy is a great time to maintain your fitness level, it's probably not a time to increase it (you can set new personal bests after baby arrives).

Get off to a slow start every time you start. Warm-ups can be a drag when you're eager to get your workout started—and over with. But as every athlete knows, they're an essential part of any exercise program. They ensure that the heart and circulation aren't taxed suddenly and reduce the chances of injury to muscles and joints, which are more vulnerable when cold—and particularly during pregnancy. So walk before you run, swim slowly or jog in place in the pool before you start your laps.

Finish as slowly as you start. Collapse may seem like the logical conclusion to a workout, but it isn't physiologically sound. Stopping abruptly traps blood in the muscles, reducing blood supply to other parts of your body and to your baby. Dizziness, faintness, extra heartbeats, or nausea may result. So finish your exercise with exercise: about 5 minutes of walking after running, easy paddling after a vigorous swim, light stretching exercises after almost any activity. Top off your cool down with a few minutes of relaxation. You can help avoid dizziness (and a possible fall) if you get up slowly when you've been exercising on the floor or on the stationary bike.

Watch the clock. Too little exercise won't be effective, too much can be debilitating. A full workout, from warm up to cool down, can take anywhere from 30 minutes to an hour. But keep the level of exertion mild to moderate.

Keep it up. Exercising erratically (4 times one week and none the next) won't get you or keep you in shape. Exercising regularly (at least 4 times, preferably 5 to 7 times a week, every week) will. If you're too tired for a strenuous workout, don't push yourself, but do try to do the warm-ups so that your muscles will stay limber and your discipline won't dissolve. Many women find they feel better if they do some exercise—if not necessarily their full workout—every day. Besides, daily (or mostly daily) exercise is, after all, what the doctors of ACOG ordered.

Consider classes. For many moms-to-be, taking a group fitness class can provide camaraderie, support, and feedback—not to mention a motivating kick in the yoga pants when self-discipline lags. Any class you take should be specifically designed for moms-to-be and taught by an instructor who has pregnancy fitness cred. Look for a program that's fun, maintains moderate intensity, meets at least 3 times weekly, and individualizes according to abilities. If you can, try a class out before you buy a whole series. Can't commit to a regularly scheduled class? Bring one into your own home, at your own convenience, with the *What to Expect When You're Expecting: The Workout* DVD.

Make it fun. The right workout will be one that you really enjoy instead of really dread. A workout that's fun (not torture) will be easier to stick with—particularly on days when you have no energy, feel the size of an SUV, or both.

Do everything in moderation. Never exercise to the point of exhaustion when you're expecting (and even if you're a trained athlete, ask your practitioner whether it's wise to work out to your fullest capacity during pregnancy, whether it exhausts you or not). There are several ways of checking to see whether you're overdoing it—and checking your pulse isn't one of them, so lose that habit. First, if it feels good, it's probably okay. If there's any pain or strain, it's probably not. A little sweat is fine, a drenching sweat is a sign to slow down. So is being unable to carry on a conversation as you go. Work hard enough so you feel yourself breathing more heavily, but not so out of breath that you aren't able to talk, sing, or whistle while you work(out). Needing a nap after completing a workout means you've likely worked too hard. You should feel energized, not drained, after exercising.

Know when to stop. Your body will signal when it's time by saying, "Hey, I'm tired." Take the hint right away, and throw in the towel. Minor aches and pains that aren't necessarily dangerous (like round ligament pain; see page 255) but that pop up every time you work out are a sign that you should take it a little slower (don't run as fast, for instance, or walk instead of run). More serious signals suggest a call to your practitioner: unusual pain anywhere (hip, back, pelvis, chest, head, and so on), a cramp or stitch that doesn't go away when you stop exercising, uterine contractions and chest pain, lightheadedness or dizziness, very rapid heartbeat, severe breathlessness, difficulty walking or loss of muscle control, sudden headache, increased swelling, amniotic fluid leakage or vaginal bleeding, or, after the 28th week, a slowing down or total absence of fetal movement.

Taper off in the last trimester. Most women find that they need to slack off somewhat in the third trimester, particularly during the 9th month, when stretching routines and brisk walking or water workouts will probably provide enough exercise. If you feel up to sticking with a more vigorous program (and you're fit enough to handle it), your practitioner may green-light your usual workout routine right up until delivery, but definitely ask first.

Don't just sit there. Sitting for an extended period without a break causes blood to pool in your leg veins and can cause your feet to swell. If your work entails a lot of sitting, or if you have a long daily commute, or travel long distances frequently, be sure to break up every hour or so of sitting with 5 or 10 minutes of walking. And while at your seat, periodically do some exercises that enhance circulation, such as taking a few deep breaths, extending your lower legs, flexing your feet, and wiggling your toes. Also try contracting the muscles in your abdomen and buttocks (a sort of sitting pelvic tilt). If your hands tend to swell, periodically stretch your arms above your head, opening and closing your fists several times as you do.

Choosing the Right Pregnancy Workouts

While it's true that pregnancy isn't the time to learn to water ski, snowboard, or enter a horse-jumping competition, you'll still be able to enjoy most fitness activities—and use many of the machines at the gym (with a few caveats). You can select, too, from the growing number of exercise programs specifically designed for expecting moms (pregnancy water aerobics, pregnancy Pilates, and prenatal yoga classes, for example). But be sure to ask your practitioner about what's okay and what's not when it comes to choosing an exercise program or sport. You'll probably find that most of the activities that are off-limits when you're expecting are ones you'd probably have a hard time doing well anyway once you have a basketball-size belly (like competitive basketball . . . or football or scuba diving or downhill racing or mountain biking). Here are the do's and don'ts of pregnancy workouts:

Walking. Just about anyone can do it—and do it just about anywhere, anytime. There's no easier exercise to fit into your busy schedule than walking (don't forget, all the walking you do counts, even if it's walking 2 blocks to the market or 10 minutes while the dog does her business). And you can continue to fit it in right up until delivery day (and even on delivery day if you're eager to get those contractions moving along). Best of all, there's no equipment necessary—and no gym membership or classes to pay for, either. All you need is a supportive pair of sneakers and comfortable, breathable clothes. If you're just beginning a walking routine, go slowly at first (start out at a stroll before you move on to a brisk pace). Weather's not cooperative? Do a power mall walk.

Jogging. Experienced runners can stay on track during pregnancy—but you may want to limit your distances and stick to level terrain or use a treadmill (if you weren't a runner prepregnancy, stick to brisk walking for now). Keep in mind that loosening ligaments and joints during pregnancy can literally be a pain, make running harder on your knees, and also make you more prone to injury—all good reasons to listen to your pregnant body and adjust your runs accordingly

Exercise machines. Treadmills, ellipticals, and stair-climbers are all good bets during pregnancy. Adjust speed, incline, and tension to a level that's comfortable for you (starting out slowly if you're a rookie). Toward the end of your pregnancy, though, you may find a machine workout too strenuous (or maybe not—as always, take your cues from your body). You may also have to be more conscious of avoiding stumbles on the machine when you're no longer able to see your feet.

Swimming and water workouts. Consider this: In the water, you weigh just a tenth of what you do on land (how often do you have the chance to be close to weightless these days?), making water workouts the perfect choice for a pregnant woman. Working out in the water boosts your strength and flexibility but is gentle on your joints—plus there's much less risk of overheating (unless the pool is overheated). What's more, many pregnant women report that water workouts help ease swelling in their legs and feet and relieve sciatic pain. Most gyms with a pool offer water aerobics, and many have classes specifically designed for expectant moms. Just be careful when walking on slippery pool sides, and don't dive in.

Yoga. Yoga encourages relaxation, focus, and paying attention to your breathing—so it's just about perfect for

30 Minutes Plus?

Is more (exercise) more—or less? That depends. If you're really ambitious (or just really fit), and you've been green-lighted by your practitioner (based on your fitness level), it's safe to work out for up to an hour or even more, as long as you listen to your body. Moms-to-be tend to tire out sooner than they used to, and tired bodies are more apt to injure themselves. Plus, overexertion could lead to other problems—for instance, dehydration if you don't take in enough fluids, or lack of oxygen to the baby if you're short of breath for long periods. Burning more calories during your marathon sessions also means you'll need to take in more, so be sure to compensate appropriately (the best part of a workout, wouldn't you say?).

pregnancy (and great preparation for childbirth, as well as for parenting). It also increases oxygenation (bringing more oxygen to the baby) and increases flexibility, possibly making pregnancy—and delivery—easier. Select a class that's specifically tailored to expectant women or ask your instructor how to modify poses so that they're safe for you. For instance, you probably shouldn't exercise on your back after the 4th month, and as pregnancy progresses your center of gravity changes, so you'll have to adjust your favorite poses accordingly. And unless you're an experienced yoga inversion practitioner, you should probably avoid full inversions (handstand, supported shoulder stand, and supported headstand) after the 3rd month—not only because your balance will be off, but also because of potential blood pressure issues. Some doctors and midwives say half inversions—like downward facing dog—are okay during pregnancy.

Another important caveat: Avoid Bikram or hot yoga. It's done in a very warm room (one that's generally 90°F to 100°F), and you'll need to take a pass during pregnancy on any workouts that heat you up too much.

Pilates. Pilates is similar to yoga in that it's a discipline that improves your flexibility, strength, and muscle tone with no- to low-impact. The focus is on strengthening your core, which will ease backaches and improve your posture (important for preventing aches and pains when you're toting a baby in your belly, but also when you're toting one in your arms). Look for a class specifically tailored to pregnant women, or let your instructor know that you're expecting so you can avoid pregnancy-inappropriate moves (including those that overstretch) or equipment that isn't compatible with pregnancy.

Dance/Aerobics. Zumba, mama? Experienced athletes in good shape can continue all types of dance (like belly dancing, ballroom dancing, hip-hop or salsa, Zumba, and so on) and aerobic workouts during pregnancy. But dance with care. Tone down the intensity level, avoid jumping or high-impact movements, and never exert yourself to the point of exhaustion. If you're a beginner, choose low-impact aerobics or consider the water version, which is uniquely suited to the pregnant set.

Barre classes. These ballet-inspired workouts are great when you're expecting because they include lots of legwork with minimal jumping. The balance exercises and core strengthening are pregnancy perfect, too, especially when your swelling belly slackens the core and throws you off balance. So belly up to the barre, but with a little mom-to-be modification: Since some of the lower-body movements may put strain on your back, especially as your belly gets bigger, adapt movements (such as by getting to your hands and knees for certain positions) as needed.

Step routines. As long as you're already in good shape and have experience doing step routines, it's usually fine to stay in step with them now. Just remember that your joints are more prone to injury when you're pregnant, so stretch out well beforehand and don't overexert yourself. And of course, don't step on something too high off the ground. As your abdomen expands, avoid any activities that require careful balance.

Spinning. Is spinning in when you're expecting? If you've been spinning for at least 6 months before pregnancy, you should be able to continue, but tone down the workout (and let the instructor know you're expecting so you're not pushed too hard). Remember to take it down a notch if you're panting or gasping for breath. And for maximum comfort, adjust the handlebars so they're closer to you, allowing you to sit back instead of leaning forward, which could make your lower back ache more than it likely already does. Stay seated, since standing while spinning is too intense for a mama-to-be. If spinning suddenly seems exhausting, take a bike break until after the baby's born (and after you've recovered from childbirth).

Kickboxing. Kickboxing takes grace and speed—two things pregnant women don't typically possess lots of. Many pregnant kickboxers find they can't kick as high or move as quickly, but if you're still comfortable getting your exercise from getting your kicks, and you have plenty of experience (no novices now), it's okay to continue while you're expecting. Just be sure to avoid any movements that you have difficulty with or cause you to strain. Make sure you keep a safe distance from other kickboxers (you don't want to be kicked in the belly by accident) by leaving 2 leg lengths of space between you and those around you. Be sure, too, that everyone in the class knows you're pregnant, or look for pregnancy-specific classes (where everyone around you is pregnant—and far away).

Weight training. Using weights can increase your muscle tone (and get your biceps ready for lifing baby), but it's important to avoid heavy weights or those that require grunting or breath holding, which may compromise blood flow to the uterus. Use light weights with multiple repetitions instead. Ask your practitioner about what modifications you'll need to make to your TRX routine (or whether you should retire the equipment for the duration) and skip those CrossFit routines for now (unless you've been at it for years and your practitioner gives you the thumbs-up).

Outdoor sports (hiking, skating, bicycling, skiing). Pregnancy isn't the time to take up a new sport—especially one that challenges your balance—but experienced athletes should be able to continue these activities with their practitioner's approval and some sensible precautions. When hiking, be sure to avoid uneven terrain (especially later on in pregnancy when it won't be easy to see that rock in your path), high altitudes, and slippery conditions—and of course, rock climbing is out. When biking, be extra careful—wear a helmet, don't ride on wet pavement, winding paths, or bumpy surfaces (falling is never a good idea but especially not when you're pregnant), and don't lean forward into racing posture (it can tax your lower back, plus this isn't the time for speeding—slow and steady should win all your races now). As for ice skating, you can give it a whirl (and a figure 8) early in pregnancy if you're experienced and careful—later on, you'll probably face balance issues, so stop as soon as you get more bulky than graceful. Ditto for in-line skating and horseback riding. Avoid downhill skiing or snowboarding altogether, even if you've got years of double black diamonds under your belt—the risk of a serious fall or collision is too great (even pros take the occasional tumble—and there's no gauging the skill of others around you). Cross-country skiing and snowshoeing are okay for the experienced, but you'll have to be extra careful to avoid falling.

Tai chi. An ancient form of meditative exercises, tai chi's basic slow movements allow even the least limber the opportunity to relax and strengthen the body without the risk of injury. If you're comfortable with it and have experience, it's fine to continue tai chi now. Look for pregnancy-specific classes, or just stick to moves you can easily complete—take extra care with the balancing poses.

Basic Pregnancy Exercises

Never been to a gym? Don't know a lunge from a squat? Or just unsure where to begin when exercising for two? Here are some simple and safe exercises you can do when you're expecting.

Shoulder Stretch. To ease tension in your shoulders (especially helpful if you spend a lot of time at the computer), try this simple move: Stand with your feet shoulder-width apart and knees slightly bent. Bring your left arm out in front of you at chest height and bend it slightly. Take your right hand, place it on your left elbow, and then gently pull your left elbow toward your right shoulder as you exhale. Hold the stretch for 5 to 10 seconds, then switch sides.

Shoulder Stretch ▶

Dromedary Droop ▶

Standing Leg Stretch. Give your legs a much-needed break with this easy stretch: Stand and hold on to a countertop, the back of a heavy chair, or another sturdy object for support. Bend your right knee and bring your right foot back and up toward your buttocks. Grasp your foot with your right hand and bring your heel toward your buttocks while extending your thigh backward from the hip joint. Keep your back straight and hold the stretch for 10 to 30 seconds. Repeat with the left leg.

Standing Leg Stretch ▶

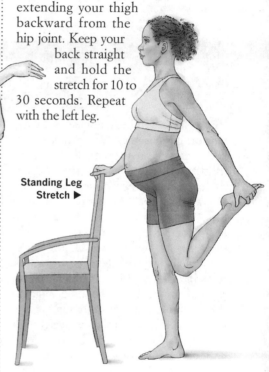

Dromedary Droop (or Cat/Cow Pose). A great way to relieve back pressure is to get down on your hands and knees and relax your back, keeping your head straight and making sure your neck is lined up with your spine. Then arch your back—you'll feel your abs and buttocks tighten. Let your head gently droop down. Slowly return to your original position. Repeat several times—and do this stretch several times a day if you can, especially if you're standing or sitting a lot on the job.

Neck Relaxer ▼

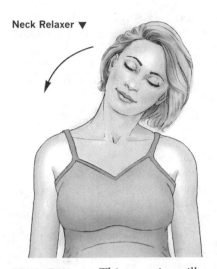

Neck Relaxer. This exercise will ease tension in your neck. Sit up tall. Close your eyes and breathe deeply, then gently tilt your head to one side and let it slowly drop toward your shoulder. Don't raise your shoulder to meet your head, and don't force your head down. Hold for 3 to 6 seconds, then switch sides. Repeat 3 or 4 times. Gently bring your head forward, letting your chin relax into your chest. Roll your cheek to the right toward your shoulder (again, don't force the motion, and don't move your shoulder toward your head) and hold for 3 to 6 seconds. Switch sides and repeat. Do 3 or 4 sets per day.

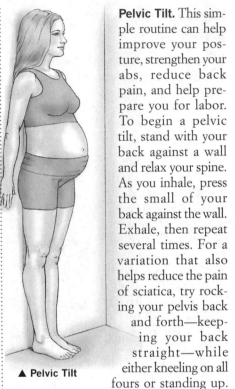

▲ **Pelvic Tilt**

Pelvic Tilt. This simple routine can help improve your posture, strengthen your abs, reduce back pain, and help prepare you for labor. To begin a pelvic tilt, stand with your back against a wall and relax your spine. As you inhale, press the small of your back against the wall. Exhale, then repeat several times. For a variation that also helps reduce the pain of sciatica, try rocking your pelvis back and forth—keeping your back straight—while either kneeling on all fours or standing up. Do pelvic tilts regularly (take a 5-minute pelvic-tilt break several times during your workday).

Leg Lifts. Leg lifts use your body's own weight to tone your thigh muscles (no infomercial equipment necessary). Simply lie on your left side with your shoulders, hips, and knees lined up straight. Support yourself by holding your head with your left arm and placing your right arm on the floor in front of you. Then slowly lift your right leg as high as you comfortably can (remember to breathe). Do 10 reps, then switch sides and repeat.

▼ **Leg Lifts**

Biceps Curl. Start by selecting light weights (3- or 5-pound weights if you're a beginner, and never more than 12 pounds even if you're a pro). Stand with your legs shoulder-width apart, making sure not to lock your knees. Keep your elbows in and your chest up. Slowly raise both weights toward your shoulders by bending your elbows and keeping your arms in front of you (remember to breathe), stopping when your hands have reached your shoulders. Lower slowly and repeat. Try to do 8 to 10 repetitions, but take breaks if needed and don't overdo it. You'll feel a burn in your muscles, but you should never strain or start holding your breath.

Biceps Curl ▲

Tailor Stretch. Sitting cross-legged and stretching will help you relax and get in touch with your body (the more familiar you are with your body as you move into labor and delivery, the better). Experiment with different arm stretches while sitting—try placing your hands on your shoulders, then try reaching them over your head and stretching toward the ceiling. You can also alternate stretching one arm higher than the other or leaning to one side. (Don't bounce as you stretch.)

▲ Tailor Stretch

Clamming. Lie on your right side with legs slightly forward and knees bent and stacked on top of each other. Place a pillow under your head and a flat pillow under your belly for support. Stack your hips, and keep your spine straight and abs drawn in (as best you can). Keeping your toes touching, rotate at your left hip and lift the left knee, taking your knees apart as far as possible. Slowly lower and repeat for 8 to 10 reps, then switch sides.

Clamming ▶

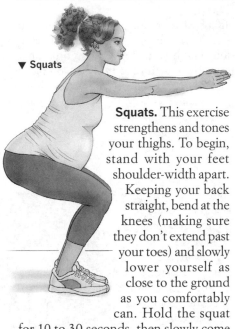

▼ Squats

Squats. This exercise strengthens and tones your thighs. To begin, stand with your feet shoulder-width apart. Keeping your back straight, bend at the knees (making sure they don't extend past your toes) and slowly lower yourself as close to the ground as you comfortably can. Hold the squat for 10 to 30 seconds, then slowly come back to a standing position. Repeat 5 times. (Note: Avoid lunges and deep knee bends, since your joints are more prone to injury.)

Waist Twists. If you've been sitting for a while or just feel generally tensed up or uncomfortable, try this easy circulation-boosting move. Stand up and place your feet shoulder-width apart. Twist gently from the waist, slowly turning from side to side. Keep your back straight and let your arms swing freely. Can't get up? You can do this exercise even while you're sitting.

◀ Waist Twists

Hip Flexors. Stretching the hip flexor muscles periodically will help keep you limber and make it easier for you to open your legs wide when it's time for the baby to exit. To flex your flexors, stand at the bottom of a flight of stairs as though you were about to climb them. (Hang on to the railing with one hand for support if you need to.) Place one foot on the first or second stair up (whatever you can comfortably reach) and bend your knee. Keep your other leg behind you, knee straight, foot flat on the floor. Lean into your bent leg, keeping your back straight. You'll feel the stretch in your straight leg. Switch legs and repeat.

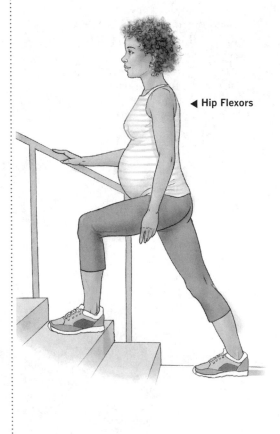

◀ Hip Flexors

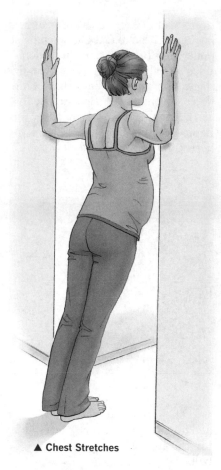

▲ Chest Stretches

Triangle Pose. This pose works the legs, stretches the side of the body, energizes the hips, and opens up the shoulders (which might be drooping these days). Stand with your feet wider than hip distance apart and turn your right foot outward to 90 degrees and your left foot inward slightly so you are comfortably balanced. Raise your arms sideways to shoulder level, keeping them parallel to the floor with your palms facing downward. Resist the urge to let your shoulders rise up to your ears. Take a deep breath in. Exhale slowly and bend at the waist as much as is comfortable to your right side. Extend your right hand downward toward your right ankle. (No need to touch your ankle when you're contending with a big belly—getting to your shin is just fine.) Lift your left arm up, bringing it in line with your lowered right arm. Try to keep both your arms and legs straight. Stay in this position for as long as is comfortable, breathing normally. Return to your starting position and rest a moment before repeating on the other side.

Chest Stretches. Gently stretching your chest muscles will help you feel more comfortable while improving your circulation. Here's how: With your arms at shoulder level and bent, grasp both sides of a doorway. Lean forward, feeling the stretch in your chest. Hold this position for 10 to 20 seconds and release. Do 5 reps.

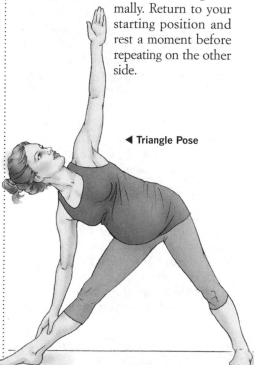

◀ Triangle Pose

Forearm Plank. Get on your hands and knees, then lower yourself onto your elbows and place your forearms on the floor. Lace your fingers together, keeping your elbows wide. Straighten one leg at a time until your body forms a straight line from head to feet. Lengthen your body from your head to tailbone, keeping abs pulled in as best you can (illustration A). If it's too difficult, keep your knees bent slightly (or put your knees back on the floor, illustration B). Breathe deeply as you hold the position for 5 to 10 seconds. Repeat. Need a rest? Sit back on your heels with your back straight.

▲ Forearm Plank A

▶ Forearm Plank B

Ball Exercises. Working out with a fitness (aka birthing) ball not only strengthens your abs, but helps maintain balance and stability as your belly grows. Here's one ball exercise to try: Sit upright on top of the ball, arms relaxed by your sides and feet flat on the floor a comfortable distance from the ball and about hip-width apart. After balancing for a few seconds, lift your arms out to the sides up to around shoulder height, and then straighten your right leg and lift it up to hip level (if extending your leg is difficult, keep your knee bent and just lift your foot off the floor). Lower your leg and then your arms, balance on the ball again, and repeat with your left leg. Do 6 to 8 reps, alternating legs.

The pelvic tilt, shoulder stretch, and forearm plank can also be modified for the fitness ball.

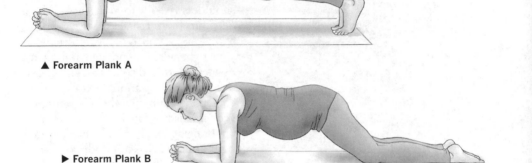

◀ Ball Exercise

When Workouts Are Out

Exercising during pregnancy can certainly do the average pregnant body (and her baby) good. But sometimes complications require a mom to sit pregnancy out—and in that case, taking it easy is the best prescription. If your practitioner has restricted exercise for you during part or all of your pregnancy, ask if there are any workouts you can still work in—say, arm-only exercises or stretches—so you can stay in shape while you stay on the sofa, or even in bed. See page 576 for more.

CHAPTER 9

The Fifth Month

What was once completely abstract is getting real . . . fast. Chances are that sometime this month or the beginning of the next, you will feel your baby's movements for the first time. That miraculous sensation, along with the serious rounding of your belly, will finally make pregnancy feel more like a reality. Though your baby is far from ready to make a personal appearance in your arms, it's really nice to know for sure there's actually someone in there.

Your Baby This Month

Week 18 At 5½ inches long and about 5 to 6½ ounces in weight (about the size of that chicken breast you're having for dinner, but a lot cuter), your baby is filling out nicely and getting large enough that you might even be feeling those twists, rolls, kicks, and punches he or she is perfecting. Another set of skills your baby is mastering now: yawning and hiccupping (you might even begin to feel those hiccups soon, as well as watch them shake your belly!). And your one-of-a-kind baby is truly one of a kind now, complete with unique fingerprints on those tiny fingertips and toes.

Week 19 This week your baby is hitting the growth charts at 6 inches long and just over a full half pound in weight. What fruit is it this week? Your baby's about the size of a large mango. A mango dipped in greasy cheese, actually. Vernix caseosa—a greasy white protective substance that resembles cheese—now covers your baby's sensitive skin, protecting it from that long soak in an amniotic bath. Without that protection, your baby would look very wrinkled at birth. The coating sheds as delivery approaches, but some babies born early are still covered with vernix when they arrive.

Week 20 You've got a baby the size of a small cantaloupe in your melon-size belly this week, about 10 ounces and 6½ inches (crown to rump). Your ultrasound this month should be able to detect—if you want to know—whether your baby is a boy or a girl. And oh boy—or oh girl—has that baby been busy. If you're having a girl, her uterus is fully formed, her ovaries are holding about 7 million primitive eggs (though at birth, the number of eggs will have dropped to closer to 2 million—more than enough to keep her covered during her reproductive years), and her vaginal canal is starting to develop. If you're having a boy, his testicles have begun their descent from the abdomen. In a few months, they'll drop into the scrotum (which is still under construction). Luckily for your baby, there's still plenty of room in your womb for twisting, turning, kicking, punching, and even an occasional somersault. If you haven't felt these acrobatics yet, you almost certainly will in the coming weeks.

Week 21 How big is baby this week? Switching from crown-to-rump to crown-to-heel length, about 10½ inches in length (think large carrot) and almost 11 to 12½ ounces in weight. And speaking of carrots, you might want to eat some this week if you'd like your baby to have a taste for them. That's because the flavor of amniotic fluid differs from day to day, depending on what you've eaten (hot chili one day, mild carrot another), and now that your baby is swallowing amniotic fluid each day (for hydration, nutrition, and also to get practice swallowing and digesting), he or she will be getting a virtual taste of—and a taste for—whatever's on your menu. Here's another baby update: Arms and legs are finally in proportion, neurons are now connected between the brain and muscles, and cartilage throughout the

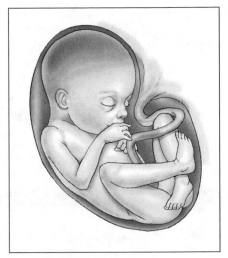

Your Baby, Month 5

body is turning to bone. Which means that when your baby makes those moves (which you're probably feeling by now), they're much more coordinated—no more jerky twitches.

Week 22 Forget about ounces, baby. This week, we're talking a whopping weight of 1 pound and a crown-to-heel length of approximately 11 inches, about the size of a small doll. But your doll is a living one—with developing senses, including touch, sight, hearing, and taste. What's your baby touching? He or she may grab on to the umbilical cord (there's not much else to hang on to in there) and practice the strong grip that will soon be clutching your fingers (and pulling on your hair). What's your baby seeing? Though it's dark in the uterine cocoon—and even with fused eyelids—fetuses this age can perceive light and dark. If you shine a flashlight over your belly, you might feel your baby react, perhaps trying to turn away from the jarring light. What's your baby hearing? The sound of your voice and that of your partner, your heart beating, the whoosh-whoosh of your blood circulating through your body, those gastric gurgles produced by your stomach and intestines, the dog barking, sirens, a loud TV. And what's your baby tasting? Pretty much everything you're tasting (so pass the salad).

Your Body This Month

Here are some symptoms you may experience this month (or may not experience, since every pregnancy is different). Some of these symptoms may be continuing from last month, while others may be brand new. Some may be easing up, others intensifying:

Physically

- More energy

- Fetal movement (probably by the end of the month)

- Increasing vaginal discharge

- Achiness in the lower abdomen and along one side or the other, or sometimes on both sides (from stretching of the ligaments supporting the uterus)

- Constipation

- Heartburn, indigestion, flatulence, bloating

- Occasional headaches

- Occasional lightheadedness or dizziness, especially when getting up quickly or when your blood sugar dips

- Backache

- Nasal congestion and occasional nosebleeds; ear stuffiness

- Sensitive gums that may bleed when you brush

- Hearty appetite

- Leg cramps

- Mild swelling of ankles and feet, and occasionally of hands and face

Your Body This Month

You're halfway through your pregnancy now—and the top of your uterus will hit your belly button sometime around the 20th week. By the end of this month, your uterus will be about an inch above your belly button. Chances are, there's no hiding the fact that you're pregnant now (though some women may still not be showing noticeably).

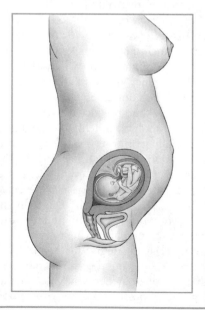

- Varicose veins of legs and/or of vulva
- Hemorrhoids
- Skin color changes on belly and/or face
- A protruding navel (a popped-out belly button)
- Faster pulse (heart rate)
- Easier—or more difficult—orgasm

Emotionally

- A growing sense of reality about the pregnancy
- Fewer mood swings, though you'll likely still be weepy and irritable occasionally
- Forgetfulness, absentmindedness, aka "placenta brain"

What You Can Expect at This Month's Checkup

This month, you can expect your practitioner to check the following, though there may be variations, depending on your particular needs and your practitioner's style of practice:

- Weight and blood pressure
- Urine, for sugar and protein
- Fetal heartbeat

- Size and shape of uterus, by external palpation (feeling from the outside)
- Height of fundus (top of uterus)
- Feet and hands for swelling, and legs for varicose veins
- Symptoms you have been experiencing, especially unusual ones
- Questions or problems you want to discuss—have a list ready

What You May Be Wondering About

Heating Up

"I feel hot and sweaty all the time these days, even when everybody else is cool. What's that about?"

Feeling like hot stuff these days? You can thank your hormones (as always) plus increased blood flow to the skin and a hopped-up pregnancy metabolism for that perpetually damp feeling. Throw in a warm climate or a record hot summer (or even just an overheated office in the middle of

winter), and the heat is on—big time. Luckily, there are plenty of ways to stay comfortable when the temperature inside you is soaring. To stay cool while you're heating for two:

- Wear loose, light clothing in cotton or other breathable fabrics, and dress in layers so you can peel them off as you heat up.
- Sleep smart, not sweaty. Besides turning the thermostat down while you're sleeping, consider switching to

natural fibers when you sleep, too—from your pj's to your pillow.

- To chill out fast, put ice packs, cold compresses, or cold running water on your inner wrists. Since it's a pulse point, the cold temp on the outside will help cool the blood inside. You can also try cold compresses on other pulse points whenever you're heating up: your neck, ankles, and behind the knees.

- Put any lotions you use in the fridge for at least 30 minutes before you apply. When you rub the cold creams on your skin, it'll help cool you down.

- No time for a cold shower? You can wet your hands with cold water and then run your fingers through your hair (assuming you don't mind your hair being wet). A cooler head will prevail in cooling down your body. Or keep a spray bottle of water in the fridge (at home and on the job) for a cold spritz.

- Munch on a bunch of frozen grapes. Not only will you net some vitamin C and K, this delicious chilled snack will help cool you down (and it's a whole lot lower in fat than ice cream). Not a grape lover? You can freeze any type of cut up fruit (think mango, banana, berries, and so on) and grab it when you're heating up. Or stay hydrated and cool by freezing your water bottle and sipping the icy water as it melts.

    And speaking of munching, remember that the 6-Meal Solution is the solution for overheating problems, too. Eating lightly more frequently will require less effort to digest. Spicy food may heat you up in the short term, but because it'll get you sweating, it'll cool you down later.

- A sprinkle of cornstarch-based powder can help absorb moisture (plus help to prevent heat rash). Sprinkle it on your skin while it's still dry.

    On the plus side, while you'll be more sweaty—you'll be less smelly. That's because the production of apocrine perspiration (the stinkier kind produced by glands under the arms and breasts and in the genital area) slows down when you're expecting.

Dizziness

"I feel dizzy when I get up from a sitting position. And yesterday while I was shopping, I almost felt like I was going to black out for a minute. Am I okay?"

Feeling a little dizzy can definitely be unsettling when you're pregnant (especially because you might already be having a hard enough time staying on your feet or keeping your balance), but it isn't dangerous. In fact, it's a pretty common—and almost always normal—symptom of pregnancy. Here's why:

- Throughout your pregnancy, high levels of your old friend progesterone cause your blood vessels to relax and widen, increasing the flow of blood to your baby (good for baby) but slowing the return of blood to you (not so good for mom). Less blood flow to you means lower blood pressure and reduced blood flow to your brain, which can contribute to that lightheaded, dizzy feeling. In the second trimester, that faint feeling may be caused by the pressure of your expanding uterus on your blood vessels. It can also be a sign of anemia (see next question).

- Getting up too quickly, which causes a sudden blood pressure drop, can trigger an especially lightheaded moment. The cure for that kind of dizziness (also known as postural hypotension) is simple: Just get up gradually. Jumping up in a hurry to answer a text on the phone you left across the room is likely to land you right back on the sofa.

- Low blood sugar—something expectant moms are particularly prone to, since they're fueling a baby factory—might also send the room spinning. To avoid those blood sugar dips, get some protein and complex carbs at every meal (this combo helps maintain even blood sugar levels) and eat more frequently (choosing the mini-meal approach or snacking in between meals). Carry trail mix, some freeze-dried fruit, nuts, a granola bar, or some whole-grain chips in your bag for quick blood sugar lifts.

- Dizziness can be a sign of dehydration, so be sure you're getting enough fluids—and that you're chug-a-lugging more if you've been sweating.

- A dizzy spell can also be triggered by indoor stuffiness—in an overheated or crowded store, office, or bus—especially if you're overdressed. In that case, getting some fresh air by stepping outside or opening a window may bring relief. Taking off your coat and loosening your clothes—especially around the neck and waist—should help, too.

If you feel dizzy or like you're about to faint, lie down on your left side—with your legs elevated, if you can—or sit with your head lowered between your knees. Take deep breaths, and loosen any tight clothing (like that button on your jeans). As soon as you feel a little better, get something to eat and drink.

Tell your practitioner about the dizzy spells. He or she may want to check your iron levels to rule out anemia.

When Too Much Is Too Much

Feel breathless or exhausted when you're jogging? What about when you're doing heavy cleaning—does the vacuum cleaner suddenly feel as if it weighs a ton? Stop before you drop. Exerting yourself to the point of exhaustion is never a good idea. During pregnancy it's a particularly bad one, because overwork takes its toll not only on you but on your baby as well. Instead of marathon activity sessions, pace yourself. Work or exercise a bit, then rest a bit. Ultimately, the work or the workout gets done, and you won't feel drained afterward. If occasionally something doesn't get done, consider it good training for the days when the demands of parenthood will frequently keep you from finishing what you started.

Actual fainting is rare, but if you do faint, there is no need for concern—it won't affect your baby. But do call your practitioner as soon as possible.

Anemia

"A friend of mine became anemic during pregnancy—is that common?"

Iron-deficiency anemia is common during pregnancy—but it's also incredibly easy to prevent. And when it comes to prevention, your practitioner almost certainly has your back. You were already tested for anemia at your first prenatal visit, though it's unlikely you were low on iron then. That's because iron stores are quickly replenished once those monthly periods stop.

Symptoms of Anemia

Pregnant women with mild iron deficiency rarely have noticeable symptoms—or symptoms that are easily distinguished from pregnancy symptoms (most expectant moms are tired whether they're anemic or not). But as oxygen-carrying red blood cells are further depleted, an anemic mother-to-be becomes pale, extremely weak, and easily tired or very breathless (beyond what's normal in pregnancy), and might even experience fainting spells. She may experience strange cravings for nonfood items, like clay, or a compulsion to chew ice. There's also a possibility that RLS, or restless leg syndrome, may be linked to low iron stores. This may be one of the few instances where fetal nutritional needs are met before a mom's, since babies are rarely iron deficient at birth.

Though the increased demand for blood production during pregnancy makes all moms-to-be susceptible to iron-deficiency anemia, some are at particularly high risk: those who've had back-to-back pregnancies, those who have been vomiting a lot or eating little because of morning sickness, and those who came to pregnancy undernourished (possibly because of an eating disorder) and/or have been eating poorly since they conceived. Daily iron supplementation, as prescribed by your practitioner, should prevent (or treat) anemia.

As your pregnancy progresses and you hit the halfway mark (around 20 weeks, coming right up), your blood volume expands significantly and the amount of iron needed for producing red blood cells dramatically increases, depleting those stores once again. Fortunately, refilling those stores—and effectively preventing anemia—is as easy as taking a daily iron supplement (in addition to your prenatal vitamin), which your practitioner may prescribe starting midway through pregnancy. You should also pump up your diet by eating foods loaded with iron. Though dietary sources, such as the ones listed on page 97, may not do the job alone, they provide a great backup for an iron supplement. For extra absorption, chase your iron (and iron-rich foods) down with your morning OJ (or another vitamin C-rich food or drink) but not with your morning java, which will actually reduce the amount of iron absorbed. Is your iron supplement making your tummy miserable (causing nausea or constipation)? Ask about switching to a time-release formula.

Backache

"I'm having a lot of back pain. I'm afraid I won't be able to stand up at all by the 9th month."

The aches and discomforts of pregnancy aren't designed to make you miserable, though that's often the upshot. They're the side effects of the preparations your body is making for that momentous moment when your baby is born. Backache is no exception. During pregnancy, the usually stable joints of the pelvis begin to loosen up to allow easier (hopefully) passage for the baby at delivery. This, along with your oversize abdomen, throws your body off balance. To compensate, you tend to bring your shoulders back and arch your neck. Standing with your belly thrust forward—to be sure that no one who passes fails to notice you're pregnant,

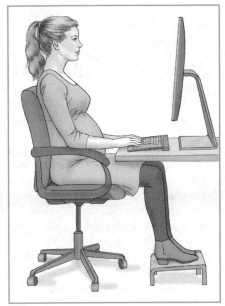

Give your feet a leg up

not just bloated—compounds the problem. The result: a deeply curved lower back, strained back muscles, and pain.

Even pain with a purpose hurts. But without defeating the purpose, you can conquer (or at least subdue) the pain. The following should help:

- Sit smart. Sitting puts more stress on your spine than almost any other activity, so it pays to do it right. At home and at work, make sure the chairs you use most provide good support, preferably with firm cushioning and arms. A chair back that reclines slightly can also help take the pressure off. Use a footrest to elevate your feet slightly (see illustration, above), and don't cross your legs, which can cause your pelvis to tilt forward, exacerbating those strained back muscles.

- Don't sit too long. Sitting for long periods can be as bad for your back as sitting the wrong way. Try not to sit for more than an hour without taking

a walking and stretching break—setting a half-hour limit would be even better.

- Try not to stand too long, either. If you work on your feet, keep one foot on a low stool to take some pressure off your lower back. When you're standing on a hard surface—in the kitchen while cooking or washing dishes, for example—put on supportive shoes or use a small skid-proof cushioned rug underfoot to ease the pressure.

- Be a slow lifter. Avoid lifting heavy loads, but if you must, do it slowly. First, stabilize yourself by assuming a wide stance. Next, bend at the knees, not at the waist. And finally, lift with your arms and legs, not your back (see illustration, below). If you have to carry a heavy load when you're shopping, split it evenly between 2 shopping bags and carry one in each arm rather than carrying it all in front of you.

- Try to keep weight gain within the recommended parameters (see page

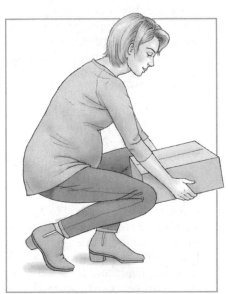

Bend at the knees when you lift

Carrying Older Children

Wondering if you need to put the mommy taxi service you've been running off duty until after delivery? Carrying moderately heavy loads (even some 35 or 40 pounds of preschooler) is safe throughout pregnancy unless your practitioner has told you otherwise.

What about your aching back? Save it some strain by learning to lift your tot properly (see page 253).

178). Excess pounds will only add to the load your back is struggling under.

- Wear the right shoes. Extremely high heels are a pain for your back—as are very unsupportive flat ones. Experts recommend a chunky 2-inch heel, a low wedge, or flats with good arch support to keep your body in proper alignment. You might also consider orthotics, orthopedic shoe inserts designed for muscle support. As for those posture-improving shoes, some women find them helpful, while others find they increase back pain. Wearing them may also exacerbate your off-balance factor.

- Sleep right. A comfortable sleeping position will help minimize aches and pains (see page 264). When getting out of bed, swing your legs over the side of the bed to the floor rather than twisting to get up.

- Consider belly support. Think of it as support hose for your bump, designed to help take the burden of your belly's weight off your lower back and hips, helping relieve those aches and pains. Belly-support garments come in stretchy bands and sleeves as well as in belts, slings, braces, compression shorts, and cradles—choose one that's comfortable for you (and works best under the kinds of clothes you wear, since some are belly smoothing and others are a little lumpy). Whichever style you opt for, try not to wear your support band or belt 24/7. That's because with prolonged use of a belly support, your body will start to rely on it (instead of your abdominal and back muscles) to hold up your bump, resulting in further weakening of your core muscles and ultimately worsening back and hip pain. Take steps to strengthen your back and core muscles with pregnancy-safe exercise (see page 239) so your belly band isn't doing all the work all the time.

- No reaching for the stars—or the salad bowl you stored on the top shelf. Minimize strain by using a low, stable step stool (or a taller friend) to retrieve items from high places.

- Alternate cold and heat to temporarily relieve sore back muscles. Use a towel-wrapped ice pack for 15 minutes, followed by a towel-wrapped heating pad for 15 minutes. Ask your practitioner before using heat patches (like Salonpas or ThermaCare) directly on your skin. Some recommend that you place such patches on your clothes instead of on your skin because they can get very hot—and very irritating to pregnancy-sensitive skin (definitely don't apply them to your belly). Ask, too, before slathering on Bengay, Icy Hot, or BioFreeze creams for your pain. Not all practitioners give the green light to these muscle soothers, especially in the last trimester. If yours does, go for it—but watch for signs of irritation (and don't use on your bump). Arnica products (like Traumeel) should not be used during pregnancy.

Pregnant with Scoliosis

You're probably no stranger to back pain if you have scoliosis, but pregnancy can make those aches even more annoyingly familiar, especially if your condition involves your hips, pelvis, or shoulders. Weight-bearing difficulties may increase as your weight increases, too. A potential pain for you, but very happily, rarely anything that might seriously impact your pregnancy.

If you find your back pain increases during pregnancy, try the tips starting on page 253, including using a belly support. You can also ask your practitioner for the name of an obstetric physiotherapist who may be able to help you with some exercises specific to your scoliosis-related pain. Also discuss which CAM approaches (page 78) might be helpful. Hydrotherapy and exercising in water (which is zero impact) may be especially beneficial.

Wondering how scoliosis will affect your baby's birth? Chances are it won't—most moms with scoliosis are able to have a vaginal delivery (check with your practitioner). Thinking about an epidural? Talk to your practitioner about finding an anesthesiologist who has experience with moms with scoliosis. Though the condition usually does not interfere with the epidural, it may make it a little more difficult to place. An experienced anesthesiologist, however, should have no problem getting the needle where it needs to go.

Also talk to your practitioner if you have severe curvature, which may affect your breathing as pregnancy progresses, and may require extra monitoring.

- Take a warm bath. Or turn the showerhead to pulsating (if yours has that feature) and enjoy the back massage.

- Rub your back the right way. Treat yourself to a therapeutic massage (with a massage therapist who knows you're pregnant and is trained in prenatal massage).

- Learn to relax. Many back problems are aggravated by stress. If you think yours might be, try some relaxation exercises when pain strikes. Also follow the suggestions beginning on page 145 for dealing with stress.

- Do simple exercises that strengthen your abs, such as the Dromedary Droop (page 239) and the Pelvic Tilt (page 240). Or sit on an exercise ball and rock back and forth (or lie back on it to ease back discomfort as well as hip pain). Join a pregnancy yoga or water aerobics class, or consider water therapy if you can find a medically (and pregnancy) savvy water therapist.

- If pain is significant, ask your practitioner about prescribing physical therapy or recommending alternative therapies, like acupuncture, chiropractic, or biofeedback.

Abdominal Aches (Round Ligament Pain)

"What are those aches and pains I've been getting on the lower sides of my abdomen?"

What you're probably feeling is the pregnancy equivalent of growing pains: the stretching of muscles and ligaments supporting your enlarging uterus. Technically, it's known as round ligament pain, and most expectant moms experience it. But there's a wide variety of ways to experience it. The pain may be crampy, sharp and stabbing, or achy, and it may be more noticeable when you're working out (or even when you're just walking), getting up from bed or from a chair, when you cough or sneeze—in fact, any kind of sudden movement can bring it on. It can be brief, or it may last for several hours. And it's completely normal. As long as it is occasional, and there are no other symptoms accompanying it (such as fever, chills, bleeding, or lightheadedness), this kind of pain is absolutely nothing to be concerned about.

Kicking up your feet (though not literally) and resting in a comfortable position should bring some relief. You can also wear a belly band, belt, or support system designed for pregnancy to ease the pain. Avoiding sudden movements can help prevent the pains in the first place (so get up from bed or a chair more slowly next time), though you may find that no matter what you do, you'll get them occasionally. If the pain really bothers you when you're working out, it's probably best to decrease the intensity of your workouts (run more slowly or walk instead, for instance). Of course, mention the pain—like all pains—to your practitioner at your next visit so you can be reassured that this is just another normal, if annoying, part of pregnancy.

Foot Growth

"All my shoes are beginning to feel tight. Could my feet be growing, too?"

The belly isn't the only part of the pregnant body that's prone to expansion. If you're like many expectant moms, you'll discover that your feet are growing, too. Good news if you're looking to revamp your entire shoe collection—not so good if you've already sized out of your favorites and shopping for baby has left you cash crunched.

What causes your feet to go through a growth spurt? While some expansion can be attributed to the normal fluid retention and swelling of pregnancy (or to new fat in your feet if your weight gain has been substantial or quick), there's another reason, too. Relaxin, the pregnancy hormone that loosens the ligaments and joints around your pelvis so your baby can fit through the exit, doesn't discriminate between the ligaments you'd want loosened up (like those pelvic ones) and those you'd rather it just leave alone (like those in your feet). The result: When those ligaments in the feet loosen, the bones under them tend to spread slightly, often resulting in an added half or even a whole shoe size. Though the joints will tighten back up again after delivery, it's possible that your feet will be permanently larger.

In the meantime, try the tips for reducing excessive swelling (see page 312) if that seems to be your problem, and get a couple of pairs of shoes that fit you comfortably now and will meet your "growing" needs (so you won't end up barefoot and pregnant). When shoe shopping, put comfort before style—even if it's just this once. Look for shoes with heels that are no more than 2 inches high and have both non-skid soles and plenty of space for your feet to spread out (shop for them at the end of the day when your feet are the most swollen). The shoes should be made from a material that will allow your swollen, sweaty dogs to breathe (nothing synthetic).

Are your feet and legs achy, especially at the end of the day? Shoes and orthotic inserts specially designed to correct the distorted center of pregnancy gravity can not only make your feet more comfortable but can reduce back and leg pain as well. Getting off your feet periodically during the day can (obviously) help with swelling

An Itchy Situation

Feeling flaky? You might, now that you're expecting. Normal pregnancy hormonal fluctuations can lead to an itchy, flaky scalp. Dandruff can be the result of a scalp that's either too dry or too oily. Yeast (a common fungus among expectant moms) can also scale up flaking. How to treat dandruff during pregnancy depends on what's behind it. Dry flakes (the kind that rain down onto your shoulders) can be eased by rubbing coconut or olive oil on your scalp before shampooing. Oily, scaly, or yeasty dandruff can be treated with a pregnancy-approved dandruff shampoo (like Head and Shoulders). Ask your practitioner before reaching for other dandruff shampoos (like T-Gel), since the stronger ones may not be pregnancy safe. Ask, too, before using shampoos that contain tea tree oil, since not all practitioners give it the all clear.

Cutting down on sugar and refined grains, and stepping up healthy fat sources (like avocados and nuts) may also help clear up your scalp—and your shoulders.

and pain, as can elevating (and periodically flexing) your feet when you get the chance. You can also try slipping on elasticized slippers while you're at home. Wearing them for several hours a day may not make a great fashion statement—but it can make for happier feet, easing fatigue and achiness.

Fast-Growing Hair and Nails

"It seems to me that my hair and nails have never grown so fast before."

Though it may seem as if pregnancy hormones team up only to make you miserable during your 9 months (constipation, heartburn, and nausea come to mind), those same hormones are actually responsible for a substantial pregnancy perk: nails that grow faster than you can manicure them and hair that grows before you can secure appointments with your stylist (and if you're really lucky, hair that is thicker and more lustrous). Those pregnancy hormones trigger a surge in circulation and a boost in metabolism that nourish hair and nail cells, making them healthier than ever before.

Of course, every perk has its price. That extra nourishment can, unfortunately, have less than happy effects, too: It can cause hair to grow in places you would rather it didn't (and probably didn't know it could, at least on a woman). Facial areas (lips, cheeks, and that chinny-chin-chin) are most commonly plagued with this pregnancy-induced hairiness, but arms, legs, chest, back, and belly can feel the fur, too. (To read about which hair removal treatments are safe during pregnancy, see page 150.) And though your nails might be long, they can also turn dry and brittle.

Remember that these hair and nail changes are only temporary. Your good hair day run ends with delivery—when the normal daily hair loss that's suppressed during pregnancy (thus the thicker hair) resumes with a vengeance. And your nails will likely go back to their slower growth schedule postpartum, too (probably not such a bad thing—you'll want to keep your nails short anyway, with a new baby around).

The New Skin You're In

If you haven't already noticed, pregnancy impacts just about every inch of your body—from head (that forgetfulness!) to toes (those expanding feet!). So it's not surprising that your skin is also showing the effects of pregnancy. Here are some changes you may expect from your expectant skin:

Linea nigra. Sporting a zipper down the center of your swelling belly? Just as those pregnancy hormones caused the hyperpigmentation, or darkening, of the areolas, they are now responsible for the darkening of the linea alba, the white line you probably never noticed that runs between your belly button and your pubic area. During pregnancy, it's renamed the linea nigra, or black line, and may be more noticeable in dark-skinned women than in those who are fair-skinned. It usually starts to appear during the second trimester and most often will begin to fade a few months after delivery (though it may never go away entirely—you may, in fact, wear traces of it into old age). Interested in a round of guess-the-sex-of-my-baby? According to an old wives' tale (Not Backed By Science Edition), if the linea nigra runs only up to the belly button, you're having a girl. If it runs past the navel up to the xiphoid process (near your ribs), it's a boy.

Mask of pregnancy (chloasma). These brownish-bluish-grayish discolorations appear in a masklike, confetti pattern on around 50 to 75 percent of moms-to-be, particularly those with darker complexions (since they have more pigment in their skin to start with), as well as those who have a genetic predisposition to it (if your mom had it, there's a good chance you'll have it, too). Not a fan of the blotchy look? Since exposure to sunlight can make chloasma worse, be faithful about applying sunscreen with an SPF of at least 30, and avoid direct sun when possible. Fill up on folic acid, too, since a folate deficiency can be related to hyperpigmentation. Still blotchy? Some moms-to-be strike back at the mask of pregnancy with homemade masks made from lemon juice, apple cider vinegar, or even mashed banana. No luck with those? Never fear—chloasma usually fades within a few months after delivery. If it doesn't, a dermatologist can prescribe a bleaching cream or Retin-A (but not while you're breastfeeding) or recommend another treatment (such as a laser or a peel). Because those treatments are no-no's for now, bring on the concealer and foundation in the meantime.

Other skin hyperpigmentation. Many women also find that freckles and moles become darker and more noticeable and that darkening of the skin occurs in high-friction areas, such as between the thighs. All this hyperpigmentation should fade after delivery. Sun can intensify the discoloration, so use a sunscreen with an SPF of 30 or more on exposed skin, and avoid spending long hours in the sun (even with sunscreen on).

Red palms and soles. It's your hormones at work again (plus an increase in blood flow), and they're causing red, itchy palms (and sometimes soles of the feet) in more than two-thirds of white women and one-third of women of color. There's no specific treatment, but some women find relief by soaking their hands and/or feet in cold water or applying an ice bag for a few minutes a couple of times a day. Steer clear of anything that heats up your hands and feet (such as taking hot baths, washing dishes, wearing wool gloves). The dishpan look will disappear soon after delivery.

Bluish, blotchy legs. Because of stepped-up estrogen production, many expectant women experience this kind of mottled discoloration on their legs (and sometimes their arms) when they're chilly. It comes and goes, is harmless, and will disappear postpartum.

Skin tags. A skin tag, which is essentially a tiny piece of excess skin, is another harmless (if annoying) skin complaint common in pregnant women. Skin tags usually grow on areas of the body that are warmer and moister or are frequently rubbed by other skin or by clothing, including the folds of your neck, your armpits, your torso, beneath your breasts, or on your genitals. The (only) good news: They're completely benign and most will disappear after delivery. If your skin tags stick around, your doctor can remove them.

Heat rash. Think babies when you think heat rash? Think women expecting babies, too. Caused by the combination of an already overheated pregnant body, dampness from all that extra perspiration, and the friction of skin rubbing against itself or against clothing (as it tends to do when there's more skin to rub), heat rash is both super common and super irritating among the expectant set. You can find it anywhere, but it's most likely to creep up in the crease between and beneath the breasts, in the crease where the bulge of the lower abdomen rubs against the top of the pubic area, and on the inner thighs. A cool, damp compress can take some of the heat out of your heat rash. Patting on some cornstarch-based powder after your shower, wearing loose, breathable clothes, and trying to keep as cool as possible will help minimize discomfort and recurrence. A dab of calamine lotion can also be soothing and is safe to use, but check with your practitioner before you apply any other medicated lotions. If a rash or irritation lasts longer than a couple of days, ask your practitioner about next steps.

Tinea versicolor. Tinea is a fungal infection that causes small, oval or round, flat, itchy, and flaky spots on the skin. The fungus causing the infection disrupts the normal pigmentation of the skin, resulting in discolored, scaly patches. It usually pops up on the oily parts of the body like the chest and back, but can appear anywhere. Though it's not technically considered a pregnancy skin condition, it can appear for the first time during pregnancy or become exacerbated when you're expecting. Treatment usually includes antifungal shampoos like Head and Shoulders (yes, on your body!) or antifungal creams, but be sure to ask your practitioner for a recommendation now that you've got a baby on board.

Irritated skin rashes. Often, rashes are triggered by pregnancy-sensitive skin reacting to a product you've used prepregnancy without a reaction. Switching to a gentler product often relieves these contact rashes, but still do let your practitioner know about any persistent rash.

But wait, there's more. Believe it or not, there are a host of other skin changes you might experience. For information on stretch marks, see page 190; acne, see page 166; itchy pimples, see page 313; dry or oily skin, see page 166; spider veins, see page 164.

Keep in mind, too, that while the hair on your head will almost certainly be thicker, not all women experience the scary part of this hairy situation during pregnancy (the part where you find hair in all the wrong places). Some mamas-to-be find that the hair on their legs, underarms, or even eyebrows grows especially slowly during pregnancy—giving them a welcome break from the razor or the wax. Count yourself lucky if you fall into this less furry camp.

Vision

"My eyesight seems to be getting worse since I got pregnant. And my contact lenses don't seem to fit anymore. Am I imagining it?"

Nope, you're not seeing things—that is, you really aren't seeing things as well as you used to now that you're expecting. The eyes are just another of the seemingly unrelated body parts that can fall prey to pregnancy hormones. Not only can your vision seem less sharp, but your contact lenses, if you wear them, may suddenly feel uncomfortable. Eye dryness, which is caused by a hormone-induced decrease in tear production, may be at least partially to blame for irritation and discomfort. Another cause is extra fluid (it's everywhere!), that can change the shape of eye lenses—actually making some pregnant women more near- or farsighted. Your vision should clear up and your eyes return to normal after delivery (so don't bother to get a new prescription unless the change is so pronounced that you really can't see well anymore).

In case you were thinking about it, now isn't the time to consider corrective laser eye surgery. Though the procedure wouldn't harm the baby, it could overcorrect your vision and take longer to heal, possibly requiring a second corrective surgery later on (plus the eye drops used aren't recommended for pregnant women). Ophthalmologists recommend avoiding the surgery during pregnancy, in the 6 months preconception, and for at least 6 months postpartum (and if you're nursing, 6 months postweaning).

Though a slight deterioration in vision is not unusual in pregnancy, other symptoms do warrant a call to your practitioner. If you experience blurring or dimming vision or often see spots or floaters, or have double vision that persists for more than 2 or 3 hours, don't wait to see if it passes—call your practitioner at once. Briefly seeing spots after you have been standing for a while or when you get up suddenly from a sitting position is fairly common and nothing to worry about, though you should report it at your next visit.

Fetal Movement Patterns

"I felt little movements every day last week, but I haven't felt anything at all today. What's wrong?"

Feeling your baby twist, wriggle, punch, kick, and hiccup is simply one of pregnancy's biggest thrills (it sure beats heartburn and puffy feet). There may be no better proof that a brand-new—and impressively energetic—life is developing within you. But fetal movements can also drive a mom-to-be to distraction with questions and doubts: Is my baby moving enough? Too much? Moving at all? One minute you're sure those were kicks you were feeling, the next you're second-guessing yourself (maybe it was just gas?). One day you feel your baby's twists and turns nonstop. The next day your little athlete seems to have been benched, and you barely feel a thing.

Not to worry. At this stage of pregnancy, concerns about your baby's movements—while understandable—are usually unnecessary. The frequency of noticeable movements at this point varies a great deal, and patterns of movement are erratic at best. Though your baby is almost certainly on the move much of the time, you probably won't be feeling it consistently until he or she is packing a more powerful punch. Some of those dance moves may be missed because of the fetal position (facing and kicking inward, for instance, instead of outward). Or because of your own activity: When you're walking or moving about a lot, your baby may be rocked to sleep—or you may be too busy to notice the movements. It's also possible that you're sleeping right through your baby's most active period, which for many fetuses is in the middle of the night. (Even at this stage, babies are most likely to kick up when their moms are lying down.)

One way to prompt fetal movement if you haven't noticed any all day is to lie down for an hour or two in the evening, preferably after a glass of milk, orange juice, or a snack. The combination of your inactivity and the jolt of food energy may be able to get your fetus going. If that doesn't work, try again in a few hours, but don't worry. Many moms-to-be find they don't notice movement for a day or two at a time, or even for 3 or 4 days, this early on. If you're still worried, call your practitioner for reassurance.

After the 28th week, fetal movements become more consistent, and it's a good idea to get into the habit of checking on your baby's activity daily (see page 315).

Finding Out Baby's Sex

"I'm going for my 20-week ultrasound, and we're not sure whether to find out the baby's sex or not."

Team Pink? Team Blue? Or Team Wait and See? Ball's in your court when it comes to deciding whether or not to find out baby's sex—and there's no right or wrong way to play it. Some parents opt for a heads-up on baby's gender for practical reasons: It makes layette shopping, nursery painting, and name selection (only one to pick!) a lot easier. Others decide to get the baby gender bulletin early because they just can't stand the suspense. But a significant minority of parents still prefer to play the guessing game right up until the end—and to find out baby's sex the old-fashioned way, when his (or her) lower half finally makes its way into the world. The choice is yours.

If you do decide to find out now, keep in mind that determining the sex of a baby through ultrasound is not an exact science (unlike amniocentesis, which determines the gender through chromosomal analysis). Rarely, parents are told they're expecting a girl only to hear at delivery, "It's a boy!" (or far less often, the other way around—after all, it's easier to miss a penis than to see a penis where there isn't one). Also occasionally, a baby won't cooperate with the gender reveal—instead, keeping those privates private with stubbornly crossed legs. So if you do choose to find out your baby's gender when you go for your ultrasound, remember that it's a very educated guess—but still, a guess.

What if one of you wants to find out the sex and one of you doesn't? It's not easy to make that arrangement work

Second Trimester Ultrasound

Get ready for the big reveal (of your baby's adorable features, at least). Moms-to-be are routinely scheduled for an anatomy scan (also called a level 2 ultrasound) in the second trimester, usually between 18 and 20 weeks. That's because a second trimester ultrasound is a great way to see how a baby is developing—and to offer reassurance that everything is going exactly the way it should be. One of its most exciting functions as far as many parents are concerned: It can give you the 411 on baby's sex, on a want-to-know basis, of course (that is, unless you've already scored those results via an earlier chromosomal analysis). Plus, it's fun to get a sneak peek at your baby—especially now that he or she actually looks like a baby!

This more detailed scan will also give your practitioner additional valuable information about what's going on in that belly of yours. For example, it can measure the size of your baby and check all the major organs. It can measure the amount of amniotic fluid to make sure there's just the right amount, and evaluate the location of your placenta. In short, the second trimester ultrasound—besides being fun to watch—will give you and your practitioner a clear picture (literally) of the overall health of your baby and your pregnancy. Eager to make some sense of what you're seeing on the screen?

Your cutie's beating heart will be easy to locate, but ask the sonographer to point out baby's face, hands, feet, and even some of those tiny but amazing organs, like the stomach and kidneys.

Routine second trimester ultrasounds are usually done in 2D—which will provide just a flat profile of baby's features, if a very cute one (suitable for framing, or uploading). Most practitioners reserve the more detailed 3D (which takes multiple 2D images and pieces them together to form a 3D rendering that shows the whole surface, resembling a photo) and 4D scans (which shows baby moving in real time, like a video) to more closely examine a fetus for a suspected anomaly, such as cleft lip or spinal cord problems, or to monitor something specific that has to be seen more clearly. Currently, these more sophisticated (and, admittedly fun-to-watch) scans are officially recommended only when they're considered medically necessary. That's because studies evaluating the safety of ultrasound technology show mixed results and as yet unclear potential risks.

Thinking about springing for an upgraded in-womb experience at your local prenatal portrait center (Baby, the Movie), so you can get up-close-and-personal with your little one before he or she arrives? Ask your practitioner first and see page 322.

(especially if the one who knows has problems keeping a poker face . . . or resisting hint dropping . . . or blurting out to friends and family), but it can be done. Another choice you'll have to make if you opt to know the news: whether (and how, and when) to go public with it. Some parents like to save their little secret as long as they can. Others choose to live-stream the scan, making their discovery and their announcement simultaneously. Still others decide to milk the momentous moment for all its worth, while celebrating with family and friends at the same time via a gender reveal (see box, facing page).

It's a . . . Gender Reveal

Want to find out your little one's sex in the biggest way (think one part Oscars, one part game show, all parts excitement, celebration, fun, and fanfare)? Then join the ranks of parents making that big news bigger than ever, finding out and announcing baby's sex during a gender reveal, either at a party or on social media.

There are plenty of ways to do a gender reveal—and you can get as creative as you like. If you're planning to reveal the gender to yourselves at the same time you reveal it to friends, family, and the social media stratosphere, don't peek at the ultrasound. Instead, ask the technician to write baby's sex down and seal it in a closed envelope. Then, let your imagination run wild. Some ideas: Drop the news off at a bakery, where a cake can be baked in the appropriate color and frosted to hide the news—when you cut into the sweet treat, you and your guests will see whether it's blue for a boy or pink for a girl. Or have a piñata filled with pink or blue confetti or pink or blue candy to reveal your big news—or a box filled with blue or pink helium-filled balloons that get released when everyone has gathered around (and with someone capturing on video, of course). Looking for more inspiration? You'll find plenty on Pinterest, Instagram, and YouTube.

Not feeling the trend? Prefer to keep the news about your little one's privates, well, private for now—instead of vying for viral? Don't feel compelled to join the gender reveal party. Share, overshare, or don't share at all (until delivery day, that is)—it's your baby and your call.

Placenta Position

"The doctor said my ultrasound showed that the placenta was down near the cervix. She said that it was too early to worry about it, but of course I started worrying."

Think your baby is the only thing moving around in your uterus? Not so. Like a fetus, a placenta can move around during pregnancy, too. It doesn't actually pick up and relocate, but it does appear to migrate upward as the lower segment of the uterus stretches and grows. Though an estimated 10 percent of placentas are in the lower segment in the second trimester (and an even larger percentage before 14 weeks), the vast majority move into the upper segment by the time delivery nears. If this doesn't happen and the placenta remains low in the uterus, partially or completely covering the cervix (the mouth of the uterus), a diagnosis of "placenta previa" is made. This complication occurs in very few full-term pregnancies (about 1 in 200). In other words, your doctor is right. It's too early to worry about the position of your baby's placenta—and statistically speaking, the chances are slim that you'll ever have to worry about it. Another reason not to worry: If you do end up being diagnosed with placenta previa, your baby will simply be delivered via a scheduled cesarean.

"During my ultrasound, the technician told us that I have an anterior placenta. What does that mean?"

It means your baby is taking a backseat to the placenta. Usually, a fertilized egg situates itself in the posterior uterus—the part closest to your spine, which is where the placenta eventually develops. Sometimes, though, the egg implants on the opposite side of the uterus, closest to your belly button. When the placenta develops, it grows on the front (or anterior) side of your uterus, with the baby behind it. And that, apparently, is what happened with your little bundle.

Happily, your baby doesn't care which side of the uterus he or she is lying on, and where the placenta is located certainly makes no difference to development. The downside for you is that you might be less able to feel those early kicks and punches because the placenta will serve as a cushion between your baby and your tummy—and that could lead to unnecessary worrying. For the same reason, your doctor or midwife may find it a bit harder to pick up your baby's heartbeat, especially early on (and it could make amniocentesis, if you need it, a little more challenging). But despite those slight inconveniences—which are no big deal—an anterior placenta is inconsequential. What's more, it's very likely that the placenta will move into a more posterior position later on (as anterior placentas commonly do).

Sleeping Position

"I've always slept on my stomach. Now I'm afraid to. And I just can't seem to get comfortable any other way."

Unfortunately, two common favorite sleeping positions—on the belly and on the back—are not the best (and certainly not the most comfortable) choices during pregnancy. The belly position, for obvious reasons: As your stomach grows, it's like sleeping on a watermelon. The back position, though more comfortable, rests the entire weight of your pregnant uterus on your back, your intestines, and

major blood vessels. This pressure can aggravate backaches and hemorrhoids, make digestion less efficient, interfere with optimum circulation, and possibly cause hypotension (low blood pressure), which can make you dizzy. The less-than-optimum circulation can also reduce blood flow to the fetus, giving your baby less oxygen and nutrients. It's not unsafe for your fetus if you find yourself on your back every once in a while, but being on your back for prolonged periods of time over weeks and months can be problematic.

This doesn't mean you have to sleep standing up. Curling up or stretching out on your side—preferably the left side, though either side is fine—with one leg crossed over the other and with a pillow between them (see illustration, below), is ideal for both you and your baby-to-be. It not only allows maximum flow of blood and nutrients to the placenta but also enhances kidney function, which means better elimination of waste products and fluids and less swelling of ankles, feet, and hands.

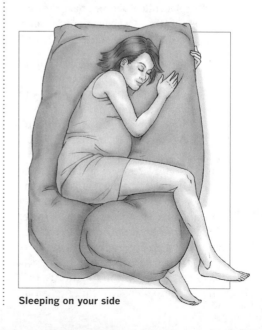

Sleeping on your side

Very few people, however, manage to stay in one position through the night. Don't worry (repeat: do not worry) if you wake up and find yourself on your back or abdomen. No harm done (repeat: no harm done); just turn back to your side. You may feel uncomfortable for a few nights—or even a few weeks—but your body will most likely adjust to the new position. A body pillow that's at least 5 feet long or a wedge-shaped pillow can offer support, making side sleeping much more comfortable and staying on your side much easier. If you don't have either of these, you can improvise with any extra pillows, placing them against your body in different positions until you're comfortable. Confirmed tummy sleeper? Try a pregnancy blow-up pillow with a cutout for your belly. Still not comfy? Try lying semi-upright in a recliner instead of a bed.

Class Womb?

"I've heard of people reading to their bellies or playing music to give their babies a head start in learning. Should I be trying to stimulate my baby, too?"

Now hear this: While your baby can hear by the end of the second trimester—and will even start learning from what he or she hears—there's no need to start piping in any kind of curriculum during pregnancy. Not only is promoting this early head start in music or language or literature not necessary, it can come with a potential downside—especially if it signals the start of extremely premature parental pushiness and begins placing too much emphasis on achievement at a too-tender age (and before birth is definitely too tender an age). Fetuses (like the babies and children they'll become before you know it) develop—and later, learn—best at their own pace, no prodding necessary.

There's also the chance that when parents attempt to turn the womb into a classroom, they may unknowingly disrupt the natural sleep patterns of their baby-to-be, hampering development instead of nurturing it (just as waking up a newborn for a game of name-this-letter might).

That said, there's nothing wrong—and a lot right—with providing a uterine environment that's rich in language and music, and, much more important, about finding ways to get close to your little one long before you even have that first cuddle. Talking, reading, or singing to your baby while he or she is in the womb (no amplification necessary) won't guarantee straight A's (or faster ABCs), but it will ensure that your baby will know your voice (and dad's voice) at birth—and will give you both a head start on bonding.

Playing music now may mean that your newborn will recognize, appreciate, and even be soothed by these sounds later on. Same thing with lullabies sung or nursery rhymes recited. And don't underestimate the power of touch. Since this sense also begins to develop in utero, stroking your belly now may also help strengthen the bond between you and your baby later. Plus it feels good.

So turn on the Mozart, bring on the Bach, pull out those dusty Shakespeare sonnets (or pull them up online), and read away to your belly if you like—and if you can without cracking up. Just make sure you're doing it all to get closer to your baby—not to get him or her closer to a spot in the school orchestra or an academic scholarship.

Of course, if you feel silly performing for your belly, there's no reason to worry that your baby will miss out on getting to know you. He or she is getting used to the sound of your voice—and dad's—every time you speak to each other or someone else. So enjoy making baby contact now, but definitely don't worry about early learning this early. As you'll discover, kids grow up all too soon anyway. There's no need to rush the process, particularly before birth.

Approaching Parenthood

"I keep wondering if I will be happy with this whole parenthood thing. I have no clue what it'll really be like."

Most people approach any major change in their lives—and there's no more major change than becoming a parent—wondering whether it will be a change they'll be happy with. And it's always much more likely to be a happy change if you keep your expectations realistic.

So, first of all: Reality check . . . check . . . and recheck. If you have images of bringing a cooing, smiling, picture-perfect baby home from the hospital, you may want to read up on what newborns are really like. Not only won't your newborn be smiling or cooing for weeks, but he or she may hardly communicate with you at all, except to cry—and this will almost invariably be when you're sitting down to dinner or starting to get busy in bed, have to pee, or are so tired you can't move.

And if your visions of parenthood consist of leisurely morning walks through the park, sunny days at the zoo, and hours coordinating baby's wardrobe, another reality check is probably in order. You'll have your share of walks in the park (that is, if you have one nearby), but there will also be many mornings that turn into evenings before you and your baby have the chance to see the light of day, many sunny days that will be spent largely in the laundry room, and very few tiny

Feeling Left Out

Let's face it. No matter how much the gender roles have evolved, biology still has its limitations. Which means that pregnancy is—and will always be—women's work, at least physically. It's mom who's carrying the baby, mom who's connected to the baby (and has the bump to back it up), mom who's doing the prenatal nourishing and nurturing, as well as the one taking most of the hits for Team Baby. She's also the one getting the bulk of the pregnancy attention (from friends, from family, from the doctor or midwife, even from solicitous strangers). And that can sometimes leave you feeling like you're on the outside of pregnancy looking in.

Not to worry. Just because the pregnancy's not taking place in your body doesn't mean you can't share it. And the best way to keep from feeling left out is to get involved. Here's how:

- Talk it over. Your partner may not realize that you're feeling left out—or she may even have the impression that you're just as happy staying on the sidelines. Let her know you'd not only like to be let in, but that you are all in.

- Be a prenatal regular. Whenever you can (and if you're not already), join her at her prenatal appointments. She'll appreciate the moral support, but you'll appreciate the chance to hear the practitioner's recommendations for

outfits that will escape unstained by spit-up, pureed sweet potatoes, and baby vitamins.

What you can expect realistically, however, are some pretty magical moments and some epically awesome experiences. That feeling you'll get when cuddling a warm, sleeping bundle of baby (even if that cherub was howling moments before) will be like yourself. Plus you'll get to ask all those questions you have. The visits will also give you much-needed insight into the miraculous changes going on in your spouse's body. Best of all, you'll get to experience those momentous milestones with her (hearing the heartbeat, seeing those tiny limbs on ultrasound).

- Act pregnant. You don't have to start sporting a baby-on-board t-shirt or a milk mustache. But you can become a true partner in pregnancy: Exercise with her. Take a pass on the alcohol and be her comrade in club soda. Make an extra effort to eat well (at least when you're around her). And if you smoke, quit.

- Get an education. Even dads with advanced degrees (including those with MDs) have a lot to learn when it comes to pregnancy, childbirth, and baby care, just as moms do the first time. Read this book and follow it up with *What to Expect the First Year*. Check in with daddy bloggers and join online and local dads' groups. Download the What To Expect app, so you can get updates and tips and watch the weekly videos together. Attend childbirth classes as a team, and attend baby care classes for dads, if they're available locally. Chat up new dad friends and colleagues.

- Make a baby love connection. A mom-to-be may have the edge in prenatal bonding because baby's living inside her, but dads can get close, too. Talk, read, sing to your baby frequently—a fetus can hear from about the end of the 6th month on, and hearing your voice often now will help your newborn recognize it after delivery. Enjoy baby's kicks and squirms by resting your hand or your cheek or chest on your partner's bare belly for a few minutes each night. It's a nice way to get close with her, too. And baby can feel your belly rubs— even hear your heart beating if you get near enough.

- Gear up as a team. Decorate the nursery together. Pore over baby-name apps. Research prospective baby doctors and attend any consults. Become active in every aspect of planning and prepping for the baby's arrival if you haven't already.

- Consider taking off. Start looking into your company's paternity leave policy, if there is one. That way, you'll be sure not to be left out of all the fun after the baby is born. If there isn't one, consider mobilizing other dads and dads-to-be around the issue (an idea, like paid maternity leave, whose time has come in the U.S.).

nothing else you've ever felt. Ditto that first toothless smile meant just for you. The coo that finally comes, all breathy and sweet. Sticky hugs and wet kisses and fresh-from-the-bath snuggles. The reality is, they'll make all those sleepless nights, delayed dinners, mountains of laundry, and frustrated romance more than worth it.

Happy? Just you wait, mommy.

Wearing a Seat Belt

"Is it safe to wear a seat belt when you're pregnant? And what about the air bag?"

There's no safer way for an expectant mom—and her baby—to travel than buckled up. Plus, it's the law in most places. For maximum safety and minimum discomfort, fasten the belt below your belly, across your pelvis and

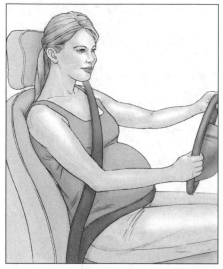

Buckling up for two

upper thighs. Wear the shoulder harness over your shoulder (not under your arm), diagonally between your breasts and to the side of your belly. And don't worry that the pressure of an abrupt stop will hurt your baby—he or she is well cushioned by amniotic fluid and uterine muscle, among the world's best shock-absorbing materials. Skip seatbelt positioners designed for moms-to-be—many (such as those secured with Velcro) won't hold up in a crash anyway, and other designs haven't been found to be any safer for mom and baby.

As for air bags, don't think about disabling them. If you get into an accident, you'll be much safer if you have a functional air bag than if you don't. In fact, studies have shown that not only do air bags save pregnant women's lives (and the lives of their babies), they don't cause harm, either—when deployed during an accident they don't increase the risk of fetal distress, placental separation, or c-section. To make sure your air bag is keeping you safe, keep your distance. If you're sitting in the passenger seat, set the seat as far back as

you can (your legs will appreciate the stretching room, too). If you're driving, tilt the wheel up toward your chest, away from your bump, and try to sit at least 10 inches from the steering wheel.

Travel

"We had booked a vacation before we got pregnant—is it still safe to go?"

Never again will it be so easy to vacation with your baby. Fast-forward to next year when you'll be lugging along a car seat, diapers, toys, and child-proofing kits, and you'll see why.

So don't have reservations about those reservations you've made. But before you pack your suitcase, do get the go-ahead from your practitioner. Chances are your vacation plans will be green-lighted, since travel is rarely restricted during pregnancy unless there's a complication (or if you're super close to term).

Once you've been cleared for take-off, you'll need to do a little planning to ensure a safe and comfortable expectant voyage, whether it's a quick business trip or a leisurely babymoon:

Time it right. When you're planning pregnancy travel, timing it right is the ticket—with the mostly easygoing second trimester typically travel-friendliest. By then, first trimester queasiness and fatigue (less than ideal travel companions) should have eased up—but you won't yet be so big that dragging yourself around is harder than dragging your bags. Traveling down-to-the-delivery-wire also might mean risking going into labor far from your practitioner—and depending on your destination, far from a reliable hospital. Contemplating a cruise? Most cruise lines won't let you board if you've reached your 24th week.

Choose a destination that fits. A hot, humid climate may be hard for your

Mosquitoes Find Pregnant Women Delicious

If mosquitoes seem to love snacking on you more than ever now that you're pregnant, it's not just your imagination. Scientists have found that pregnant women attract twice as many mosquitoes as nonpregnant women, possibly because those pesky bugs are fond of carbon dioxide and pregnant women tend to take more frequent breaths, thereby releasing more of this mosquito-friendly gas. Another reason why mosquitoes make a beeline for expectant mothers: They're heat-seeking, and expectant mothers generally have higher body temperatures, what with all that baby making going on. Most of the time, all this added attention from mosquitoes is merely an itchy nuisance. But when mosquito-borne illnesses are involved, bites can spread disease that might be dangerous to you and your baby (as with the Zika virus; see page 536). That's why it's important to take precautions if you live in or must travel to an area where mosquitoes pose a health risk (including checking with your practitioner—and current travel warnings—before considering a trip to such an area): Stay indoors as much as possible in heavily mosquito-infested areas, use tight-fitting screens on windows to keep mosquitoes out, wear protective clothing sprayed with permethrin (just don't get any on your skin), and apply insect repellent on exposed skin. Repellents containing DEET or picaridin offer the best defense against mosquitoes. These EPA-registered ingredients are considered both effective and safe during pregnancy. Repellents with purified forms of plants like citronella and cedar can help ward off bugs, but since they're not as effective as DEET or picaridin, don't rely on them in high-risk areas.

Always apply repellent after you've applied sunscreen, and be prepared to reapply sunscreen more frequently, since DEET decreases SPF. Products that combine repellent and sunscreen aren't recommended.

hopped-up metabolism to handle, but if you do opt for tropical, make sure your hotel and transport are air-conditioned, and that you stay hydrated and out of the sun. Get your practitioner's okay before booking a trip to a high altitude (see page 272). Also get the go-ahead before venturing into any region requiring extra vaccinations (some may not be pregnancy safe), as well as other areas that are hotbeds of potentially dangerous infections (including water-, food-, and mosquito-borne disease, such as Zika virus). For information on traveler's health, visit cdc.gov/travel.

Plan a trip that's relaxing. A single destination beats a whirlwind tour that takes you to 6 cities in 6 days. A trip that lets you (and your pregnant body) set the pace is a lot better than one that's set by a group tour guide. A few hours of sightseeing or shopping (or meetings) should be alternated with time spent with your feet up.

Insure yourself. Sign up for reliable travel insurance, in case a pregnancy complication requires you to change your plans. Consider medical evacuation insurance as well if you're traveling abroad (or just far from reliable medical services), in case you need to return home quickly under medical supervision. Medical travel insurance may also be useful if your regular insurance plan does not include foreign medical care. Check your policy ahead of time.

Over the (Baby) Moon

Of course you're over the moon about your baby making three (or more). But maybe you're also wondering how that particular life change will impact your future as a twosome—especially when it comes to the kind of carefree couple's time that will soon be in short supply.

Enter, the babymoon. Call it a last (for now) hurrah—a chance to be happy-go-lucky (or happy-and-get-lucky) together before you hunker down with baby.

Whether it's a week on the beach, a weekend in the country, a night at a local hotel, or a day at a spa, more and more parents-to-be are booking a babymoon—that is, time, schedule, finances, and practitioner's approval permitting. The best time for a babymoon? Clearly, when you're feeling your best and most energetic—which for most mamas-to-be is in the relatively comfortable second trimester.

Can't fit a babymoon in, or just can't afford one? Or maybe you'd both rather spend the extra cash on baby shopping than babymooning? Or your pregnancy is high risk and you're not allowed to leave town? Consider a staycation-style babymoon instead. Pick a weekend and plan just-for-two activities you might not get around to for a while once baby arrives on the scene: breakfast in bed, dinner and a movie, and, well, you get the picture.

Have medical backup. If you're traveling far, have the name of a local ob handy, just in case. If you're traveling abroad, contact the International Association for Medical Assistance to Travelers at iamat.org, which can provide you with a directory of English-speaking physicians throughout the world. Some major hotel chains can also provide you with this kind of information. If you find yourself in need of a doctor in a hurry and your hotel can't provide you with one, you can call the U.S. Embassy or the American Consulate for a recommendation. Or you can head to the nearest ER. If you have medical travel insurance, there should be a number to call for help.

Pack a pregnancy survival kit. Make sure you take enough prenatal vitamins to last the trip, some healthy snacks, Sea-Bands if you're susceptible to motion sickness, and a medication for traveler's stomach recommended by your practitioner. Something to leave out of your kit: jet lag remedies (including melatonin) that aren't practitioner-approved.

Take healthy eating habits with you. Have fun eating while you're away (you're on vacation!), but also try to eat regularly and well, and to snack as needed—the energy-boosting combo of complex carbs and protein will be especially helpful if you're dragging from jet lag. Also don't forget to bring your hydration habit along on the trip. Getting enough fluids is always essential during pregnancy, but key for jet-setters (dehydration steps up jet lag symptoms, such as fatigue).

Try to stay regular on the road. Changes in schedule and diet can compound constipation problems. So make sure you get plenty of the three most effective constipation combaters: fiber, fluids, and exercise.

When you've gotta go, go. Don't encourage a UTI or constipation by postponing trips to the bathroom. Go as soon as you feel the urge (and can find a toilet).

Get the support you need. Support hose, that is, particularly if you already suffer from varicose veins. But even if you only suspect you may be predisposed to them, consider wearing support hose when you'll be doing a lot of sitting (in cars, planes, or trains, for example) and when you'll be doing a lot of standing (in museums, in airport lines). They'll also help minimize swelling in your feet and ankles.

Don't be stationary on the move. Sitting for hours—especially in a cramped space, like an airplane seat—can restrict circulation, and even lead to a blood clot, something moms-to-be are already at higher risk of (see page 565). So be sure to shift in your seat frequently, do foot circles and stretch, flex, wiggle, and massage your legs often—and avoid crossing your legs. If possible, take your shoes off and elevate your feet a bit. Get up at least every hour or two to walk the aisles when you are on a plane or train. When traveling by car, don't go for more than 2 hours without stopping for a stretch.

Will getting there be half the fun when you're expecting? Probably not, but to make sure it's not twice as uncomfortable:

- If you're traveling by plane, check with the airline to see if there are any special regulations concerning pregnant women. Book a seat in the bulkhead (preferably on the aisle, so you can get up and stretch or use the restroom as needed), or if seating is not reserved, ask for preboarding. On board, wear your seat belt comfortably fastened below your belly.

Don't Drink the Water?

Yes, staying hydrated is important for expectant travelers. But if the purity of the water is questionable at your destination, plan to use bottled water for drinking and brushing your teeth. Make sure the seal on the bottle top is intact when opening it. Avoid ice, too, unless you're certain it was made with purified water.

Also at such locales, you'll want to be as wary of food safety as water purity. Avoid raw fruits, vegetables, and salad (unless you know it has been washed in purified water). If you're craving fresh fruit, wash it with bottled water and peel it yourself. No matter where you roam, steer clear of cooked foods that are lukewarm or at room temperature (as on a buffet) and anything sold by street vendors (even if it's hot). Of course, skip juice or dairy you aren't positively sure is pasteurized.

Stay safe when you're dipping (not just sipping and eating), too. Check ahead about the safety of local lakes, rivers, and ocean you might be swimming in (some may be polluted or contaminated with dangerous bacteria). Any pool you swim in should be chlorinated or be purified by ozone, saline, or ionizing—ask before you dip.

For more info on safe and healthy travel, visit cdc.gov/travel.

More and more often, the so-called friendly skies are also the go-hungry skies. Even if you will be scoring a meal or will be able to purchase one on board, keep in mind that it may be (a) tiny (b) inedible (c) a long time coming because of delays or (d)

Mile-High Pregnancy

Wondering if the thinner air at higher altitudes is safe for everyday breathing when you're expecting? It likely is if you've lived at a high altitude for a long time. But altitude-induced pregnancy problems (such as hypertension, water retention, a somewhat smaller-than-average baby) can occur in women who have just moved to a high-altitude area after a lifetime at sea level. For that reason, many practitioners suggest postponing such a move until after delivery if possible.

What about visiting from a low altitude to a high one during pregnancy? Clearly, scaling Mount Rainier is out for now—but also think twice (and ask your practitioner) before booking that trip to a resort in the Rockies. If you must make a trip to a high altitude destination, try to make the ascent gradually so you can adjust to the thinning air. If you're driving and there are places to stay along the way, try to go up 2,000 feet a day, rather than climbing all 7,000 feet at once or fly to a city that's at 5,000 feet, spend a few days to acclimate, then drive the rest of the way up. To minimize the risk of developing acute mountain sickness (the headache, nausea, and fatigue that can happen to anyone at altitudes over 8,000 feet, but can also produce symptoms at somewhat lower altitudes), plan on taking it easy for a few days after your arrival, drink lots of water, eat frequent small meals, and seek to sleep, if possible, at a somewhat lower altitude.

all of the above. So plan ahead. Pack a nonperishable sandwich or buy a sandwich, salad, or yogurt and fruit at the airport (just make sure you'll be eating it while it's still fresh). Stash some snacks in your carry-on, too. Drink plenty of water to counter dehydration caused by air travel (this will also ensure that you'll get plenty of leg-stretching during frequent bathroom trips), but don't drink airline tap water, since it's often contaminated with bacteria.

- If you're traveling by car, keep nutritious snacks and water handy. For long trips, be sure your seat is comfortable. If it isn't, consider buying or borrowing a special cushion for back support, available in auto supply or specialty stores or online. For car safety tips, see page 267.

- If you're traveling by train, check to be sure there's a dining car with a full menu. If there's not, pack enough meals and snacks for the ride. If you're traveling overnight, book a sleeper car, if you can. You don't want to start your trip exhausted.

- If you're traveling by boat, check with the cruise line about restrictions (there are many for pregnant women), as well as about medical facilities on board. Check in with your practitioner for trip clearance, too, and to see if there are any meds you should bring along (onboard medical staff may not be able to dispense to expectant moms). And of course, keep in mind when considering a cruise that morning sickness plus motion sickness could make for a trip-ruining combo. Also be aware that outbreaks of gastrointestinal illness are not uncommon on cruise ships, and may be especially dangerous if you're expecting.

How Safe Is Security?

Getting through airport security may be a pain, but fortunately it's not a safety risk when you're traveling for two. The very low levels of electromagnetic waves emitted by metal detectors are perfectly safe (you're exposed to them all the time at home, from your appliances, for instance). Ditto the wands sometimes used by security agents. And those full body scans? The TSA says they pose no risk, including to pregnant women and their unborn babies, with the radiation from a scan equal to 2 minutes of flying at a high altitude. Pat-downs may or may not be an alternative to the scan (you can always ask if you're concerned).

If you qualify for TSA PreCheck (apply at tsa.gov), you may be able to avoid the body scan altogether (as well as the hassle of taking off your shoes and jacket and pulling out your bag of liquids)—assuming it's available at the airport you're flying from.

ALL ABOUT:

Sex and the Pregnant Couple

Religious and medical miracles aside, every pregnancy starts with sex. So why does what probably got you here in the first place become so complicated now that you're here?

Whether you're having it more often or less often, whether you're enjoying it more or less or not at all—or whether you're not even doing it—chances are that making a baby has changed the way you make love. From sorting out what is and isn't safe in bed (or on the living room rug or on the kitchen counter) to figuring out which positions best accommodate your ever-bigger belly, from mismatched moods (you're turned on, he's turned off, he's turned on, you're turned off) to hormones gone wild (leaving your breasts more enticing than ever, yet too tender to touch), pregnancy sex is full of challenges on both sides of the bed. But not to worry. A little creativity, a good sense of humor, plenty of patience (and practice), and lots of love will conquer all when it comes to pregnancy sex.

Sex Through the Trimesters

Down-up-down. While that might sound like a new sex move, it's actually a good description of the roller-coaster pattern most couples can expect their sex lives to follow during their 9 months of pregnancy. In the first trimester, many women find that their libidos take a nosedive, plummeting promptly as soon as pregnancy hormones kick in. And that slowdown in sexual interest should come as no shocker. After all, fatigue, nausea, vomiting, and painfully tender nipples don't make for great sex partners. But as with all things pregnancy, no two women are alike, which means no two libidos are alike, either. If you're lucky, you might find that the first trimester makes you hotter than

The Ins and Outs of Sex During Pregnancy

Wondering what's safe and what's not when it comes to making love during pregnancy? Here's the lowdown:

Oral sex. Cunnilingus ("going down" on a woman) is as safe as it is potentially pleasurable throughout pregnancy, so don't hesitate to go for it. Just make sure your partner doesn't forcefully blow air into your vagina. Fellatio ("going down" on him) is always safe during pregnancy—as is swallowing semen, in case you're curious—and for some couples is a nice way to stay close when intercourse isn't permitted.

Anal sex. Anal sex is probably safe during pregnancy, but proceed to the back door with caution. First, it probably won't be comfortable if you have hemorrhoids—an occupational hazard of pregnancy—and it can make them bleed (which can really spoil the moment). Second, you'll need to remember the same safety rule of anal sex whether you're pregnant or not, but be especially fastidious about following it now: Never go from anal to vaginal sex without cleaning up first. Doing so may introduce harmful bacteria into your vaginal canal, setting you up for infection and risk to the baby.

Masturbation. Unless orgasm is off-limits because of a high-risk pregnancy, masturbating (with or without a vibrator) during pregnancy is perfectly safe—and a great way to release all that tension you're feeling.

Sex toys. As long as your practitioner has okayed sex, sex toys (like dildos and vibrators) are a go, too—after all, they're just mechanical versions of the real thing. But be sure any sex toy you use is clean, and be careful not to penetrate the vagina too deeply with it.

ever, thanks to the happy side of hormonal changes: genitals that are ultrasensitive and ever-tingly, and breasts that are extra big and extra fun.

Interest often (though not always) picks up during the second trimester, when early pregnancy symptoms have subsided and there's more energy to put into lovemaking (and when less time in the bathroom leaves more time in the bedroom). Never had multiple orgasms before (or any orgasms)? This may be your lucky break—and your chance to get lucky again and again. That's because extra blood flow to the labia, clitoris, and vagina can make it easier to climax than ever before—and to have orgasms that are stronger and longer lasting, too. But again, nothing's a given during pregnancy. Some women

actually lose that loving feeling in the second trimester—or never end up finding it at all during their 9 months, and that's normal, too.

As delivery nears, libido usually wanes again, sometimes even more drastically than in the first trimester, for obvious reasons: First, your watermelon-size abdomen makes the target more difficult for your partner to reach, even with creative positioning. Second, the aches and discomforts of advancing pregnancy can cool even the hottest passion. And third, late in the trimester it's hard to concentrate on anything but that eagerly and anxiously awaited event. Still, some couples manage to overcome those late pregnancy obstacles and keep up the action until that first contraction.

FOR FATHERS

The Sex Fear Factor

Worried that sex might hurt your partner or your baby-to-be? Worry no more. As long as the doctor or midwife has issued the green light on all red-light activities during pregnancy (and most of the time, that's exactly what'll happen), sex is completely safe up to delivery. Your baby is way out of your reach (even for the particularly gifted), well secured and safely sealed off in the uterus, unable to watch or be aware of the adult action—in short, perfectly oblivious to what's going on when you're getting it on. Even those mild contractions your partner might feel after orgasm are nothing to worry about, since they're not the kind that trigger premature labor in a normal pregnancy.

In fact, research shows that low-risk women who stay sexually active during pregnancy are actually less likely to deliver early (so get busy!). And not only will making love to your spouse do her no harm, it can do her a world of good by filling her increased needs for physical and emotional closeness, and by letting her know that she's desired at a time when she may not be feeling her most desirable. Though you should proceed with care (take your cues from her and keep her needs top priority), you can certainly proceed—and feel good about it.

Still concerned? Let her know. Remember, open and honest communication about everything, including sex, is the best policy.

What's Turning You On (or Off)?

Maybe pregnancy agrees with your sex life . . . maybe it strongly disagrees. Either way, all the physical changes you're experiencing are bound to have an impact of some kind on the sex you have (or don't have)—for better, for worse, or for a little of both. Symptoms that can turn you on, or turn you off, include:

Nausea and vomiting. Morning sickness can certainly come between you and a good time. After all, it's hard to purr with pleasure when you're busy gagging up dinner. So use your time wisely. If your morning sickness rises with the sun, put after-dark hours to good use. If your evenings are queasy, hop on the morning love train. If morning sickness stays with you day and night, you and your spouse may just have to wait out its symptoms, which typically taper off by the end of the first trimester. Whatever you do, don't pressure yourself to feel sexy when you're feeling sick—the result won't be satisfying for anyone.

Fatigue. It's hard to get busy when you barely have the energy to get undressed. Happily, the worst of pregnancy fatigue should pass by the 4th month (though exhaustion will probably return in the last trimester). Until then, make love while the sun shines (when the opportunity presents itself) instead of trying to force yourself to stay up for late night romance. Cap off a weekend afternoon of lovemaking with a nap or the other way around. Have the kind of breakfast in bed that doesn't leave crumbs.

Your changing shape. Maybe the recent rounding of your body has made you

Sexercise

Though you can do them anytime, anywhere, there's no better way to mix business with pleasure than performing Kegels during sex. Get the lowdown on everyone's favorite exercise on page 229.

feel sexier than ever. Or maybe you're having a hard time embracing your new shape. If so, wrapping yourself up in some lacy, racy lingerie (yes, they make it for pregnant lovers, too) may help you wrap yourself around those curves. If it's the physical challenges of pregnancy sex that have you down (as pregnancy progresses, the gymnastics required to scale Bump Mountain may seem too much like hard work), you can conquer those, too. Read on.

Your engorged genitals. Increased blood flow to the pelvic area, caused by hormonal changes of pregnancy, can make some lucky women more sexually eager and responsive than ever. But it can also make sex less satisfying (especially later in pregnancy) if a residual fullness persists after orgasm, leaving you feeling as though you didn't quite make it. For your partner, too, the swelling of your sweet spot may increase pleasure (if he feels snugly caressed) or decrease it (if the fit is too tight). If swelling is accompanied by pain during intercourse, that could be a sign of varicose veins in your pelvic region (they can happen in the vulva, the vagina, and the surrounding area). Check with your practitioner and see page 165.

Leakage of colostrum. Late in pregnancy, some women begin producing the premilk called colostrum (see page 377), which can leak from the breasts during sexual stimulation and can be a little distracting (and messy) in the middle of foreplay. It's nothing to worry about, of course, but if it bothers you or your partner, concentrate on other parts of the body (like that possibly trigger-happy clitoris of yours!).

Breast tenderness. For some couples, pregnant breasts (full, firm, and maybe larger than life) are favorites that can't get enough playtime. But for many, that early pregnancy swelling comes with a high price—painful tenderness—and along with it, a look-but-don't-touch policy. If your breasts are bringing you more pain than pleasure, make sure your partner gets the message—and remind him that the tenderness will ease up by the end of the first trimester, at which point you'll both be able to enjoy a hands-on approach.

Changes in vaginal secretions. Wet isn't always wild when you're expecting. Normal vaginal secretions increase during pregnancy and also change in consistency, odor, and taste. If you've always been on the dry or narrow side, that extra lubrication may make sex more enjoyable. But sometimes, too much of a good thing can make the vaginal canal so wet and slippery that it actually decreases sensation for both of you—and even make it more difficult for your partner to keep his erection or reach orgasm. (A little extra foreplay for him may help him out in that department.) The heavier scent and taste of the secretions may also make oral sex off-putting.

Some expectant moms experience vaginal dryness during sex, even with all those extra secretions. Unscented water-based lubricants, such as K-Y or Astroglide, are safe to use as needed when you're having a dry spell.

Bleeding caused by the sensitivity of the cervix. The mouth of the uterus also

Expectant Sex Explained

Sure, you've done it before. But have you done it pregnancy-style? Though the basic rules of the game apply when you're expecting, you'll find that pregnant sex requires a few adjustments, a little finessing, and a lot of flexibility—literally. Here are some suggestions to get you going in the right direction:

- Wait for the nod. She was hot to trot yesterday, but today she's cold as ice to your advances? As a pregnant woman's moods swing, so does her sex drive. You'll have to learn to swing along (and to hold on tight).

- Warm her up before you start your engine. This may go without saying (always), but it's a must when she's expecting. Go as slowly as she needs you to, making sure she's fully charged on foreplay before you get in gear.

- Stop for directions. The road map of what feels good and what doesn't may have changed (even since last week), so don't rely on a possibly outdated GPS. Always ask before going in. For instance, you may need to tread especially lightly when it comes to those probably supersize breasts. Though they may have swelled to thrilling proportions, they can be tender to even the gentlest touch, especially in the first trimester. Which means you may have to look but not touch for a while.

- Put her in the driver's seat. Choose positions with her comfort in mind. A top pregnancy favorite is her on top (mom on pop?), since this position gives her the most control over depth and speed of penetration. Another is spooning (she faces away on her side). And when her belly starts getting between you, get around it creatively: Try it from behind with her on her knees or sitting on your lap while you lie down.

- Be prepared for rerouting. All roads aren't leading to intercourse? Find alternate paths to pleasure that you both can enjoy—masturbation, oral sex, two-way massage.

becomes engorged during pregnancy—crisscrossed with many additional blood vessels to accommodate increased blood flow—and is much softer than before pregnancy. This means that sex (especially deep penetration) can occasionally cause spotting, particularly late in pregnancy when the cervix begins to ripen for delivery (but also at any time during pregnancy). This spotting is usually nothing to be concerned about, though do mention it to your practitioner for extra reassurance.

There are also plenty of psychological hang-ups that can get between you, your partner, and your pregnancy sex life. These, too, can be eased:

Fear that sex will cause a miscarriage. Stop worrying and start enjoying. In normal pregnancies, sex isn't harmful. Your practitioner will tell you if there's a reason why you shouldn't have sex during your pregnancy. If not, go for it.

Fear that having an orgasm will trigger miscarriage. Although the uterus does contract after orgasm, sometimes quite powerfully and for as long as half an hour, these post-climax contractions are not a sign of labor and aren't harmful in a normal pregnancy. Again, if

Position Matters

When you're making love at this point in your pregnancy (and later on, too), position matters. Side-lying positions (front-to-front or front-to-back, aka spooning) are often most comfortable because they keep you off your back. Ditto woman on top (which allows you more control over penetration). Rear entry can work well, too, with you on your knees or sitting on his lap facing his legs while he lies down (aka reverse cowgirl). Him on top is fine for quickies (as long as he keeps his weight off you by supporting himself with his arms), but after the 4th month, it's not a good idea to spend too much time flat on your back.

there's a reason why you should avoid orgasm (because you're at high risk for miscarriage or preterm labor, or have a placenta problem, for instance), your practitioner will let you know. If you haven't broached the subject and aren't sure, ask.

Fear that the baby is "watching." Not possible. Though your baby may enjoy the gentle rocking during sex and orgasm, he or she can't see what you're doing, has no clue what's happening, and will certainly have no memory of it. Fetal reactions (slowed movement during sex, then furious kicking and squirming and a speeded-up heartbeat after orgasm) are just natural responses to uterine activity.

Fear of "bumping into" the baby. Though your partner may not want to admit it, no penis is big enough to get close to your baby. Your little one is completely sealed off in your cozy uterine home—perfectly protected even once baby's head drops into your pelvis as delivery nears.

Fear that sex will cause infection. The amniotic sac seals baby off safely from both semen and infectious organisms. Unless your membranes have ruptured (your water has broken), the seal is intact.

Anxiety over the coming attraction. Sure, you're both preoccupied and maybe a little (or a lot) stressed out. You might be experiencing mixed feelings, too, over your baby's imminent arrival. And it's sometimes hard to have sexy thoughts when your mind's cluttered with worries about all those upcoming financial responsibilities and lifestyle changes, not to mention all those baby prep to-do lists. Your best move? Talk about these feelings openly and often—and don't bring them to bed.

Your changing relationship. Maybe you're having a little trouble adjusting to the upcoming changes in your family dynamics—the idea that you'll no longer be just a couple, but a couple of parents, too. Talk it over and you'll begin to see: Change can be good. The extra dimension in your relationship can actually bring deeper intimacy—and even deeper sexual satisfaction.

Feelings of resentment. Maybe he's feeling a little resentful because you seem more into the baby, less into him. Maybe you're feeling a little resentful because you're doing all the heavy lifting for a baby you'll both get to enjoy. Such feelings can keep things chilly under the sheets, so talk them out—again, before you hit the sack.

Worry that sex later in pregnancy will cause preterm labor. Unless the cervix is ripe and ready, sex does not appear to trigger labor (as many hopeful overdue couples have discovered). In fact, studies show that couples with low-risk pregnancies who are sexually active during late pregnancy are more likely to carry to term.

Of course, psychological factors can also add to pregnancy-sex pleasure (good news!). For one, some couples who worked hard at becoming pregnant may be happy to switch from procreational to recreational sex. Instead of being slaves to ovulation predictor kits, charts, calendars, and monthly anxiety, they can enjoy spontaneous sex for pleasure's sake. For another, many couples find that creating a baby brings them closer together than ever before, and they find the belly a symbol of that closeness—instead of an awkward obstacle.

Enjoying It More, Even If You're Doing It Less

Good, lasting sexual relationships are rarely built in a day (or even a really hot night). They grow with practice, patience, understanding, and love. This is true, too, of an already established sexual relationship that undergoes the emotional and physical changes of pregnancy. Here are a few ways to "stay on top":

- Enjoy your sex life instead of analyzing it to death. Seize the moment as you seize each other. Don't focus on how frequently or infrequently you're having sex (quality beats quantity, but especially when you're expecting) or compare prepregnancy sex with your sex life now (they're two different animals and, for that matter, so are both of you).

- Accentuate all the positives. Think of sex as relaxing—and remember relaxation is good for all involved (including baby). Think of the roundness of your pregnant body as sensual and sexy. Think of every embrace as a chance to get closer as a couple, not just a chance to get closer to closing the deal.

- Get adventurous. The old positions don't fit anymore? Look at this as an opportunity to try something new (or a lot of somethings new). But give yourselves time to adjust to each position you try. You might even consider a "dry run," trying out a new position fully clothed first, so that it'll be more familiar (and you'll be more successful) when you try it for real.

- Keep it real. Your expectations, that is. Pregnant sex presents plenty of challenges, so cut yourself some slack in the sack. Though some women achieve orgasm for the first time during pregnancy, other women find the big O more elusive than ever. Your goal doesn't always have to be mutual fireworks, perfectly synced up. Remind yourself that getting close is sometimes the best, and most satisfying, part of getting it on.

- Don't forget the other kind of intercourse (talking, that is). Communication is the foundation of every relationship, particularly one that's going through life-changing adjustments. Discuss any problems you're facing as a couple openly instead of trying to sweep them under the bed (and instead of taking them to bed). If any problems seem too big to handle by yourselves, consider couples counseling. There's never been a better time to work on your twosome than now that it's about to become a threesome.

Good, bad, or indifferent, remember, too, that every couple feels differently about sex during pregnancy,

When Sex Is Off the Table

Clearly, there are plenty of perks to pregnancy sex, for all involved. But what if sex is restricted during part or all of pregnancy—or off the table altogether? If your practitioner has told you to abstain (often called "pelvic rest") but hasn't issued specifics, ask for a breakdown. Is it a temporary restriction or a full 9-month ban? Is foreplay fine? Oral okay, but penetration prohibited? Anything goes except orgasm for you? Or anything goes but with a condom? Knowing precisely what is safe and when it's safe is essential, so make sure you get a list of do's and don'ts.

Sex will probably be restricted under the following, and possibly other, circumstances:

- If you are experiencing signs of preterm labor or, possibly, if you have a history of preterm labor

- If you've gotten a diagnosis of cervical insufficiency or placenta previa

- Possibly, if you are experiencing bleeding or have a history of miscarriages

- If your partner has been (or possibly has been) infected with a dangerous-for-pregnancy virus (such as Zika) or an STD. Your practitioner might suggest using a condom during intercourse, or abstaining completely.

If penetration is off-limits, but orgasm's allowed, consider mutual masturbation. If orgasm's taboo for you, you might get pleasure out of pleasuring your partner this way (he probably won't object). If intercourse has been okayed—but orgasm's prohibited—you could try making love without you reaching climax. Though this definitely won't be completely satisfying for you (and may be way easier said than done if you climax easily), you'll still get some of the intimacy you're both craving while providing pleasure for your partner. If all lovemaking activities have been banned for the duration, try not to let that come between you as a couple. Focus on other ways of getting close—the romantic, G-rated kinds you might not have tapped into since early on in your relationship (like holding hands, cuddling, and old-fashioned making out).

both physically and emotionally. The bottom line (whether you're on top, on bottom, side to side, or not doing it at all): What's normal, as is almost always the case when you're expecting, is what's normal for you and your partner. Embrace that, embrace each other—and try not to sweat the rest.

CHAPTER 10

The Sixth Month

Approximately 23 to 27 Weeks

No doubt about those tummy moves these days: They're all baby, not gas (though you're probably still having plenty of that, too). And as those little arms and legs start to pack more of a punch, these baby gymnastics—and sometimes bouts of baby hiccups—will become visible from the outside (talk about a built-in entertainment center!). This month marks the last of second trimester, which means you're almost two-thirds of the way to the pregnancy finish line. Still, you've got a ways to go and a ways to grow—as does baby, who's a relatively light load compared with what you'll be carrying around in a month or two. Take advantage—and while you can still see your feet (if not touch your toes), kick up your sensible heels a little.

Your Baby This Month

Week 23 A window into your womb would reveal that your baby's skin is a bit saggy, hanging loosely from that little body. That's because skin grows faster than fat develops, and there's not much fat to fill that skin out yet. But don't worry—the fat is about to start catching up. Beginning this week, your baby (who is around 11 inches long and just over a pound in weight) begins to pack on the pounds (which means you will, too!). In fact, during the next month your baby will actually double in weight (fortunately, you won't). Once those fat deposits are made, your baby will be less transparent, too. Right now, the organs and bones can still be seen through the skin, which has a red hue thanks to the developing veins and arteries just underneath. But by month 8, no more see-through baby!

Week 24 At a weight of 1⅓ pounds and a length of about 11½ inches, your baby

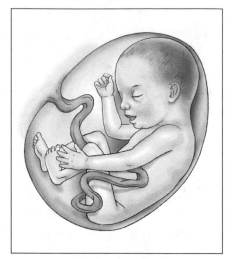

Your Baby, Month 6

is now the size of an ear of corn (sweet corn, of course). Baby's weekly weight gain is now about 6 ounces—not quite as much as you're putting on, but getting a lot closer. Much of that weight is coming from accumulating baby fat, as well as from growing organs, bones, and muscle. By now, your baby's tiny face is almost fully formed and achingly adorable—complete with a full set of eyelashes and eyebrows and a good sprinkling of hair on that head. Is your baby a brunette, a blond, or a redhead? Actually, right now he or she's snow white, since there's no pigment in that hair just yet.

Week 25 Baby's growing by leaps and bounds (and inches and ounces), this week reaching 13 inches (over a foot long!) in length and more than 1½ pounds in weight. And there are exciting developments on the horizon, too. Capillaries are forming under the skin and filling with blood. By week's end, air sacs lined with capillaries will also develop in your baby's lungs, getting them ready for that first breath of air. Mind you, those lungs aren't ready for prime-time breathing yet—and they have a lot of maturing left to do before

they will be. Though they're already beginning to develop surfactant, a substance that will help them expand after birth, your baby's lungs are still too undeveloped to sufficiently send oxygen to the bloodstream and release carbon dioxide from the blood (aka breathe). And speaking of breathing, your baby's nostrils, which have been plugged up until now, are starting to open up this week. This enables your little one to begin taking practice "breaths." Vocal cords are functioning now, too, leading to occasional hiccups (which you'll certainly be feeling).

Week 26 Next time you're browsing through the meat department, pick up a 2-pound chuck roast. No, not for dinner—just so you can get a sense of how big your baby almost is this week. That's right—your baby now weighs nearly a full 2 pounds and measures in at 14-plus inches long. Another momentous development this week: Your baby's eyes are beginning to open. The eyelids have been fused for the past few months (so the retina, the part of the eye that allows images to come into focus, could develop). The colored part of the eye (the iris) still doesn't have much pigmentation, so it's too early to start guessing your baby's eye color. Still, your baby is now able to see—a huge development. Sure, there's not much to see in the dark confines of the womb. But with heightening of those senses, you may notice an increase in activity when your baby perceives a bright light or hears a loud noise. In fact, if a loud vibrating noise is brought close to your belly, your baby will respond by blinking and startling (a good reason not to pump up the volume too much).

Week 27 This week your baby's head-to-toe length is about 14½ inches. Your baby's weight is creeping up the charts as well, coming in at just about 2 pounds this week. And here's an interesting fetal factoid: Your little one has more taste buds now than he or she will have at birth (and beyond). Which means that not only is your baby able to taste the difference in the amniotic fluid when you eat different foods, but he or she might even react to it. For instance, some moms report that their babies respond to spicy foods by hiccupping—or by kicking when they get that spicy kick. Will baby arrive with a taste for Tabasco? Time will tell!

Your Body This Month

Here are some symptoms you may experience this month (or may not experience, since every pregnancy is different). Some of these symptoms may be continuing from last month, while others may be brand new. Some may be easing up, others intensifying.

Physically

- More definite fetal activity
- Continued vaginal discharge
- Achiness in the lower abdomen and along the sides (from stretching of ligaments supporting the uterus)
- Constipation
- Heartburn, indigestion, flatulence, bloating
- Occasional headaches
- Occasional lightheadedness or dizziness, especially when getting up quickly or when your blood sugar dips
- Nasal congestion and occasional nosebleeds; ear stuffiness
- Sensitive gums that may bleed when you brush
- Hearty appetite

Your Body This Month

At the beginning of this month, the top of your uterus is around 1½ inches above your belly button. By the end of the month, your uterus has grown an inch higher and the top can be felt approximately 2½ inches above your belly button. Your uterus is the size of a basketball now, and you might even look like that's what you're carrying around in your belly.

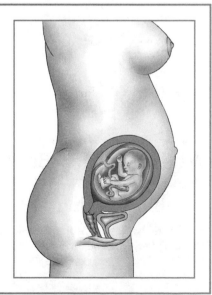

- Leg cramps
- Mild swelling of ankles and feet, and occasionally of hands and face
- Hemorrhoids
- Varicose veins in legs and/or vulva
- Itchy belly
- A protruding navel (a popped-out belly button)
- Backache
- Patchy skin discoloration on belly and/or face

- Stretch marks
- Enlarged breasts

Emotionally

- Fewer mood swings
- Forgetfulness, absentmindedness (aka "placenta brain")
- A feeling like pregnancy is endless
- Plenty of excitement about the future
- Some worry about the future

What You Can Expect at This Month's Checkup

It will probably be business pretty much as usual at this month's checkup. As you end your second trimester, you can expect your practitioner to check the following, though there may be variations, depending on your particular needs and on your practitioner's style of practice:

- Weight and blood pressure
- Urine, for sugar and protein
- Fetal heartbeat
- Height of fundus (top of uterus)

- Size of uterus and position of fetus, by external palpation (feeling from the outside)
- Feet and hands for swelling, and legs for varicose veins
- Glucose screening test (usually given between 24 and 28 weeks)
- Symptoms you may have been experiencing, especially unusual ones
- Questions and problems you want to discuss—have a list ready

What You May Be Wondering About

Trouble Sleeping

"I've never had a sleep problem in my life—until now. I can't seem to settle down at night."

Between midnight bathroom runs, a racing mind, cramping/restless legs, heartburn that's keeping you upright, a hopped-up metabolism that's keeping the heat on even when it's off, and the impossibility of getting comfortable when you're sporting a basketball in your midsection, it's no wonder you can't settle in for a good night's sleep. While this insomnia is definitely good preparation for the sleepless nights you'll encounter as a new parent, that doesn't mean you have to take it lying down . . . or even propped up. Try the following tips for summoning the sandman:

- Move your body during the day. A body that gets a workout by day will be sleepier at night. But don't exercise too close to bedtime, since the post-exercise high could keep you from crashing when your head hits the pillow.

- Clear your mind. If you've been losing sleep over stress at work or at home, unload it on your spouse or a friend earlier in the evening so it doesn't weigh you down at bedtime. If no one's around to vent to, writing your concerns down can be therapeutic. As bedtime approaches, put those worries aside, empty your head, and try thinking happy thoughts only. Meditation can help, too.

- Be an early bird diner. A full meal (and a full tummy) can keep you from falling asleep and staying asleep. So try to eat your evening meal earlier in the evening.

- Top off before you turn in. A too-empty tummy can also keep you up. To keep low blood sugar (and the midnight munchies) from waking you, have a light snack as part of your bedtime routine. That sleepy-standard, warm milk, may be especially effective (even if you no longer get tucked in with your teddy). Add a whole-grain muffin for blood-sugar-sustaining complex carbs, and substitute almond milk if heartburn strikes you at night. Or nibble on some cheese and crackers.

When She Can't Sleep

She's making a baby, but chances are she isn't sleeping like one. So instead of snoring up a storm next time your partner's pregnancy insomnia strikes, consider keeping her company while she waits for the sandman to show. Buy her a body pillow to help get her comfy, or build her a cozy fort of support with your extra pillows. Relax her with a back rub, run her a bath, bring her a warm cup of milk and a muffin. Do a little pillow talking. Cuddle as needed and as wanted. And if one thing leads to another—and she's up for a sexual nightcap—you might both sleep better.

- Slow the flow. If frequent trips to the bathroom are standing between you and a good night's sleep, limit fluids after 6 p.m. (just get enough fluids before then). Drink if you're thirsty, but don't guzzle a 16-ounce bottle of water right before bedtime.

- Don't get buzzed. Avoid caffeine in the afternoon and evening (its effects can keep you buzzing into the night). Ditto for sugar (especially combined with caffeine, as in a white chocolate mocha), which will give you an energy boost when you least want one and then leave your blood sugar levels wobbly during the night.

- Give yourself a bedtime routine. It's not just for kids. The relaxing repetition of the right bedtime rituals can help adults settle down for a good night's sleep, too. Easy does it, so focus on activities that slow you down, practiced in a predictable order. Good options to consider adding to your routine: light reading (but nothing you can't put down) or soothing music, serene yoga poses or relaxation exercises, a warm bath, a back rub, plus, that other bedtime snack—sex.

- Download. Sleep? There are plenty of apps for that, too. Explore some of the better-rated sleep apps—from those that rely on self-guided meditation to those that use nature sounds and other white noise. And while you're at it, try meditating to relieve daily stress that might be keeping you up.

- Wean off the screen. Using your phone, tablet, e-reader, laptop, or other electronic device before bed (for anything other than a sleep or white noise app) can mess with your z's. Light from the screen alters sleepiness and alertness, and also suppresses levels of melatonin, the hormone that regulates your internal clock and plays a role in your sleep cycle. Experts say you should power down your devices at least an hour before turning in.

- Get comfy. There is no such thing as too many pillows when you're pregnant. Use them to prop you up, support you where you need it, or just cozy up to. Be sure, too, that your bedroom isn't too hot or too cold. Just can't get comfy in your bed? Try snoozing semi-upright in a recliner, which will allow you to stay on your back without actually lying flat on your back.

- Get some air. It's hard to get sleepy when it's stuffy. Weather permitting, crack a window—if not, run a fan to circulate the air. And don't sleep with the covers over your head. This will decrease the oxygen and increase the carbon dioxide you breathe in, which can cause headaches.

- Ask before you pop. While there are sleep aids that are safe for occasional use in pregnancy, don't take any sleep aid (prescription, over-the-counter, or herbal) unless it's been prescribed or okayed by your practitioner. If your practitioner has recommended that you take a magnesium supplement (or a calcium-magnesium supplement) to combat constipation or leg cramps, it makes sense to take it before bed because magnesium—touted for its natural muscle relaxing powers—may help lull you to sleep.

- Smell your way to sleep. A lavender-scented pillow that you tuck into bed with you or a lavender sachet slipped between the pillowcase and pillow can help relax you and bring on sleep faster.

- Save your bed for sleep, cuddling, and sex. Don't invite activities you associate with being wide awake and wired (work, paying bills, even shopping for baby gear) into your bed.

- Avoid clock-watching. Judge whether you're getting enough sleep by how you feel, not by how many hours you stay in bed. You're getting enough rest if you're not chronically tired (beyond the normal fatigue of pregnancy). And speaking of midnight hours: If the sight of those glowing numbers (and the hours ticking by) on the clock stresses you out, turn it so you can't see it.

- Don't just lie there. When sleep's eluding you—and you've run out of baby sheep to count—do something relaxing (read, listen to music, meditate) until you feel sleepy.

- Don't lose sleep over losing sleep. Stressing about your lack of shut-eye will only make it harder to grab any. In fact, sometimes just letting go of that "will I ever fall asleep?" worry is all it takes to drop off into dreamland.

An Umbilical Hernia

Most mamas-to-be expect their belly buttons to pop when their bumps do. But for some women, that popping navel is more than a sign there's a baby on board—it's an umbilical hernia.

An umbilical hernia happens when there is a small hole in the abdominal wall, which allows abdominal tissue (like loops of the small intestine) to protrude through the umbilical area. Most umbilical hernias are congenital (meaning present at birth). In fact, umbilical hernias are common in newborns (you can read all about that in *What to Expect the First Year*), usually closing up quickly on their own. Even when a small hole doesn't close up, it's not likely to cause problems or even be noticeable—that is, until a growing uterus starts applying pressure, causing the hernia to get bigger, sometimes leading to a painful bulging around the belly button. Expecting multiples can multiply your odds of an umbilical hernia (after all, there's more growing going on in your uterus).

How will you know if you have an umbilical hernia? You might feel a soft lump around your belly button (it might be more noticeable when you lie down), and you might see a bulge under the skin. You might also have a dull achy pain in the belly button area that becomes more noticeable when you're active, bend over, sneeze, cough, or laugh hard.

You can wear a belly band to help keep the hernia from bulging and causing pain. Some women find relief by gently massaging the lump until the bulging goes back in. Or, if it's not bothering you, you can choose to do nothing at all.

If, once you deliver your baby, the hernia doesn't recede on its own (or with the help of special exercises recommended by your practitioner), surgery may be required to repair it. Surgery is not recommended during pregnancy unless a loop of bowel slips through the hole and becomes trapped (herniated), risking a loss of blood supply to that area. In that case, your practitioner may recommend that you have a simple operation to repair the hernia—usually during the second trimester.

The same applies to the far less common inguinal hernia—when tissue pushes through a weak spot in your groin muscle, resulting in a bulge in the groin—which can be caused by the pressure from your growing uterus. A belly band can help keep your growing abdomen from pressing on the inguinal hernia during pregnancy, and if the hernia doesn't recede on its own after you deliver, surgery can repair it (though surgery may need to be performed during the second trimester if a loop of bowel gets trapped).

Popped Belly Button

"My belly button used to be a perfect innie. Now it's sticking all the way out. Will it stay that way even after I deliver?"

Has your innie been outed? Is it poking straight through your clothes these days? Taking on a life of its own? Don't worry: There's nothing novel about navels that pop during pregnancy. Just about every belly button does at some point. As the swelling uterus pushes forward, even the deepest innie is sure to pop like a timer on a turkey (except, on most women, the navel pops well before baby's "done"). Your belly button should revert to its regular position a few months after delivery, though it may bear the mommy mark: that somewhat stretched-out, lived-in look. Until then, you can look at the bright side of your protruding navel—it gives you a chance to clean out all the lint that's accumulated there since you were a kid. If you find that the outie look doesn't quite work with the clingy fashion statement you're trying to make—or if your poor outie's getting irritated from rubbing against your clothes—you can use a specially designed belly button cover to smooth and protect it. Pregnancy support products (like tummy sleeves or tummy shapers) can also hide that popped-out navel. Or just wear it out and proud, as yet another pregnancy badge of honor.

Wondering about your navel piercing? See page 169 for the lowdown on belly rings.

Baby Kicking

"Some days the baby is kicking all the time, other days he seems very quiet. Is this normal?"

Fetuses are only human. Just like us, they have "up" days, when they feel like kicking up their heels (and elbows and knees), and "down" days, when they'd rather lie back and take it easy. Most often, their activity is related to your activities. Like babies out of the womb, fetuses are lulled by rocking. So when you're on the go all day, your baby is likely to be pacified by the rhythm of your routine, and you're likely not to notice much kicking—partly because baby has slowed down, partly because you're so busy. As soon as you slow down or relax, your little one's bound to start acting up (a pattern babies tend to continue even after they're born). That's why you're more apt to feel fetal movement in bed at night or when you're resting during the day. Activity may increase, too, after you've had a meal or snack, perhaps in reaction to the surge of sugar in your blood. You may also notice increased fetal activity when you're excited or nervous—about to give a presentation, for example—possibly because the baby is stimulated by your adrenaline response. Or when baby gets a jolt of caffeine from your morning latte, or hears an already-familiar song playing.

Babies are actually most active between weeks 24 and 28, when they're small enough to belly dance, somersault, kickbox, and do a full aerobic step class in their roomy uterine home. But their movements are erratic and usually brief, so they aren't always felt by a busy mother-to-be, even though they are visible on ultrasound. Fetal activity usually becomes more organized and consistent, with more clearly defined periods of rest and activity, between weeks 28 and 32. It's definitely felt later and less emphatically when there's an anterior placenta getting in the way (see page 263), and sometimes when a mom has a lot of abdominal fat muffling the kicks.

Don't be tempted to compare baby movement notes with other pregnant women. Each fetus, like each newborn, has an individual pattern of activity and development. Some seem always active, others mostly quiet. The activity of some fetuses is so regular, their moms could set their watches by it—in others there's no discernible activity pattern at all. As long as movements don't suddenly slow down significantly or stop entirely, all variations are normal.

Keeping track of your baby's kicks isn't necessary until week 28 (see page 315), so don't worry if you haven't felt your baby's movements for a day or two at this point in the pregnancy.

"Sometimes the baby kicks so hard, it hurts."

Posting Pregnancy

If sharing is caring, there's a whole lot of caring going on when it comes to baby bumps. Mommy social media is loaded with uploaded baby bump selfies, belly-baring pregnancy portraits, and ultrasound pics. And as your own bump grows, maybe you're wondering whether you, too, should hop (carefully) onto the pregnancy selfie bandwagon—and push "share."

Capturing your bump on camera as it grows, grows, grows is priceless—it'll ensure you'll have pregnancy images to reminisce about long after your baby has made the move from your belly to your arms. So as they say—take a picture, it'll last longer. But should you share those most-special of selfies with the world of social media—or even with family and friends on Facebook? Or post those first ultrasound glimpses of your baby (yes, including the money shot)?

Going public—or staying private—is a personal choice. If you do opt to showcase your baby bump and baby-to-be's first pictures online, remember that whatever you put online lives online forever—and in this case you've begun to build your little one's digital footprint before he or she is even born. Ask yourself if you're okay with that. While you're asking, make sure your spouse is happy with all the social media sharing, too. Pay attention to who can see the images that you've posted, and be sure both of you are on board with any images you post on an open network that anyone can access.

As babies mature in the uterus, they grow stronger and stronger, and those once butterfly-like fetal movements pack more and more punch. Which is why you shouldn't be surprised if you get kicked in the ribs or poked in the abdomen with such force that it hurts. When you seem to be under a particularly fierce attack, try changing your position. It may knock your little linebacker off balance and temporarily stem the assault.

Measuring Large or Small

"According to my pregnancy app and the due date my midwife gave me, I'm supposed to be 26 weeks. But at this appointment, she told me my uterus is measuring only 24 weeks. Does that mean there's something wrong with the baby?"

Your uterus (like your baby) is one-of-a-kind—and so is its growth. Some moms measure a little bigger, some a little smaller, just like the baby inside them—with an average uterine size for a certain date just that: an average. What's more, measuring your uterus (or your baby), especially from the outside, isn't a precise science—which means your practitioner's measurement won't always correlate with your dates. And that's perfectly okay.

At each prenatal visit, your practitioner checks your fundal height—the distance from your pubic bone to the top of your uterus—with a tape measure (see why the science isn't so precise?). That number in centimeters is approximately equal to the number of weeks of pregnancy you are—but 1 or 2 centimeters in either direction is no big deal. In fact, a discrepancy of a couple of weeks (again, in either direction) is

When Something Just Doesn't Feel Right

Maybe it's a twinge of abdominal pain that feels too much like a cramp to ignore, a sudden change in your vaginal discharge, an aching in your lower back or in your pelvic floor—or maybe it's something so vague, you can't even put your finger on it. Chances are, it's just par for the pregnancy course, but to play it safe, check page 140 to see if a call to your practitioner is in order. If you can't find your symptoms on the list, it's probably a good idea to call anyway. Remember, you know your body better than anyone. Listen up when it's trying to tell you something.

pretty typical because fundal height can be affected by many factors other than baby's size, including your body type, the baby's position, the volume of fluid on a particular day, and so on. High tech, this process isn't. (And the truth is, even far higher tech measurements, done via ultrasound, aren't super accurate after the first trimester.)

If your measurements show a discrepancy of 3 weeks or more at any point, your practitioner will do a little investigating to try to learn why. Most of the time, there's a harmless explanation—maybe your baby is genetically destined to be larger or smaller than average or your EDD is off by a week (due dates are also an estimate, remember?). Or perhaps there's something that requires more looking into, like a uterine fibroid, extra (or too little) amniotic fluid, or a baby that's not growing as expected (IUGR, see page

553) or is growing bigger than expected (sometimes due to gestational diabetes).

Itchy Belly

"My belly itches constantly. It's driving me crazy."

Join the club. Pregnant bellies are itchy bellies, and they can become progressively itchier as the months pass. That's because as your belly grows, the skin stretches rapidly, becoming increasingly moisture deprived—leaving it itchy and uncomfortable. Try not to scratch, which will only make you itchier and could cause irritation. Moisturizing can temporarily curb the itching, so massage that bump frequently and liberally with a pure cream, lotion, or oil (shea butter or cocoa butter are favorites, and ones made with aloe can also be soothing). An oatmeal bath can soothe itchiness, too, but before you reach for anti-itching lotions, check with your practitioner.

If you have an all-over itch that doesn't seem to be related to dry or sensitive skin or you develop a rash on your abdomen, check with your practitioner.

Clumsiness

"Lately I've been dropping everything I pick up. Why am I suddenly so clumsy?"

Like the extra inches on your belly, the extra thumbs on your hands are part of the pregnancy package. This real (and, unfortunately, plain for everyone to see) pregnancy-induced clumsiness is caused by the loosening of joints and ligaments and the retention of water, both of which can make your grasp on objects less firm and sure. A lack of concentration (as a result of pregnancy forgetfulness; see page 228) can contribute to clumsiness, too, as can brain circuits overloaded by baby prep and baby daydreams. So can a decline in dexterity caused by swollen fingers and carpal tunnel syndrome (see next question).

There's not much you can do to counter your expectant klutz factor— you can, in fact, expect to get only clumsier in the coming months (particularly at the end of each day, when your mind is least focused and your hands are most puffy). The best strategy: Avoid handling breakables (especially ones you don't own—like the precious porcelain frame for baby's room you were eyeing at the store). Keep your grandmother's crystal safely tucked into the cabinet for now, don't volunteer to clear the table at your pal's dinner party when she's using the good china, and have someone else load and unload the dishwasher.

Is pregnancy tripping you up, too? See page 318.

Numbness in the Hands

"I keep waking up in the middle of the night because some of the fingers on my right hand are numb. Does that have anything to do with being pregnant?"

Feeling all a-tingle these days? Chances are it isn't romance or even excitement about the baby—it's the normal numbness and tingling in the fingers and toes that many expectant moms experience, probably the result of swelling tissues pressing on nerves. If the numbness and pain are confined to your thumb, index finger, middle finger, and half of your ring finger, you probably have carpal tunnel syndrome (CTS). Though CTS is most common in people who regularly perform repetitive motions of the hand or wrist (like typing or piano playing), it's also extremely common in pregnant women—even in those who don't do a lot of repetitive hand motions. That's because the carpal

tunnel in the wrist, through which the nerve to the affected fingers runs, becomes swollen during pregnancy (as do so many other tissues in the body, you might have noticed), with the resultant pressure causing numbness, tingling, burning, and pain. The symptoms can also affect the hand and wrist, and they can radiate up the arm.

Though CTS symptoms can strike at any time of the day, you might feel yourself wrestling with wrist pain more at night. That's because fluids accumulated in your feet and legs during the day are redistributed to the rest of your body (including your hands) when you lie down at night. Sleeping on your hands can make the problem worse, so try elevating them on a separate pillow.

Typically, CTS symptoms resolve sometime after delivery, once all that pregnancy swelling goes down. In the meantime, acupuncture may bring relief, as can a wrist splint (though you may find wearing one more uncomfortable than the CTS itself). As for the nonsteroidal anti-inflammatory drugs and steroids usually prescribed for CTS, ask your practitioner—they may not be recommended during pregnancy. If you think the CTS is related to your work habits (or other keyboard use) as well as your pregnancy, see page 204.

Leg Cramps

"I have leg cramps at night that keep me awake."

Between your overloaded mind and your bulging belly, you probably have enough trouble catching those z's without leg cramps cramping your sleeping style. Unfortunately, these painful spasms that radiate up and down your calves and occur most often at night are very common among the

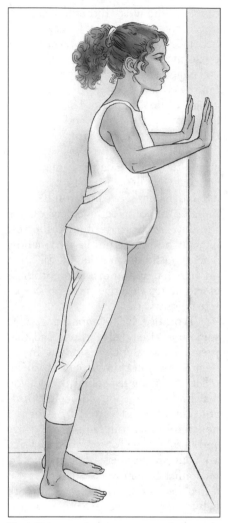

Stretching away leg cramps

expectant set in the second and third trimesters.

No one's quite sure what causes leg cramps. Various theories blame fatigue from carrying pregnancy weight, compression of the blood vessels in the legs, and possibly diet (an excess of phosphorus and a shortage of calcium or magnesium). You might as well blame hormones, too (what are the odds they're not to blame?). But whatever the cause of leg cramps in your case,

there are ways of both preventing and alleviating them:

- When a leg cramp strikes, straighten your leg right away and flex your ankle and toes slowly up toward your nose (don't point your toes). You can do this in bed, but you may find faster relief if you get up and do it on your feet. This should soon ease the pain. Doing this several times with each leg before turning in at night may even help ward off the cramps later.

- Stretching exercises can also help stop cramps before they strike. Before you head to bed, stand about 2 feet away from a wall and put your palms flat against it. Lean forward, keeping your heels on the floor. Hold the stretch for 10 seconds, then relax for 5. Repeat 3 times. (See the illustration.)

- To ease the daily load on your legs, put your feet up as often as you can, alternate periods of activity with periods of rest, and wear support hose during the day. Flex your feet periodically.

- Try standing on a cool surface, which can sometimes stop a spasm. An ice pack or a cool compress may also help.

- You can add massage or local heat for added relief if the pain has subsided (do not massage or add heat if pain persists).

- Make sure you're drinking enough fluids.

- Eat a well-balanced diet that includes plenty of calcium and magnesium, but also check with your practitioner to see if you should add a magnesium supplement before bed.

Really bad leg cramps can cause muscle soreness (like a charley horse) that lasts a few days. That's nothing to worry about. But if the pain is severe and persists, contact your practitioner,

---

Bleeding in Mid or Late Pregnancy

It's always unsettling to see pink or red on your underwear when you're expecting, but spotting in the second or third trimester is often not a cause for concern. Sometimes it's the result of bruising to the increasingly sensitive cervix during an internal exam or sex, or it could simply be triggered by causes unknown and innocuous.

Still, it's important to let your practitioner know about any spotting or bleeding because it could also be a sign of preterm delivery, placental abruption, or another serious condition. If you're bleeding heavily or if the spotting is accompanied by pain or discomfort, call your practitioner right away. Ultrasound, a physical exam, lab work, and/or fetal monitoring can often determine whether there's a problem and if so, how to treat or manage it.

---

because there's a slight possibility that a blood clot may have developed in a vein, making medical treatment necessary (see page 564).

Hemorrhoids

"I'm dreading getting hemorrhoids—I've heard they're common during pregnancy. Is there anything I can do to prevent them?"

It's a big pain in the butt, but more than half of all expectant moms develop hemorrhoids, which are just veins in the rectum that become swollen (like so many other things during pregnancy). Pressure from your enlarging uterus, plus increased blood flow to the pelvic area, not only causes those veins to swell, but to bulge and itch (how's that for a pleasant thought?). Because they can resemble a pile of grapes or marbles, hemorrhoids also go by the nickname "piles."

Thinking pile prevention? Your best strategy may be to avoid piling on extra pounds, since added weight means added pressure on your rectal veins. Constipation (and straining to poop when you're constipated) can contribute to hemorrhoids, too, so do your best to stay regular (see page 185). Doing your Kegels (see page 229) can also ward off hemorrhoids by improving circulation to the area, as can taking the pressure off by sleeping on your side (not your back) and avoiding standing or sitting for long periods of time or lingering on the toilet. Sitting with your feet on a low stool when you're on the toilet may make that other stool easier to pass, so pushing is less of a strain.

So, prevention didn't do the trick? To soothe the sting of hemorrhoids, try applying witch hazel pads, cool compresses, or ice packs. A warm bath (or a bottom-only sitz bath, which you can do with a basin that fits over the toilet seat) may ease discomfort, too, and wiping gently with damp toilet paper can reduce irritation. If sitting is a pain, use a donut-shaped pillow to ease pressure. Ask your practitioner before using any medication, topical or otherwise.

Hemorrhoids can sometimes bleed, especially when you're bearing down during a bowel movement, though anal fissures (painful cracks in the skin of the anus caused by straining from constipation) can also be the cause of rectal bleeding. (To rule out any less likely

Diagnosing Preeclampsia

Chances are you've heard of (or know) someone who developed preeclampsia during pregnancy. But the reality is, preeclampsia isn't that common, occurring in only about 3 to 8 percent of pregnancies, even in its mildest form. And luckily, in women who are receiving regular prenatal care, preeclampsia can be diagnosed and treated early, preventing needless complications. Though routine office visits sometime seem a waste of time in a healthy pregnancy ("I have to pee in a cup again?"), that's when the earliest signs of preeclampsia are usually picked up.

Early symptoms of preeclampsia include a rise in blood pressure, protein in the urine, severe swelling of the hands and face, persistent severe headaches, pain in the stomach or the esophagus, and/or vision disturbances. If you experience any of these, call your practitioner. Otherwise, assuming you are getting regular medical care, there's no reason to worry about preeclampsia. See pages 221 and 550 for more information on and tips for dealing with high blood pressure and preeclampsia.

cause, check in with your practitioner about any rectal bleeding.)

If there's good news about hemorrhoids, it's that they're not dangerous, just uncomfortable. They usually go away sometime after delivery—though they can occasionally be aggravated or even develop for the first time postpartum as a result of pushing during childbirth.

Breast Lump

"I'm worried about a small, tender lump on the side of my breast. What could it be?"

Though they're still months away from being able to feed your baby, it sounds like your breasts are already gearing up. The result: a clogged milk duct. These red, tender-to-the-touch, hard lumps in the breast are very common even this early in pregnancy, especially in second and subsequent pregnancies. Warm compresses (or letting warm water run on it in the shower) and gentle massage will probably clear up the duct in a few days, just as they will during lactation. Some experts suggest that avoiding underwire bras also helps, but make sure you get ample support from the bra you do wear.

Keep in mind that monthly self-exams of your breasts shouldn't stop when you're pregnant. Though checking for lumps is trickier when you're expecting because of the changes in your breasts (they're naturally lumpier, firmer, and heavier than before), it's still important to try. Show any lump to your practitioner at your next visit, or check in sooner if you're concerned.

Glucose Screening Test

"My practitioner says I need to take a glucose screening test. Why would I need it, and what does it involve?"

Don't feel too picked on. Almost all practitioners screen for gestational diabetes (GD) in almost all expectant moms at about 24 to 28 weeks. Moms who are at higher risk for GD (including older or obese mothers or those with a family history of diabetes) are screened even earlier in their pregnancies. So chances are, the test your practitioner ordered is just routine.

And it's simple, too, especially if you have a sweet tooth. You'll drink a very sweet glucose drink, which usually tastes like flat orange soda, an hour before having some blood drawn—happily, you don't have to be fasting when you do this. The drink is definitely not delicious but most women are able to chugalug the stuff with no problem and no side effects. A few, especially those who don't have a taste for sweet liquids, feel a little queasy afterward.

If the blood work comes back with elevated numbers, which suggests the possibility that you might not be producing enough insulin to process the extra glucose in your system, the next level of test—the glucose tolerance test—is ordered. This 3-hour test, which involves fasting and then drinking a higher-concentration glucose drink, is used to diagnose GD.

GD occurs in about 7 to 9 percent of expectant moms, which makes it one of the most common pregnancy complications. Fortunately, it's also one of the most easily managed. When blood sugar is closely controlled through diet, exercise, and, if necessary, medication, women with GD are likely to have perfectly normal pregnancies and healthy babies. See page 548 for more.

Cord Blood Banking

"I've seen a lot of ads about cord blood banking. Should I consider doing it?"

As if you don't have enough to think about before baby's born, here's something else to consider: Should you save your baby's umbilical cord blood—and if so, how?

Cord blood harvesting is a simple, painless procedure that takes less than 5 minutes and is performed after the cord has been clamped and cut. It's completely safe for both mom and baby (as long as the cord is not clamped and cut prematurely). Why collect and store cord blood, instead of tossing it as is usually done? Because a newborn's cord blood contains many types of stem cells (including cells with the incredible capacity to turn into any other kind of blood and immune system cells) that can, in some cases, be used to treat certain immune system disorders or blood diseases. The stem cells in cord blood are already considered a standard treatment for a variety of diseases, including leukemias (cancers of the blood immune system), bone marrow cancers, lymphomas, and neuroblastoma; inherited red-blood-cell abnormalities such as sickle cell disease and anemias; Gaucher disease and Hurler syndrome; and inherited immune system and immune-cell disorders. What's more, cord blood stem cells are also being investigated as possible treatments for other conditions and diseases, ranging from diabetes and cerebral palsy to autism and certain heart defects present at birth. You can also save placental tissue and blood from placental cells, which may contain even more stem cells.

There are two ways to store the blood: You can pay for private storage or you can donate the blood to a public storage bank. Private storage can be expensive—costing a couple of thousand dollars or more for the collection of the blood, plus yearly maintenance fees (plus the fee for the doctor and hospital if they offer cord blood collection). Some private banks offer free or discounted banking if there is a family medical need (such as a family member who's in need of a transplant) or a family history of a condition that qualifies them to participate in a trial (autism, for instance). Discounts are also often given for military families and those of first responders. And you can check whether your health insurance company offers

Home Birth and Cord Blood Banking

If you've decided to bank your baby's cord blood (privately or publicly) but are delivering at home, you'll have to think through the logistics well ahead of time. First ask your home-birth midwife if he or she is on board with banking. Next, arrange to have the kit on hand and ready to go before those contractions strike. Finally, be sure you understand how cord blood collecting may impact your birth. For instance, if you're planning a water birth you'll need to leave the water when birthing the placenta to minimize the unnecessary loss of cord blood.

Be sure, too, to notify the company you're storing the cord blood with that you're having a home birth in case there are any special storage and shipping instructions you'll need to know about.

discounts or partial reimbursement for private banking.

The benefits of private cord blood banking, if your family has no history of immune disorders currently being treated with cord blood stem cells, isn't completely clear. Also not clear is how many years the frozen units will remain viable (different companies make different claims about their storage equipment). If you can afford the price of private banking, there's no downside—though realistically, it's very unlikely that your baby or another family member will ever end up with a condition that can be treated with the stored cells.

What are the official recommendations? ACOG doesn't take a stand, but recommends that doctors present parents with the pros and cons of both private and public banking. The American Academy of Pediatrics (AAP) doesn't recommend private cord blood storage unless a family member has a medical condition that might be helped by a stem cell transplant now or in the near future. The AAP does, however, support parents donating the cord blood to a bank for general use by the public.

As of now, studies show that the likelihood that a child will ever tap into his or her own saved cord blood later is very low (1 in 2,700 to 1 in 20,000 by some estimates). In fact, experts point out that a baby's own cord blood cells are often unsuitable for treating a condition that shows up later in the child's life (like leukemia), because the mutations ultimately responsible for the condition are present at birth, and can be found in those cells. What about treating an adult family member with the stored cells later on? The likelihood of that is also low, since most stored units of cord blood don't contain enough stem cells to treat anyone weighing more than 90 pounds. The chances are somewhat higher that you'd be able to use the stored cord blood to help treat a young sibling who has or develops a certain disease.

Public banking is open to any family (as long as the hospital where you're delivering offers it). The upside is that it's free and could ultimately save a life (including your own child's, since the more cord blood donations there are, the higher the chances that you'll be able to find a suitable match if your child should need one). In fact, the odds of finding a suitably matched, publicly donated, unrelated cord blood unit are already quite high and continue to improve as inventories of public cord blood banks grow (a good reason to think about donating your baby's).

The downside is that you can't access your own child's cord blood cells once they're donated.

One thing is for sure: There's no benefit to letting your baby's cord blood get tossed. To make sure that those precious blood cells don't go to waste (or into the medical waste bin), talk about the options available to you with your practitioner. Maybe you'll decide that private banking makes sense for your family, either because of a family history or because you can easily afford the extra price. Maybe you'll decide that public banking is the way to go. Either way, just remember that you'll need to make this decision well before those first contractions strike, and to make sure everyone on your birth team is in on your plan and ready to implement it.

"I'm considering storing my baby's umbilical cord blood in a private bank—but I'm not sure how to go about doing it."

The first step is to partner up with your practitioner on your plan. Not only so you can get your practitioner's take on cord blood banking, but also so you can make sure he or she is willing and able to collect the cord blood. It's rare that a doctor or midwife couldn't (or wouldn't) perform this simple and quick procedure, but a fee may be involved.

Then it's time to hit the books— or at least the internet—to do your research, so you can find the right cord blood bank for you. Any bank you're considering should be accredited with the American Association of Blood Banks (AABB). Once you've narrowed your choices, it's worth calling each one to find out more about their services. You'll want the bank's representative to explain key things: how the bank collects and stores the blood (there are different collection and storage methods,

and you'll want to make sure the bank complies with federal standards), how viable the bank's cord blood samples are compared with other banks (you'll want to choose a bank that has demonstrated good odds of getting a usable blood sample), how stable the company is (you don't want the bank to go out of business, so explore the pros and cons of choosing a lesser-known, smaller bank versus a larger, well-known bank that has been operating for longer), and what they actually store (some banks store only cord blood, while others store the blood and cord tissue from around the blood vessels in the cord that contain different types of stem cells).

Once you've made your pick, it's time to enroll with your bank of choice. Aim to sign up by the end of your second trimester—or at least before week 34. Once you sign up, the cord blood bank will mail you a collection kit so that you'll have it on hand for the big day. The kit will probably have a medical form for you to fill out, plus sealed medical supplies your practitioner will use to collect the cord blood. Fill out the form, sign it, and put it back in the kit (but leave the kit's medical supplies sealed). Pack the kit away in your hospital bag so you won't have to scramble to find it when those contractions hit.

Once you're in labor, it's time to give the cord blood kit to your practitioner (or the staff). This will remind him or her about your cord blood banking decision, and it will alert the medical staff that they'll need to collect a blood sample from you before delivery (the kit comes with the materials your practitioner will need to collect and send in your blood). Right after you deliver (whether it's a vaginal or cesarean delivery), your practitioner will clamp the umbilical cord (he or she can and should wait until the cord stops pulsating to allow for delayed cord clamping) and collect the cord blood with the supplies provided in your kit. Your partner can still cut the cord, because that doesn't affect the collection process. When the collection is complete, it's time for you (or more likely your partner, since you'll be a bit distracted) or your practitioner (or staff) to call the bank. Once the call is made, the bank will arrange for a courier to pick up the cord blood kit and send it off to the laboratory for storage. The kit will arrive at the lab no later than 36 hours after you deliver your precious bundle. The bank will contact you to let you know that your cord blood arrived safely and to tell you how much they were able to collect and process. They will also, of course, send you a yearly bill for storage fees.

Keep in mind that you may not be able to collect and store enough of your baby's cord blood if he or she is born preterm (even if you've planned for it) or if your twins share a placenta (though check with your chosen bank for guidelines to be certain). You may also find cord blood banking a struggle to arrange if you are based overseas but would like to bank or donate your baby's blood in the U.S.

"I'd like to donate my baby's cord blood to a public bank. What's the best way to do that?"

First, know that the decision you've made might save a life someday. Cord blood contains stem cells that can treat a host of diseases, and most major medical organizations (including the AAP) encourage public donation of umbilical-cord blood cells so they can be used for actual transplants or for valuable medical research—a far better option than letting that precious cord blood be thrown away.

Then, it's time to share your decision with your practitioner. Together,

you can determine if you qualify for public donation (which you most likely will unless you are HIV-positive or have an STD, hepatitis, or cancer) and start making the arrangements necessary to bank publicly. You may also want to find out whether your practitioner charges a fee for collecting the cord blood, even if it's being donated to a public bank that accepts all donations free of charge. Donating your baby's cord blood will be easiest if you'll be delivering at a hospital that participates in the national cord blood donation program run through the National Marrow Donor Program (to check if your hospital does, go to marrow.org/cord). If your hospital doesn't participate, find out if there's a public bank nearby that will accept your donation, or one that will allow mail-in donations, by visiting parentsguidecordblood.org. Be sure to register with your bank of choice before week 34, since you won't be able to arrange this at the last minute (say, when you're about to start pushing).

Remember to keep your practitioner in the loop about the plans you make for your baby's cord blood. The cord blood bank will ask for your medical history, a blood sample (which will be taken right before you deliver), and a signed consent form. The bank may send you a collection kit to bring to the hospital, or may work directly with your practitioner or the hospital for the collection. (Just double-check to see if this is the case if you don't receive a kit.)

If you're working with a public cord blood bank that's not affiliated with your hospital or birthing center, your partner may have to call the bank once you're in labor to arrange for a courier to pick up the cord blood. Depending on the public bank you use, you may be able to keep track of your donation and find out if it was accepted and stored.

Childbirth Pain

"I'm eager to become a mother, but not so eager to experience childbirth. Mostly, I worry about the pain."

Almost every expectant mom eagerly awaits the birth of her child, but few look forward to labor and delivery—and far fewer still to the pain of labor and delivery. And many, like you, spend a fair amount of time in the months leading up to this momentous event worrying about the pain. That's not surprising. The fear of labor pain—which is, after all, an unknown quantity of pain—is very real and very understandable.

But it's important to keep in mind the following: Childbirth is a normal life process, which women have been experiencing as long as there have been women. Sure, it comes with pain, but it's a pain with a positive purpose (though it won't necessarily feel positive when you're in it): to thin and open your cervix, and bring your baby into your arms. And it's also a pain with a built-in time limit. You might not believe it (especially somewhere around the 5-cm mark), but labor won't last forever. Not only that, but the pain of childbirth is optional (no pain, no gain doesn't apply to labor and delivery). An epidural or another form of pain relief is always just a request away, should you end up wanting it or needing it—or both. And if you're sure you'll want and need it, you can even sign up for that epidural ahead of time and get it as early in labor as you like—at least, once you arrive at the hospital.

So there's no point in dreading the pain, but there's a lot to be said for being prepared for it. Preparing now (both your body and mind—since both are involved in how you experience pain) should help reduce the anxiety you're feeling now and the amount of discomfort (okay, pain) you'll feel once those contractions kick in.

Get educated. A good childbirth education class can ease your anxiety (and ultimately pain) by increasing knowledge, preparing you and your coach, stage by stage and phase by phase, for labor and delivery. If you can't take a class or if you just don't want to, read up on childbirth as much as you can. What you don't know can worry you more than it has to. Taking classes makes sense, by the way, even if you're planning to have an epidural—or even if you have a cesarean delivery scheduled. Just make sure that the curriculum in the class you choose covers all the birthing bases.

Get moving. You wouldn't consider running a marathon without the proper physical training—and you shouldn't consider heading into labor untrained, either. Work out with all the breathing, stretching, and toning-up exercises your practitioner and/or childbirth educator recommends, plus plenty of Kegels.

Team up. Whether you have your partner there to comfort you and feed you ice chips, a doula (see page 328) to massage your back, or a friend to wipe your brow—or if you really like company, all three—a little support can go a long way in easing your fears. Even if you don't end up feeling very chatty during labor, it will be comforting to know that you're not going it alone. And make sure your coach is trained, too—not only by taking classes with you, but by reading the section on labor and delivery beginning on page 418.

Have a pain plan—and a backup plan. Maybe you've already decided that an epidural has your name on it. Maybe you're hoping to breathe your way through those contractions—or use

Labor and Delivery Worries

Excited about witnessing your baby's birth but worried you won't be able to keep it together? Few fathers enter the birthing room without a little trepidation—or a lot. Even obs, nurses, and other medical professionals who've assisted at the births of thousands of other people's babies can experience a sudden loss of self-confidence when confronted with the delivery of their own.

Yet very few of those dad-to-be fears—of freezing, falling apart, fainting, getting sick, and otherwise humiliating themselves or their spouses or falling short of their expectations—are ever realized. In fact, most dads handle childbirth with surprising ease, keeping their composure, their cool, and their lunch (if they managed to grab some). But like anything new and unknown, childbirth becomes less scary and intimidating if you know what to expect. So become an expert on the subject. Read the section on labor and delivery, beginning on page 418. Read up online, too. Attend childbirth education classes, watching the labor and delivery videos with your eyes wide open. Visit the hospital or birthing center ahead of time so it'll be familiar ground on labor day. Talk to friends (or online buddies) who've attended the births of their children—you'll probably find that they were stressed out about the birth beforehand, too, but that they came through it like pros.

Though it's important to get an education, remember that childbirth isn't pregnancy's final exam. Don't feel you're under any pressure to perform. The doctor or midwife and the nurses won't be evaluating your every move or comparing you with the coach next door. More important, neither will your spouse. She won't care if you forget every coaching technique you learned in class. Your being beside her, holding her hand, urging her on, and providing the comfort of a familiar face and touch is what she'll need—and appreciate—most of all. (Though she may also push you away at certain painful or frustrating points, so be prepared for that, too.) Still having performance anxiety? Some couples find that having a doula present during birth helps them both to get through labor and delivery with less stress and more comfort (see page 328).

hypnobirthing for pain management. Maybe you're waiting to make that decision until you see how much pain you're facing. Either way, think ahead, and then keep your mind open (because labor has a way of not always following plans). See page 330 for more on pain relief.

Labor Inhibitions

"I'm afraid I'll do something embarrassing during labor."

That's because you're not in labor yet. Sure, the idea of screaming, cursing, or involuntarily peeing or pooping on the birthing bed (which you will, because everybody does) might seem embarrassing now. But during labor, embarrassment (or appearances) will be the last thing on your mind. Besides, nothing you can do or say during labor will shock your birth attendants, who've seen and heard it all before—and then some. So check your inhibitions when you check into the hospital or birthing center, and feel free to do what comes naturally, as well as what makes you most comfortable. If you're ordinarily a person who tells (or yells) it like it is, don't try to hold in your moans or hold back your grunts and groans—and, yes, screams and howls. But if you're normally soft-spoken or stoic and would prefer to whimper quietly into your pillow, don't feel obligated to out-yell the mom next door.

Hospital Tours

"I've always associated hospitals with sick people. How can I get more comfortable with the idea of giving birth in one?"

The labor and delivery floor is by far the happiest in the hospital. Still, if you don't know what to expect, you can arrive with not only contractions, but apprehension. That's why the vast majority of hospitals and birthing centers encourage expectant couples to take advance tours of maternity facilities. Ask about such tours when you preregister, and look online, too. Some hospitals and birthing centers have websites that offer virtual tours.

Chances are, you'll be happily surprised by what you see during your visit, and that it will make you more comfortable about the surroundings you'll be giving birth in. Facilities vary, but the range of amenities and services offered in many hospitals and birthing centers has become more and more impressive—and family-friendly.

ALL ABOUT:
Childbirth Education

The countdown to cuddles is on—all that stands between you and the bundle of baby joy you can't wait to welcome is a single trimester. That, of course, and labor and delivery.

So, you're not quite as excited about labor and delivery as you are about your baby's arrival? Maybe you have a healthy dose of apprehension about childbirth? Maybe even a whole lot of nerves?

Relax. It's normal to be nervous about childbirth—especially if you're a first-timer, but even if you're a second- or third-timer (every labor and delivery is different, after all). But fortunately, there's a great way to ease jitters, to calm worries, and to feel less anxious and more confident when that first contraction strikes: by getting educated.

A little knowledge and a lot of preparation can go a long way in helping you feel more comfortable when you enter the birthing room. Reading all about childbirth can definitely give you an idea of what to expect (see page 418), but a good childbirth education class can fill in even more blanks. So it's back to school time.

Benefits of Taking a Childbirth Class

What's in a childbirth education class for you and your coach? That depends, on the course you take, the instructor who teaches it, as well as you and your coach (the more you put in, the more you tend to get out of a childbirth education class). No matter what, there's something in it for every soon-to-be-laboring team. Some potential benefits include:

Another Class to Take

B esides studying up on childbirth techniques, there's another class you should consider signing up for now: infant CPR and first aid. Even though you don't actually have the baby yet, there's no better time to learn how to keep that little bundle you're about to deliver safe and sound. First, because you won't have to line up a babysitter to attend class now. And second—and more important—because you'll be able to bring baby home secure in the knowledge that you have all the necessary know-how at your fingertips in case of an emergency. You can find a course by contacting the American Red Cross (redcross.org) or the American Heart Association (americanheart .org/cpr), or check with your local hospital. Private classes can also be arranged—a great option if you can afford the higher price, and especially if there are grandparents or other relatives, a babysitter, or others you'd like to see certified before they care for your little one.

- A chance to spend time with other expectant couples who are at the same stage of pregnancy—to share experiences and tips, compare progress, and symptoms, and swap notes on baby gear, nursery gear, pediatricians, and childcare. In other words, a chance to cash in on lots of expectant camaraderie and empathy. It's also a chance to make friends with other couples who, like you, will soon be parents (a definite plus if your current crowd of friends hasn't taken the baby plunge yet). Keep in touch with these classmates after delivery and you've got yourself a ready-to-go parents'

group—and a playgroup for the little ones. Many classes hold "reunions" once everyone has delivered.

- A chance for your partner to join in. Much of pregnancy revolves around mom, which can sometimes leave an expectant father feeling like he's on the outside looking in. Childbirth education classes are aimed at both parents and help to get dad feeling like the valued member of the baby team he is—particularly important if he hasn't been able to attend all the prenatal visits. Classes will also get dad up to speed on labor and delivery so that he can be a more effective coach when those contractions start coming. Best of all, perhaps, he'll be able to hang out with other guys who can relate to—among other things—those maternal mood swings he's been on the receiving end of and those normal nagging feelings of daddy self-doubt. Some courses include a special session for fathers only, which gives them the chance to open up about concerns they might otherwise not feel comfortable expressing.

- A chance to ask questions that come up between prenatal visits or that you don't feel comfortable asking your practitioner (or that you never seem to have the time to during those quickie checkups).

- A chance to learn all about it—labor and delivery, that is. Through lessons, discussion, models, and video, you'll get an inside peek at what childbirth's all about—from prelabor to crowning to cutting the cord. The more you know, the more comfortable you'll feel when it's actually happening to you.

- A chance to learn all about your pain relief options, from an epidural to hypnosis.

- A chance to get hands-on instruction in breathing, relaxation, and other alternative approaches to pain relief and to get feedback from an expert as you learn. Mastering these coping strategies—and coaching techniques—may help you be more relaxed during labor and delivery, while somewhat decreasing your perception of pain. They'll also come in handy if you're planning to sign up for an epidural.

- A chance to become familiar with the interventions sometimes used during labor and delivery, including fetal monitoring, IVs, vacuum extraction and forceps delivery, and c-sections. You may not end up encountering any of these interventions, but knowing about them all ahead of time will boost your confidence quotient.

- A chance to have a relatively more enjoyable labor—and a relatively less stressful one—thanks to all of the above. Couples who've had childbirth preparation generally rate their childbirth experiences as more satisfying overall than those who haven't.

Choosing a Childbirth Class

So you've decided to take a childbirth class. But where do you begin looking for one? And how do you choose?

In some communities, where childbirth class options are limited, the choice of which class to take is a relatively simple one. In others, the variety of offerings can be overwhelming and confusing. Courses are run by hospitals, by private instructors, by practitioners through their offices. There are "early bird" prenatal classes, taken in the first or second trimester, which cover all things pregnancy: nutrition, exercise,

fetal development, and sex. And there are down-to-the-wire 6- to 10-week childbirth preparation classes, usually beginning in the 7th or 8th month, which concentrate on labor, delivery, and postpartum mother and baby care. There are even weekend getaway classes. No time for an in-person course? Check out the offerings on DVD or online.

If the pickings are slim, any childbirth class is probably better than none at all. If there is a selection of courses where you live, it may help to consider the following when making your decision:

Who sponsors the class? A class that is run by or recommended by your practitioner often works out best. Also useful could be a class provided by the hospital or birthing center where you'll be delivering. If the laboring and delivering philosophy of your childbirth education teacher varies a lot from that of your birth attendants, you're bound to run into contradictions and conflicts. If differences of opinion do come up, make sure you address them with your practitioner well before your delivery date.

What's the size of the class? Small is best. Five or six moms-to-be and their coaches per class is ideal—more than 10 or 12 may be too large. Not only can a teacher provide extra time and individual attention in an intimate group—particularly important during the breathing and relaxation technique practice sessions—but the camaraderie in a small group tends to be stronger.

What's the curriculum like? Whichever type of class you choose, you can expect to learn about the stages of a normal labor and delivery as well as possible complications and how they might be handled. A comprehensive class should also cover postpartum care, basic newborn care, and breastfeeding. Most

304   THE SIXTH MONTH

For Information on Pregnancy/ Childbirth Classes

Ask your practitioner about classes in your area, or call the hospital where you plan to deliver. The following organizations can also give you referrals to local classes:

Lamaze International: lamaze.org

The Bradley Method: bradleybirth.com

International Childbirth Education Association: icea.org

Hypnobirthing International (the Mongan Method): hypnobirthing.com

Alexander Technique: alexandertechnique.com

Birthing from Within: birthingfromwithin.com

Birthworks: birthworks.org

---

classes will enlighten you about birth plans, doulas, hospital births versus delivering in a birthing center or at home, and medical interventions (such as a c-section or induction) that could (but probably won't) be necessary. Be sure to find out, too, if the course covers natural ways to reduce or cope with pain (such as massage, acupressure, aromatherapy, or using a birthing ball) as well as provides an overview of pain-relief options.

How is the class taught? Is it hands-on, interactive instruction? Are videos of actual childbirths shown? Will you hear from moms and dads who've recently delivered? Will there be ample opportunity for parents-to-be to ask questions?

Childbirth Education Options

Childbirth education classes in your area may be taught by certified teachers, doulas, nurses, or midwives. Approaches may vary from class to class, even among those trained in the same programs. The most common classes include:

Lamaze. The Lamaze approach to childbirth education is probably the most widely used in the U.S. Though it's known best for the breathing and relaxation techniques it teaches expectant couples, the philosophy has grown to encompass more than that. Now at the core of Lamaze childbirth education are the Lamaze 6 Healthy Birth Practices: letting labor begin on its own, moving and changing positions throughout labor, avoiding interventions that are not medically necessary, avoiding giving birth on your back, following your body's urges to push, and keeping you and your baby together after birth. While advocating for the healthiest, safest, and most natural birth possible, Lamaze teachers also cover birth options, including pain relief, as well as commonly used interventions—and a good class won't judge those options or interventions, or your choices. In a Lamaze class, you and your coach will learn to use relaxation and rhythmic breathing techniques that (along with continuous support from your coach) will help you achieve a state of "active concentration." You'll also practice directing your attention to a focal point to increase your concentration. A traditional Lamaze course consists of six 2- to 2½-hour sessions, and may be taught as a group class or one-on-one.

Bradley. The Bradley method teaches deep abdominal breathing and other relaxation techniques that focus the laboring mom's attention inward, to her body, rather than at a "focal point" outside the body, as in Lamaze. The course is also designed to help mom accept pain as a natural part of the birthing process—as a result, most Bradley graduates don't use pain medication during a vaginal delivery. In a Bradley class, you'll learn to mimic your nighttime sleeping positions and breathing (deep and slow) and use relaxation techniques to make labor more comfortable. The typical Bradley course runs 12 weeks, beginning in the 5th month, and most are taught by married couples. "Early bird" Bradley classes, which focus on a variety of pregnancy topics, are also available.

International Childbirth Education Association (ICEA) classes. These classes tend to be broader in scope, covering more of the many options available today to expectant parents in maternity and newborn care. They also recognize the importance of freedom of choice, and so classes focus on a wide range of possibilities rather than on a single approach to childbirth. Teachers are certified through ICEA.

Hypnobirthing. No zombie-like trances here. Hypnobirthing (also known as the Mongan Method) provides techniques that help laboring women achieve a highly relaxed state. The goal: to reduce discomfort, pain, and anxiety during childbirth (and during other stressful situations). And for some moms, the results are pretty amazing. For more on hypnobirthing, see page 335.

Alexander Technique. It's often used by actors to get the body and mind working in sync, but when it comes to labor and delivery, the Alexander Technique focuses on countering your body's natural tendency to tense up during pain.

Classes for Second-Timers

Been there, done that? Pregnant with your second (or third or more) baby? Even seasoned pros stand to benefit from taking a childbirth education class. First of all, every labor and delivery is different, so what you experienced last time may not be what you can expect this time. Second, you may want to do things differently this time around—perhaps you delivered with an ob in the hospital last time and this time you'd like to try a birthing center with a midwife (or vice versa). Or you want to try out Lamaze breathing for this baby because hypnobirthing didn't quite turn out the way you had hoped last time—or the other way around. Finally, things change quickly in the delivery business, and they may have changed quite a bit, even if it's been only a couple of years since you were last on a birthing bed. There may be different childbirth options available than there were last time—say, water birth. Certain procedures that were routine on your last visit to the birthing room may now be uncommon, while certain procedures that were uncommon then may now be routine. Chances are, however, that you won't have to sit in with the rookies. "Refresher" courses are available in most areas.

The instructor will emphasize coping with pain by exerting conscious control over posture and movement. Students learn how to sit and squat comfortably to release the pelvic floor and work with gravity as the baby descends through the birth canal.

Birthing from Within. In this holistic and spiritual approach to childbirth preparation, parents-to-be learn to cope with the intensity of birth while also focusing on how their journey through childbirth will be unique. Sessions focus on normal labor and what to expect during the natural birth process, but expectant couples also learn ways to deal with the unexpected and to navigate modern medicine without being traumatized by it. Couples spend 2½ hours every week concentrating on their transition into parenthood with a self-discovery multisensory approach that engages mind and body.

BirthWorks. This holistic method promotes birth as an instinctive process that doesn't need to be learned. The techniques aim to help a mom-to-be feel empowered by developing her self-confidence and helping her trust in her ability to give birth.

Other childbirth classes. There are also classes designed to prepare parents to deliver in a particular hospital, and classes sponsored by medical groups, HMOs, or other health care provider groups.

Home study. If you can't or don't want to attend a group class, you can look into the online Lamaze program. There are also other online courses and childbirth education classes that you can tap into, just a search away.

Private classes. Not interested in being part of a crowd, or your work schedule is too unpredictable to stick to a certain class time? You can look into private childbirth education classes that can be tailored to fit your schedule and your specific preferences—while letting you ask all the questions you'd like. With more flexibility and individualization, of course, comes a higher price.

Weekend classes at resorts. These offer the same curriculum as typical classes, packed into a single weekend. In addition to promoting extra camaraderie among expectant parents, these weekends can promote romance, too—a nice plus for twosomes who are about to become threesomes. Plus, they're a great opportunity for some pre-baby pampering if they're held at a hotel that offers prenatal spa options.

CHAPTER 11

The Seventh Month

Approximately 28 to 31 Weeks

Welcome to your third—and final!—trimester. Believe it or not, you're just 3 months away from holding (and kissing, and cuddling) your precious prize. With eyes on that prize in this last stretch of pregnancy (definitely the biggest stretch, at least as far as your belly is concerned), you'll probably find the excitement and anticipation mounting—along with your pregnancy aches and pains, which tend to multiply as the load you're lugging gets heavier and heavier. Drawing near to the end of pregnancy also means you're closing in on labor and delivery, an event you've been preparing for, thinking about, and maybe stressing out a little bit about. Now's a great time to sign up for those classes, if you haven't already.

Your Baby This Month

Week 28 This week, your amazing baby has reached 2¼ pounds and may be almost 15 inches long. Baby's skill of the week: blinking. Yes, along with the other tricks in a growing repertoire that already includes coughing, sucking, hiccupping, and taking practice breaths, your baby can now blink those sweet little eyes. Dreaming about your baby? Baby may be dreaming, too, courtesy of the REM (rapid eye movement) sleep he or she has started getting. But this little dreamer isn't ready for birth day just yet. Though those lungs are nearly fully mature by now (making it easier for your baby—and you—to breathe a little easier if he or she were born now), your little bundle still has a lot of growing to do.

Week 29 Your baby may be as tall as 15½ to 16 inches now and may weigh 2½ to 3 pounds—almost as much as that extra large bottle of water you're sipping on. But baby still has lots to gain. In fact, over the next 11 weeks, your baby will more than double—and may even come close to tripling—in weight. Much of that weight will come from the fat accumulating under his or her skin right now. And as your baby plumps up, the room in your womb will start to feel a little cramped, making it less likely that you'll feel hard kicks from your little one, and more likely that you'll be feeling jabs and pokes from elbows and knees.

Week 30 What's about 16 inches long, 3 pounds in weight, and cute all over? It's your baby—who's getting bigger by the day (in case you couldn't tell from the size of your belly). Also getting bigger daily is baby's brain, which is preparing for life outside the womb—and for a lifetime of learning. Starting this week, your baby's brain is starting to look like one, taking on those characteristic grooves and indentations. These wrinkles allow for future expansion of brain tissue that is crucial as

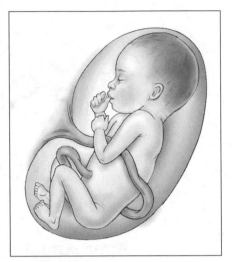

Your Baby, Month 7

your baby goes from helpless newborn to responsive infant to verbal toddler to curious preschooler and beyond. Your baby's bigger and better brain is also starting to take on tasks previously delegated to other parts of the body, like temperature regulation. Now that the brain is capable of turning up the heat (with the help of that growing supply of baby fat), your little one will start shedding lanugo, the downy, soft body hair that has been keeping him or her warm up to this point. Which means that by the time your baby is born, he or she probably won't be fuzzy anymore.

Week 31 Though your baby still has 3 to 5 pounds more to gain before delivery, he or she is weighing in at an impressive 3-plus pounds this week. And at 16 inches long (give or take a couple, because fetuses this age come in all sizes), your baby is quickly approaching birth length. Also developing at an impressive clip these days: your baby's brain connections (trillions of them must be made). He or she is able to put that complex web of brain

Baby Brain Food

Have you been feeding your baby's brain? Getting enough of those fabulous fats, the omega-3s, is more important than ever in the third trimester, when your baby's brain development is being fast-tracked. See page 98 for all the good-fat facts.

connections to good use, too—already processing information, tracking light, and perceiving signals from all 5 senses. Your brainy baby is also a sleepy one, putting in longer stretches of snooze time, specifically in REM sleep—which is why you're probably noticing more defined patterns of awake (and kicking) and sleeping (quiet) times from your little one.

Your Body This Month

Here are some symptoms you may experience this month (or may not experience, since every pregnancy is different). Some of these symptoms may be continuing from last month, while others may be brand new. With the start of the last trimester, symptoms that may have just been pesky to this point may be becoming more and more uncomfortable:

Physically

- Stronger and more regular fetal activity
- Increasing vaginal discharge

- Achiness in the lower abdomen or along the sides
- Constipation
- Heartburn, indigestion, flatulence, bloating
- Occasional headaches
- Occasional lightheadedness or dizziness, especially when getting up quickly or when your blood sugar dips
- Nasal congestion and occasional nosebleeds; ear stuffiness
- Sensitive gums that may bleed when you brush

Your Body This Month

At the beginning of this month, the top of your uterus is approximately 11 inches from the top of your pubic bone. By the end of the month, your baby's home has grown another inch in height and can be felt around 4½ inches above your belly button. You may think that there's no more room for your womb to grow (it seems to have already filled up your abdomen), but you still have 8 to 10 more weeks of expansion ahead of you!

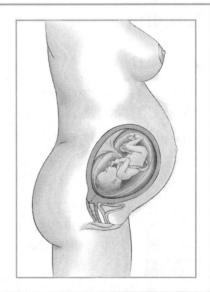

- Leg cramps

- Backache

- Mild swelling of ankles and feet, and occasionally of hands and face

- Hemorrhoids

- Varicose veins in the legs and/or vulva

- Itchy belly

- Protruding navel (a popped-out belly button)

- Stretch marks

- Shortness of breath

- Difficulty sleeping

- Scattered Braxton-Hicks contractions

- Occasional, sudden sharp or shocklike sensations in the pelvic area (aka "lightning crotch")

- Clumsiness

- Enlarged breasts

- Colostrum, leaking from nipples (though this premilk substance may not appear until after delivery)

Emotionally

- Increasing excitement (the baby's coming soon!)

- Increasing apprehension (the baby's coming soon!)

- Forgetfulness, absentmindedness (aka "placenta brain")

- Strange and vivid dreams

- Pregnancy fatigue (as in, you're tired of being pregnant) or a sense of contentment

What You Can Expect at This Month's Checkup

As you enter your last trimester, a couple of new items are added to the agenda you've come to expect:

- Weight and blood pressure

- Urine, for protein

- Fetal heartbeat

- Height of fundus (top of uterus)

- Size and position of fetus, by palpating (feeling from the outside)

- Feet and hands for swelling, and legs for varicose veins

- Glucose screening test, if you haven't had one yet (see page 294)

- Blood test for anemia

- Tdap vaccine (see page 328)

- Symptoms you have been experiencing, especially unusual ones

- Questions and problems you want to discuss—have a list ready

What You May Be Wondering About

Fatigue Revisited

"I was feeling really energetic for the last few months, and now I'm starting to drag again. Is this what I have to look forward to in the third trimester?"

Pregnancy is full of ups and downs—not only when it comes to moods (and libidos) but when it comes to energy levels. That trademark first-trimester fatigue is often followed by a second-trimester energy high, making those typically comfortable middle months the ideal time to pursue just about any activity. (Exercise! Sex! Travel! All of them in one weekend!). But by the third trimester, many moms-to-be find themselves once again dragging—and eyeing the sofa longingly.

And that's not surprising. Though some women continue to sprint as they close in on the pregnancy finish line (remember, every pregnancy is different, even when it comes to energy levels), there are lots more good reasons why you might be lagging behind. The best reason can be found around your midsection. After all, you're carrying much more weight there (and other places) than you were earlier on—and carting those extra pounds can be exhausting. Another reason: These days, that extra bulk may be lying (literally) between you and a good night's sleep, leaving you less rested each morning. Your baby-overloaded mind (jam-packed with shopping lists, to-do lists, baby-name lists, questions-to-ask-the-doctor lists, decisions to be made) may also be costing you z's—and energy. Add other, unrelated life responsibilities to the mix—a job, the care and feeding of other children, and so on—and the fatigue factors multiply exponentially.

As always, fatigue is a signal from your body, so pay attention. If you've been living life in the maternity fast lane (too much baby prep, not enough rest), slow down the pace a bit. Cut back on nonessential essentials in your day (no fair calling them all essentials). Get your exercise high but take the intensity down a notch, and time it so it's not too close to bedtime (when it can mess with sleep). And since running on empty can bench you in a hurry, fuel your energy levels with frequent healthy snacks. Most of all, remember that

Picking Up the Slack(s)

If you think you're tired at the end of the day, think about this: Your baby mama expends more energy lying on the sofa building a baby than you do bodybuilding at the gym. Which makes her a lot more tired than you've ever known her to be—and a lot more tired than you can even imagine. So pick up the slack. And your slacks. And the trail of socks and sneakers in the hallway. Beat her to the vacuuming and the laundry and the toilet cleaning—the fumes from the cleaning products will make her feel sicker anyway. Encourage her to watch your cleanup routine from a fully reclining position on the sofa—even if that's always been your favorite position.

third-trimester fatigue is nature's way of telling mamas-to-be to conserve energy. You'll need every bit of strength you can save up now for labor, delivery, and (of course) what follows. For more energy-saving tips, revisit the ones on page 130.

If you do get the extra rest your body is calling for but still feel consistently run-down, talk to your practitioner. Sometimes, extreme fatigue that doesn't ease up is triggered by third-trimester anemia (see page 251), which is why most practitioners repeat a routine blood test to check iron stores in the 7th month.

Swelling

"My ankles and feet are puffy, especially at the end of the day. Is that supposed to happen?"

Your belly's not the only thing that's swelling these days. That puff mama look often extends to the extremities, too. And although all that swelling's not so swell—especially as your shoes

---

Take Them Off, While You Can

Have your rings been getting snugger and snugger? Before they get too tight for comfort (and much too tight to remove), you might want to consider taking them off and putting them away for safe-keeping until your fingers depuff postpartum. Having trouble prying them off already? Try taking them off in the morning and after cooling down your hands in icy cold water. Some liquid soap can make the rings slippery and easier to slide off, too (just be sure to keep the drain covered if you'll be yanking your rings off over the sink).

---

and watch get uncomfortably tight and your rings become harder and harder to pry off your fingers—mild swelling (aka edema) of the ankles, feet, and hands is completely normal, related to the necessary increase in body fluids in pregnancy. In fact, 75 percent of women develop swelling at some point in their pregnancies, usually around this point (the other 25 percent never notice any at all, which is normal, too). As you've probably already noticed, the puffiness is likely to be more pronounced late in the day, in warm weather, or after spending too much time sitting or standing. In fact, you may find that much of the swelling disappears overnight or after several hours spent lying down (another good reason to get that rest).

Generally, this type of swelling means nothing more than a little discomfort—and a few fashion compromises if you can no longer squeeze your ankles into those super cute boots or strappy sandals. Still, you'll want to find ways to deflate, if you can. To spell swell relief, keep these tips in mind:

- Stay off your feet and off your butt. If long periods of standing or sitting are part of your job description—at home or at the office—take periodic breaks. Have a seat if you've been standing, and get up if you've been sitting. Or for best results, take a brisk 5-minute walk to rev up your circulation (which should get those pooled fluids flowing).

- Put 'em up. Elevate your legs when you're sitting. If anyone deserves to put her feet up, it's you.

- Get some rest on your side. If you're not already in the side-lying habit, it's time to try it now. Lying on your side helps keep your kidneys working at peak efficiency, enhancing waste elimination and reducing swelling.

- Choose comfort. Now's the time to make a comfort statement, not a fashion statement. Favor shoes that are accommodating (those slinky slingbacks don't fit now, anyway).

- Move it. Keeping up your practitioner-approved workouts will keep down the swelling. Walking (you'll probably soon call it waddling) is swell for swollen feet since it'll keep blood flowing instead of pooling. Swimming or water aerobics are even better, because the water pressure pushes tissue fluid back into your veins. From there it goes into your kidneys, after which you'll pee it out.

- Salt to taste. It was once believed that salt restriction would help keep the swelling down, but it is now known that limiting salt too much increases swelling. Just make moderation your motto.

- Get the support you need. You may not think "sexy" when you think maternity support hose, but they've come a long way in style and innovation—and most important, they're very effective in relieving swelling. Comfortable compression comes in basic full panty hose, knee highs and thigh highs (just avoid ones with tight elastic tops), and even fashion-forward tights and footless/legging varieties. When possible, opt for cotton blends for breathability. Putting compression hose on first thing in the morning, before the day's swelling begins, can keep those fluids from pooling in the first place.

The good news about edema, besides that it's normal, is that it's temporary. You can look forward to your ankles deflating and your fingers depuffing soon after you give birth (though some moms find it can take up to a month or more for swelling to disappear completely). In the meantime, look on the bright side: Soon your belly will be so big, you won't be able to see how swollen your feet are.

If the swelling seems to be more than mild, let your practitioner know. Severe swelling can be one of the symptoms of preeclampsia, but it isn't considered a reliable one (since pregnancy swelling is common and varies so much from mom to mom). So unless severe swelling is accompanied by protein in the urine and elevated blood pressure (both are screened for at each prenatal appointment), or by other symptoms of preeclampsia (which may include severe headaches, vision disturbances, and increasing shortness of breath), it's likely just a normal part of the pregnancy package. Still, when in doubt, get it checked out.

Strange Skin Bumps

"As if it's not bad enough that I have stretch marks, now I seem to have some kind of itchy bumps breaking out in them."

Cheer up. You have less than 3 months left until delivery, when you'll be able to bid a grateful good-bye to most of the unpleasant side effects of pregnancy—among them, these late-breaking-out bumps. Until then, it may help to know that although they may be uncomfortable (and slightly unsightly), the bumps aren't concerning. Known medically—and unpronounceably—as pruritic urticarial papules and plaques of pregnancy (try saying that fast 3 times), aka PUPPP, or PEP (polymorphic eruption of pregnancy), the condition generally disappears after delivery and doesn't recur in subsequent pregnancies. Though PUPPP most often develops in abdominal stretch marks, it sometimes also appears on the thighs, buttocks, or arms of expectant moms. Show your rash to your practitioner, who may prescribe topical medication, an antihistamine, or a shot to ease any discomfort.

A variety of other skin conditions and rashes can develop during pregnancy (lucky you!), making you less than happy with the skin you're in. Though you should always show any rash that crops up to your practitioner, keep in mind that rashes are rarely cause for concern. See page 258 for more.

Lower Back and Leg Pain (Sciatica)

"I've been having pain on the side of my lower back, running right down my hip and leg. What's that about?"

Sounds like your sweet little baby may be getting on your nerves—your sciatic nerve, that is. Toward the middle to end of your pregnancy, your baby begins to settle into the proper position for birth (a big positive). In doing that, however, his or her head—and the weight of your ever-enlarging uterus—may settle on the sciatic nerve in the lower part of your spine (a big negative). Such so-called sciatica can less frequently be caused by a herniated or slipped disk (also due to the extra pressure of that growing uterus). Either way, sciatica can result in sharp, shooting, sometimes intense pain, tingling or numbness that starts in your buttocks or lower back and radiates down the back of either of your legs. Though sciatica may pass if your baby shifts positions, it can also linger until you've delivered—and sometimes even linger a little postpartum.

How can you get baby off your nerves and relieve the pain of sciatica? Try these tips:

- Take a seat. Getting off your feet may ease the pain (but avoid sitting on the floor, which can intensify pain). Lying down on the side that doesn't hurt can also relieve pressure—and it's smart to sleep on that side, too.

- Get support. A belly band or other support garment can take the pressure of your growing uterus off your lower back and hips.

- Warm it. A warm heating pad applied on the spot where you feel the pain can help ease it, as can a long soak in a warm bath. Have jets in your tub? Keep them focused on your aching lower back and legs.

- Work it out. The right kind of exercises can ease the pain of sciatica (your practitioner and/or a physical therapist will be able to recommend others as well):

  ◆ Pelvic tilts (see page 240)

  ◆ Child's pose. Kneel on the floor, sitting on your heels, with your big toes touching each other. Spread your thighs and lean forward, resting your belly, outstretched arms, and forehead on the floor. Stay in this position for 2 minutes, and repeat a few times a day.

  ◆ Ball exercises. Sit on (or lie back on) an exercise ball and rock back and forth for relief.

  ◆ Water workouts. Swimming and water aerobics stretch and strengthen back muscles, helping to ease that searing pain—plus they're not weight bearing, a plus when it's the pressure that's causing the pain.

- Seek an alternative. Ask your practitioner about CAM therapies that might help ease sciatic pain, such as physical therapy, therapeutic massage, acupuncture, and chiropractic medicine.

Count Your Kicks

From the 28th week on, it may be a good idea to test for fetal movements twice a day—once in the morning, when activity tends to be quieter, and once in the more active evening hours. Your practitioner may recommend a test, or you can use this one: Note the time on the clock and start counting. Count movements of any kind (kicks, flutters, swishes, rolls), but don't include hiccups in your tally. Stop counting when you reach 10, and note the time. (If you like, you can use the fetal movement tracker in the *What to Expect Pregnancy Journal and Organizer* or on the What To Expect app or Apple Watch app). Often, you will feel 10 movements within 10 minutes or so—sometimes it will take longer.

If you haven't counted 10 movements by the end of an hour, have some juice or a snack, walk a bit, even jiggle your belly a little—then lie down, relax, and continue counting. If 2 hours go by without 10 movements, call your practitioner. Though such an absence of activity doesn't necessarily mean something's wrong, it can occasionally be a red flag that needs quick evaluation.

The closer you are to your due date, the more important regular checking of fetal movements becomes.

It's a good idea to check in with your practitioner if you're having symptoms of sciatic pain, not only for suggested therapies and treatments (including medication, if needed), but for a proper diagnosis. Another condition with similar symptoms (pelvic girdle pain, or PGP) is sometimes misdiagnosed as sciatica. See page 561 for more.

Lightning Crotch

"Once in a while I get this sudden sharp pain deep inside my crotch—almost like I'm being stabbed down there. It doesn't last long but it's so intense it takes my breath away. What is it?"

Sounds like you've been struck by lightning crotch—a surprisingly common, yet little discussed, symptom of late pregnancy that can be a real pain. This sensation can be felt deep in the pelvis or vagina—sometimes like an electric shock, sometimes like a sharp jabbing, sometimes with a little stinging and burning or pins and needles added in. It typically comes on suddenly and unexpectedly and with such intensity that it can nearly knock you off your feet (and have you shrieking out loud in public).

There's no definitive medical evidence that pinpoints why lightning crotch happens—there isn't even a medical term for it—but there are plenty of theories on what triggers that punched-in-the-pants feeling. Some experts say it happens when baby presses on or kicks a nerve that runs to the cervix. Others suggest that your little one might be using your sensitive cervix and lower uterus as a punching bag or that your baby-on-the-move is pushing down as he or she changes positions. Or that the very normal stretching and pulling of the ligaments surrounding and supporting your uterus as your belly grows (and grows) is switching on those electric-like shocks in your pelvis. One thing that is clear is that lightning crotch is not a result of cervical dilation, which means if you're feeling that telltale stabbing feeling down below, there's no reason to worry that you might be going into labor anytime soon. It isn't dangerous and it isn't a sign of pregnancy problems.

There's probably not much you can do when lightning crotch strikes, other than perhaps moving positions to try to knock baby off your nerves (or maybe, lightening the load on your pelvis with a belly support garment). Still, it makes sense to ask about those painful twinges at your next prenatal visit. Sometimes pelvic pain can also be linked to varicose veins in the vulva, a vaginal infection, sciatica, or even a magnesium deficiency, and it's a good idea to get your practitioner's opinion on what's going on down there.

Restless Leg Syndrome

"As tired as I am at night, I can't seem to settle down because my legs feel so restless. I've tried all the tips for leg cramps, but they don't work. What else can I do?"

With so many other things coming between you and a good night's sleep in your last trimester, it hardly seems fair that your legs are, too. But for the 15 percent or so of pregnant women who experience restless leg syndrome (RLS), that's exactly what happens. The name captures it all—that restless, creeping, crawling, tingling, burning, prickling, itchy feeling inside the foot and/or leg that keeps the rest of your body from settling down. It's most common at night, but it can also strike in the late afternoon or pretty much any time you're lying or sitting down.

Experts aren't certain what causes RLS in some pregnant women (though there does seem to be a genetic component to it), and they're even less sure how to treat it. None of the tricks of the leg cramp trade—including rubbing or flexing—seem to bring relief.

Medications used to treat RLS aren't safe for use during pregnancy (check with your practitioner), so they're most likely off the table, too. And speaking of medications, certain ones (like antinausea meds or antihistamines, drugs expectant moms often take to relieve morning sickness) can make RLS worse for some moms.

How can you stop those restless legs from messing with your rest? Though there are no sure bets, it may pay to try any of the following:

- Keep track of triggers. It's possible that diet and other lifestyle habits may contribute to RLS, so it may help to keep a journal of what you eat, what you do, and how you feel each day so you can see what habits, if any, bring on symptoms. Some women, for instance, find that eating carbohydrates late in the day can set off restless legs, and others find that caffeine can pull the trigger. Look at the meds you take, too, to see if there might be a connection to your RLS.

- Turn to CAM. Acupuncture may help turn off RLS, as may yoga, meditation, or other relaxation techniques. Even distraction (doing something to take your mind off the discomfort) may help ease that restless feeling.

- Check your levels. Iron-deficiency anemia (common in the third trimester anyway) sometimes triggers RLS, so ask your practitioner about getting your levels tested. If your stores do turn out to be low, taking the right iron supplement can relieve the symptoms. Other possible triggers of RLS that a blood test can reveal: a deficiency in magnesium or vitamin D, either of which can be treated with a supplement. While you're at it, ask your practitioner about other suggested treatments.

■ Get active. For some mamas-to-be, getting those legs moving during the day can keep them from wanting to move all night. Try pregnancy-safe moderate cardio exercise and lower-body strength training, but not too close to bedtime (since that can exacerbate RLS, plus keep you from sleeping, period). Simple stretches may also work—try calf stretches or a standing leg stretch (see page 292).

■ Try these at home. Applying hot or cold packs to your legs or even taking a cold shower (or soaking your legs in cold water) before bed may ward off that restless feeling. You can also try wearing compression socks or stockings during the day.

And, of course, it couldn't hurt to try the sleep tips on page 284. In fact, because fatigue can worsen RLS symptoms, do what you can to get the sleep your body is craving.

Hopefully, you'll find at least some relief from RLS in the strategies listed here. Unfortunately, some moms-to-be with RLS find that nothing works for them and their only option is waiting it out until delivery brings relief (if not a good night's sleep—after all, a new baby rarely brings that). If you came into pregnancy with the condition, you'll probably have to wait until after delivery (and possibly after weaning, if you're nursing) to resume any drug treatment you were using.

Fetal Hiccups

"I sometimes feel regular little spasms in my abdomen. Is this kicking, or a twitch, or what?"

Believe it or not, your baby's probably got hiccups. Many fetuses have bouts of hiccups in the last half of pregnancy, with some getting them every

---

Snap, Crackle, Pop, Mom?

So, you were definitely expecting to see your baby's movements—but hear them? Apparently, it's possible. Some moms-to-be hear a mysterious clicking, snapping, popping, or knuckle cracking sound coming from their bellies, and while no one really knows for sure why, there are a few theories. Maybe it's hiccup related, or the sound of amniotic fluid swooshing as your baby moves and somersaults. Maybe it's the clicking of your baby's joints as he or she wiggles, punches, or kicks. Or perhaps the sounds aren't coming from your baby at all, but from your looser-than-normal joints, popping and clicking as they rub against each other or stretch out.

You'll probably never know what's causing all the snapping, crackling, and popping, though you can always ask your practitioner to venture a guess. One thing is for sure, though: It's nothing to worry about, just something else to enjoy (or endure) while you're expecting.

---

day, even several times a day. Others never seem to get them at all. The same pattern may continue after birth.

But before you start holding your breath or trying other hiccup tricks, you should know that hiccups don't cause discomfort in babies—in or out of the uterus—even when they last 20 minutes or more. So just sit back, relax, and enjoy the show. As entertaining as they are, though, keep in mind that fetal hiccups don't count when you're doing your kick counts (see page 315).

Orgasm and Baby's Kicking

"After I have an orgasm, my baby usually stops kicking for about half an hour. Does that mean that sex isn't safe at this point in pregnancy?"

No matter what you do these days, your baby's along for the ride. And when it comes to lovemaking, the ride can make baby very sleepy. The rocking motion of sex and the rhythmic uterine contractions that follow orgasm often lull fetuses to dreamland. Some babies, on the other hand (because every baby's an individual), become more lively after sex. Either reaction is normal and healthy, and it is in no way a sign that sex isn't safe. Nor, in case you're wondering, is it a sign that baby's in the know about what's going on between those sheets (baby's completely in the dark, literally).

In fact, unless your practitioner has prescribed otherwise, you can continue enjoying sex of all varieties—and orgasms of all intensities—until delivery. And you might as well get that sex in while you can. Let's face it—it may be a while before it's this convenient to make love again (at least, with your baby in the house).

Accidental Falls

"I missed the curb today when I was out walking and belly-flopped onto the pavement. Could the fall have hurt the baby?"

Is pregnancy tripping you up? That's not surprising—after all, once you enter the third trimester, there are plenty of factors that can combine to literally put you head over heels. For one, your impaired sense of balance, which has been thrown off-kilter as your center of gravity keeps shifting forward, along with your belly. For another, your looser, less stable joints, which add to awkwardness and make you prone to minor falls, especially those belly flops. Also contributing to clumsiness are your tendency to tire easily, your predisposition to distraction and daydreaming, and the difficulty you may be having seeing past your belly to your feet—all of which make those curbs and other stumbling blocks easy to miss . . . and easy to stumble over.

Once again, nature has baby's back (if not yours). Your little one is protected by one of the world's most sophisticated shock absorption systems, made up of amniotic fluid, tough membranes, the elastic, muscular uterus, and the sturdy abdominal cavity, which is girded with muscles and bones. For it to be penetrated, and your baby hurt, you'd have to sustain very serious injuries, the kind that would very likely land you in the hospital.

Still concerned? Call your practitioner for extra reassurance—and to ask if you can pop over for a quick check of baby's heartbeat to ease your mind.

Of course, it's always best to avoid falls. So as you become more and more prone to tripping and slipping, try to become more cautious, too. Avoid walking in slippery socks or on slippery surfaces in shoes that don't have stabilizing traction (or anywhere in shoes you can easily slip out of, like flip flops or open-back sandals). Stay off ladders and other precarious places. And take extra care with stairs and curbs.

Dreams and Fantasies

"I've been having so many vivid, really crazy dreams lately that I'm beginning to think I'm losing my mind."

Feel like you've been streaming some pretty strange Netflix while you're sleeping lately? Pregnancy dreams—and

Daddy Dreams

So your dream life has been more interesting than your real life these days? You've got lots of company. For just about all expectant mothers and fathers, pregnancy is a time of intense feelings, feelings that run the roller coaster from joyful anticipation to panic-stricken anxiety and back again. It's not surprising that many of these feelings find their way into dreams, where the subconscious can act them out and work them through safely. Dreams about sex, for instance, might be your subconscious telling you what you probably already know: You're worried about how pregnancy and having a baby is affecting and will continue to affect your sex life. Such fears are not only normal, but valid. Acknowledging that your relationship is in for some changes now that baby's making three is the first step in making sure your twosome stays cozy. Another strong possibility: You're dreaming about sex more because you're having it less.

R-rated dreams are most common in early pregnancy. Later on, you may notice a family theme in your dreams. You may dream about your parents or grandparents as your subconscious attempts to link past generations to the future one. You may dream about being a child again, which may express an understandable fear of the responsibilities to come and a longing for the carefree years of the past. You may even dream about being pregnant yourself, which may express sympathy for the load your partner is carrying, jealousy of the attention she's getting, or just

a desire to connect with your unborn baby. Dreams about dropping the baby or forgetting to strap your newborn into the car seat can express your insecurities about becoming a father (the same insecurities every expectant parent shares). Uncharacteristically testosterone-charged dreams—scoring a touchdown or driving a race car, even if you've never come close to doing either one—can communicate the subconscious fear that becoming a nurturer will chip away at your manliness. Dreams about loneliness and being left out are extremely common—these speak to those feelings of exclusion that so many expectant fathers experience.

Not all of your dreams will express anxiety, of course. The flip side of your subconscious may also get equal time (sometimes even in the same night): Dreaming about taking care of your baby helps prepare you for your new role as doting dad. Other nurturing dreams—of being handed or finding a baby, of baby showers or family strolls through the park—show how excited you are about the imminent arrival.

One thing is for sure: You're not dreaming alone. The expectant mom in your life (for the same reasons) is subject to strange dreams, too—plus the heavier load of hormones she's carrying can make them even more vivid. Sharing dreams with your partner in the morning can be an intimate, enlightening, and therapeutic ritual, as long as neither one of you takes them too seriously. After all, they're just dreams.

daydreams and fantasies—can be big productions, with plenty of special (and sometimes scary) effects, and so vivid and lifelike that they may leave you pinching yourself when you wake up. What's more, they can come in a

variety of genres, from horror (like the one about leaving the baby on the bus) to heartwarming (snuggling chubby cheeks, pushing strollers through a sunny park), to stranger-than-science-fiction (giving birth to an alien baby with a tail or to a

Preparing Fido and Whiskers

Already a parent—to the kind of baby that has 4 legs, fur, and a tail? Concerned that your pet, who's used to ruling the roost (and curling up on your bed and your lap), will suffer from a bad (and possibly risky) case of sibling rivalry when you show up with a new baby? Taking steps to prepare your dog or cat for when baby makes three (people, that is) is crucial. See *What to Expect the First Year* for tips and recommendations on preparing the family pet for baby's arrival. You'll also find a video about preparing your pet on WhatToExpect.com.

litter of puppies). And though they may make you feel as though you're losing your mind (was that really a giant salami that chased you around the parking lot of Babies "R" Us last night?), they're healthy, normal—and actually helping you stay sane. These dreams (and nightmares) are just one of the many ways that your subconscious works through your mind's overload of pre-baby anxieties, fears, hopes, and insecurities, helping you come to terms with the impending upheaval in your life. An outlet for the 1,001 conflicting emotions (from ambivalence to trepidation to overwhelming excitement and joy) you're almost certainly feeling but may be uneasy expressing any other way. Think of it as therapy you can sleep through.

Hormones contribute, also, to your heavier-than-usual dream schedule (what don't they contribute to?). Plus, they can make your dreams much more intense. The lighter sleep you've been getting also plays a part in your ability to recall your dreams—and recall

them in high definition. Because you're waking up more often than you used to, whether to use the bathroom, kick off some blankets, or just toss, turn, and try to get comfortable, you have more opportunities to wake up in the middle of a REM dream cycle. With the dreams so fresh in your mind each time you wake up, you're able to remember them in greater—and sometimes unnerving—detail:

Here are some of the most commonly reported dream and fantasy themes during pregnancy. Some probably sound familiar.

- Oops! dreams. Dreaming about losing or misplacing things (from your car keys to your baby), forgetting to feed the baby, leaving baby home alone or in the car, or being completely unprepared for baby's arrival can reveal the common (and understandable) fear that you're not up to being a mom.

- Ouch! dreams. Being attacked (by intruders, burglars, animals) or hurt (by falling down the stairs after a push or a slip) may represent a sense of vulnerability—and what pregnant woman doesn't feel vulnerable sometimes?

- Help! dreams. Dreams of being enclosed or unable to escape—trapped in a tunnel, a car, or a small room, or drowning in a pool, a lake of snowy slush, a car wash—can signify the fear of being tied down by the expected new family member, of losing your once carefree life to a demanding newborn.

- Oh no! dreams. Dreams of gaining no weight or gaining a lot of weight overnight, or of eating or drinking the wrong things (a tray of tuna sashimi washed down with a pitcher of martinis) are common among those trying to stick to the kind of dietary restrictions moms-to-be are stuck with.

- Ugh! dreams. Dreaming about becoming unattractive or repulsive to your partner or about him taking up with someone else expresses the common fear that pregnancy will destroy your looks forever and make you unappealing to your partner.

- Sex dreams. Dreams about sex can run the X-rated gamut during pregnancy, expressing everything from lust you've been repressing to fantasies you've been closeting to guilt and ambivalence you've been feeling. It's those hormones talking—and just as they can while you're conscious, they can trigger intense sexual arousal (sometimes including orgasm) while you sleep or even daydream.

- Memory dreams. Dreaming of death and resurrection—lost parents or grandparents or other relatives reappearing—may be the subconscious mind's way of linking old and new generations.

- Life-with-baby dreams. Dreaming about getting ready for the baby and loving and playing with the baby is practice parenting, a way that your subconscious bonds you with your baby before delivery.

- Imagining-baby dreams. Dreaming about what your baby will be like can reveal a wide variety of feelings. Dreams about the baby being deformed, sick, or too large or too small express anxieties that just about all parents-to-be harbor deep down inside. Fantasies about the infant having unusual skills (like talking or walking at birth) may indicate concern about the baby's intelligence and ambition for his or her future. Premonitions that the baby will be a boy or a girl could mean your heart's set on one or the other. So could dreams about the baby's hair or eye color or resemblance to one parent or the other. Nightmares of the baby being born fully grown could signify your fear of handling a newborn.

- Labor dreams. Dreaming about labor pain—or lack of it—or about not being able to push the baby out may reflect your anxieties about labor (and who doesn't have those?).

Bottom line about your dreams and fantasies—don't lose any sleep over them. They're completely normal and as common among expectant moms as heartburn and stretch marks (just ask around and you'll get an interesting earful). Keep in mind, too, that you may not be the only one in your bed who's dreaming up a sometimes unsettling storm. Expectant dads may also have strange dreams and fantasies as they attempt to work out their conscious and subconscious anxieties about impending fatherhood (it's also their hormones talking, if more quietly). Swapping dreams in the morning can be fun (can you top this one?) as well as therapeutic, making that transition into real-life parenthood easier—plus it can help bring you closer together. Starting a dream journal so you can work out your feelings now—and one day look back and laugh (or analyze)—can also be good therapy. So dream on!

Handling It All

"I'm beginning to worry that I won't be able to manage my job, my house, my marriage—and the baby, too."

Here's the first thing you should know about doing it all: You can't do it all—at least, you can't do it all well, all the time. Many new mothers have tried to don the Super Mom cape—handling a full workload on the job, keeping the house spotless, the laundry

Baby, the 3D Movie

So you've probably already had your standard level 2 ultrasound, and your baby's adorable profile has been your phone's wallpaper for weeks. But with a couple of months or so before you can actually hold that bundle of sweetness in your arms, maybe you're hankering for a closer peek at that button nose, that kissable mouth, that little chin (not to mention those tiny baby feet and hands that have been pummeling you day and night). And maybe you're wondering whether it's time to book an appointment for a 3D or 4D scan at your local prenatal portrait center.

It's tempting, for sure, especially if you've seen these stunning baby portraits and vivid videos online (complete with thumb sucking, yawning, blinking and cord tugging!). But check with your practitioner before you leap (or heave yourself) onto the exam table at the mall. Experts (including ACOG) recommend that 3D and 4D ultrasounds (especially long or multiple ones) be performed only when medically necessary, by qualified technicians or practitioners using well-maintained equipment. The concern? Just-for-fun ultrasounds (though definitely fun) are often done using higher powered machines that are not necessarily operated or maintained by skilled staff. Some of the sessions last a much longer time than a medical scan would—up to 45 minutes—which means more (unnecessary) ultrasound exposure. Sign up for multiple sessions to build a prenatal scrapbook of images and videos, as many centers offer, and baby's exposure is exponentially increased. Another concern experts have: Without a skilled medical professional to perform the scan and interpret the results, parents-to-be may walk away convinced there's something wrong with their baby, or worse, that the less-trained wand wavers will miss real problems that a pro would detect. Plus, a long session or repeated sessions can be intrusive and disruptive for a fetus, who's using womb time to grow, develop, and get the sleep he or she needs—free of interruptions. Finally, while there are no proven risks to extra ultrasound exams, there's no definitive proof that risks don't exist—potential risks that can be avoided by skipping unnecessary scans.

Remember, there will be plenty of opportunities to take photos and videos, and make memories when your baby is born. In the meantime, think about keeping ultrasounds to the number and type prescribed by your practitioner (currently, ACOG recommends a total of 1 to 2 in low-risk, complication-free pregnancies).

Have your practitioner's clearance and an appointment scheduled? Consider limiting your visits to 1 or 2, with each scan no more than 15 minutes in length. And bring your wallet. The image may be priceless, but some studios charge a hefty price for that photo, CD, and DVD of your baby.

---

basket empty, the refrigerator stocked, and home-cooked meals on the table, being a sexy partner and an exemplary parent, and leaping the occasional building in a single bound—but most have realized somewhere in midflight that something's got to give.

Just how well you'll manage your new life will probably depend on how quickly you come to that real-life realization. And there's no better time than now to start—before your latest (and cutest) life challenge arrives.

First, you'll need to give some

thought to what your priorities are so you can begin arranging them in order of importance (and not everything can make that top spot). If baby, spouse, and job are priorities, perhaps keeping the house clean will have to take a (messy) backseat. Maybe home cooked will sometimes give way to home delivered, or the laundry basket will become someone else's responsibility. If you're thinking that full-time motherhood might have your name on it, and you can afford to stay home for a while, maybe you can pause your career. Or you might consider working part-time or job sharing with another mom, if you can swing it, or working from home. Or maybe dad will stay home while you work.

Once you've settled on your priorities, you'll need to let go of your unrealistic expectations (you know, the ones your daydreams are filled with). Check in with experienced moms, and you'll get a reality check fast. As every mother finds out sooner or later—and you'll save yourself a lot of stress if you find out sooner—nobody's perfect, not even moms. As much as you'll want to do everything right, you won't be able to—and there will be those days when it seems like you can't do anything right. Despite your best efforts, beds may go unmade and laundry undone, takeout may take over your dinner table, and getting your "sexy" back may mean finally getting around to washing your hair. Set your standards too high—even if you were able to meet them in your preparenting days—and you'll set yourself up for a whole lot of disappointment.

However you decide to rearrange your life, it will be easier if you don't have to go it alone. Beside most successful moms is a dad (or other partner) who not only shares equally in household chores but also is a full partner in parenting. If dad's not available as much

as you'd like (or is deployed, or isn't in the picture at all), tap into whatever help you can find and/or afford, including babysitting co-ops.

A Birth Plan

"My midwife suggested I come up with a birth plan, but I'm not sure what's supposed to be on it."

Decisions, decisions. Childbirth involves more decisions than ever, and expectant moms and their partners are involved in making more of those decisions. But how can you and your practitioner keep track of all those decisions—from how you'll manage the pain and what position you'll push in to who'll catch your baby and cut the cord? Enter: the birth plan.

A birth plan is just that—a plan (or more aptly, a wish list). In it, parents-to-be can offer up their best-case birthing scenario: how they'd ideally like

---

Passing the Birth Plan (to a New Shift)

Once you've passed your approved birth plan on to your practitioner, it should become part of your chart and find its way to your delivery. But just in case it doesn't make it in time, you might want to print up several copies of the plan to bring along to the hospital or birthing center, just so there's no confusion about your preferences. Your coach or doula can make sure that each new shift (with any luck, you won't have to labor through too many of them) has a copy for reference.

Signs of Preterm Labor

It's a good idea for every expectant mom to be familiar with the signs of premature labor, since early detection can have a tremendous impact on outcome. Think of the following as information you'll probably never use but should know, just to be on the safe side. Read this list over, and if you experience any of these symptoms before 37 weeks (or think you might be experiencing them but aren't sure), call your practitioner immediately:

- Persistent cramps that are menstrual-like, with or without diarrhea, nausea, or indigestion

- Regular painful contractions coming every 10 minutes (or sooner) that do not subside when you change positions or drink water (not to be confused with the Braxton Hicks contractions you might be already feeling, which don't indicate early labor; see page 340)

- Constant lower back pain or pressure or a change in the nature of lower backache

- A change in your vaginal discharge, particularly if it is watery or tinged or streaked pinkish or brownish with blood

- An achiness or feeling of pressure in the pelvic floor, the thighs, or the groin

- Leaking from your vagina (a steady trickle or a gush)

Keep in mind that you can have some or all of these symptoms and not be in labor (most pregnant women experience pelvic pressure or lower back pain at some point). In fact, the majority of women who have symptoms of preterm labor do not deliver early. But only your practitioner can tell for sure, so pick up the phone and call. After all, it's always best to play it safe.

For information on preterm labor risk factors and prevention, see page 31. For information on the management of preterm labor, see page 559.

labor and delivery to play out if all goes according to "plan." Besides listing those preferences, the typical birth plan factors in what's practical, what's feasible, and what the practitioner and hospital or birthing center will accommodate (not everything on a birth plan may fly with them) or have available. It isn't a contract but a written understanding between a patient and her practitioner and/or hospital or birthing center. Not only can a good birth plan deliver a better birth experience, but it can also head off unrealistic expectations, minimize disappointment, and eliminate major conflict and miscommunication between

a birthing mom and her birth attendants. Some practitioners routinely ask an expectant couple to fill out a birth plan, while others are happy to oblige if one is requested. A birth plan is also a springboard for dialog between patient and practitioner. Not sure how your practitioner feels about some of your birth preferences? Now, well before labor starts, is the time to find out.

Some birth plans cover just the basics, while others are extremely detailed (down to the birthing room music, lighting, and guest list). And because every expectant woman is different—not only in what she'd like out of the birth experience but what she can likely expect given her particular pregnancy profile and history—a birth plan should be individualized (so don't fill yours out based on one you saw on another mom's blog). Some of the issues you may want to tackle in your birth plan, should you decide to fill one out, are listed below. You can use it as a general guideline, then flesh it out as needed. For a sample birth plan, see the *What to Expect Pregnancy Journal and Organizer*.

- How far into labor you'd prefer to remain at home

- Eating and/or drinking during active labor (page 406)

- Being out of bed (walking around or sitting up) during labor

- Being in a tub for labor and/or birth (page 326)

- Personalizing the atmosphere with music, lighting, items from home

- Who you'd like to have with you (besides your partner) during labor and/or at delivery—including a doula (page 328), your other children, friends, family

- Taking pictures and videos

- The use of a mirror so you can see the birth

- The use of an IV (intravenous fluid; page 407)

- The use of a catheter

- The use of pain medication and the type you'd prefer (page 331)—or wishes about alternatives to pain meds (page 334)

- Artificial rupture of the membranes (page 409) and/or leaving membranes intact

- External fetal monitoring (continuous

Don't Hold It In

Do you often hold in your pee to avoid making yet another run for the bathroom? Not going when you've got the urge can inflame your bladder, which can irritate your uterus and cause contractions. It can also lead to a urinary tract infection, another cause of preterm contractions. So don't hold it in. When you gotta go, go . . . promptly.

---

or intermittent) or internal fetal monitoring (page 407)

- The use of oxytocin to induce or augment contractions (page 424)

- Delivery positions (page 412), use of a birthing bar (page 414), and so on

- Use of warm compresses and perineal massage (pages 432 and 384)

- Episiotomy (page 408)

- The option of "laboring down" (page 429)

- Vacuum extraction or forceps use (page 410)

- Cesarean delivery, including option of "gentle cesarean" (page 438)

- Special requests around suctioning baby, such as suctioning by the father

- Holding the baby immediately after birth, allowing baby time to creep from belly to breast (page 434)

- Plans for breastfeeding right away, having a lactation consultant there to help

- Delayed cord clamping (page 416)

- Dad catching the baby and/or cutting the cord (page 434)

Water Birth

Your baby spends 9 blissful months doing water ballet in a warm pool of amniotic fluid, and then makes a sudden, harsh entrance into a cold, dry world. Advocates of water birth say that allowing a baby to arrive in conditions that mimic those of the womb—warm and wet—can ease the transition and make that entry more peaceful, reducing a newborn's stress.

If you choose to have a water birth, you'll not only spend your labor in a warm tub or pool, but you'll also deliver your newborn while you're still in the water (your baby will be pulled gently into the soothing water and then slowly lifted into your arms). Your partner can be in the water with you during labor to support you and he can play catch (literally) with the baby during delivery. During labor, cold cloths, spray bottles, and plenty of water will keep you refreshed (as much as possible—you're having a baby, after all) while the midwife or other medical personnel monitors your baby's condition with an underwater Doppler device.

Water births are really an option only for low-risk pregnancies, but they're available in more and more settings. Most birthing centers and some hospitals offer the option of water births and most birthing centers have large tubs or Jacuzzis in the birthing rooms (or portable birthing tubs on wheels that can be rolled into your room) that can also be used for soothing soaks or hydrotherapy, even if you ultimately decide against actually giving birth in water (or if it turns out not to be possible in your case). It's less likely that a hospital will have a tub large enough to accommodate a water birth, so if you prefer a water birth but are delivering in a hospital that doesn't offer the option or doesn't have tubs, ask whether it might be possible to bring your own birthing tub that you've rented or purchased (see below).

You can also choose to have a water birth at home—as long as you have your midwife's approval and the right equipment on hand. Most home water birth tubs look like deep kiddie pools—they're inflatable, large enough to allow you to move around freely, deep enough so your pregnant belly can stay fully submerged, and have soft sides, allowing

---

- Cord blood banking (page 295)

- Postponing weighing the baby and/or administering eye drops until after you and your baby greet each other

- Special requests around the placenta (seeing it, preserving it; see page 362)

You may also want to include some postpartum items on your birth plan, such as:

- Your presence (and/or dad's) at baby's weigh-in, the pediatric exam, and baby's first bath

- Baby feeding in the hospital (see page 478)

- Circumcision (see *What to Expect the First Year*)

- Rooming-in (usually required by hospital when mom and baby are both doing well; see page 474)

- Other children visiting with you and/or with the new baby

- Postpartum medication or treatments for you or your baby

you to lean against (or over) the edges comfortably. You can purchase or rent a birthing tub online or from your midwife (some midwives loan out tubs at no cost—or you might also be able to borrow one from a friend who's been there, done that). If you're purchasing, expect to shell out a few hundred dollars for the tub and all the equipment that goes along with it, including liners, heater, filter, and tarp. On a tighter budget? You can also use your home's bathtub (assuming it's deep enough for your big belly and with enough room around the tub for your midwife to reach you during delivery or if an emergency arises). Of course, you'll have to make sure it's cleaned and sterilized (with a water-bleach mixture) before the big day arrives. You'll also have to make sure you have a floating thermometer to monitor the water temperature and keep it stable at approximate body temperature (95°F to about 100°F, but no more than 101°F, because your body temperature could rise, causing the baby's heart rate to increase). Birthing tubs come with heaters, so that's one less thing to worry about if you do end up using one.

Since a baby's breathing will not start until he or she comes out of the water and into the air (babies don't breathe in utero), drowning is not considered a risk of water births. For several reasons, however, a baby's underwater entry should be limited to no more than a few moments (10 seconds is the norm in the U.S.). First, because the umbilical cord can tear, cutting off the baby's oxygen lifeline unexpectedly. Second, because once the placenta separates from the uterus—which can happen at any time after delivery—it can no longer provide the baby with sufficient oxygen. And finally, because the fluid your baby will be born into isn't sterile. Remember, birth is a messy business. Most women will poop when pushing (the midwife will scoop the feces out of the tub), and there will also be blood and urine in the water you're sitting in. If the baby aspirates (inhales) the fluid—unlikely except in the case of fetal stress during labor—he or she could be at risk of a serious infection.

Thinking you'd like your baby to make an underwater appearance into the world? Though it's a personal decision to make (like so many other birth decisions), it's one best made in consultation with your practitioner, so you can be sure it's a safe option for you and your baby. For more information on water births, go to waterbirth.org.

- Arrangements for newborn screening (page 360)

- The length of the hospital stay, barring complications (page 468)

Of course, the most important feature of a good birth plan is flexibility. Since childbirth—like most forces of nature—is unpredictable, the best-laid plans don't always go, well, according to plan. Though chances are very good that your plan can be carried out just the way you drew it up, there's always the chance that it won't. There is no way to predict precisely how labor and delivery will progress (or not progress) until it gets underway—or how you'll really feel about those contractions once they get started. A birth plan you design ahead of time may not end up being medically advisable—or what works for you in the moment—and may have to be adjusted at the last minute for your baby's wellbeing and yours. A change of mind (yours) can also prompt a change of plan (you were dead set against having an epidural, but somewhere around 5 cm, you become dead set on having one).

Doulas: Best Medicine for Labor?

Think three's a crowd? For many couples, not when it comes to labor and delivery. More and more are opting to share their birth experience with a doula, a woman trained as a labor companion. And for good reason. Some studies have shown that women supported by doulas are less likely to require cesarean deliveries, induction, and pain relief. Births attended by doulas may also be shorter, with a lower rate of complications.

The term "doula" comes from ancient Greece, where it was used to describe the most important female servant in the household, the one who probably helped mom out the most during childbirth. What exactly can a doula do for you and your birth experience? That depends on the doula you choose, at what point in your pregnancy you hire her, and what your preferences are. Some doulas become involved well before that first contraction strikes, helping with the design of a birth plan and easing prelabor jitters. Many will come to the house to help a couple through early labor. Once at the hospital or birthing center, the doula takes on a variety of responsibilities, again depending on your needs and wishes.

Typically, her primary role is as a continuous source of comfort, encouragement, and support (both emotional and physical) during labor. She'll serve as a soothing voice of experience (especially valuable if you're first-timers), help with relaxation techniques and breathing exercises, offer advice on labor positions, and do her share of massage, hand holding, pillow plumping, and bed adjusting. A doula can also act as a mediator and an advocate, ready to speak for you as needed, translate medical terms and explain procedures, and generally run interference with hospital personnel. She won't take the place of your coach (and a good doula won't make him feel like she's taking his place, either) or the nurse on duty—instead, she will augment their support and services (especially important if the nurse assigned to you has several other patients in labor at the same time or if labor is long and nurses come and go as shifts change). She will also likely be the only person (besides your coach) who will stay by your side throughout labor and delivery—a friendly and familiar face from start to finish. And many doulas don't stop there. They can also offer support and advice postpartum

Bottom line: Birth plans, though by no means necessary (you can definitely decide to go with the childbirth flow), are a great option, one that more and more expectant parents are taking advantage of. To figure out whether a birth plan is right for you and what should be in it, talk it over with your practitioner at your next visit.

Tdap Vaccine

"My practitioner told me I need to get the Tdap vaccine this month. But I thought I already had that shot as a child."

Time to roll up that sleeve again, mama. The CDC recommends that every pregnant woman get the Tdap vaccine (which prevents diphtheria, tetanus, and pertussis) between 27 and 36 weeks of each pregnancy, regardless of when she was last vaccinated with on everything from breastfeeding to baby care.

Though an expectant father may worry that hiring a doula will relegate him to third-wheel status, that isn't the case. A good doula is also there to help your coach relax so he can help you relax. She'll be there to answer questions he might not feel comfortable broaching with a doctor or nurse. She'll be there to provide an extra set of hands when you need your legs and back massaged at the same time, or when you need both a refill on ice chips and help breathing through a contraction. She'll be an obliging and cooperative member of your labor team—ready to pitch in, but not to push dad (or the medical team) aside and take over. And if dad's not in the picture, a doula can be an especially helpful helping hand by your side throughout the entire labor, delivery, and even postpartum period.

How do you locate a doula? Doulas don't need to be certified, but many birthing centers and hospitals keep lists of doulas, and so do some practitioners. Ask friends who've recently used a doula for recommendations, or check online for local doulas. Once you've tracked down a candidate, arrange a consultation before you hire her. Ask her about her experience, her training, what she will do and what she won't do, what her philosophies are about childbirth (if you're planning on asking for an epidural, for instance, you won't want to hire a doula who discourages the use of pain relief), and whether she will be on call at all times and who covers for her if she isn't. Ask whether she provides pregnancy and/or postpartum services, and what her fees are—a consideration for many couples, since doulas aren't covered by insurance. Some doulas offer discounts or even donate their services to those who can't afford their services or to military families (especially when the partner is deployed and won't be at the birth). For more information or to locate a doula in your area, contact Doulas of North America at dona.org.

An alternative to a doula is a female friend or relative who has gone through pregnancy and delivery herself and who you feel totally comfortable with. The plus: Her services will definitely be free. The drawback: She probably won't be quite as knowledgeable. One way to remedy that is having a "lay doula," a female friend who goes through 4 hours of training in doula techniques (ask if your hospital has such a training course). Researchers have found that a lay doula can provide many of the same benefits as a professional one.

---

the Tdap or Td vaccine. That's because immunity from pertussis (and tetanus and diphtheria) wanes after several years. If you've never been vaccinated against tetanus (either with the DTaP series as a child or with Td or Tdap as an adult), you'll need to receive 2 doses of Td early in pregnancy in addition to the regularly scheduled Tdap in the third trimester.

Why the recommendation? It's to protect your baby when he or she is born. Very young babies are vulnerable to pertussis (also called whooping cough), a contagious respiratory illness that can lead to pneumonia and even death. Until your baby is vaccinated against the disease with the full series of the DTaP vaccine (the childhood version of the Tdap, given beginning at 2 months), the antibodies that your body makes after receiving your Tdap shot will be passed along to your little one, effectively protecting him or her from

Take One
for the Team

Are your immunizations up to date? Get your Tdap booster shot if you haven't already (and other booster shots you may need) as well as a seasonal flu vaccine to protect the precious baby who's joining the family. Seventy percent of babies who get whooping cough are infected by immediate family members—and that includes dads. Good news for the needle-phobic: unlike moms, dads don't need a Tdap booster during each pregnancy—one time only.

the disease. And the studies back this up. Research has found that when moms receive the recommended Tdap booster during pregnancy, their babies are 50 percent less likely to catch pertussis than babies whose moms aren't vaccinated. And it's not just you who needs the vaccine. It's important that anyone else who will be in close contact with your newborn—baby's dad, baby's grandparents, the babysitter—get a booster, too. That way they won't contract the disease and spread it to baby, and your little one will be "cocooned" against pertussis.

And here's some great news for busy moms-to-be: If the beginning of your third trimester (when you're scheduled for your Tdap vaccine) coincides with flu season (when you'll need a flu shot) you won't have to schedule two appointments. Research shows that it's completely safe to be vaccinated with both at the same time—making getting the vaccines you need to protect yourself and your baby-to-be a whole lot easier.

Speaking of vaccines, now's the perfect time to begin learning about all the vaccines your little one will be on the receiving end of during his or her first few years of life. There's no better or safer way to protect your precious bundle from preventable, sometimes life-threatening childhood diseases than by making sure he or she is vaccinated completely and on time, according to the recommended schedule. See *What to Expect the First Year* for more information about vaccines, their benefits, and their safety.

ALL ABOUT:
Easing Labor Pain

Let's face it. Those 15 or so hours it takes to birth a baby aren't called labor because they're a walk in the park. Labor (and delivery) is hard work—hard work that can hurt, big time. And if you actually consider what's going on down there, it's really no wonder that labor's a pain. During childbirth, your uterus contracts over and over again to squeeze a relatively big baby through one relatively tight space (your cervix) and out through an even tighter one (your vagina, the same opening you probably once thought was too small for a tampon). Like they say, it's pain with a purpose—a really cute and cuddly purpose—but it's still pain.

But while there may be no getting around the pain of labor altogether (unless you're scheduled for a cesarean delivery, in which case you'll be skipping labor and labor pain), there are plenty of ways to get through it. As a laboring mom, you can select from a wide menu of pain management and relief options, both medicated and nonmedicated (and you can even opt for a combo from both columns). You can choose to go unmedicated throughout your entire labor or just through part of labor (like those relatively easy first centimeters). You can use the breathing and relaxation techniques you learned in childbirth education classes (Lamaze, for instance, or Bradley), or you can turn to alternative approaches (like acupuncture, hypnosis, or hydrotherapy). Or you can birth your baby with a little help—or a lot of help—from medicated pain relief, such as the very popular epidural (which leaves you with little or no pain during labor but allows you to remain awake during the entire process).

Which option is for you? To figure that out, look into them all. Read up on childbirth pain management (this section covers the gamut). Talk to your practitioner. Get insights from friends who have recently labored. Chat about it online. And then do some thinking. Remember that the right option for you might not be one option but a combination of several (reflexology with an epidural chaser, or a variety of relaxation techniques topped off with a round of acupuncture). Remember, too, the value of staying flexible—and not just so you can stretch yourself into some of those pretzel-like pushing positions you learned in childbirth class. After all, the option or options you settle on now may not sit well later, and may need to be adjusted mid-labor (you were planning on an epidural but found you could handle the pain—or vice versa). Most of all, remember that (assuming no medical circumstances end up getting in the way), it's your choice to make—your birth, your way. So read on before you belly up to the birthing bar.

Managing Your Pain With Medications

Here are the most commonly used labor and delivery pain medications:

Epidural. A full two-thirds of women delivering at hospitals choose to relieve their labor pain with an epidural. Why do so many laboring moms request the epidural by name? For one, it's an extremely safe way to net good pain relief—only a small amount of medication is needed to achieve the desired effect, and the drug barely reaches the bloodstream (unlike general anesthesia or tranquilizers), meaning your baby isn't affected. For another, it's relatively easy to administer (it's injected directly into the epidural space, which is between the ligament that sheathes the vertebrae and the membrane that covers the spinal cord) and it's very patient friendly (you'll likely get that sweet relief within 10 to 15 minutes). The pain relief is local, focused on the lower part of the body (where the pain is the greatest), allowing you to be an active participant during childbirth and completely alert when it's time to greet your baby bundle. What's more, an epidural can be given to you as soon as you ask for one (and an anesthesiologist is available to administer it)—no need to wait until you're dilated a certain amount. Happily, studies show that an early epidural doesn't increase the chances of a c-section.

Here's what you can expect if you're having an epidural:

- First, an IV of fluids is started to prevent a drop in blood pressure.

- In some hospitals (policies vary), a catheter (tube) is inserted into the bladder just before or just after the epidural is administered and stays in place to drain urine while the epidural is in effect (since you may not feel the urge

Pushing Without the Pain

Does pushing have to be a pain? Not always. In fact, many women find they can push very effectively with an epidural, relying on their coach or a nurse to tell them when a contraction is coming on so they can get busy pushing. But if pain-free pushing isn't getting you (or your baby) anywhere—with the lack of sensation hampering your efforts—the epidural can be stopped so you can feel the contractions. The medication can then be easily restarted after delivery to numb the repair of a tear, if necessary.

to pee). In other hospitals, the bladder is drained with a catheter as needed.

- Your lower and midback are wiped with an antiseptic solution, and a small area of the back is numbed with a local anesthetic. A needle is placed through the numbed area into the epidural space of the spine, usually while you're lying on your side or sitting up and leaning over a table or being supported by your coach or nurse. You may feel a little pressure as the needle is inserted or a little tingling or a momentary shooting pain. If you're lucky (and many women are), you might not feel a thing. Besides, compared to the pain of contractions, any discomfort from a needle poke is likely to be pretty minimal.

- The needle is removed, leaving a fine, flexible catheter tube in place. The tube is taped to your back so you can move from side to side. Three to 5 minutes after the initial dose, the nerves of the uterus begin to numb. Usually after 10 minutes, you'll begin to feel the full effect. The medication numbs the

nerves in the entire lower part of the body, making it hard to feel any contractions at all (and that's the point).

- Your blood pressure will be checked frequently to make sure it's not dropping too low. IV fluids and lying on your side will help counteract a drop.

- Because an epidural is sometimes associated with the slowing of a baby's heartbeat, continuous fetal monitoring is usually required. Though such monitoring limits your movements somewhat, it allows your practitioner to monitor the baby's heartbeat and allows you to "see" the frequency and intensity of your contractions (because, ideally, you won't be feeling them).

There are few side effects with an epidural, though some women might experience numbness on one side of the body only (as opposed to complete pain relief). Epidurals also might not offer complete pain control if you're experiencing back labor (when the fetus is in a posterior position, with its head pressing against your back). And keep in mind that you won't be able to labor (or deliver) in water if you have an epidural.

Combined spinal epidural (aka "walking epidural"). The combined spinal epidural delivers the same level of pain relief as a traditional epidural, but uses a smaller amount of medication to reach that goal. Not all anesthesiologists or hospitals offer this type of epidural (ask your practitioner if it'll be available to you). The anesthesiologist will start you off with a shot of analgesic directly into the spinal fluid to help relieve some pain, but because the medication is delivered only in the spinal fluid, you'll still feel and be able to use the muscles in your legs, at least somewhat. When you feel you need more pain relief, more medication is placed into the epidural space (through a catheter inserted at the same time the spinal medication was administered).

Keep in mind that the nickname walking epidural is misleading. Though you'll be able to move your legs, they'll probably feel weak, so it'll be unlikely you'll actually want to walk around.

Spinal block. Similar to the epidural, the spinal block is usually given just before delivery. It's faster acting and stronger than an epidural, but also lasts for a shorter time. Though it is primarily reserved for cesarean deliveries (if an epidural hasn't already been started and there's less time to spare) it can also be used in a vaginal birth if mom is in the market for speedy pain relief as she closes in on delivery. Like the epidural, this regional block is administered by an anesthesiologist while you're sitting or lying on your side, but unlike the epidural, no catheter is left in place—it's given as a 1-dose injection directly into the fluid surrounding the spinal cord.

Pudendal block. A pudendal block is usually reserved for the vaginal delivery itself. Administered through a needle inserted into the vaginal area, the medication reduces pain in the region but not uterine discomfort. It's useful when forceps or vacuum extraction is used, and its effect can last through the repair of a tear or an episiotomy (if needed).

General anesthesia. General anesthesia is used rarely, only in specific cases for emergency surgical births. An anesthesiologist injects drugs that put you to sleep into an IV.

The major downside to general anesthesia (besides the fact that mom has to miss the birth) is that it sedates the baby along with the mother. The medical team will minimize those sedative effects by administering the anesthesia as close to the actual birth as possible. That way the baby can be delivered before the anesthetic has reached him or her in amounts large enough to have an effect. When you come to, you may be groggy, disoriented, and restless. You may also have a cough and sore throat (due to the tube that's routinely inserted through the mouth into the throat) and experience nausea and vomiting (though it's less likely if you were given anti-nausea medications in your IV).

Demerol. This IV-administered drug, which dulls pain and induces a relaxed state, isn't often used anymore, but can be useful in certain circumstances—as when a laboring mom needs short-term help coping with contractions. Demerol can be repeated every 2 to 4 hours, as needed. Keep in mind, though, that if you want to be "present" during labor, this probably isn't the pain relief for you. Many women don't like that drugged, drowsy feeling, and some find they are actually less able to cope with labor pain while under the effects of Demerol. There may also be some side effects, including nausea, vomiting, and a drop in blood pressure. And if Demerol is given to a mom too close to delivery, her baby may be sleepy and unable to suck at birth. Less frequently, baby's breathing may be depressed and supplemental oxygen may be required. Any effects on the newborn are generally short term and can be treated.

Nitrous oxide. This dentist office staple, more commonly known as laughing gas, doesn't eliminate pain (and it definitely won't make you break out in giggles), but it does take the edge off contractions and could be a good alternative for women who choose not to go for an epidural. You're able to self-administer the laughing gas during labor—taking a few puffs when you feel you need a little relief and setting it aside when you don't. Not all doctors and hospitals offer laughing gas, so ask ahead if you're considering it.

Moms in Recovery

If you're in recovery, you'll want to discuss the best pain-relief strategy during labor, delivery, and postpartum, and to make sure hospital staff is aware that medications should be administered judiciously.

Tranquilizers. These drugs (such as Phenergan and Vistaril) are used to calm and relax an extremely anxious mom-to-be so that she can actively participate in the process of labor instead of fighting it. Like analgesics, tranquilizers are usually administered once labor is well established, and well before delivery. But they are occasionally used in early labor if a mother's anxiety is slowing down the progress of her labor. Some women welcome the gentle drowsiness, while others find it keeps them from feeling in control, and also dims the memory of this memorable experience. Dosage definitely makes a difference. A small dose may relieve anxiety without impairing alertness. A larger dose may cause slurring of speech and dozing between contraction peaks, making it difficult to use breathing and relaxation techniques learned in childbirth class. Though the risks to a fetus or newborn from them are minimal, most practitioners prefer to stay away from tranquilizers unless they're really necessary. If you think you might be extremely anxious during labor, you may want to try learning some nondrug relaxation techniques now, so you won't end up needing this kind of medication.

Managing Your Pain with CAM

Not every mom-to-be wants traditional pain medication, but most still want their labor to be as comfortable as possible. And that's where natural childbirth techniques (see page 304) or complementary and alternative medicine (CAM) therapies (or both!) can come in—either as alternatives to pain medication or as relaxing supplements to it. Even if you're sure there's an epidural with your name on it waiting at the hospital, you may want to explore the world of CAM, too. (And to explore it well before your due date, since many of the techniques take practice—or even classes—to perfect.) But remember to seek out CAM practitioners who are licensed, certified, and have plenty of labor and delivery experience.

Acupuncture and acupressure. These techniques can be effective forms of pain relief. Researchers have found that acupuncture, through the use of needles inserted in specific locations, triggers the release of several brain chemicals, including endorphins, which block pain signals, relieving labor pain—and maybe even helping boost labor progress. Acupressure works on the same principle as acupuncture, except that instead of poking you with needles, your practitioner will use finger pressure to stimulate the points. Acupressure on the center of the ball of the foot is said to help back labor. If you're planning to use either during labor, let your prenatal practitioner know that your CAM practitioner will be attending, too (these techniques are not DIY).

Reflexology. Reflexologists believe that the internal organs can be accessed through points on the feet. By massaging the feet during childbirth, a reflexologist can relax the uterus and stimulate the pituitary gland, apparently reducing the pain of childbirth and even shortening labor. Some of the pressure points are so powerful that you should avoid stimulating them unless you are in labor (or are overdue). Again, if you're using reflexology you'll need to let your prenatal practitioner know that your reflexology practitioner will be joining you in labor.

Physical therapy. From massage and hot compresses to ice packs and intense counterpressure on your sore spots, physical therapy during labor can ease a lot of the pain you're feeling. Massage at the hands of a caring coach or doula or a skilled health professional can bring relaxing relief and help diminish pain.

Hydrotherapy. This one's easy: Just settle into a jetted tub (or a soaking tub) for a session of hydrotherapy during your labor to reduce pain and relax. Many hospitals and birthing centers provide tubs to labor—or even deliver—in. No tub available? You can try a warm shower for some relief. For more on water births, see page 326.

Hypnobirthing. Though hypnosis won't mask your pain, it can get you so deeply relaxed that you are totally unaware of any discomfort. Hypnosis doesn't work for everyone—for the fullest effect, you have to be highly suggestible. Some clues that your mind will be open to hypnosis: You have a long attention span and a rich imagination, you're able to tune out activity and noise around you, and you enjoy alone time. More and more expectant moms are signing up for hypnobirthing classes so they can learn the techniques necessary to self-hypnotize themselves through labor and delivery, though you can also hire a medically trained hypnotherapist to be by your side through childbirth. Just keep in mind that hypnobirthing isn't something you can opt into when that first contraction hits. You'll have to practice plenty during pregnancy to be able to achieve total relaxation, even

---

Just Breathe

Hoping to skip the meds but can't—or don't want to—go the CAM route? Lamaze (or other kinds of natural childbirth techniques) can be very effective in managing the pain of contractions. See page 304 for more.

---

with a therapist guiding you. One big benefit of hypnobirthing: While you're completely relaxed, you're also completely aware of every moment of your baby's birth. For more information, go to hypnobirthing.com.

Distraction. If you took a childbirth education class such as Lamaze, you may have learned about directing your attention to a focal point to manage your pain. The idea is to concentrate on something other than the contractions, so that you're not focused on the pain. Distraction works the same way. Anything that takes your mind off the pain—watching TV, playing games on your phone, listening to music, meditating—can decrease your perception of it. So can focusing on an object (an ultrasound picture of your baby, a soothing landscape, a photo of a favorite place). Visualization exercises can help, too (for instance, picturing your baby being pushed gently by contractions, moving peacefully through your birth canal).

Transcutaneous electrical nerve stimulation (TENS). This technique uses electrodes that deliver low-voltage pulses to stimulate nerve pathways to the uterus and cervix, in theory blocking pain. Studies aren't clear on whether TENS is really effective at reducing labor pain, but if you're interested, ask your practitioner if it's an option for you.

Labor Disputes

Maybe you're not technically a mommy yet—or a daddy—but that probably doesn't mean you don't already have some pretty definite ideas about how you'd like to parent when the time comes (soon!): Breast or bottle? Stay-at-home or back-to-work? Baby-wearing or strollers? Separate sleep or co-sleep? And you've probably also noticed that these and other hot button topics capture a lot of social media attention, the good, the bad, and especially, the judgey. But you may also find that these so-called mommy wars extend to labor choices, too, pitting home-birth moms against hospital-birth moms, unmedicated-birth moms against moms who opt for an epidural, VBAC moms against moms who sign up for a second c-section. Guilt? There's plenty of that to go around ("You didn't even *try* to labor first?"), plus a fair amount of shaming and finger wagging ("What? You let your doctor induce you?").

But the truth is—and it's a truth that really deserves to go viral—there's room for every safe childbirth choice in the birthing room, but there should be no room for judging. Every mom and dad, every labor, every situation is different—and what works for one doesn't necessarily fly with the next. The bottom line that matters, as always, is a healthy mom-and-baby bottom line—and any choice or circumstance that delivers a safe delivery is a good one. And there's no disputing that.

Making the Decision

You now have the lowdown on pain management and pain relief options for labor and delivery—the information you'll need to make an informed decision. But before you decide what's best for you and your baby, you should:

- Discuss pain management and relief options with your practitioner well before that first contraction kicks in. Ask about the options you're considering, what side effects may be experienced when using medication options, under what circumstances medication may be absolutely necessary, and when the choice is all yours.

- Consider keeping an open mind. Though it's smart to think ahead about what might be best for you under certain circumstances, it's impossible to predict what kind of labor and delivery you'll have, and whether or not you'll want or need medication—or even if you'll have access to the type of pain relief you're hoping for. Even if you're absolutely convinced that you'll want an epidural, you may not want to close the door on some CAM approaches. After all, your labor may turn out to be more manageable (or a lot shorter) than you'd thought. And even if you're sold on a med-free delivery, you may want to think about leaving the medication window open—even just a crack—in case your labor turns out to be tougher than you'd bargained for.

Most important, remember, as you sort through all your options, to keep your eye on the bottom line—a bottom line that has a really cute bottom. After all, no matter how you end up managing the pain of childbirth—and even if you don't end up managing it the way you'd planned to or the way you'd really hoped to—you'll still manage to give birth to your baby. And what could be a better bottom line than that?

CHAPTER 12

The Eighth Month

Approximately 32 to 35 Weeks

I n this next-to-last month, you may still be loving every expectant moment, or you may be growing weary of, well, growing. Either way, you're sure to be preoccupied with—and super excited about—the much-anticipated arrival of your baby. Of course, along with that heaping serving of excitement, you and your partner may also be experiencing a side of trepidation—especially if this is your first foray into parenthood. Talking those very normal feelings through—and tapping into the insights of friends and family members who've preceded you into parenthood—will help you realize that everyone feels that way, particularly the first time around.

Your Baby This Month

Week 32 This week your baby is tipping the scales at almost 3½ to 4 pounds (about a half gallon of milk) and topping out anywhere from 15 to 17 inches. And growing isn't the only thing on your little one's agenda these days. While you're busy getting everything ready for baby's arrival, baby's busy prepping for that big debut, too.

In these last few weeks, it's all about practice, practice, practice, as baby hones the skills needed to survive outside the womb, from swallowing and breathing to kicking and sucking. And speaking of sucking, your little one has been able to suck on a sweet little thumb for a while now. Another change this week: Your baby's skin is

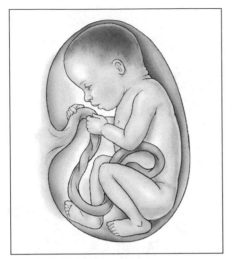

Your Baby, Month 8

no longer transparent. As more and more fat accumulates under the skin, it's finally opaque.

Week 33 Baby's gaining weight almost as fast as you are these days (averaging out to about half a pound a week), which puts the grand total so far at more than 4¼ pounds. Still, your baby has plenty of growing to do. He or she may grow a full inch this week alone and may come close to doubling in weight by birth day. And with that much baby inside your uterus now, your amniotic fluid level has maxed out (there's no room for more fluid). Which explains why those pokes and kicks are sometimes extremely uncomfortable: There's less fluid to cushion the pushing. Antibodies are also being passed from you to baby as your little one continues to develop an immune system of his or her very own. These antibodies will definitely come in handy on the outside and will protect your baby-to-be from a world of germs.

Week 34 Your baby could be as tall as 17 to 18 inches right now and weigh nearly 5 pounds—as much as a bag of sugar, only much sweeter. Got male (a male baby, that is)? If you do, then this is the week that his testicles are making their way down from his abdomen to their final destination: his scrotum. (About 3 to 4 percent of boys are born with undescended testicles, which is nothing to worry about—they usually make the trip down south before the first birthday.) And in other baby-related news, those tiny fingernails have probably reached the tip of those little fingers by this week, so make sure you have baby nail clippers on your shopping list!

Week 35 Your baby stands tall this week—if he or she could stand, that is—at about 18 inches, and continues to follow the half-pound-a-week plan, weighing in at about 5¼ big ones. While growth will gradually taper off when it comes to height (the average full-termer is born at about 20 inches), your baby will continue to pack on the pounds until delivery day. Something else he or she will be packing on in the few weeks that remain are brain cells. Brain development continues at a mind-boggling pace, making baby a little on the top-heavy side. And speaking of tops, it's likely your baby's bottom is. Most babies have settled into a head-down, bottoms-up position in mom's pelvis by now, or will soon. That's a good thing, since it's easier on you if baby's head (the biggest part of his or her body) exits first during delivery. Here's another plus: Baby's head may be big, but it's still soft (at least, the skull is), allowing that tight squeeze through the birth canal to be a little less tight.

Your Body This Month

Here are some symptoms you may experience this month (or may not experience, since every pregnancy is different). Some of these symptoms may be continuing from last month, while others may be new to the list. Chances are as your baby load grows and grows, so will your symptom load (or overload)—with the discomforts of late pregnancy multiplying.

Physically

- Strong, regular fetal activity

- Increasing vaginal discharge

- Constipation

- Heartburn, indigestion, flatulence, bloating

- Occasional headaches

- Occasional lightheadedness or dizziness, especially when getting up quickly or when your blood sugar dips

- Nasal congestion and occasional nosebleeds; ear stuffiness

- Sensitive gums that may bleed when you brush

- Leg cramps

- Backache

- Achiness in the lower abdomen or along both or either sides

- Occasional, sudden sharp or shock-like sensations in the pelvic area (aka "lightning crotch")

- Mild swelling of ankles and feet, and occasionally of hands and face

- Varicose veins in legs and/or vulva

- Hemorrhoids

- Itchy belly

- Protruding navel (a popped-out belly button)

- Stretch marks

- Increasing shortness of breath as the uterus crowds the lungs

Your Body This Month

An interesting bit of pregnancy trivia: Measurement in centimeters from the top of your pubic bone to the top of your uterus roughly correlates with the number of weeks you're up to—so, at 34 weeks, your uterus measures close to 34 cm from the pubic bone.

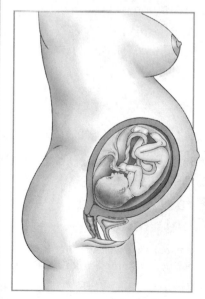

- Difficulty sleeping
- Increasing Braxton Hicks contractions (see question, below)
- Clumsiness
- Enlarged breasts
- Colostrum, leaking from nipples (though this premilk may not appear until after delivery)

Emotionally

- Increasing eagerness for the pregnancy to be over
- Apprehension about labor and delivery
- Increasing absentmindedness
- Jitters about becoming a parent
- Excitement—at the realization that it won't be long now

What You Can Expect at This Month's Checkup

After the 32nd week, your practitioner may ask you to come in every 2 weeks so your progress and your baby's can be more closely watched. You can probably expect the following:

- Weight and blood pressure
- Urine, for protein
- Fetal heartbeat
- Height of fundus (top of uterus)

- Size (you may get a rough weight estimate) and position of the fetus, by palpation (feeling from the outside)
- Feet and hands for swelling, and legs for varicose veins
- Group B strep culture at 35 to 37 weeks (see page 359)
- Symptoms you have been experiencing, especially unusual ones
- Questions and problems you want to discuss—have a list ready

What You May Be Wondering About

Braxton Hicks Contractions

"Every once in a while my uterus seems to bunch up and harden. What's going on?"

It's practicing. With delivery right around the corner, your body is warming up for the big day by flexing its

muscles—literally. Those uterine calisthenics you're feeling are called Braxton Hicks contractions—practice-for-labor contractions that usually begin sometime after the 20th week (though they're more noticeable in the last few months of pregnancy). They play a part in pumping up blood flow to the placenta (get ready), toning the muscles of the uterus (get set), and softening the cervix (go . . . soon). These rehearsal contractions (typically experienced earlier and with more intensity in second and subsequent pregnancies) feel like a tightening sensation that begins at the top of your uterus and then spreads downward, lasting from 15 to 30 seconds, though they can sometimes last as long as 2 minutes or more. If you check out your bump while you're having a Braxton Hicks, you might even be able to see what you're feeling: Your usually round belly might appear pointy or strangely bunched up. Weird to watch, but normal.

Though Braxton Hicks contractions are not true labor, they may be difficult to distinguish from real labor—especially as they become more intense, which they often do as pregnancy edges to a close. You may notice them more often when you've got a full bladder, if you're dehydrated, after sex, when you or baby are very active, or even when someone touches your belly. And though they're not efficient enough to deliver your baby (even when they get really uncomfortable), they may give you a leg up on labor by getting effacement and early dilation of the cervix started when the time is right.

To relieve any discomfort you may feel when you're getting a Braxton Hicks, try changing your position—lying down and relaxing if you've been on your feet, or getting up and walking around if you've been sitting. A warm bath may also help relieve discomfort. A drink of water may help, too. You can also use this labor rehearsal to practice your breathing exercises and the various other childbirth techniques you've learned, which can make the real contractions easier to deal with when they do arrive.

If the contractions don't subside with a change in activity, and if they become progressively stronger and more regular (especially if you feel pressure in your lower back), you may be in real labor, so be sure to put in a call to your practitioner. A good rule of thumb: If you have more than 4 Braxton Hicks in an hour, call your practitioner and let him or her know. If you're having a hard time distinguishing Braxton Hicks contractions from the real thing—especially if this is your first pregnancy and you've never experienced the real thing—give your practitioner a call, being sure to describe exactly what you're feeling.

Aching Ribs

"I keep feeling a dull achy pain on my side, near my rib cage—almost like my ribs are bruised. Is that because the baby is kicking me?"

It may be yet another in the long list of pregnancy pains that have been kicking you in the butt these days—but you can't blame baby's kicking for this pain in your ribs. No, those achy-breaky ribs are courtesy of pregnancy hormones, which have been loosening the joints in the area. In some moms-to-be this loosening causes the ribs to bow out (called subluxated ribs), to make room for expanded lungs (which need extra oxygen) and an ever-expanding uterus. You may also be feeling the ache because of inflammation of the cartilage attached to the ribs as they loosen and expand (and possibly because of the pressure placed on the ribs by your uterus or larger-than-usual breasts), or rarely, because of a dislocated rib (again, because of rib expansion to accommodate your pregnancy).

There is some relief in sight: Your ribs may feel less stretched—and less achy—during the last few weeks of pregnancy, when your baby moves down into position for birth—and of course once you deliver. Until then, keep the clothes you're wearing loose so you're not putting more pressure on those aching ribs, especially when you're sleeping (or trying to sleep). A pregnancy belly-support band can help to evenly distribute the weight of your growing belly, removing the strain off the muscles of the abdomen, which pull on the ribs and cause rib pain. Shifting positions may also lessen your discomfort, as may a warm bath or a heating pad placed over your clothes. Nothing working? Acetaminophen (Tylenol) can help ease the ache. And be sure to avoid heavy lifting, which can make it worse (and which you shouldn't be doing now anyway).

"Sometimes I get the feeling like my baby has jammed his feet up into my rib cage, and it hurts."

Occasionally, a baby will manage to wedge a foot into his mama's ribs—and that's one kind of rib tickling that doesn't tickle. You may be able to change baby's position by changing yours, or by bouncing on a birthing ball. Or, you can also try a gentle nudge or a few pelvic tilts to dislodge that little foot. Or try this mama move: Sit up straight and take a deep breath while you raise one arm over your head, then exhale while you drop your arm and repeat with the other arm. Baby's not budging, at least not for long? Sometimes the rib jamming becomes chronic, lasting until your little pain-in-the-ribs engages, or drops into your pelvis, which usually happens 2 or 3 weeks before delivery in first pregnancies (though often not until labor begins in subsequent ones).

Shortness of Breath

"Sometimes I have trouble breathing, even when I'm just sitting doing nothing. Does that mean my baby isn't getting enough oxygen?"

It's not surprising you're feeling a little spare on air these days. Your ever-expanding uterus is now crowding out all your other internal organs in an effort to provide spacious-enough accommodations for your ever-growing baby. Among those organs feeling the crunch are your lungs, which your uterus has compressed, limiting their ability to expand fully when you take a breath. This, teamed with the extra progesterone that has already been leaving you breathless for months, explains why a trip upstairs these days can make you feel as if you've just run a marathon (winded, big time). Fortunately, while this shortness of breath may feel uncomfortable to you, it doesn't bother your baby in the least. Your little one is kept well stocked with all the oxygen he or she needs through the placenta—no breathing, deep or otherwise, needed.

Some relief from that winded feeling usually arrives toward the end of pregnancy, when your baby drops into your pelvis in preparation for birth (in first pregnancies this generally occurs 2 to 3 weeks before delivery, in subsequent deliveries often not until labor begins). Until then, be sure to take it easy and slow down, decreasing the amount of work your lungs have to do. You may find it easier to breathe if you sit straight up instead of slumped over and sleep in a semi-propped position, bolstered by 2 or 3 pillows. When you're feeling especially breathless, lift your arms over your head to take pressure off your rib cage so you can breathe in more air. Try some breathing exercises as well: Breathe in slowly and deeply, making sure your rib cage—not your abdomen—is expanding (put your hands on the sides of your rib cage and make sure the ribs push out against your hands as you inhale deeply). Breathe out slowly and deeply, feeling the contraction of your rib cage. Return to this type

Choosing a Pediatrician

Choosing a pediatrician (or a family practitioner) is one of the most important decisions you'll make as a parent—and actually, one you shouldn't wait until you become a parent to make. Sifting through your choices and making your selection now, before your baby starts crying inexplicably at 3 a.m., will ensure that your transition to parenthood is that much easier. It will also allow for an informed—not rushed—decision.

If you're not sure where to begin your search, ask your practitioner for a referral (if you've been generally happy with the care you've been getting during pregnancy) or poll friends, neighbors, or coworkers who have young children for their favorite pediatricians. You can also look online for local pediatrician groups (though online listings of physicians are not always accurate) or local parent groups to ask for their recommendations. Or contact the hospital or birthing center where you'll be delivering (you can call the labor and delivery floor or pediatrics, and ask a nurse on duty for some suggestions—no one gets a better look at doctors than nurses do). Of course, if you're on a health insurance plan that limits your choices, you'll have to pick from that list.

Once you've narrowed your options to 2 or 3, call for consultations—most pediatricians or family practitioners will oblige. Bring a list of questions about issues that are important to you, such as office protocol (for instance, whether there are call-in hours for parents or when you can expect calls to be returned), breastfeeding support, circumcision, the use of antibiotics, whether the doctor handles all well-baby visits or if they're typically handled by nurse-practitioners in the practice. Also important to know: Is the doctor board certified? Which hospital is the doctor affiliated with, and will he or she be able to care for the newborn in the hospital? For more questions to ask and issues to consider, check out *What to Expect the First Year*.

of deep breathing whenever you feel a little breathless.

Sometimes breathlessness can be a sign that iron stores are low, so check in with your practitioner about it. Call 911 or head to the ER if shortness of breath is severe and accompanied by rapid breathing, blueness of the lips and fingertips, sweating, chest pain, and/or rapid pulse.

Morning Sickness, Again

"I've been feeling nauseous again recently, but I thought that was only a first trimester pregnancy symptom."

Feel like you've seen this movie before—and aren't happy to see a sequel? While first trimester morning sickness definitely gets more attention (and more expectant sufferers), for some mamas-to-be, the third trimester variety can cause just as much misery, sometimes even more. Especially discouraging if you thought you'd seen the last of that nausea and vomiting, at least in this pregnancy.

Remember those pregnancy hormones you blamed for your first trimester morning sickness? You can blame them again—along with your ever-growing uterus, which has been crowding out your digestive tract, causing stomach acids to bubble back up the esophagus, leading to reflux and a return of nausea. With less space to hold your meals and no easy way to digest them, extra food often has nowhere to go, other than up and out (another case for grazing on mini-meals). Braxton Hicks contractions can also unsettle your stomach, sometimes causing stomach cramps and even vomiting.

Try combating this pregnancy queasiness with the tips for early pregnancy morning sickness (see page 132) and heartburn (page 159). And be sure to stay hydrated—especially if you've been vomiting. Dehydration is never safe when you're expecting, but it's especially unsafe in late pregnancy, since dehydration can lead to preterm contractions.

Mention your queasiness to your practitioner, too. He or she might suggest antacids or anti-nausea meds if it's really bad. Your practitioner should also be able to rule out other, less likely reasons for this late-onset nausea and vomiting, including preeclampsia and preterm labor.

Lack of Bladder Control

"I watched a funny movie last night and noticed I was peeing myself a little every time I laughed. What is that about?"

It's called stress incontinence—appropriately, since it can really stress a mama out. This sudden, often inconvenient, and embarrassing loss of bladder control—which can cause you to spring a small leak when you cough, sneeze, lift something heavy, or even laugh (though there's nothing funny about that)—is the result of the mounting pressure of your growing uterus on your bladder. Some expectant moms also experience urge incontinence, the overwhelming, seemingly out-of-nowhere need to pee

(gotta go *now*!) during late pregnancy. Try these tips to help prevent or control stress or urge incontinence:

- Empty your bladder as completely as possible by leaning forward each time you pee.

- Practice your Kegels. Being faithful to your Kegels will help prevent or correct most cases of pregnancy-induced incontinence—plus, looking ahead, they'll also help prevent postpartum incontinence of both the urinary and fecal variety. For a Kegel how-to, see page 229.

- Do Kegels or cross your legs when you feel a cough, sneeze, or laugh coming on, or the urge to pee coming on.

- Wear a panty liner if you need one or you're afraid you'll need one. Graduate to a maxipad (or bladder control pad) when leaks might be especially inconvenient.

- Stay as regular as you can, because impacted stool can put pressure on the bladder. Also, straining hard when you're pooping can weaken pelvic floor muscles. For tips on fighting constipation, see page 185.

- If it's the urge that's driving you crazy (and always sending you to the bathroom in a hurry), try training your bladder. Urinate more frequently— about every 30 minutes to an hour— so that you go before you feel that uncontrollable need. After a week, try to gradually stretch the time between bathroom visits, adding 15 minutes more at a time.

- Continue drinking enough fluids, even if you experience stress incontinence or frequent urges. Limiting your fluid intake will not limit leaks, and it may lead to a UTI and/or dehydration. Not only can both of these lead to a lot of other problems (including preterm contractions), but UTIs can make stress and urge incontinence worse. See page 528 for tips on keeping your urinary tract healthy.

To be sure that the leak you've sprung is urine (which it almost certainly is) and not amniotic fluid, it's smart to give it the sniff test. If the liquid that has leaked doesn't smell like urine (urine smells ammonia-like, while amniotic fluid has a sweet smell), let your practitioner know as soon as possible.

How You're Carrying

"Everyone says I seem to be carrying small for the 8th month. My midwife says everything's fine, but is it possible my baby's not growing as fast as she should?"

The truth is, you can't tell a baby by her mom's belly. How you're carrying has much less to do with the size of your baby and much more to do with these factors:

- Your own size, shape, and bone structure. Bumps come in all sizes, just like expectant moms do. A petite mom may carry more compactly (small, low, and out in front) than a larger mom—or she may seem to be carrying "larger" in comparison to her slighter scale. A bigger-boned mom may have less to show bump-wise, simply because there's more area for her uterus and her baby to spread out in. Same for some very obese women—with so much room in an already ample abdomen, these moms-to-be may never seem to "pop" at all.

- Your muscle tone. A mom-to-be with very tight muscles may not show as soon or as much as one whose muscles are slacker. For that reason, and because each baby tends to end up a little larger than the last, second- and

---

Oh, My Aching Pelvic Bones

Does your pelvis sometimes feel as if it's coming apart at the seams— with wrenching pain in the pubic area (or in the perineum or upper thighs) that makes walking agonizing and climbing stairs or getting in and out of the car excruciating? You may have what's called pelvic girdle pain or symphysis pubis dysfunction—a surprisingly common and unexpectedly painful condition that affects up to 25 percent of moms-to-be, usually late in the last trimester, as ligaments that normally keep the pelvic bone aligned become over-relaxed and stretchy in preparation for labor. To find out how to deal with this often debilitating pain, see page 561.

---

more-time moms tend to end up a bit larger, too.

- Your baby's position. How your fetus is positioned on the inside may also affect how big or small you look on the outside.

- Your weight gain. A bigger weight gain doesn't necessarily predict a bigger baby, just a bigger mom. If you've kept your weight gain within recommended guidelines, you may appear smaller because you're sporting less fat, not because you're carrying less baby.

The only assessments of a baby's size that are worth paying attention to are the ones you get from your practitioner—not the ones you get from your sister-in-law, your coworkers, social media buddies commenting on your bump selfies, or know-it-all nosey-bodies in the supermarket checkout line.

The Gender Guessing Game

All belly and glowing skin? You're having a boy. Spreading hips, nose, and zits? It's a baby girl on board. If you've opted out of the gender reveal, you've probably generated plenty of predictions on your baby's sex based entirely on how you're carrying, how you're feeling, and how you're looking. Just remember that those predictions—by old wives or others—have about a 50 percent chance of coming true. (Actually, a little better than that if a boy is predicted, since 105 boys are born for every 100 girls.)

In other words, keep them guessing.

In other words, it's what's inside that counts—and apparently, what's inside your little bump is a baby who's plenty big enough.

Your Size and Your Delivery

"I'm tiny, just 5 feet tall—and I'm wondering whether that'll make it harder for me to deliver vaginally."

Size matters when it comes to birthing your baby—but inside size, not outside size. It's the internal numbers—the size and shape of your pelvis in relation to the size of your baby's head—that determine how difficult (or easy) your labor will be, not your height or your build. A petite mom can have a roomier (or more accommodatingly configured) pelvis than a plus-size mom—or she can have a baby with an easier-to-fit head.

How will you know what size your pelvis is (after all, it doesn't come labeled)? Your practitioner can make an educated guess about its size, usually using rough measurements taken at your first prenatal exam. Your baby's size will be approximated, too, as your due date approaches. If there's some concern that your baby's head is too large to fit through your pelvis, ultrasound may be used to get a better view (and measurement).

Of course, in general, the overall size of the pelvis, as of all bony structures, is smaller in people of smaller stature. But that's the genius of genetics: Nature doesn't typically present a tiny mom with giant offspring. Instead, babies are usually pretty well matched to mom's size and the size of her pelvis—even if they are destined for bigger things later on. And chances are, your baby will be just the right size for you.

Your Weight Gain and the Baby's Size

"I've gained so much weight that I'm afraid my baby will be huge and hard to deliver."

Just because you've gained a lot of weight doesn't necessarily mean your baby has. Your baby's weight is determined by a number of variables: genetics, your own birthweight (if you were born large, your baby is more likely to be, too), your prepregnancy weight (heavier women tend to have heavier babies), and the quality of your pregnancy diet. Depending on those variables, a 35- to 40-pound weight gain can yield a 6- or 7-pound baby and a 25-pound weight gain can net an 8-pounder. On average, however, the more substantial the weight gain, the bigger the baby. Moms who have GD that isn't well controlled may also be more likely to have a very large baby.

By palpating your abdomen and measuring the height of your fundus (the top of the uterus), your practitioner will be able to give you some idea of your baby's size, though such guesstimates can be off by a pound or more. An ultrasound can gauge size more accurately, but it may be off the mark, too.

Even if your baby does turn out to be on the big side, that doesn't automatically predict a difficult delivery. Though a 7-pound baby often makes its way out faster than a 10-pounder, most women are able to deliver a large baby (or even an extra-large baby) vaginally and without complications. The determining factor, as in any delivery, is whether your baby's head (the largest part) can fit through your pelvis.

Baby's Position

"How can I tell which way my baby is facing? I want to make sure he's the right way for delivery."

Playing "name that bump" (trying to figure out which are shoulders, elbows, bottom) may be endlessly entertaining, but it's not the most accurate way of figuring out your baby's position. Your practitioner will be able to give you a better idea by palpating your abdomen for recognizable baby parts. The location of the baby's heartbeat is another clue to its position: If the baby's presentation is head first, the heartbeat will usually be heard in the lower half of your abdomen—and it will be loudest if the baby's back is toward your front. If there's still some doubt, an ultrasound offers the most reliable view of your baby's position.

Still can't resist a round of your favorite evening pastime (or resist patting those round little parts)? Play away—and to make the game more interesting (and to help clue you in), try looking for these markers next time:

- Baby's back is usually a smooth, convex contour opposite a bunch of little irregularities, which are the "small parts"—hands, feet, elbows.

- Sometime around the 8th month, baby's head usually settles near mom's pelvis—it is round, firm, and when pushed down bounces back without the rest of the body moving.

- Baby's bottom is a less regular shape, and softer, than the head.

Bottoms up—hopefully!

Breech Baby

"At my last prenatal visit, my doctor said he felt my baby's head up near my ribs. Does that mean she's breech?"

Even as her accommodations become ever more cramped, your baby will still manage to perform some pretty remarkable gymnastics during the last weeks of her stay. In fact, although most fetuses settle into a head-down position between weeks 32 and 38 (breech presentations occur in fewer than 5 percent of full term pregnancies), some don't let on which end will ultimately be up until a few days before birth. Which means that just because your baby is bottoms down now doesn't mean she will be breech when it comes time for delivery.

What if your baby does stubbornly remain breech as delivery approaches? Keep reading to find out.

"If my baby is breech, can anything be done to turn him?"

There are several ways to try to coax a bottoms-down baby bottoms up. On the low-tech side, your practitioner may recommend simple exercises (like

Face Forward

It's not just up or down that's important when it comes to your baby's position—it's also front or back. If baby's facing your back, chin tucked onto chest (as most babies end up), you're in luck. This so-called occiput anterior position is ideal for birth, because your baby's head is lined up to fit through your pelvis as easily and comfortably as possible, smallest head part first. If baby's facing your tummy (called occiput posterior, but also known by the much cuter term "sunny-side up"), it's a setup for back labor (see page 401), because his or her skull will be pressing on your spine. It also means your baby's exit might take a little longer.

As delivery day approaches, your practitioner will try to determine which way (front or back) your baby's head is facing—but if you're in a hurry to find out, you can look for these clues: When your baby is occiput anterior (face toward your back), your belly will feel hard and smooth (that's your baby's back). If your little one is posterior, your tummy may look flatter and softer because your baby's arms and legs are facing forward, so there's no hard, smooth back to feel.

Do you think—or have you been told—that your baby is posterior? Don't worry about back labor yet. Most babies turn accommodatingly to the anterior position during labor. Some midwives recommend giving baby a nudge before labor begins by getting on all fours and doing pelvic rocks. Others suggest placing warm towels on mom's back and cold ones on her tummy because babies naturally turn away from cold. These tactics can also be tried during labor. Whether they can successfully flip a baby is unclear, but they can't hurt. And who knows—they could help relieve any back pain you have now.

---

the ones described in the box on page 350). Two other options come from the CAM camp. One is moxibustion (see page 79), which uses a form of acupuncture and burning herbs to help turn a fetus (although, studies show, with a low success rate). The other is the Webster technique (as well as other chiropractic maneuvers; see page 79). Clearly, it's important to use a CAM practitioner who is experienced and has had plenty of success using these therapies to turn breech babies, and to make sure your practitioner is on board with the therapy you're considering.

If your baby seems determined not to budge, your practitioner may suggest a somewhat higher-tech yet hands-on approach to manipulating your baby into the coveted heads-down position: external cephalic version (ECV). ECV is usually performed around weeks 36 to 38 or very early in labor when the uterus is still relatively relaxed and before mom's membranes have ruptured. It's always done in a hospital, in case an emergency c-section is needed (which happens rarely). Since an ample amount of amniotic fluid is necessary to help facilitate a safe ECV, levels are checked first via ultrasound. Ultrasound may also be used to guide the doctor during ECV, and baby's heart rate will be watched with an electronic fetal monitor to make sure he's doing well before and after the procedure. Medication may be given to prevent contractions, so the uterus stays relaxed, and you may also get an epidural (which not only prevents any pain but also keeps the uterus relaxed, apparently boosting the odds of ECV success). Your practitioner will apply his or her hands to your abdomen, one near baby's head, one near baby's bottom (you'll feel some pressure, and possibly some discomfort, though not if you've had an epidural) and try to gently turn your little one around.

ECV is successful in nearly two-thirds of attempts. The success rate is even higher for those who have an epidural as well as those who have delivered before (thanks to those more lax uterine and abdominal muscles), but it's slightly lower for obese women, since abdominal padding can make maneuvering baby more challenging. The more experience a doctor has in turning babies, the better the success rate generally is (some doctors have a rate as high as 90 percent). And happily the complications rate is low across the board (less than 1 percent for serious complications that might lead to an emergency c-section). Some babies refuse to turn at all (though often a doctor will suggest multiple attempts), and a small number of contrary fetuses turn and then flip back into a breech position (in which case, your doctor might also suggest trying again).

Having multiples? You're most likely not a candidate for ECV. Ditto if you had a prior c-section.

"If my baby stays in a breech position, will I still be able to try for a vaginal birth?"

Whether you'll be able to give vaginal birth a chance will depend on a variety of factors, including your practitioner's policy and your situation. Most obs routinely perform a c-section when a baby refuses to budge out of a breech position, because many studies have suggested it's a safer way to go. There are some doctors and midwives, however, who feel it's reasonable to attempt a vaginal delivery in certain circumstances, especially if they're experienced delivering breech babies vaginally. The best-case circumstance: when a baby is in a frank breech position (buttocks first, with legs straight up and flat against his or her face) and it's clear that mom's pelvis is roomy enough to accommodate a vaginal delivery.

The bottom line if your baby remains bottom down: You'll need to be flexible in your childbirth plans. Even if your practitioner green-lights a trial of labor, it's just that—a trial. If your breech baby doesn't move down the birth canal, or if other problems come up, you'll likely wind up having a c-section. Talk the options over with your practitioner now so you'll be prepared for any possibility come delivery day.

Other Unusual Presentations

"My doctor said that my baby's in an oblique position. What's that, and what does it mean for delivery?"

Babies can squirm their way into all kinds of unusual positions, and oblique is one of them. What this means is that your baby's head (though down) is pointed toward one of your hips, rather than squarely on your cervix. An oblique position makes a vaginal exit difficult, so your practitioner might do ECV (see facing page) or suggest other techniques to try to coax your baby's head straight down. If none of those work (even after multiple attempts), he or she will probably opt for a c-section.

Turn, Baby, Turn

Some practitioners recommend simple exercises to help turn a breech baby into a delivery-friendly, heads-down position. Though there isn't much medical evidence to prove they work, they're probably worth a shot. Ask your practitioner if you should be trying any of these baby-moving moves at home:

- Rock back and forth a few times on your hands and knees several times a day, with your buttocks higher than your head (see illustration, top right).

- Forward-leaning inverse. Have someone help you with this position: Kneel on the edge of a couch and carefully lower yourself to your hands on the floor and then lower yourself to your forearms, head propped on your arms or hanging freely (see illustration, below). Take 3 breaths, then return to a kneeling position. (Do this 3 or 4 times a day.)

- Knee-to-chest position. If you're alone (with no one around to spot you for safety's sake), you can do a modified version of the forward-leaning inverse: Get on your knees (keep them slightly apart), and then bend over so your butt's up and your belly's almost touching the floor (stay in that position for 20 minutes 3 times a day if you can, for best results); see illustration, middle right.

- Breech pelvic tilts. Lie on your back on a mat or carpeted surface, then lift your hips off the floor (use your heels to push your lower body up), keeping your hands, arms, and shoulders flat on the floor. The idea is to get your hips above your head (see illustration, bottom right). Not feeling the

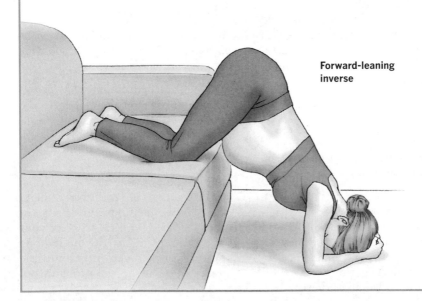

Forward-leaning inverse

pelvic tilt? For a simpler version, lie on your back and prop up your hips with pillows.

- Hot and cold. Put a cold pack (or a bag of frozen vegetables) on the top of your belly where your baby's head is and place a warm compress on your lower belly (or submerge your lower half in a warm tub). Some say

this will encourage baby to seek the warmth and move his or her head away from the cold sensation.

- Music to baby's ears. Playing soothing music or singing near mom's pelvis may coax a baby to flip for a better listen. Again, no proof it works, but certainly no harm trying.

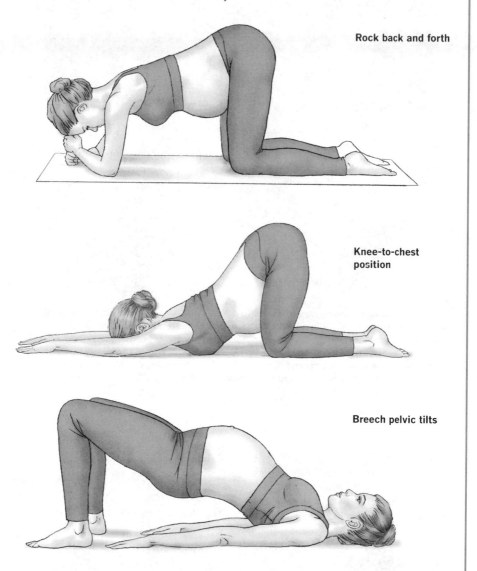

Rock back and forth

Knee-to-chest position

Breech pelvic tilts

How Does Your Baby Lie?

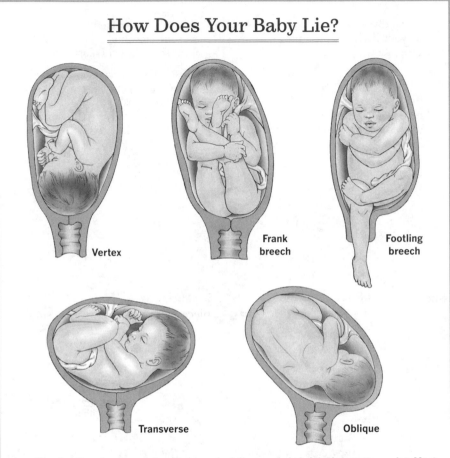

Vertex

Frank
breech

Footling
breech

Transverse

Oblique

Location, location, location—when it comes to delivery, a baby's location matters a lot. Most babies present head first, or in a vertex position. Breech presentations can come in many forms: A frank breech is when the baby is buttocks first, with his or her legs facing straight up and flat against the face. A footling breech is when one or both of the legs are pointing down. During labor, the first presenting part is baby's foot and leg. A transverse lie is when the baby is lying sideways in the uterus. An oblique lie is when the baby's head is pointing toward mom's hip instead of toward the cervix.

Yet another tight spot a baby can get into is a transverse position. This is when your baby's lying sideways, across your uterus, instead of vertically. Again, an ECV or other techniques will be done to try to turn baby up and down. If that doesn't work, your baby will be delivered via cesarean.

Cesarean Delivery

"I was hoping for a vaginal birth, but my doctor just told me I'll probably have to have a c-section. I'm really disappointed."

Even though it's still considered major surgery (and by far the happiest kind), a cesarean is a very safe way to deliver, and in some cases, the safest way. It's also a pretty common way—and in the view of many experts, too common. About 32 percent of women are having c-sections these days, which means the chances that your baby will end up arriving via the surgical route are just under 1 in 3, even if you don't have any predisposing factors.

That said, if you had your heart set on a vaginal delivery, the news that your baby may need to arrive surgically instead can be understandably disappointing. Visions of pushing your baby out the way nature intended—and perhaps the way you'd always pictured—can be displaced by concerns about the surgery, about being stuck in the hospital longer, about the tougher recovery, and about the scar that comes standard issue.

First, make sure you've had a discussion with your practitioner about why a cesarean delivery might be necessary in your case (see box, page 354, for reasons why it might be). Ask if there are potential options that can be tried, like attempting to turn your breech baby or doing a trial of labor to see how things progress. If ultimately your practitioner determines that your baby's safest exit strategy is through your abdomen, then consider the following: Most hospitals now strive to make a cesarean delivery as family friendly as possible, with mom awake (but appropriately numb), dad by her side, and a chance to meet, greet, cuddle, and possibly breastfeed baby right after delivery if there's no medical reason why not. In fact, a growing number of hospitals now offer (or may be open to facilitating) a "gentle cesarean." In a gentle cesarean, noise is kept to a minimum and clear drapes are set up so mom can watch as her baby emerges (an option in some hospitals: a drape with a built-in portal so baby can be handed directly to mom without compromising the sterile surgical environment).

EKG electrodes are placed toward mom's back so there's room for baby to snuggle on her chest, and one arm is left free of cuffs, monitors, and IVs so she can hold her freshly delivered baby and even breastfeed. Cord clamping is delayed, as it ideally is in a vaginal birth (see page 416). Have a doula (or a midwife who has cared for you during your pregnancy)? You may be able to invite her into the OR, too.

In other words, a surgical birth experience may be more satisfying (and less disappointing) than you're imagining. And while the recovery will be longer (in hospital and out) and the scar unavoidable (though usually placed unobtrusively), you'll also be delivering with your perineum intact and your vaginal muscles unstretched. One more piece of good news: Studies show that having a c-section doesn't negatively impact your future fertility or how many babies you can have (see page 357). And there's an upside for baby that's purely cosmetic—and temporary. Because there's no tight squeeze through the birth canal, he or she will have an initial edge in appearance over vaginally delivered babies (think round head, not pointy).

But by far the most important thing to keep in mind as your baby's arrival approaches: The best birth is the one that's safest—and when it's definitely medically necessary, a cesarean birth is definitely safest. And after all, any delivery that brings a healthy baby into the world and into your arms is a perfect delivery.

"Why does it seem everyone is having c-sections these days?"

There has actually been quite a push to lower the rate of cesarean delivery in the U.S. Experts are encouraging more trials of labor to promote

Reasons for a Scheduled C

While some women won't find out whether they're having a c-section until they're well into labor, others will get the heads-up ahead of time—joining the ranks of moms-to-be who are scheduled for a cesarean delivery. Though the following don't automatically mean you'll need a c-section, these are the most common reasons why one might be scheduled in advance:

- A previous c-section, when VBAC is not an option (see page 357).

- When a fetus's head is estimated to be too large to fit through mom's pelvis (cephalopelvic disproportion). But since a baby's size can be overestimated, attempting a trial of labor may be possible first (baby may fit more easily than believed).

- Higher-order multiples. Almost all triplets, quads, and more (and many twins) are delivered by c-section.

- Breech or other unusual presentation. Studies show that a cesarean delivery is usually safest when efforts to turn a breech baby haven't succeeded. Many midwives and some doctors may attempt a vaginal breech birth in some circumstances (see page 348).

- A condition in mom or baby that may make labor and vaginal delivery risky.

- Obesity in mom. Obesity increases the odds of a c-section for several reasons. For one, obese moms tend to have ineffective contractions in early labor, which means they don't make progress as quickly. For another, extra abdominal padding makes it harder to monitor a baby during a vaginal delivery. Another factor: Both ECV (to turn a breech baby to a vaginal delivery-friendly position) and VBAC are less successful in obese moms than in average-weight moms. And finally, obese moms often have larger-than-average babies, making cesarean deliveries a safer bet in many (but not all) cases.

- An active herpes infection, especially a primary one, or poorly controlled HIV infection that can be transmitted to the baby during a vaginal delivery.

- Placenta previa (when the placenta partially or completely blocks the cervical opening) or placental abruption (when the placenta separates from the uterine wall too soon).

If your practitioner says you'll need a scheduled c-section, ask for a detailed explanation of the reason (or reasons) why. Ask, too, if any alternatives, such as a trial of labor, are open to you.

---

vaginal birth after prior cesarean delivery (VBACs; see page 357) and more widespread use of vacuum and forceps delivery to prevent unnecessary surgical deliveries. They're also suggesting that moms be given more time to labor and to push and/or that doctors use Pitocin as needed to nudge nature along (assuming all is going well) before they move on to a c-section. Finally, there's a growing recognition that

while c-sections are very safe, they're still major surgery, which comes with greater risk (including that a mom will end up needing a repeat next time). In other words, experts agree: C-sections shouldn't be the delivery of choice, at least when there is a choice.

Still, while rates of c-section have declined about 2 percent over the last few years, and even a little more among low-risk moms, the numbers are still very high and in the minds of many (including most doctors), too high. Why? There are a number of reasons:

Bigger babies. With more expectant moms exceeding the recommended weight gain of 25 to 35 pounds, and with the rate of GD increasing, more large babies, who may be more difficult to deliver vaginally, are arriving. A wrinkle: Since estimates of a baby's birthweight based on ultrasound measurements can be unreliable (in about 20 percent of cases, estimates are high), a baby who's predicted to be too large to deliver vaginally may end up not so big after all. These over-estimates sometimes result in unnecessary scheduled c-sections.

Bigger moms. The c-section rate has also risen with the obesity rate. Being obese (or gaining too much weight during pregnancy) significantly increases a woman's chance of needing a c-section, partly because of other risk factors that accompany obesity (diabetes, for instance, or hypertension), partly because obese women tend to have longer labors, and longer labors are more likely to end up on the operating table.

Older mothers. More and more women in their late 30s (and well into their 40s) are now able to have successful pregnancies, and though their rates of c-sections have been dropping, older moms are still more likely to require a surgical delivery. The same is true of women with chronic health problems.

Multiples. More and more multiples are being born these days, and there's a higher chance of delivering via cesarean if you're birthing multiple babies (though a vaginal birth with twins is often possible; see page 455).

Repeat c-sections. Though VBAC is still considered a viable option in many

> # C-Section Decision During Labor
>
> Often the decision to perform a c-section is made only once labor is well under way—and it's usually to ensure the safety of the mom and her baby. Sometimes it's because labor fails to progress (the cervix isn't dilating, even after attempts have been made to give sluggish contractions a boost with oxytocin, or it's taking too long to push the baby out, and delivery with vacuum extractor or forceps has failed or isn't appropriate). Sometimes it's because there's fetal distress (the baby's heart rate has plummeted to a dangerously low level), or because the uterus has ruptured, or because of a prolapsed umbilical cord (when the cord slips out the birth canal before the baby does, running the risk of being compressed and depriving the baby of oxygen). As always, the safety of both mom and baby will be the prime consideration in whether to turn to a surgical delivery.

cases, and though more and more experts are encouraging VBACs, fewer doctors and hospitals are allowing moms to try one, and more are scheduling surgeries instead of attempting a trial of labor (see page 357 for reasons why).

Fewer instrumental deliveries. Fewer babies are being born with the help of vacuum extraction and even fewer with forceps. That's largely because training in these instrumental deliveries dropped off as c-section rates took off—so many doctors feel more comfortable going straight for the surgical option, when they might have (back in

Prepping for a C-Section

Wondering if your partner's scheduled c-section means your coaching days are over—even before they've started? No, not at all. While you won't be able to pitch in quite as actively during a surgical delivery as you would during a vaginal birth, your coaching will still be more valuable than you might think. A dad's reaction at a cesarean delivery can actually have an impact on mom's level of anxiety—meaning, a less-stressed father contributes greatly to a less-stressed mother. And there's no better way to reduce your stress than knowing what to expect. So sign up together for a childbirth education class that includes c-sections in the curriculum, read up on surgical deliveries and recoveries (see page 438 and 473), and get as prepped as you can. Be prepared to help her through breathing and relaxing techniques so she stays calm during

the c-section, and remember that you'll be by her side to support her as you both welcome your baby into this world.

Any kind of surgery can seem like a scary proposition, but c-sections are extremely safe for both mom and baby. Plus, most hospitals now strive to make them as family friendly as possible, allowing you to watch if you want to (either by lowering the drape or using a clear drape), sit by your spouse's side, hold her hand (which, in most hospitals will not be strapped down), and hold and cuddle the baby right after birth—just like the couples delivering vaginally down the hall. If the hospital where you'll be delivering doesn't officially offer a "gentle cesarean" policy (see page 353), it definitely doesn't hurt to ask the doctor and hospital staff whether some or all of the measures can be applied at your baby's birth.

the day) routinely tried an instrument-assisted birth first. This may change as ob training begins to reflect changing attitudes about these delivery options.

Requests by moms. Since cesarean deliveries are safe and can prevent the pain of labor while keeping the perineum neatly intact, some women (particularly those who've had a c-section before) still prefer them to vaginal deliveries and actually ask ahead for one (see page 359). These numbers are dropping, however, especially as many practitioners have begun discouraging medically unnecessary c-sections. That's because unnecessary c-sections come with unnecessary risks, while vaginal deliveries—when they're possible—are safer, especially for mom.

Time limits in labor. Some doctors put time limits on how long labor should last—how long it "should" take for the cervix to dilate, for instance, or how long a mom "should" push. When artificial time limits are placed on the length of labor, doctors may proceed to a surgical delivery before giving the laboring mom (and her baby) a fair chance to progress. See the box on page 424 for more on these time limits. Happily there are now strong efforts under way to change the recommendations on how long to let a mom labor and push before resorting to a c-section (assuming everything is still proceeding safely)—and that's a "push" that may do a lot to help bring the rate of cesarean deliveries down. Another change that may push c-section rates down:

having moms stays at home a little longer. Moms who show up at the hospital very early in labor may be somewhat more likely to end up having a c-section.

C-section rates are much lower for patients of midwives, not only because midwives attend only low-risk births, but because they tend to let moms take their time with labor and delivery (again, assuming all is well). But even with c-section rates as high as they are these days for doctor-attended births, keep in mind that surgical deliveries still comprise the minority of births. After all, 2 out of 3 women can expect to deliver their babies vaginally.

Repeat Cesareans

"I've had two c-sections and want to go for my third—and maybe my fourth. Is there a limit on how many c-sections you can have?"

Thinking of having lots of babies—but not sure whether you'll be allowed to make multiple trips to the hospital's happiest operating room? Chances are, you'll be able to. There are no arbitrary limits placed on the number of cesarean deliveries a woman can undergo, and having numerous c-sections is generally considered a safe option. Just how safe depends on the type of incision made during the previous surgeries, as well as on the scars that form after the procedures, so discuss the particulars of your case with your ob.

Depending on how many incisions you've had, where you've had them, and how they've healed, multiple c-sections can put you at higher risk for certain complications. These include uterine rupture, placenta previa (a low-lying placenta), and placenta accreta (an abnormally attached placenta). So you'll need to be particularly alert for any

---

Scheduled Classes for Scheduled C's

Think a scheduled c-section means you won't have to schedule childbirth classes—or that you should drop out of the ones you signed up for? Not so fast. Childbirth education classes still have plenty to offer you and your partner (including plenty on what to expect with a c-section—and with an epidural). Most classes also offer invaluable advice on taking care of your newborn (which you'll have to master no matter which exit your baby takes), breastfeeding, and possibly getting back into shape postpartum. And don't tune out when the teacher's going over the labor breathing routine with the other couples. You might find those skills come in handy when you're trying to stay relaxed in the OR—or after delivery, when you're confronted with both post-op pain and assorted postpartum aches.

---

bright red bleeding during your pregnancies, as well as the signs of oncoming labor (contractions, bloody show, your water breaking). If any of these occur, notify your practitioner right away.

Vaginal Birth After Cesarean (VBAC)

"I had a cesarean delivery with my first baby. Should I try for a vaginal delivery now that I'm expecting baby number 2?"

If you asked the experts, the answer to your question would probably be yes. In fact, ACOG guidelines say that attempting a VBAC (pronounced vee-back) is both a safe and appropriate choice for most women who had a prior cesarean delivery (or even 2, in some cases). Research shows that the very low risk of uterine rupture (less than 1 percent) is only elevated during VBAC under certain less common circumstances (see below). What's more, VBAC attempts are successful a full two-thirds of the time—meaning that a mom who tries VBAC is just as likely to end up with a vaginal delivery as a mom who never had a c-section.

Yet, with all the mounting evidence—and all the experts—backing up VBAC, many doctors and hospitals won't even consider a vaginal delivery for a mom who has already had a c-section. More than 90 percent of women eligible for trying VBAC end up having a scheduled cesarean delivery instead.

Why are VBAC rates so low? The answer lies more in hospital policies and high malpractice insurance rates than in the safety of VBAC. Some hospitals have stopped offering VBACs because of safety and liability concerns and a shortage of staff and resources to handle emergencies.

That said, there are still plenty of hospitals and doctors, some birthing centers, and many midwives who are open to (and enthusiastically encourage) VBACs. So your first step, if you do decide you'd like to attempt a VBAC, is to find a practitioner who is open to it. And then, taking into account the many factors that are predictive of a successful VBAC, you and your practitioner can decide whether it's the best choice in your case. Here are a few of those factors:

VBAC is recommended only if labor starts spontaneously. If you have to be induced (especially with prostaglandins), VBAC is generally not considered an option. That's because induction (and the stronger contractions it triggers) ups the risk of uterine rupture.

VBAC is recommended only if you have a low-transverse uterine scar. And there's over a 90 percent chance that you do. Vertical uterine incisions (which are more likely to result in a uterine rupture and usually take VBAC off the table) are rarely used.

VBAC is more likely to succeed if the reason for your last c-section no longer exists. For instance, if you had a c-section because of something unique to your previous pregnancy that isn't affecting your current pregnancy—maybe your baby was breech last time but is head-down this time—then a successful VBAC becomes more likely. On the other hand, if you needed a c-section because the size or shape of your pelvis led to an especially slow or stalled labor the first time around, you may encounter the same problem the next time you try to deliver vaginally, making the chances of successful VBAC lower.

VBAC is more likely to succeed if you start out pregnancy at a healthy weight and if you kept your pregnancy weight gain on target. Research shows that VBAC success is 40 percent lower among women who gained more than 40 pounds during pregnancy compared to women who gained less than that. Overweight and obese women who attempt VBACs are also less likely to successfully deliver vaginally in general, even after accounting for baby's larger size (a large baby is more common in overweight women).

VBAC is more likely to succeed if your baby is average size. Research shows that the chance of VBAC failure is 50 percent higher when babies weigh more than 8 pounds 13 ounces at delivery, compared to babies weighing less than 7 pounds 11 ounces. A large baby may also increase the risk of uterine rupture and perineal tears—which is one reason why some doctors won't perform a VBAC on a mom who's more than a week past her due date (older babies may be larger babies). Second and subsequent babies are, on average, larger than first babies—still, having a too-large-to-fit baby before doesn't mean you'll definitely have one this time.

VBAC can be an excellent choice if you've had a vaginal birth before. Research suggests that if you've already delivered a baby vaginally before having one or more by c-section, your likelihood of having a safe and successful VBAC is greater than 90 percent.

If, despite best efforts, you end up having a repeat c-section instead of a VBAC, try not to be disappointed. Remember that even a mom who has never had a cesarean delivery before has a nearly 1 in 3 chance of having one. No regrets, either, if you decide ahead of delivery (in consultation with your practitioner) that you'd rather schedule an elective repeat c-section than attempt VBAC. Again, what's best for your baby—and best for you—is what matters.

"My ob is encouraging me to try for a VBAC, but I'm not sure why I should bother going through labor when I might end up needing a c-section anyway."

Your feelings definitely factor in to the decision of whether or not to give VBAC a chance. Still, your ob has a point. The risks of VBAC are very low, while a c-section, after all, is still major surgery. A vaginal birth means a shorter hospital stay, a lower risk of infection, and a faster recovery—all good reasons to consider VBAC. What's more, if you were hoping to get an epidural during labor, you still can—even if a VBAC is in the works. There are even perks for baby if you give labor a try (see box, this page).

Elective Cesareans

Considering a scheduled cesarean that's not medically necessary (or opting out of a trial of labor)? Here's something to consider first: The best time for your baby to arrive is when he or she is ready. When an elective delivery is planned, there's the possibility that baby will inadvertently be born too soon (particularly if the dates are off to begin with). Another potential perk for your baby if you elect to let labor take its course (or try VBAC instead of scheduling a repeat cesarean delivery): There's evidence to suggest that babies who have gone through at least some labor have fewer health problems than those who never did—even if mom ultimately ends up with a medically necessary c-section.

The best strategy: Weigh the pros and cons of VBAC, factor in your feelings, and then make the decision that feels right for you—whether it's to give labor a try or head straight for the OR—without regret.

Group B Strep

"My doctor is going to test me for group B strep infection. What does this mean?"

It means that your doctor's playing it safe, and when it comes to group B strep, safe is a very good way to play it.

Group B strep (GBS) is a strain of bacteria that lives quietly in the vaginas of between 10 and 35 percent of healthy women—which makes them "carriers" of GBS (or GBS-positive). That's no problem for them, since being GBS-positive doesn't cause symptoms of any kind (and it isn't related to group A

Lifesaving Screenings for Newborns

Most babies are born healthy and stay that way. But a very small percentage of infants are born apparently healthy and then suddenly sicken due to a metabolic disorder. Though most of these conditions are very rare, they can be life-threatening if they go undetected and untreated. Testing for these and other metabolic disorders is inexpensive, and in the very unlikely event that your baby tests positive for any of them, the pediatrician can verify the results and begin treatment immediately—which can make a tremendous difference in the prognosis.

Luckily, there are ways to screen for such metabolic disorders. Drops of blood, taken routinely from an infant's heel after birth, are used to test for 21 (or more) serious genetic, metabolic, hormonal, and functional disorders, including PKU, hypothyroidism, congenital adrenal hyperplasia, biotinidase deficiency, maple syrup urine disease, galactosemia, homocystinuria, medium-chain acyl-CoA dehydrogenase deficiency, and sickle cell anemia.

All 50 states and the District of Columbia require newborn screening for at least 21 disorders, and more than half of all states screen newborns for all 29 disorders for which the American College of Medical Genetics (ACMG) recommends testing.

Check with your practitioner or your local board of health to find out what tests are done in your state. You can also look up your state's requirements at the National Newborn Screening & Genetics Resource Center's (NNSGRC) website: genes-r-us.uthscsa.edu. If your hospital doesn't automatically provide all 29 tests, you can arrange to have them done. For more information about newborn screening, check with the March of Dimes: marchofdimes.com.

The CDC also recommends, and some states require, screening tests soon after birth for congenital heart disease (CHD). This condition, which affects 1 in 100 babies, can lead to disability or death if not caught and treated early. Happily, when a baby gets a diagnosis early and is treated early, those risks are reduced significantly—and in most cases, completely. Screening for CHD is simple and painless: A sensor is placed on your baby's skin to measure your little one's pulse and the amount of oxygen in his or her blood. If the results of the screening test seem questionable, the doctor will be able to do further testing (echocardiogram—an ultrasound of the heart, for instance) to determine if anything is wrong. If your state doesn't require the test, ask the pediatrician if it could be given to your baby anyway.

strep, the kind that causes throat infections), but it can be a problem for their babies. That's because a baby who picks up GBS when exiting a mom's vagina is at risk of developing a serious infection—about 1 in every 200 babies born to GBS-positive mothers will.

And that's why expectant moms are routinely tested for GBS—usually between 35 and 37 weeks (testing

before 35 weeks isn't accurate in predicting who will be carrying GBS at the time of delivery). Some hospitals and birthing centers offer a rapid GBS test that can screen women during labor and provide results within the hour, taking the place of the screen routinely done between weeks 35 and 37. Ask your practitioner if that's an option at the facility where you'll be delivering.

How's the test done? It's performed using vaginal and rectal swabs. If you test positive (meaning you're a carrier), you'll be given IV antibiotics during labor—and this treatment virtually eliminates any risk to your baby. (GBS can also show up in a urine culture obtained at a prenatal checkup. If it does, it'll be treated right away with oral antibiotics and again in labor with IV antibiotics.)

If your practitioner doesn't offer the GBS test during late pregnancy, you should request it. Even if you weren't tested but end up in labor with certain risk factors that point to GBS (like preterm labor, a fever during labor, or water breaking more than 18 hours before delivery), your practitioner will just treat you with IV antibiotics to be sure you don't pass any infection you might have on to your baby. If you've previously delivered a baby with GBS, your practitioner may also skip the test and proceed straight to treatment during labor.

Playing it safe through testing—and, if necessary, treatment—means that your baby will be protected from a GBS infection. And that's a very good thing.

Taking Baths Now

"Is it okay for me to take a bath this late in pregnancy?"

Run that tub—and carefully hop (or hoist yourself) in. A warm bath is not only safe in late pregnancy, but can be just the ticket for soaking away those aches and pains and stresses after a long day (and what day isn't long when you're 8 months pregnant?).

If you're worried about bathwater entering your vagina (you may have heard that one through the pregnancy grapevine), don't be. Unless it's forced—as with douching, something you shouldn't be doing anyway—water can't get where it shouldn't go. And even if a little water does make its way up, the cervical mucous plug that seals the entrance to the uterus effectively protects its precious contents from an invasion of infectious organisms, should there be any floating around in your tub.

Even once you're in labor and the mucous plug is dislodged, you can still spend time in the bath. In fact, hydrotherapy during labor can provide welcome pain relief. You can even opt to give birth in a tub (see page 326).

One caveat when you're tubbing for two, especially this late in the pregnancy game: Make sure the tub has a nonslip surface or mat on the bottom so you don't take a tumble—and easy does it getting in and out. And as always, avoid irritating bubble baths.

Driving Now

"I can barely fit behind the wheel. Should I still be driving?"

You can stay in the driver's seat as long as you fit there—and if it's become a tight squeeze, moving the seat back and tilting the wheel up should help. Assuming you've got the room—and you're feeling up to it (and aren't too distracted)—driving short distances is fine up until delivery day.

Car trips lasting more than an hour, however, might be hard to sit through late in pregnancy—and can restrict circulation—no matter who's driving. If you must drive a longer distance, be sure to shift around in your seat frequently and stop every hour to get up and walk around. Doing some neck and back stretches may also keep you more comfortable.

Don't, however, try to drive yourself to the hospital while in labor (a

Popping Placenta

Animals do it. Tribal women do it. Chinese medicine has advocated for it for hundreds of years. And now it seems half of Hollywood is doing it—along with plenty of other American moms. Eating your placenta after giving birth (called placentophagy) may not sound particularly appetizing, but it's an option more moms are putting in their birth plans. And maybe you're wondering whether you should order it up, too.

The placenta, the incredible organ that nourished and nurtured your baby during his or her 9-month stay in your uterine home, is usually just discarded after delivery. But proponents of placentophagy say that tossing your placenta is a waste—that consuming it instead can raise your energy levels, ward off anemia, give your milk supply a boost, balance hormones, and lower your chances of postpartum depression.

Not game to gobble up your placenta, say, in a smoothie? Not to worry—few new moms do. The most common way to eat your placenta—and undoubtedly the easiest to swallow—is in pill form. In a process called placenta encapsulation, your placenta is dried, powdered, and sealed into vitamin-size capsules (there are companies who will do it for you), but it comes at a price. Some moms opt to do it themselves at home, for free (DIY kits—or instructions—are available online). The placenta can also be distilled into an alcohol-based solution for you to take in drop form in your smoothies or other drinks.

There are no clinical trials or scientific research to back the effectiveness of these placenta preparations, and most medical experts are skeptical about the perks of eating the afterbirth. They point out that the touted benefits may be the result of a placebo effect (if you expect to feel good after eating your placenta, you'll probably feel that way)—and also point to women who end up sick after they've popped placenta pills or snacked on placenta. Another major potential downside to downing placenta, according to experts: There's the very real possibility of spreading infection when you're handling a raw, blood-filled organ, easily contaminated by bacteria. A possibly better use of your placenta? Storing its blood and cells (see page 295).

If you're considering using your placenta after delivery, be sure to find out if the hospital or birthing center you're delivering in will allow you to pack it up and take it home (or send it off for processing). Not all will. Of course, you won't have to contend with hospital protocols if you're delivering at home.

really strong contraction might prove dangerous on the road). And don't forget the most important road rule on any car trip, whether you are driver or passenger (and even if you're a passenger being driven to the hospital or birthing center in labor): Buckle up. See how to buckle your pregnant self up safely—as well as what to do about those air bags—on page 267.

Traveling Now

"I may have to travel for business this month. Is it safe this late in pregnancy, or should I cancel?"

Before you schedule your trip, schedule a call or visit to your practitioner. Different practitioners have differing points of view on last trimester travel. Whether yours will encourage you or discourage you from hitting the road—or the rails or the skies—at this point in your pregnancy will probably depend on that point of view, as well as on several other factors. Most important is the kind of pregnancy you've been having: You're more likely to get the green light if yours has been uncomplicated. How far along you are (most practitioners advise against flying after the 36th week) and whether you are at any increased risk at all for premature labor will weigh into the recommendation, too. Also very important is how you've been feeling. Pregnancy symptoms that multiply as the months pass also tend to multiply as the miles pass, and traveling can lead to increased backache, aggravate varicose veins and hemorrhoids (if you'll be sitting in a cramped airplane seat), and restrict circulation, increasing the risk of a blood clot. Other considerations include how far and for how long you will be traveling (and how long you will actually be in transit), how physically demanding the trip will be, and how necessary the trip is (optional trips or trips that can be easily postponed may not be worth making now). If you're traveling by air, you'll also need to factor in any restrictions of the airline you choose. Some will not let you travel in the last month or two without a letter from your practitioner stating that you're not going into labor imminently (as in, during the flight). Others offer more wiggle room (if not seat or leg room). And some may practice an unofficial don't-ask-don't-tell policy (after all, it's hard to judge how pregnant a woman is just from a glance at the check-in desk).

If your practitioner gives you the go-ahead, there are still plenty of other arrangements you'll need to make besides the travel ones. See page 268 for tips to ensure happy (and safer and more comfortable) travels for the pregnant you. Getting plenty of rest and staying well hydrated will be especially key. But most important on your to-do list will be making sure you have the name, phone number, and address of a recommended practitioner (and the hospital or birthing center where he or she delivers) at your destination—one, of course, whose services will be covered by your insurance plan should you end up requiring them. If you're traveling a long distance, you may also want to consider the possibility of bringing along your partner on the remote chance that if you do end up going into labor at your destination, at least you won't have to deliver without him. And you might want to look into travel insurance, just in case an unexpected complication forces you to cancel your trip.

Sex Now

"I hear a lot of conflicting opinions on whether sex in the last weeks of pregnancy is safe—and whether it triggers labor."

Still have the get-up-and-go you need to get it on? Then get up and go for it. The research that's been done (both by scientists and by those playing doctor at home) indicates that sex (and orgasm, for one or both partners) doesn't trigger labor unless conditions for labor are ripe—that is, the cervix is ready for action. Then, it's theorized, the prostaglandins in semen (like the prostaglandins sometimes used to help induce labor), and perhaps the oxytocin released with orgasm, might be able to help get the labor party started. But even then, under the right and ripest circumstances, you can't bank on sex taking you to the birthing room—as many overdue do-it-yourselfers have discovered. In fact, one study found that low-risk women who had sex in the

Preparing for the Unexpected

Birth plan? Done! Childbirth education classes? Doing! Disaster readiness? Ummm . . . say what? In all your pre-baby prep you probably haven't given much thought to disaster preparedness, but experts say every expectant mom should. Disasters, whether natural or human-made, are fortunately uncommon—but they almost always strike unexpectedly. With a little bit of advance planning, you and your baby-to-be can weather the storm (perhaps literally) of any disaster. Some things to think about:

■ Have a communication plan. Landlines can go out and wireless networks can become overloaded during a disaster, making it impossible to reach your partner and other family by phone. Plan ahead to text and use social networks and messaging apps you share with family to get in touch during and after a disaster.

■ Have a plan for medical emergencies and emergency delivery (see page 400 for a how-to). Talk to your practitioner now about emergency options in case you go into labor or are having bleeding or other symptoms of a complication when phone lines are down, the practitioner's office isn't open, or you can't get to the hospital. And be sure you have a copy of your electronic health record handy in case you find yourself with an unfamiliar care provider in an emergency.

■ Prepare an emergency kit and bag. Experts recommend having an emergency kit with at least 3 days' worth of non-perishable food on hand (think nuts, freeze-dried fruit, whole grain crackers, peanut butter, granola bars, and canned goods with pull tabs, water (at least 1 gallon per person or pet for 3 days), prenatal vitamins, prescription medication, external cell phone batteries, a battery operated radio, a blanket, a first aid kit, flashlight, extra batteries, hand sanitizer, and other things you may need). Have an emergency kit in your car, too. Visit ready.gov for more tips.

Remember, too, how important it will be to take care of your baby and yourself during a disaster—to eat regularly, stay hydrated, and get the rest you need, as hard as those might be to do in such a stressful situation. And speaking of stress, try to make sure it doesn't overwhelm you—especially since extreme stress is sometimes linked to preterm labor. Tap in to the relaxation techniques you're using to stay calm during pregnancy (and if you're not using them already, prepping for just-in-case is another good reason to start). Some numbers to keep handy, if disaster does strike (and outside help is reachable): The National Disaster Distress Helpline, 1-800-985-5990, or text TalkWithUs to 66746. You can also contact your local American Red Cross chapter or public health department for more information and help.

final weeks of pregnancy carried their babies slightly longer than those who skipped sex during that time.

Bottom line on going for your bottom lines: Based on what's known, most obs and midwives allow patients with normal pregnancies to make love right up until delivery day. Check with your practitioner to see what's safe in your situation. If you get a green light (chances are, you will), then by all means hit the sheets—if you have the will and the energy (and the gymnastic skills that might be necessary at this point). If the light is red in your case (and it probably will be if you are at high risk for premature delivery, have placenta previa, or are experiencing unexplained bleeding)—or if you're just not in the mood for lovemaking—try getting intimate in other ways. While you still have some evenings to yourselves, rendezvous for a romantic candlelit dinner or a moonlit stroll. Cuddle while you watch TV, or soap each other in the shower. Or use massage as the medium. Or do everything but what's on your no-fly list (get a list of restrictions from your practitioner). This may not quite satisfy like the real thing, but try to remember you have a whole lifetime of lovemaking ahead—though the pickings may continue to be slim in that department at least until baby's sleeping through the night.

Your Twosome

"The baby isn't even born yet, and already our relationship has changed. We're both so wrapped up in the birth and the baby, instead of in each other."

Little babies bring big changes when they arrive, and often, even before they arrive. Not surprisingly, your relationship with your partner is one place where you'll notice that change, and it sounds like you've glimpsed it already. And that's actually a really good thing. When baby makes three, your twosome is bound to undergo some shifting of dynamics and reshuffling of priorities. But this predictable upheaval is usually less stressful—and easier to adapt to—when a couple begins the natural and inevitable evolution of their relationship during pregnancy. In other words, the changes to your relationship are more likely to represent a change for the better if they begin before baby's arrival. Couples who don't anticipate at least

some disruption of romance-as-usual—who don't realize that wine and roses will often give way to spit-up and strained carrots, that lovemaking marathons will place (well) behind baby-rocking marathons, that a party of three is not always as cozy as a party of two, at least not in the same way—often find the reality of life with a demanding newborn harder to handle.

So think ahead, plan ahead—and be ready for change. But as you get yourselves into nurture mode, don't forget that baby won't be the only one who'll need nurturing. As normal—and healthy—as it is to be wrapped up in your expected extra special delivery, it's also important to reserve some emotional energy for the relationship that created that bundle of joy in the first place. Now is the time to learn to combine the care and feeding of your baby with the care and feeding of your twosome. While you're busily feathering your nest, make the effort to regularly reinforce romance. Hug early and often each day. Hold hands while you're browsing for last-minute baby gear. Grab his butt, or a kiss, or a nuzzle for no reason at all. Cuddle in bed, reminiscing about your first date or dreaming about a second honeymoon (even if it won't be in the cards for many moons). Bring massage oil to bed now and then. Even if you're not in the mood for sex—or it's seeming too much like hard work these days—any kind of touching can keep you close, while reminding you both that there's more to life than Lamaze and layettes.

Keeping this very important thought in mind now will make it easier to keep the love light burning later when you're taking turns walking the floor at 2 a.m. And that love light, after all, is what will make the cozy nest you're busily preparing for your baby a happy and secure one.

ALL ABOUT:
Breastfeeding

If you've given any thought to what's going on behind those giant bra cups you've likely traded up for over the last 8 months or so, chances are, it's pretty clear: Your breasts are already on board with breastfeeding. Whether the rest of you is signed up, too, or whether you're still weighing your baby-feeding options, you'll probably want to learn more about this amazing process, a process that turns breasts (your breasts!) into the perfect purveyors of the world's most perfect infant food. You'll get some valuable highlights and insights here, but for much more on breastfeeding (from the why-to's to the how-to's), see *What to Expect the First Year*. Here are the highlights.

Why Breast Is Best

Just as goat's milk is the ideal food for kids (goat kids, that is), and cow's milk is the best meal for just-born calves, your human breast milk is the perfect meal for your human newborn. Here are the reasons why:

It's custom made. Tailored to meet the nutritional needs of human infants, breast milk contains at least 100 ingredients that aren't found in cow's milk and that can't be precisely replicated in commercial formulas. And unlike formula, the composition of breast milk changes constantly to meet a baby's ever-changing needs: It's different in the morning than it is in the late afternoon, different at the beginning of a feeding than at the end, different the 1st month than the 7th, and different for a preemie than for a full-term newborn. It even tastes different, depending on what you've been snacking on (like your amniotic fluid does when you're pregnant). A one-of-a-kind food for your one-of-a-kind baby.

It's easy to digest. Breast milk is designed for a new baby's brand new digestive system. The protein and fat in breast milk are easier to digest than those in formula, and its important micronutrients are more easily absorbed.

It's a tummy soother. Breastfed babies are almost never constipated, thanks to the easier digestibility of breast milk. They also rarely have diarrhea, since breast milk appears to reduce the risk of digestive upset both by destroying harmful microorganisms and by encouraging the growth of beneficial ones. You know the much-touted pre- and probiotics that are added to some formulas? They're naturally occurring in breast milk.

It doesn't make a stink. On a purely aesthetic note, the poops of a breastfed baby are sweeter smelling (at least until solids are introduced).

It's an infection preventer. With each and every feeding, nursers get a healthy dose of antibodies to boost their immunity to bugs of all varieties (which is why breastfeeding is sometimes referred to as a baby's first immunization). In general, breastfed babies come down with fewer colds, ear infections, lower respiratory tract infections, urinary tract infections, and other illnesses than formula-fed infants, and when they do get sick, they'll usually recover more quickly and with fewer complications. Breastfeeding also improves the immune response to vaccines for most diseases (such as tetanus, diphtheria, and polio). Plus, it may offer some protection against sudden infant death syndrome (SIDS).

It's a fat flattener. Breastfed infants are less likely to be too chubby. That is, in part, because breastfeeding lets baby's appetite call the shots (and the ounces). A breastfed baby is likely to stop feeding when full, while a bottle-fed infant may be urged to keep feeding until the bottle's emptied. What's more, breast milk is actually ingeniously calorie controlled. The lower calorie foremilk (served up at the start of a feed) is designed as a thirst-quencher. The higher calorie hindmilk (served up at the end of a feed) is a filler-upper, signaling to a nurser that it's quitting time. And research suggests that the fat-defeating benefits of breastfeeding follow a baby out of the nursery—and into high school. Studies show that former breastfeeders are less likely to battle weight as teens—and the longer they were breastfed, the lower their risk of becoming overweight. Another potential long-term health plus for nursers: Breastfeeding is linked to lower cholesterol levels and lower blood pressure later in life.

It keeps allergies on hold. Babies are almost never truly allergic to breast milk (though occasionally an infant may be sensitive to something mom has eaten). The formula flip side? More than 10 percent of babies turn out to be allergic to cow's milk formula (a switch to a soy or hydrolysate formula usually solves the problem but isn't ideal, since those stray even further in composition from the gold standard formula: breast milk). And there's more good news on the allergy front—evidence that breastfed babies may be less likely to develop asthma and eczema.

Prepping for Breastfeeding

Luckily, nature has worked out all the mechanics, so there's not much you'll need to do to get your breasts ready to feed your baby. Some lactation experts recommend that during the last months of pregnancy you skip the soap on your nipples and areolas—just rinse with water, instead. Soap can dry the nipples, which may lead to cracking and soreness early in breastfeeding. If your nipples are dry, you can apply a lanolin-based cream such as Lansinoh—otherwise, it's not necessary.

The no-prep rule applies even to women with small or flat nipples. Flat nipples don't need to be prepped for nursing with breast shells, hand manipulation, or a manual breast pump during pregnancy. Not only are these prepping techniques often less effective than no treatment, but they can do more harm than good. The shells, besides being uncomfortably bulky, can cause sweating and rashes. Hand manipulation and ahead-of-time pumping can stimulate contractions and, occasionally, even trigger breast infection.

It's a brain booster. Breastfeeding, according to some evidence, appears to slightly increase a child's IQ, at least through age 15, and possibly beyond. This may be related not only to the brain-building fatty acids (DHA) in breast milk, but also to the closeness and mother-baby interaction that is built into breastfeeding, which is believed to nurture a newborn's intellectual development.

Got Pierced?

You're all set to nurse your baby-to-be, but you're afraid there's a little something in the way: a nipple piercing. No worries. There's no evidence that nipple piercing has any effect on a mom's ability to breastfeed. Still, be sure to remove any nipple jewelry before baby opens up wide and you insert your breast. This is not only due to the potential for infection for you, but because the jewelry could pose a choking hazard for your baby or injure his or her tender gums, tongue, or palate during feedings.

It's safe. You can be sure that the milk served up from your breasts is always prepared perfectly—and never spoiled, contaminated, expired, or recalled.

It's made for suckers. It takes longer to drain a breast than a bottle, giving newborns more of the comforting sucking satisfaction they crave. Plus, a breastfed baby can continue to comfort-suck on a nearly empty breast—something an empty bottle doesn't allow.

It builds stronger mouths. Mama's nipples and baby's mouth are made for each other—a naturally perfect match. Even the most scientifically designed bottle nipple can't match up to a breast nipple, which gives a baby's jaws, gums, teeth, and palate the ultimate workout—a workout that ensures optimum oral development and some perks for baby's future teeth (like better alignment). Another mouth perk to breastfeeding: Babies who are breastfed are less likely to get cavities later on.

It expands the taste buds early on. Want to raise an adventurous eater? Start at the breast. Developing those little taste buds on breast milk, which takes on the flavor of whatever you've been eating, may acclimate a baby early on to a world of flavors. Researchers have found that nursed babies are less likely to be timid in their tastes than their formula-fed peers once they graduate to the high chair—which means they may be more likely to open wide to that spoonful of yams (or that forkful of curried chicken) later on.

Breastfeeding offers a pile of perks for mom (and dad), too:

Convenience. Breast milk is the ultimate convenience food—always in stock, ready to serve, and consistently dispensed at the perfect temperature. It's fast food, too: no formula to run out of, shop for, or lug around, no bottles to clean or refill, no powders to mix, no meals to warm (say, when you're on a conference call and baby's wailing in the background). Wherever you are—in bed, on the road, at the mall, on the beach—all the nourishment your baby needs is always on tap, no muss (or mess), no fuss. And if you and your baby aren't in the same place at the same time—you're at work, in school, at dinner, or even away for the weekend—a stash of expressed breast milk can be served up in bottles.

Money in the bank. The best things in life are free, and that includes breast milk and breast milk delivery (open baby's mouth, insert mommy's breast). On the other hand, bottle-feeding (once you factor in formula, bottles, nipples, cleaning supplies) can be a pretty pricey proposition. There's no waste with breastfeeding, either—what baby doesn't end up drinking at one feed will stay fresh for the next. And because breastfed babies are generally healthier babies—you're likely to save money on

When Father Knows Breast

Up until now, you've thought of your spouse's breasts sexually. And that's natural. But here's something that's also natural—and something you're probably well aware of already. Breasts are built the way they are for another good reason and to serve another really important purpose: baby feeding. There is no more perfect food for an infant than breast milk, and no more perfect food delivery system than a breast (make that 2 breasts). Breastfeeding offers an overwhelming number of health benefits for both babies (from preventing allergies, obesity, and illness to promoting brain development) and their moms (nursing is linked to a speedier recovery postpartum and a reduced risk of diabetes and of breast, ovarian, and uterine cancer later in life).

Without a doubt, the decision to choose breast over bottle can make a dramatic difference in your baby's life—and in your partner's. And perhaps surprisingly, your support in that decision can make a dramatic difference in breastfeeding success. So if you haven't already, give her your vote of breastfeeding confidence, which counts for a lot more than you'd think. Even though you may not know letdown from latch-on yet, knowing that you're behind her every step of the way (especially when the going gets tough, which it often does at first) will have an enormous influence on whether mom sticks with breastfeeding (and the longer she sticks with it, the more health benefits for both her and baby). In fact, researchers have found that when dads are supportive of breastfeeding, moms are likely to give it a try 96 percent of the time. When dads are ambivalent, only about 26 percent give it a try. So take your influence seriously. Read up on breastfeeding, take a class together, talk to other dads whose partners have breastfed, and ask whether a lactation consultant (basically, a nursing coach) will be available at the hospital or birthing center when baby's ready to chow down for the first time. (Lesson one: It's a natural process, but it doesn't always come naturally.) If your partner is hesitant to ask for help—or she's just too tired after delivery—be her breastfeeding advocate and make sure she gets it.

Help get your spouse started, cheer her on, and then sit back and watch in wonder as those amazing breasts of hers take on one of life's most important (and incredibly special) jobs: baby feeding. Sure, it takes only two to breastfeed, but it often takes three to make it happen.

---

health care costs (and lost wages, too, since you'll be less likely to miss work because of a sick baby).

Speedier postpartum recovery. It's only natural that breastfeeding is best for newly delivered moms, too—after all, it's the natural conclusion to the pregnancy-childbirth cycle. It'll help your uterus shrink back to prepregnancy size more quickly, which in turn will reduce your flow of lochia (the postpartum bloody discharge), decreasing blood loss. And by burning upward of 500 extra calories a day, breastfeeding can help you shed leftover pregnancy pounds faster. Some of those pounds were laid down as fat reserves earmarked specifically for milk production—now's your chance to use them.

Some protection against pregnancy. It's far from a sure bet, but breastfeeding

Breastfeeding After Breast Surgery

How does past breast surgery affect your breastfeeding future? That depends on what kind of surgery you had and how it was performed. Here's an overview:

If you've had a breast reduction or lumpectomy, you'll probably still be able to breastfeed, but you may not produce enough milk to nurse exclusively. Check with your surgeon to see if care was taken to preserve milk ducts and nerve pathways during the procedure—if so, chances are good that you'll be able to produce at least some milk.

If you've had breast augmentation, your chances of being able to breastfeed successfully are good, since augmentation is less likely to interfere with breastfeeding than a breast reduction. Still, it will depend on the technique, the incision, and the reason why it was done. While many women with implants are able to nurse exclusively, a significant minority may not produce enough milk.

No matter what kind of breast surgery you had, you can improve your chances of breastfeeding success by reading up, taking a class, and working with a lactation consultant right from the start. For much more, see *What to Expect the First Year.*

your baby may suppress ovulation (and your period) for several months. Is this a birth control bet you should take, without a backup? Probably not, unless back-to-back pregnancies are your objective (see page 27 for more).

Health benefits for mom. Plenty of perks here: Women who breastfeed have a slightly lower risk of developing uterine cancer, ovarian cancer, and premenopausal breast cancer. They're also less likely to develop Type 2 diabetes, rheumatoid arthritis, and osteoporosis than women who don't breastfeed. Another benefit for breastfeeding moms: Research suggests that women who breastfeed are somewhat less likely to suffer from postpartum depression (though PPD can strike a breastfeeding mom and can also strike a mom after she weans, as hormones fluctuate once again).

Nighttime feeds that are a (relative) breeze. Have a hungry baby at 2 a.m.? You will. And when you do, you'll appreciate how fast you'll be able to feed that baby if you're breastfeeding. No stumbling to the kitchen to prepare a bottle in the dark. Just pop a warm breast into that warm little mouth.

Eventually, easy multitasking. Sure, nursing your newborn will take both arms and a lot of focus at first. But once you and baby become nursing pros, you'll be able to do just about anything else at the same time—from eating dinner to playing with your toddler.

Built-in bonding. The benefit of breastfeeding you're likely to appreciate most is the bond it nurtures between you and your little one. There's skin-to-skin and eye-to-eye contact, and the opportunity to cuddle and coo built right into every feed. True, bottle-feeding mamas (and daddies) can get just as close to their babies—but it takes a more conscious effort (there's always the understandable temptation to prop a bottle when you're busy or hand off feedings when you're tired).

Making the Choice to Breastfeed

For more and more soon-to-be moms, the choice is clear. Some know they'll opt for breast over bottle long before they even decide to become pregnant. Others choose breastfeeding once they've read up on its many benefits. Some teeter on the brink right through pregnancy and even delivery. And even those who are pretty convinced that nursing isn't for them still can't shake the nagging feeling that they should do it anyway.

Undecided? Here's a suggestion: Try it—you may like it. You can always quit if you don't, but at least you will have cleared up those nagging doubts. Best of all, you and your baby will have reaped some of the most important benefits of breastfeeding, if only briefly.

Just be sure to give breastfeeding a fair trial. The first few weeks can be challenging, even for the most enthusiastic breastfeeders, and are always a learning process (though getting lactation support can make things much easier if you're having a hard time). A full 4 to 6 weeks of nursing is generally needed to

When You Can't (or Choose Not to) Breastfeed

Maybe you've decided that breastfeeding definitely isn't for you. Or there's a reason why you won't be able to (or end up not being able to) breastfeed, either at all or exclusively. Either way, remember that you can offer your baby as much love and nurturing when you bottle-feed as you can with breastfeeding. So reach for the formula without guilt or regret. To learn more about bottle-feeding with love, see *What to Expect the First Year.*

establish a successful feeding relationship and give a mom the chance to figure out whether breast is best after all.

Also keep in mind that breastfeeding isn't an all-or-nothing deal. For some moms, combining both breast and bottle is the best formula. For more on combining breast and bottle, see *What to Expect the First Year.*

The Ninth Month

Approximately 36 to 40 Weeks

F inally. The month you've been waiting for, working toward, and stressing about just a little bit is here at long last. Chances are you're at once very ready (to hold that baby . . . to see your toes again . . . to sleep on your stomach!) and not ready at all. Still, despite the inevitable flurry of activity (more practitioner appointments, last-minute layette and gear items to shop for, projects to finish at work, paint colors to pick for baby's room), you may find that the 9th month seems like the longest month of all. Except, of course, if you don't deliver by your due date. In that case, it's the 10th month that's the longest.

Your Baby This Month

Week 36 Weighing somewhere around 6 pounds and measuring anywhere from 18 to 19 inches tall, your baby is almost ready to be served up into your arms. Right now, most of baby's systems (from circulatory to musculoskeletal) are just about equipped for life on the outside. Though the digestive system is ready to roll, too, it hasn't really gotten a workout yet. Remember, up until this point, your baby's nutrition has been arriving via the umbilical cord—no digestion necessary. But that's soon to change. As soon as baby takes his or her first suckle at your breast (or suck from the bottle), that digestive system will be jump-started—and those diapers will start filling.

Week 37 Here's some exciting news: If your baby were born this week, he or she would be considered full term. Mind you, that doesn't mean baby is finished growing—or getting ready for life on the outside. Still gaining weight at about half a pound a week, the average fetus this age weighs about 6½ pounds (though size varies quite a bit from fetus to fetus, as it does from newborn to newborn). Fat continues to accumulate on your baby, forming kissable dimples in those cute elbows, knees, and shoulders, and adorable creases and folds in the neck and wrists. To keep busy until the big debut, your baby is practicing to make perfect: inhaling and exhaling amniotic fluid (to get the lungs ready for that first breath), sucking on his or her thumb (to prepare for that first suckle), blinking, and pivoting from side to side (which explains why yesterday you felt that sweet little butt on the left side and today it's taken a turn to the right).

Week 38 Hitting the growth charts at about 7 pounds and the 20-inch mark (give or take an inch or two), your little one isn't so little anymore. In fact, baby's big enough for the big time—and the big day. With only 2 (or 4, max) weeks left in utero, all systems are almost go. To finish getting ready for his or her close-up (and all those photo ops), baby has a few last-minute details to take care of, like shedding the vernix (the greasy white substance protecting that tender new skin) and lanugo (the fine downy hair that covered your cutie's body for warmth). Baby's also producing more surfactant, which will prevent the air sacs in the lungs from sticking to each other when breathing begins. Your little one will be here before you know it!

Week 39 Not much to report this week, at least in the height and weight department. Fortunately for you and your overstretched skin (and aching back), baby's growth has slowed down—or even taken a hiatus until after delivery. On average, a baby this week still weighs in at between 7 and 8 pounds (the size of . . . a baby!) and measures 19 to 21 inches (though yours may be a little bigger or smaller). Still, progress is being made in some other areas, especially baby's brain, which is growing and developing up a

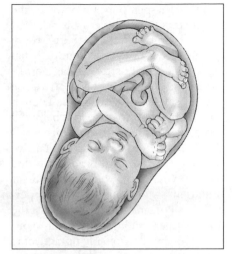

Your Baby, Month 9

storm (at a rapid pace that will continue during the first 3 years of life). What's more, your baby's pink skin has turned whitish or whitish-grayish (no matter what skin your baby will ultimately be in, since pigmentation doesn't occur until soon after birth). A development that you may have noticed by now if this is your first pregnancy: Baby's head might have dropped into your pelvis. This change of baby's locale might make for easier breathing (and less heartburn), but could also make it harder for you to walk (make that, waddle).

Week 40 Congratulations! You've reached the official end of your pregnancy (and maybe the end of your rope). For the record, your baby is fully full term and could weigh in anywhere between the 6- and 9-pound mark and measure anywhere from 19 to 22 inches, though some perfectly healthy babies check in slightly smaller or bigger than that. You may notice when your baby emerges that he or she (and you'll know for sure which at that momentous moment) is still curled into the fetal position, even though the fetal days are over. That's just sheer force of habit (after spending 9 months in the cramped confines of your uterus, your baby doesn't yet realize there's room to spread out now) and comfort (that snug-as-a-bug position feels good). When you do meet your new arrival, be sure to say hello—and more. Though it's your first face-to-face, your baby will recognize the sound of your voice—and that of dad's. And if baby doesn't arrive on time (choosing to ignore the due date on your app), you're in good—if impatient—company. About 30 percent of all pregnancies proceed past the 40-week mark, though (thankfully) your practitioner will probably not let yours continue beyond 42 weeks.

Weeks 41–42 So, looks like baby has opted for a late checkout. Fewer than 5 percent of babies are born on their actual due date—and around 10 percent decide to overstay their welcome in Hotel Uterus beyond week 41, thriving well into the 10th month (though you may have lost that "thriving" feeling long ago). Remember, too, that most of the time an overdue baby isn't overdue at all—it's just that the due date was off. Less often, a baby may be truly postmature. When a postmature baby does make a debut, it's often with dry, cracked, peeling, loose, and wrinkled skin (all completely temporary—soft new baby skin is soon to follow). That's because the protective vernix was shed weeks before, in anticipation of a delivery date that's since come and gone. An "older" fetus will also have longer nails, possibly longer hair, and definitely little or none of that baby fuzz (lanugo) at all. In general, postmature newborns tend to be more alert and open-eyed (after all, they're older and wiser). Just to be sure all is well, your practitioner will likely monitor your overdue baby closely through nonstress tests and checks of the amniotic fluid or biophysical profiles.

Your Body This Month

In your last month of pregnancy symptoms, some may be lingering from last month, while others may be brand new. Still others may hardly be noticeable because you're so used to them or because they are eclipsed by new and more exciting signs indicating that labor may not be far off:

Physically

- Changes in fetal activity (more squirming and less kicking, as your baby has progressively less room to move around)

- Vaginal discharge becomes heavier and contains more mucus, which may be streaked red with blood or tinged brown or pink after sex or a pelvic exam or as your cervix begins to dilate

- Constipation or looser stools as labor nears

- Heartburn, indigestion, flatulence, bloating

- Occasional headaches

- Occasional lightheadedness or dizziness, especially when getting up quickly or when your blood sugar dips

- Nasal congestion and occasional nosebleeds; ear stuffiness
- Sensitive gums
- Leg cramps at night
- Increased backache and heaviness
- Buttock and pelvic discomfort and achiness
- Increased swelling of ankles and feet, and occasionally of hands and face
- Itchy belly
- Protruding navel (a popped-out belly button)
- Stretch marks
- Varicose veins in the legs and/or vulva
- Hemorrhoids
- Easier breathing after baby drops
- More frequent urination after baby drops, since there's pressure on the bladder once again
- Increased difficulty sleeping
- More frequent and more intense Braxton Hicks contractions (some may be painful)
- Increasing clumsiness and difficulty getting around
- Colostrum leaking from your nipples (though this premilk substance may not appear until after delivery)
- Extra fatigue or extra energy (nesting syndrome), or alternating periods of each
- Increase in appetite or loss of appetite

Emotionally

- More excitement, more anxiety, more apprehension, more absentmindedness
- Relief that you're almost there

Your Body This Month

Your uterus is right under your ribs now, and your measurements aren't really changing that much from week to week anymore. The top of your uterus is around 38 to 40 cm from the top of your pubic bone. Your weight gain slows down or even stops as D-day approaches. Your abdominal skin is stretched as far as you think it can go, and you're probably waddling more now than ever, possibly because the baby has dropped in anticipation of impending labor.

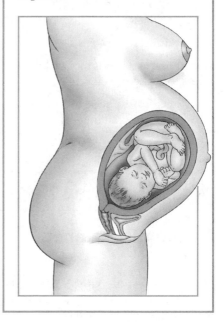

- Irritability and oversensitivity (especially with people who keep saying, "No baby yet?")
- Impatience and restlessness
- Dreaming and fantasizing about the baby

What You Can Expect at This Month's Checkup

With appointments scheduled weekly this month, you'll be spending more time than ever at your practitioner's office. These visits will be more interesting—the practitioner will estimate baby's size and may even venture a prediction about how close you are to delivery—with the excitement growing as you approach the big day. In general, you can expect your practitioner to check the following:

- Your weight (gain generally slows down or stops)

- Your blood pressure (it may be slightly higher than it was at midpregnancy)

- Your urine, for protein

- Your feet and hands for swelling, and legs for varicose veins

- Your cervix (the neck of your uterus), by internal examination, to see if effacement (thinning) and dilation (opening) have begun

- The height of the fundus

- The fetal heartbeat

- Fetal size (you may get a rough weight estimate), presentation (head or buttocks first), position (front or rear facing), and descent (is the presenting part engaged in the pelvis yet?) by palpation (feeling with the hands)

- Questions and concerns you want to discuss, particularly those related to labor and delivery—have a list ready.

You can also expect to receive a labor and delivery protocol from your practitioner (when to call if you think you are in labor, when to plan on heading to the hospital or birthing center). If you don't, be sure to ask for these instructions—you'll need them!

What You May Be Wondering About

Urinary Frequency— Again

"During the last few days, it seems like I'm in the bathroom constantly. Is it normal to be peeing this often now?"

Having a first trimester flashback? That's because your uterus is right back where it started: down low in your pelvis, pressing squarely on your bladder. And this time, the weight of your uterus is significantly greater, which means the pressure on your bladder is greater, too—as is that need to pee. So you go, girl—again, and again, and again. As long as frequency isn't accompanied by signs of infection (see page 528), it's completely normal. Don't be tempted to cut back on fluids in an attempt to cut back on your trips to the bathroom—your body needs those fluids more than ever. And as always, go as soon as you feel the urge (and can find a bathroom).

Lactating Blood

You may have expected to leak a little colostrum from your nipples later in pregnancy, but blood? Yet a bloody nipple discharge (you might notice it as spotting on the inside of your bra or red-tinged fluid when you squeeze your nipples) is not uncommon during pregnancy (usually late in pregnancy and more commonly in first-timers), and it's usually nothing to be concerned about. Why does it happen? Your breasts have been going through a lot in the last almost 9 months as they prepare for the all-important job of feeding your baby—including a lot of expansion and a lot of increased blood flow. Maybe the blood is just the very normal response to the increasing blood supply in your breasts—or it's coming from a capillary that burst as your breasts inflated their way through the cup alphabet. Or it could be a milk duct that's swollen thanks to pregnancy hormones. Or maybe it's a papilloma (a small benign lump) in a milk duct that's been irritated. Or your nipples could just be really raw (especially if you've been tweaking them a lot to see if colostrum appears, or in an effort to get labor started).

Mention the bleeding to your practitioner. To be on the safe side (always the best side to be on), as well as to put your mind at ease, he or she may suggest that you have a breast ultrasound and exam done now and a mammogram done after delivery—especially if the bleeding lasts longer than a week and/or if you've noticed a lump along with the bleeding. If everything checks out, as it almost certainly will, just avoid squeezing your nipples so you don't increase the irritation that's probably led to the bloody discharge in the first place (your nipples will get squeezed plenty when baby arrives).

Most of the time, such so-called lactating blood goes away after delivery. If it doesn't, still no worries—you can breastfeed even if you're lactating blood. The small amount of blood your baby will ingest along with the breast milk won't be harmful.

Leaky (or Not Leaky) Breasts

"A friend of mine says she had milk leaking in the 9th month. I don't. Does this mean I won't have any milk?"

Milk isn't made until baby's ready to drink it—and that's not until 3 to 4 days after delivery. What your friend was leaking was colostrum, a thin, yellowish fluid that is the precursor to breast milk. Colostrum is chock-full of antibodies to protect a newborn baby and has more protein and less fat and milk sugar (the better to digest it) than the breast milk that arrives later.

Some, but far from all, moms-to-be leak this phenomenal fluid toward the end of their pregnancies, sometimes during sex, sometimes spontaneously. But even those who aren't leaking colostrum are still producing it. Not leaking, but still curious? Squeezing your areola may allow you to express a few drops (but don't squeeze with a vengeance—that'll only result in sore nipples). Still can't get any? Don't worry. Your baby will be able to net what he or she needs when the time comes to get busy at your breast. Not leaking definitely isn't a sign that your supply won't keep up with demand.

Going Down?

You may be in for a surprise—and a treat—at this month's weigh-in. Most expectant moms who reach the end of pregnancy also reach the end of pregnancy weight gain. Instead of watching the numbers on the scale go up (and up), you may start seeing those numbers go nowhere—or even go down—over the last few weeks. What's up (or rather, down) with that? After all, your baby isn't losing weight—and your ankles are still plenty puffy, thank you very much. What's happening, actually, is perfectly normal. In fact, this weight gain standstill (or downward trend) is one way that your body gets ready for labor. Amniotic fluid starts to decrease (less water equals less weight), and loose bowels (common as labor approaches) can also send the numbers down, as can all that sweating you're doing. And if you think this weight loss is exciting, wait until delivery day. That's when you'll experience your biggest 1-day weight-loss total ever!

If you are leaking colostrum, it's probably just a few drops. But if you're leaking more than that, you may want to consider wearing nursing pads in your bra to protect your clothes (and to prevent potentially embarrassing moments). And you might as well get used to the wet t-shirt look, since this is just a glimpse of leaky breasts—and wet bras, pajamas, and blouses—to come.

Incidentally, don't worry about "wasting" colostrum if you're leaking it—you'll continue to produce it until it's time for your real milk to come in.

Spotting Now

"Right after my husband and I had sex this morning, I began to spot a little. Does this mean labor is beginning?"

Don't place the birth announcement order just yet. Pinkish-stained or red-streaked mucus appearing soon after sex or a vaginal exam, or brownish-tinged mucus or brownish spotting appearing within 48 hours after the same, is usually just a normal result of the sensitive cervix being bruised or manipulated, not a sign that labor's about to start up. But pinkish- or brownish-tinged or bloody mucus accompanied by contractions or other signs of oncoming labor, whether it follows sex or not, could be signaling the start of labor (see page 395).

If you notice bright red bleeding or persistent red spotting at any time, call your practitioner.

Prelabor Water Breaking

"How likely is it that my water's going to break before I go into labor?"

Many moms-to-be stress about springing an amniotic leak late in pregnancy, but few ever do. Contrary to popular pregnancy belief, your "water" (more accurately, your membranes) isn't likely to "break" (more accurately, rupture) before labor begins. In fact, more than 85 percent of women enter the birthing room with their membranes fully intact. In other words, it's probable that the forecast for the rest of your pregnant future will remain "mainly dry."

If you do end up being among the 15 percent who spring a prelabor leak, you'll probably notice the tell-tale gush or trickle more if you're lying down than if you're standing up. That's because when you're upright (standing, walking, even sitting), your baby's head acts like a cork in a bottle, blocking the opening of the uterus and keeping most of the amniotic fluid in.

The bright side of a prelabor water break is that it's usually followed by labor, typically within 24 hours. If labor doesn't start spontaneously within that time, your practitioner will probably start it for you. Which means your baby's arrival will be just a day away, either way.

Though it really isn't necessary, wearing a panty liner or maxipad (or if you're really stressing, a bladder control pad) in the last weeks may give you a sense of security, as well as keep you fresh as your vaginal discharge increases. You also might want to place heavy towels, a plastic sheet, or hospital bed pads under your sheets in the last few weeks, just in case your water breaks in the middle of the night.

Baby Dropping

"If I'm past my 38th week and haven't dropped, does it mean I'm going to be late?"

Just because your baby doesn't seem to be moving toward the exit doesn't mean his or her arrival will be late. Dropping, also called lightening, is what happens when a baby descends into mom's pelvic cavity, a sign that the presenting part (first part out, usually the head) is engaged in the upper portion of the bony pelvis. In first pregnancies, dropping generally takes place 2 to 4 weeks before delivery. In expectant moms who have had children previously, it usually doesn't happen until

---

Baby's Crying Already?

The most joyous sound a new parent hears is that first cry the baby makes after he or she is born. But would you believe that your little one is already crying inside you, if silently? It's true, according to researchers, who found that third-trimester fetuses show crying behaviors—quivering chin, open mouth, deep inhalations and exhalations—and startle responses when a loud noise and vibration were sounded near the mom's belly. It's known that the crying reflex is well developed even in premature infants, so it's not surprising that babies are perfecting this skill long before they're ready to emerge (and it explains why they're so good at crying once they come out!).

---

labor begins. But as with almost every aspect of pregnancy, exceptions to the rule are the rule. You can drop 4 weeks before your due date and deliver 2 weeks late, or you can go into labor without having dropped at all. You can even seemingly drop and then undrop: Your baby's head can appear to settle in and then float up again (meaning it's not really fixed in place yet).

Often, dropping is obvious. You might not only see the difference (your belly seems lower—perhaps a lot lower—and tilted farther forward), but feel the difference, too. As the upward pressure of the uterus on your diaphragm is relieved, you can breathe more easily, literally. With your stomach less crowded, you can eat more easily, too—and finish up your meals without a side of heartburn and indigestion. Of course, these welcome changes are

How Is Baby Doing?

As your pregnancy nears its end (yes, it will end), your practitioner will be keeping a closer eye on your health and your baby's—especially once you pass the 40-week mark. That's because 40 weeks is the optimum uterine stay for babies. Those who stick around much longer can face potential challenges (becoming too big to arrive vaginally, experiencing a decline in their placenta's function, or a dip in amniotic fluid levels). Luckily, your practitioner can tap into plenty of tests and assessments of fetal wellbeing to make sure all's well and will end well . . . eventually:

Kick counts. Your record of fetal movements (see page 315) can provide some indication of how your baby is doing. Ten movements in an hour or 2 is usually reassuring. If you don't notice enough activity, other tests are then performed.

The nonstress test (NST). You'll be hooked up to a fetal monitor (the same kind that's used during labor) in your practitioner's office to measure the baby's heart rate and response to movement. You will be holding a clicker (like a buzzer on *Jeopardy!*), and each time you feel the baby move, you'll click. The monitoring goes on for 20 to 40 minutes and is able to detect if the fetus is under any stress.

Fetal acoustic stimulation (FAS) or vibroacoustic stimulation (VAS). Does your baby need a little pick-me-up? If your little one isn't as active during a nonstress test as doctors would like, a sound-and-vibration-producing instrument will be placed on your tummy to give baby a little stimulus so your practitioner can more accurately measure that little heartbeat and those movements.

The contraction stress test (CST) or oxytocin challenge test (OCT). If the results of a nonstress test are unclear, your practitioner may order a stress test. This test, done at a hospital, tests how the baby responds to the "stress" of uterine contractions to get some idea of how he or she will handle full-blown labor. In this somewhat more complex and time-consuming test (it may take a number of hours), you're hooked up to a fetal monitor. If contractions are not happening on their own, you'll be given a low-dose IV of oxytocin (or you'll be asked to stimulate your nipples) to jump-start the contractions. How your baby responds to contractions indicates

often offset by a new set of discomforts, including pressure on the bladder (which will send you to the bathroom more frequently, again), pressure on the pelvic joints (which will make it harder to walk . . . or waddle), and pressure in the perineal area (sometimes causing pain). You might also experience sharp little shocks or twinges on the pelvic floor (similar to lightning crotch sensations you may have experienced earlier on in pregnancy, but this time, thanks to baby's head pressing hard on it) and a sense of being off balance (because your center of gravity has shifted once more).

It is possible, however, for baby to drop unnoticed. For instance, if you were carrying low to begin with, your pregnant profile might not change noticeably after dropping. Or if you never experienced difficulty breathing or getting a full meal down, or if you always urinate frequently, you might not detect any obvious difference.

Your practitioner will rely on two more indicators to figure out whether or his or her condition and that of the placenta. This rough simulation of the conditions of labor can allow your practitioner to make a prediction about whether or not your baby can safely remain cocooned in your uterus and whether he or she can meet the strenuous demands of true labor.

A biophysical profile (BPP). It's picture time, baby. Using an ultrasound and fetal heart rate monitor, a BPP will look at five aspects of life in the uterus: findings from a NST, fetal breathing, fetal movement, fetal tone (the ability of your baby to flex and extend an arm or leg), and amniotic fluid volume. When all these are normal, your baby is probably doing fine. If any of these are unclear, further testing (such as a CST or a VAS) will be given to provide a more accurate picture of your baby's condition.

The modified biophysical profile. The "modified" biophysical profile combines the NST with an evaluation of the quantity of amniotic fluid. A low level of amniotic fluid may indicate that a baby is not producing enough urine and the placenta may not be functioning up to par. If your baby reacts appropriately to the nonstress test and levels of amniotic fluid are adequate, it's likely that all is well.

Umbilical artery Doppler velocimetry. This test is performed when there is evidence of fetal growth lag and uses a special ultrasound to measure the flow of blood through the umbilical artery. A weak, absent, or reverse flow during the second half of the fetal cardiac cycle (when the heart is filling with blood rather than pumping it out) indicates the baby is not getting adequate nourishment and probably not growing well.

Other tests of fetal wellbeing. These include regular ultrasound exams to document fetal growth and fetal scalp stimulation (which tests how a fetus reacts to pressure on, or pinching of, the scalp) during an NST.

Most of the time, babies pass these tests with flying colors, which means they can continue to stay put until they're good and ready to make their debuts. Rarely, the NST results can be labeled "nonreactive." Because these tests yield plenty of false positives, a nonreactive result doesn't definitely diagnose distress, but it will mean that your practitioner will continue to test your baby and, if it turns out there's any indication of fetal distress, will either induce your labor (see page 567) or perform a cesarean delivery.

not your baby's head is engaged: First, he or she will do an internal exam to see whether the presenting part—ideally the head—is in the pelvis. Second, he or she will feel that part externally (by pressing on your belly) to determine whether it is fixed in position or still "floating" free.

How far the presenting part has progressed through the pelvis is measured in "stations," each a centimeter long. A fully engaged baby is said to be at "zero station"—that is, the fetal head

has descended to the level of the prominent bony landmarks on either side of the midpelvis. A baby who has just begun to descend may be at −4 or −5 station. Once delivery begins, the head continues on through the pelvis past 0 to +1, +2, and so on, until it begins to "crown" at the external vaginal opening at +5.

Though an engaged head strongly suggests that the baby can get through the pelvis without difficulty, it's no guarantee. Conversely, a fetus that is still free

What's Considered Term?

Confused about when your baby is officially considered term? Post-term? Well, ACOG comes to the rescue with his handy glossary of "term" terminology:

- Preterm. A baby born between 20 weeks and 37 weeks is considered preterm.

- Early Term. If your baby is born between 37 weeks 0 days and 38 weeks 6 days, that's considered early term.

- Full Term. Babies born between 39 weeks 0 days and 40 weeks 6 days are considered full term. (Full term in twin pregnancies is 38 weeks.)

- Late Term. Got a late termer? That means arrival at between 41 weeks 0 days and 41 weeks 6 days.

- Post-term. Who's overstayed their welcome? Babies born after 42 weeks 0 days are considered post-term.

When you first heard from your baby, way back in the 5th month or so, there was ample room in the uterus for acrobatics, kickboxing, and punching. Now that conditions are getting a little cramped, his gymnastics are curtailed. In this snug uterine straitjacket, there is little room for anything more than turning, twisting, and wiggling—which is probably what you've been feeling. And once your baby's head is firmly engaged in your pelvis, he will be even more restricted in his movements. But this late in the game, it's not important what kind of fetal movement you feel (or even if it's only on one side), as long as you feel it. If, however, you feel no activity (see next question) or significantly diminished activity, check with your practitioner.

"I've hardly felt the baby kick at all this afternoon. What does that mean?"

Chances are your baby has settled down for a nap (older fetuses, like newborns, have periodic interludes of deep sleep) or that you've been too busy or too active to notice any movements. For reassurance, check for activity using the test described on page 315. It's a good idea to repeat this test routinely twice a day throughout the last trimester. Ten or more movements during each 1 to 2 hour test period (squirms and wriggles count, but not hiccups) mean that your baby's activity level is normal. Fewer movements suggest that medical evaluation might be necessary to determine the cause of the inactivity, so put in a call to your practitioner if that's the case. Though a baby who is relatively inactive in the womb can be perfectly healthy, inactivity at this point sometimes indicates fetal distress. Picking up this distress early and taking steps to intervene can often prevent serious consequences.

floating going into labor isn't necessarily going to have trouble negotiating the exit. And in fact, the majority of babies who haven't yet engaged when labor begins come through the pelvis smoothly. This is particularly true in moms who have already delivered 1 or more babies.

Changes in Baby's Movements

"My baby used to kick so hard. I can still feel him moving, but he seems less active now."

A Push Present for Your Baby Mama?

Thinking about surprising your baby mama with a little box after she delivers your little bundle of joy? Push presents (a gift that a dad gives to a mom to commemorate the birth of their baby) are gaining popularity among new parents. Of course the baby she's birthing is the greatest gift either of you could imagine—but after all that heavy lifting (and pushing) some sort of tangible tribute might be a nice bonus.

Not sure what to get? How about gifting her with some well-deserved postpartum pampering—like a gift certificate for a facial or a massage or a mani-pedi? Or a month's worth of professional housekeeping (actually, a great present for both of you)? Is baby bling more her thing? Consider a charm necklace etched with baby's name or initials, a bracelet with baby's birthstone, or even a ring to symbolize how your love has grown with your baby's birth.

Worried that a push present might push your budget too far? Or you'd rather slide any extra cash into your little one's college fund? Remember, some of the most meaningful gifts come without a hefty price tag. Surprise her with a bouquet of balloons or flowers or a lawn sign that proclaims your new papa pride. And don't forget the card—with some heartfelt words (or if you're particularly inspired, a poem or a song) about how much your love has grown over the last 9 months, and how much you look forward to your lifetime together.

Not a fan of the push present fad? Don't feel pressured to buy anything if that's not your style or hers. After all, trends come and go—but being partnered with a coparent who's committed to doing his half is truly the gift that keeps on giving. What's more, being present is the best present of all—not only at your baby's birth, but throughout your days, months, and years together as partners in parenting and life. That's what's called priceless.

"I've read that fetal movements are supposed to slow down as delivery approaches. My baby seems as active as ever."

Every baby's different, even before he or she is born—especially when it comes to activity levels, and particularly as delivery day approaches. While some babies move a bit less as they get ready to arrive, others keep up an energetic pace right until it's time for that first face-to-face. In late pregnancy, there is generally a gradual decline in the number of movements, probably related to tighter quarters, a decrease in amniotic fluid, and improved fetal coordination. But unless you're counting every single movement, you're not likely to notice a big difference.

Nesting Instinct

"I've heard about the nesting instinct. Is it pregnancy legend, or is it for real?"

The need to nest can be as real and as powerful an instinct for some humans as it is for our feathered and four-legged friends. If you've ever witnessed the birth of puppies or kittens, you've probably noticed how restless the laboring mother becomes just before delivery—frantically running back and forth, furiously shredding papers in a corner, and finally, when she feels all is in order, settling into the spot where she will give birth. Many expectant humans do experience the uncontrollable urge to ready their nests, too, just prior to

Massage It, Mama

Got nothing but time on your hands as you wait for baby's arrival? Put your hands (or a special someone else's hands) to good use—and give yourself a rub. Perineal massage can help gently stretch a first-timer's perineum (that area of skin between your vagina and rectum), which in turn can minimize the "stinging" that occurs when baby's head crowns during childbirth. And here's another plus you'll appreciate: It may also help you avoid tearing and an episiotomy, according to some experts.

Here's how to give your perineum the right rub: With clean hands (and short nails) insert your thumbs or index fingers (lubricated with a little K-Y jelly or olive oil if you'd like— but don't use mineral oil or Vaseline) inside your vagina. Press down (toward your rectum) and slide your fingers across the bottom and sides of your perineum. Repeat daily during the last weeks of pregnancy, 5 minutes (or longer) each time. Not feeling the perineal massage concept—because it seems too weird or too time-consuming? It's certainly not a must-do. Though anecdotal evidence has long supported its effectiveness, clinical research has not yet backed it up. Even without the rubbing, your body will still stretch when the time comes. And don't bother with perineal massage if you've already popped out a baby or two. Your perineum doesn't need the extra stretching, and probably won't benefit from it either (though perineal massage during labor can help stretch out even an experienced perineum as baby's head emerges).

One word to the wise: If you do go the massage route, proceed gently. The last thing you want to do right before labor is pull too hard, scratch yourself, or irritate sensitive skin. Massage with care down there.

---

childbirth—even though they won't likely be delivering in a pile of papers or leaves and twigs. For some it's subtle. All of a sudden, it becomes vitally important to clean out and restock the refrigerator and make sure there's a 6-month supply of toilet paper in the house. For others, this unusual burst of manic energy plays itself out in behavior that is dramatic, sometimes irrational, and often funny (at least, to those watching it)—cleaning every crevice of the nursery with a toothbrush, rearranging the contents of the kitchen cabinets alphabetically, washing everything that isn't tied down or being worn, or folding and refolding baby's clothes for hours on end.

Though it isn't a reliable predictor of when labor will begin, nesting usually intensifies as the big moment approaches—perhaps as a response to increased adrenaline circulating in an expectant mom's system. Keep in mind, however, that not all women experience the nesting instinct, and that those who don't are just as successful in nurturing their nestlings as those who do. The urge to slump on the sofa during the last few weeks of pregnancy is as common as the urge to clean out closets, and just as understandable. Make that more understandable.

If a nesting urge does strike, make sure it's tempered by common sense. Suppress that overwhelming urge to paint the baby's nursery yourself—let someone else climb the ladder with the bucket and roller while you oversee

Sounds Like a Plan

How far along in labor should you be before calling your practitioner? Should you call if your water breaks? How can you make contact if the contractions start outside of regular office hours? Should you call first and then head for the hospital or birthing center? Or the other way around?

Don't wait until labor starts to get the answers to these important questions. Discuss all of these and other labor logistics with your practitioner at your next appointment (if you haven't already), and write down all the pertinent info if it's not handed to you in a printout. Otherwise, you'll be sure to forget the instructions once those contractions kick in. If you're using a doula, make sure you know when to call her, too.

Also, be sure you know the best route to your place of delivery, roughly how long it will take to get there at various times of the day, and what kind of transportation is available if you don't have someone to drive you (don't plan on driving yourself). And if there are other children at home, or an elderly relative, or a pet, be sure you've made plans for their care in advance.

from a comfy chair. Don't let overzealous home cleaning exhaust you, either—you'll need energy reserves for both labor and a new baby. Most important of all, keep the limitations of your species in mind. Although you may share this nesting instinct with members of the animal kingdom, you are still only human—and you can't expect to get everything done before that little bundle of joy arrives at your nest.

When Will You Deliver?

"I just had an internal exam and the doctor said I'll probably be going into labor very soon. Can she really tell?"

Your practitioner can make a prediction about when you'll give birth, but it's still just an educated guess—just as your original due date was. There are clues that labor is getting closer, which a practitioner looks for beginning in the 9th month, both by palpating outside and examining inside. Has lightening or engagement taken place? What level,

or station, has the baby's presenting part descended to? Have effacement (thinning of the cervix) and dilation (opening of the cervix) begun? Has the cervix begun to soften and move to the front of the vagina (another indicator that labor is getting closer) or is it still firm and positioned to the back?

But "soon" can mean anywhere from an hour to 3 weeks or more. A practitioner's prediction of "you'll be in labor by tonight" could segue into a half month more of pregnancy, while a forecast of "labor's weeks away" could be followed the next day by baby's birth. The fact is that engagement, effacement, and dilation can occur gradually, over a period of weeks or even a month or more in some moms—and overnight in others. Which means that these clues are far from sure bets when it comes to pinpointing the start of labor.

So pack your bags just in case, but definitely don't keep the car running. You'll still have to play the waiting game, knowing for certain only that your day, or night, will come—sometime.

Do-It-Yourself Labor Induction?

So what happens if you're overdue and still as pregnant as ever (make that more pregnant than ever), with your baby showing no signs of budging? Should you just let nature take its course, no matter how long that course takes? Or should you take matters into your own hands and try some DIY labor induction techniques? And if you do take matters into your own hands, will it even work?

While there are plenty of natural methods you can use to try to bring on labor (and you can search for dozens online), it's hard to prove that any of them are effective. That's at least partly due to the fact that when they do appear to work, it's difficult to establish whether they actually worked—or whether labor, coincidentally, started on its own at the same time.

Still, if you're done with being pregnant (and who isn't by 40 weeks?) but your pregnancy isn't done yet, you might want to give these a try—they won't be harmful even if they don't end up kick-starting labor:

Walking. It has been suggested that walking can help ease the baby into the pelvis, thanks perhaps to the force of gravity or the swaying of your hips. Once baby puts pressure on the cervix—literally—labor might get going. If it turns out that your stroll doesn't jumpstart labor, you'll be no worse for wear. In fact, you might be in better shape for labor, when it actually does begin.

Sex. Sure, you're the size of a small hippo (and about as agile), but hoisting yourself into bed with your partner may be an effective way to mix business with pleasure. Or not. Some research shows that semen (which contains prostaglandins) can stimulate contractions when conditions are ripe (not before), and some have suggested (hopefully) that the release of oxytocin during orgasm might nudge the process along, too, once a woman has reached term. But not only has science failed to back that happy theory up—other research has found that women who continue to have sex late in pregnancy might carry their babies even longer than those who

The Overdue Baby

"I'm a week overdue. Is it possible that I might never go into labor on my own?"

Ah, the magic date—the one you synced up on your iCloud calendars, the one you confidently handed out to family and friends, the one your pregnancy app has been counting down for weeks—has arrived. And, as in about 30 percent of all pregnancies, the baby hasn't. Anticipation dissolves into discouragement. The stroller and crib sit empty for yet another day. And then a week. And then, in about 10 percent

of pregnancies, most often those of first-time mothers, 2 weeks. Will this pregnancy never end?

Though expectant moms who have reached the 42nd week might find it hard to believe, babies are forever—but pregnancy isn't. In fact, studies show that about 70 percent of apparent post-term pregnancies aren't post-term at all. They are believed to be late only because of a miscalculation of the time of conception, usually thanks to irregular ovulation or a woman's uncertainty about the exact date of her last period. And in fact, when early ultrasound examination is used to confirm the abstain. In the mood for love, or just so desperate you're ready to try anything? Get busy if you're game to try. After all, it may be the last time in a long time that you'll actually be able (or willing) to have sex. If getting busy brings on labor, great—if it doesn't, still great.

Other natural methods have potential drawbacks (even though they've been passed down from old wives to midwives to moms on message boards). So before you try these at home, discuss them with your practitioner first:

Nipple stimulation. Interested in some nipple tweaking (ouch)? How about some nipple twisting (double ouch)? Stimulating your nipples for a few hours a day (yes, hours) can release your own natural oxytocin and bring on contractions. But here's the caveat: Nipple stimulation—as enticing as hours of it may sound (or not)—can lead to painfully long and strong uterine contractions. Not to mention very sore nipples. So unless your practitioner advises it and is monitoring your progress, you may want to think 4 times—twice for each nipple—before you or your partner attempt nipple stimulation.

Castor oil. Hoping to sip your way into labor with a castor oil cocktail? Women have been passing down this yucky-tasting tradition for generations on the theory that this powerful laxative will stimulate your bowels, which in turn will stimulate your uterus into contracting. The caveat for this one: Castor oil (even mixed with a more appetizing drink) can cause diarrhea, severe cramping, and vomiting. Before you chugalug, be sure you're ready to begin labor that way.

Herbal teas and remedies. Raspberry leaf tea, black cohosh, and evening primrose may be just what your ancestors (and message board buddies) ordered for the overdue, and some studies show that these herbal remedies may actually help trigger or speed up contractions. Ask your practitioner about whether (and how much) of these remedies you should take and how. And turn to them only when you're already at term.

And while you're pondering the effectiveness of the DIY approach, remind yourself that you will go into labor—either on your own or with a little help from your practitioner—eventually.

due date, diagnoses of post-term pregnancy drop dramatically from the long-held estimate of 10 percent to about 2 percent.

Even if you do end up among those 2 percent of women who are truly overdue, your practitioner won't let your pregnancy pass the 42-week mark. In fact, most practitioners won't even let a pregnancy continue that long, choosing instead to induce by the time your baby has clocked in 41 weeks. Inducing labor at this point, by the way, doesn't seem to pose any increased chances of c-section and may in fact be associated with significantly lower blood loss for the mom and a significantly lower rate of meconium staining (see page 398) for the baby—plus it means you'll get to hold your baby sooner. And of course, if at any point test results show that the placenta is no longer doing its job well or that the amniotic fluid levels have dipped too low—or if there are any other signs that baby might not be thriving—your practitioner will take action, and depending on the situation, either induce labor or perform a cesarean delivery. Which means that even if you don't end up going into labor on your own, you won't be pregnant forever.

What to Take to the Hospital or Birthing Center

It's smart to think ahead about what you'll want to take to the hospital or birthing center (and to pack ahead, too). But it's also smart to think about traveling on the light side, packing only what you think you'll need—and not everything on this list:

For the Birthing Room

- This book, *What to Expect the First Year*, and *The What to Expect Pregnancy Journal and Organizer*, which has ample room for labor-and-delivery and meet-the-baby note keeping. Of course, you'll also have a phone with you—which means you'll have easy access to the What To Expect app.

- Several copies of your birth plan, if you're using one (see page 323)

- The cord blood collection kit, if you're planning to have your baby's cord blood banked

- A watch with a second hand for timing contractions (or you can use the digital timer on your phone)

- A portable music device (or your phone) loaded with your favorite playlist, if music soothes and relaxes you. Don't forget your chargers.

- A camera and/or video equipment (plus chargers) if you think the camera on your phone won't cut it

- A laptop or tablet (plus chargers)

- Favorite lotions or oils for massages

- A tennis ball or back massager, for firm countermassage

- Your own pillow, for comfort

- Sugarless lollipops or candies to keep your mouth moist

- A toothbrush, toothpaste, mouthwash, face wipes, and body wipes (you may find yourself desperate for a freshen-up)

- A robe if you don't feel like walking the halls during labor in only your hospital gown

- Heavy socks, in case your feet get cold

Your Birthing Room Guest List

"I'd really love to share our baby's birth with my sisters, my best friend, and of course my mom. Can they all be in the birthing room with my husband and me?"

Already planning your labor (and delivery) party? If you're like more and more moms-to-be, the guest list is getting longer and longer. Giving birth surrounded and supported by family and friends is a trend that's pretty popular in birthing circles.

Why is more potentially merrier on labor day? For many moms-to-be delivering at home or at a birthing center, it seems only natural to have the family around—including baby's older sibs. And for moms delivering in the hospital and choosing an epidural, there's more opportunity to socialize with little or no pain to deal with—or breathe through. Moms who plan to labor unmedicated may also appreciate the support of an extended support network. What's more, hospitals and birthing centers are accommodating the maternity mob, making some birthing rooms bigger

- Comfortable slippers with nonskid bottoms

- A scrunchie, clip, or hairband, if your hair is long, to keep it out of your face and tangle-free. A hairbrush and detangling comb, too, if you think they'll come in handy.

- Snacks for your coach, so he won't have to leave your side when his stomach starts growling. And snacks for you, too, if your practitioner allows eating during labor.

For the Postpartum Room

- A robe, comfy pj's, or a nightgown (with easy breastfeeding access if you're nursing), if you'd rather not wear hospital-issue

- A change of clothes for your coach, plus a toothbrush and anything else he might need for rooming-in

- Toiletries, including shampoo and conditioner, body wash, deodorant, and any makeup you can't live (or take pictures) without

- Your preferred brand of maxipads, though the hospital will provide some

- A couple of changes of underwear and a nursing bra

- A supply of healthy snacks to supplement hospital food (food delivery is also an option)

- A going-home outfit for you, keeping in mind that you'll still be sporting a sizable belly

- A going-home outfit for baby that's weather appropriate and practical (you'll need to accommodate the car seat straps). Add a receiving blanket and a heavy bunting or blanket if it's cold. Diapers will probably be provided by the hospital, but bring along a few extra, just in case.

- Infant car seat. Most hospitals will not let you leave with the baby unless he or she is safely strapped into an approved rear-facing infant car seat. Besides, it's the only safe way to travel with a baby—and it's the law. To avoid last-minute fumbles, attach the car seat base (and practice seat installation) well before your due date.

(more equipped to handle the overflow of guests) and more comfortable (complete with sofas and extra chairs for visitors to plop down on while they're waiting for the headliner to make his or her debut). And having a gaggle of girlfriends, a set or two of in-laws, and maybe a few other assorted relatives may be a win-win for birth attendants, too. Many practitioners reason that having more distraction, support, and back-rubbing hands makes a mom-to-be happier and more relaxed during labor—always a good thing, whether it's a medicated birth or not.

Clearly, there are lots of good reasons why you might want an encouraging entourage in the birthing room with you. Still, there are a few caveats to consider before you issue the invites: You'll have to get the practitioner-powers-that-be to sign off on your guest list (not all practitioners are crowd friendly, and some hospitals and birthing centers cap the number of guests you're allowed, or ask that young children not be part of the party). You'll also have to be sure your spouse is on board with the guest list (remember, even though you'll be doing most of the work,

Can You Eat Your Way to Labor?

Hungry for labor? Ready to do—or eat—anything that might trigger that first real contraction? Though there's no science backing them up, plenty of old wives (and new moms) will tell you about a last (pregnant) supper that ended with a trip down labor lane. Among the often heard: If your tummy can take the heat, dip into something spicy. Or order something that gets your bowels—and hopefully your uterus—in an uproar (a crate of bran muffins, chased down by a bucket of prune juice, perhaps?). Not in the mood for something so stimulating? Some women swear by eggplant, tomatoes, and balsamic vinegar (not necessarily together, though it sounds like a yummy Italian salad combo or pizza topping), while others claim pineapple buys a ticket on the Labor Express. Whatever you dig into, remember that unless your baby and your body are ready to take the labor plunge, it's unlikely that dinner's going to push you over the edge.

them to view—and could their discomfort put you on edge when you most need to be relaxed? Will you want everyone standing around chatting when you're craving peace and quiet (and rest)? Will you feel obligated to entertain your guests or pay attention to your other kids when you need to be focused on birthing your baby?

If you decide you'd like the company, just remember to put flexibility on the list, too. Remember (and remind your guests) that there's always the possibility your intended uneventful vaginal birth may turn into an unexpected c-section, in which case only the expectant dad will be allowed to follow the party into the OR. Or that you'll decide—say somewhere around the second hour of pushing—that you're not up for guests anymore and they might be shown to the door for delivery. (And if you do end up regretting your decision to invite a crowd, don't worry about hurting anyone's feelings by sending the guests packing—as a woman in labor, your feelings are the only ones that matter.)

Not feeling like inviting a crowd? Don't let trends—or pushy relatives—guilt you into a full birthing room. What feels right for you and your partner is the right decision.

both of you are cohosting the birth, and he won't want to be relegated to the B-list). Think about, too, whether you'll really be comfortable with so many eyes on you during a very personal moment (there will be moaning, grunting, peeing, a little pooping—and you will be half naked). Something else to ponder: Will those you've invited (your brother, your father-in-law, or your other children, for example) be comfortable with what you're inviting

Being a Mom

"Now that the baby's almost here, I'm beginning to worry about how I'm going to take care of her. I don't know anything about babies or being a mom—I've never even held a newborn before."

Here's the very first thing you need to know about becoming a mom: Babies are born, but moms aren't. As much hype as maternal instincts get, the truth is that becoming comfortable as a mom takes more than hormones—it

Rookie Nerves

Over the moon at the thought of becoming a dad for the first time—but also more than a little overwhelmed? Worried that fatherhood won't come as naturally to you as it does to other dads (those dads you see wearing babies and pushing strollers and swings everywhere you look)? Not to worry—few men are born fathers, any more than women are born mothers. Though parental love may come naturally, parental skills (the stuff you're probably stressed out about) have to be learned. Like every other new dad and mom, you'll grow from nervous rookie to confident pro one challenge, one bath, one all-night rocking session, one cuddle and coo at a time. Gradually, with practice, patience, persistence, and a lot of love (that'll be the easy part, once you gaze into that little face), the role that seems daunting—yes, terrifying—now will become second nature.

That said, though you'll learn plenty on the job—and from your mistakes, which every new parent makes plenty of—you might feel a little more comfortable with some basic training. Fortunately, classes that teach all the baby basics—from diapering to bathing, feeding to playing—are finding their way into communities across the country. There are classes you can take as a couple, as well as ones that are just for dads (including many run by Boot Camp for New Dads) in hospitals, community centers, and military bases nationwide. Ask about local options for classes at your next prenatal appointment or at your childbirth education class, check into them at the hospital or birthing center where you'll be delivering, or search for local classes at bootcampfornewdads.org. You can also learn the ropes by reading *What to Expect the First Year*. If you have friends or coworkers who have newborns, turn to them for some hands-on instruction. Ask them to let you hold, diaper, and play with their babies while they give you new-parent pointers.

While you're learning your baby basics, keep in mind that some of the most important skills you can bring to parenting are the ones you'll hopefully never have to use: infant safety and CPR. Take a class together before baby's arrival.

And remember, too, as you learn, that just as moms have different parenting techniques, so do dads. Relax, trust your instincts (surprise . . . dads have them, too), and feel free to find the style that works for both you and your baby. Before you know it, you'll be fathering with the best of them.

takes time and practice . . . practice that can only come on the job. Which means that for the first week or two, and often longer, a new mom (just like a new dad, by the way) can feel like she's not up for the job—especially as her baby does more crying than sleeping, the diapers leak, and many tears are shed over the "no tears" shampoo (on both sides of the bottle).

Slowly but surely—one dirty diaper, one marathon feeding session, one sleepless night at a time—every new mom (even the greenest . . . even you!) begins to feel like an old pro. Trepidation turns to assurance. The baby she was afraid to hold (won't it break?) is now cradled casually in her left arm while her right pays bills online or pushes the vacuum cleaner.

Stocking Up

Your kitchen, that is. Though shopping for strollers, diapers, and pint-size clothing understandably has been your priority these days, don't forget to take a time-out at the market. Even with swollen ankles and a supersize belly weighing you down, shopping is easier 9 months pregnant than it will be again for a long time—so take advantage and stock up now so you won't have to later with baby (and car seat, and diaper bag) in tow. Fill your pantry, fridge, and freezer to the brim with healthy foods that are easy to serve—cheese sticks, individual containers of yogurt, frozen fruit bars, frozen fruit for making smoothies, cereal, granola bars, soups, freeze-dried fruit, and nuts. Don't forget the paper products, too (you'll be using paper towels by the crateful, and disposable plates and cups can fill in when you don't get around to running the dishwasher). And while you're in the kitchen—and have the time—cook up some extra servings of your favorite freezer-friendly foods (lasagna, mini meat loaves, chili, pancakes, muffins), and store them in clearly marked single-meal containers in the freezer. They'll be ready to pop in the microwave when you're pooped (and hungry) postpartum.

Feel much more like dropping than shopping? Now's also a great time to explore online grocery delivery (if you haven't already)—which could come in pretty handy once your hands are full of baby.

She can dispense vitamin drops, give baths, and slip squirming arms and legs into onesies in her sleep—literally, sometimes. As she hits her mommy stride and settles into a somewhat predictable rhythm, parenting an infant becomes second nature. She feels those instincts kicking in, sending those nagging self-doubts packing—at least, most of them. She starts to feel like the mom she is, and—difficult though it may be to imagine right now—you will, too.

Though nothing can make those first days with a first baby a cinch, starting the learning process before your newborn is placed in your arms (and in your round-the-clock care) can make them seem a little less overwhelming. Any of the following can help soon-to-be moms (and dads) ease into their new roles: holding, diapering, and soothing a friend's or family member's infant, reading up on baby basics in *What to Expect the First Year*, and watching parenting videos or taking a class in baby care (and baby CPR).

For even more reassurance, talk to friends—online or next door—who have recently become parents (no one can teach you more about being a mom than another mom). You'll be surprised—and relieved—to know that just about everybody comes into the job with the same new mom (or new dad) jitters.

ALL ABOUT:
Prelabor, False Labor, Real Labor

It always seems so simple in the movies. Somewhere around 3 a.m., the expectant mom sits up in bed, puts a knowing hand on her (perfectly proportioned) belly, and reaches over to rouse her sleeping spouse with a calm (or crazed), "Honey, it's time."

But how, you wonder, does she know it's time? How does she recognize labor with such cool, clinical confidence when she's never been in labor before? What makes her so sure she's not going to get to the hospital, be examined by the resident, found to be nowhere near her time, and be sent home, amid snickers from the night shift, just as pregnant as when she arrived? The script, of course.

On your side of the screen (with no script in hand), you're more likely to awaken at 3 a.m. with complete uncertainty. Are these really labor pains or just more Braxton Hicks? Should I turn on the light and start timing? Should I bother to wake my spouse? Do I drag my practitioner out of bed in the middle of the night to report what might really be false labor? If I do and it isn't time, will I turn out to be the mom who cried "labor" once too often, and will anybody take me seriously when it's for real? Or will I be the only one in my childbirth class not to recognize labor? Will I leave for the hospital too late, maybe giving birth in the backseat (and making media headlines)? The questions multiply faster than the contractions.

The fact is that most women, worry though they might, don't end up misjudging the onset of their labor. The vast majority, thanks to instinct, luck, or no-doubt-about-it killer contractions, show up at the hospital or birthing center neither too early nor too late, but at just about the right time. Still, there's no reason to leave your judgment up to chance. Becoming familiar in advance with the signs of prelabor, false labor, and real labor will help allay the concerns and clear up the confusion when those contractions (or are they?) begin.

Prelabor Symptoms

Before there's labor, there's prelabor—a sort of pregame show that sets things up before the main event. The physical changes of prelabor can precede real labor by a full month or more—or by only an hour or so. Prelabor is characterized by the beginning of cervical effacement and dilation, which your practitioner can confirm on examination, as well as by a wide variety of related signs that you may notice yourself (though not all moms will experience them all):

Dropping. Usually somewhere between 2 and 4 weeks before labor starts in first-time mothers, the fetus begins to settle down into the pelvis. This milestone is rarely reached in second or later births until labor is about to kick off.

Sensations of increasing pressure in the pelvis and rectum. Crampiness (similar to menstrual cramps) and groin pain are common—and particularly likely in second and later pregnancies. Persistent low backache may also be present.

Loss of weight or no gain. Weight gain might slow down in the 9th month— and as labor approaches, you might

Ready or Not

To make sure you're ready for your baby's arrival when he or she is ready to arrive, start reading up now about labor and delivery in the next chapter.

even lose a bit of weight, as much as 2 to 3 pounds.

A change in energy levels. Some 9th-monthers find that they are increasingly exhausted. Others experience energy spurts. An uncontrollable urge to scrub floors and clean out closets has been related to the "nesting instinct," in which the female of the species—that's you—prepares the nest for the impending arrival (see page 383).

A change in vaginal discharge. If you've been watching your undies closely, you may find your discharge increases and thickens.

Loss of the mucous plug. As the cervix begins to thin and open, the "cork" of mucus that seals the opening of the uterus may becomes dislodged (see page 396). This gelatinous chunk of mucus can be passed through the vagina a week or two before the first real contractions, or just as labor begins. Not everyone notices the passing of their mucous plug—but if you're watching the toilet and toilet paper closely, it's usually hard to miss if you lose it.

Pink, or bloody, show. As the cervix effaces and dilates, capillaries frequently rupture, tinting the mucus pink or streaking it with blood (see page 397). This "show" usually means labor will start within 24 hours—though it could be as much as several days away.

Intensification of Braxton Hicks contractions. These practice contractions (see page 340) may become more frequent and stronger, even very painful.

Diarrhea. Some women experience loose bowel movements just before labor starts.

False Labor Symptoms

Is it or isn't it? Real labor probably has not begun if:

- Contractions are not at all regular and don't increase in frequency or severity. Real contractions won't necessarily fall into a neat textbook pattern, but they will become more intense and more frequent over time.

- Contractions subside if you walk around or change your position (though this can sometimes be the case in early "real" labor, too).

- Show, if any, is brownish. This kind of discharge is often the result of an internal exam or intercourse within the past 48 hours.

- Fetal movements intensify briefly with contractions.

- Contractions start and stop . . . and start and stop. This frustrating form of false labor—when contractions start becoming more regular (if not closely spaced) for a period of time, then taper off, then start up again and taper off again—is also known as prodromal labor, and it can linger on and off for days.

Keep in mind that false labor isn't a waste of time—even if you've driven all the way to the hospital or birthing center only to get sent home. It's your body's way of getting pumped, primed, and prepped, so when the time comes, it'll be ready—whether you are or not.

Real Labor Symptoms

No one knows exactly what triggers real labor (and more just-about-due moms are concerned with "when" than "why"), but it's believed that a combination of factors are involved. This very intricate process begins with the fetus, whose brain sets off a relay of chemical messages (which probably loosely translate into something like, "Mom, let me out of here!") that kick off a chain reaction of hormones in the mother. These hormonal changes in turn pave the way for the work of prostaglandins and oxytocin, substances that trigger contractions when all labor systems are "go."

You'll know that the contractions of prelabor have been replaced by true labor if:

- The contractions intensify, rather than ease up, with activity and aren't relieved by a change in position.

- Contractions become progressively more frequent and painful, and generally (but not always) more regular. Each contraction won't necessarily be more painful or longer (they usually last about 30 to 70 seconds) than the last one, but the intensity does build up as real labor progresses. Frequency doesn't always increase in regular, perfectly even intervals, either—but it does increase.

- Early contractions feel like gastrointestinal upset, or like heavy menstrual cramps, or like lower abdominal pressure. Pain may be just in the lower abdomen or in the lower back and abdomen, and it may also radiate down into the legs (particularly the upper thighs). Location, however, is not as reliable an indication, because false labor contractions may also be felt in these places.

In 15 percent of labors, the water breaks—in a gush or a trickle—before labor begins. But in many others, the membranes rupture spontaneously during labor, or are ruptured artificially by the practitioner.

When to Call the Practitioner

Your practitioner has likely told you when to call if you think you're in labor (when contractions are 5 to 7 minutes apart, for instance, though your practitioner may have given you different parameters). Don't wait for perfectly even intervals—they may never come. If you're not sure you're in real labor—but the contractions are coming pretty regularly—call anyway. Your practitioner will probably be able to tell from the sound of your voice, as you talk through a contraction, whether it's the real thing—but only if you don't try to cover up the pain in the name of good phone manners. Even if you've checked and rechecked the above lists and you're still unsure, call your practitioner. Don't feel guilty about waking him or her in the middle of the night (people who deliver babies for a living don't expect to work 9 to 5) or be embarrassed if it turns out to be a false alarm (you wouldn't be the first expectant mom to misjudge her labor signs, and you won't be the last). Don't assume that if you're not sure it's real labor, it isn't. Err on the side of caution and call.

Also call your practitioner immediately if contractions are increasingly strong but your due date is still weeks away, if you notice bright red blood, if your water breaks with or without labor, if your water breaks and it has a greenish-brown tint, or if you feel something slipping out into your cervix or vagina after your water has broken (it could be the umbilical cord).

CHAPTER 14

Labor and Delivery

....

Are you counting down the days? Eager to see your feet again? Desperate to sleep on your stomach—or just plain desperate to sleep? Don't worry—the end (of pregnancy) is near. And as you contemplate that thrilling moment—when your baby will finally be in your arms instead of inside your belly—you're probably also giving a lot of thought to (and coming up with a lot of questions about) the process that will make that moment possible: labor and delivery. When will labor start? More important, when will it end? Is that pee in my pants, or did my water just break? Will I be able to handle the pain? Will I need an epidural (and when can I have one)? A fetal monitor? An IV? What if I want to labor—and deliver—in a tub? Without any meds? What if I don't make any progress? What if I progress so quickly that I don't make it to the hospital or birthing center in time?

Armed with answers to these (and other) questions—plus the support of your partner and your birth attendants—you'll be prepared for just about anything that labor and delivery might bring your way. Just remember the most important thing that labor and delivery will bring your way (even if nothing else goes according to plan): that beautiful new baby of yours.

What You May Be Wondering About

Mucous Plug

"I think I lost my mucous plug. Does that mean labor is about to start?"

It may be a rite of pregnancy passage (some might say, a slightly yucky one) but passing the mucous plug isn't a sign that labor's about to start. It's not even universally experienced among about-to-be-moms. The mucous plug—the clear, globby, gelatinous blob-like barrier that has corked your cervix throughout your pregnancy—often becomes dislodged as dilation and effacement begin. Some women notice the popping of this mucous plug (what exactly is that in the toilet?), others don't (especially if you're the flush-and-rush type). Though the passage of the plug is a sign that your body's gearing up for the big day, it's not a reliable signal that the big day has arrived—or even that it's around the corner. At this point, labor could be days, or even weeks, away, with your cervix continuing to open gradually over that time. In other words, there's no need to call your practitioner or frantically pack those last minute items into your bags just yet. There's also no need to worry about your baby's safety now that you're unplugged. In fact, your cervix continues to make mucus to protect the cervical opening and prevent infection, which means baby's still snugly sealed off—and it means that you can have sex, take a bath, and otherwise go about your business even after you've lost your plug.

No plug in your pants or your toilet? Not to worry. Many women don't lose it ahead of time, and that doesn't predict anything about the eventual progress of labor.

Bloody Show

"I have a pink mucousy discharge. Does it mean labor's about to start?"

Sounds like it's bloody show time—and happily, this particular production is a preview of labor very soon to come. Passing that bloody show, a mucousy discharge tinged pink or brown with blood, is usually a sign that the blood vessels in the cervix are rupturing as it dilates and effaces and the process that

leads to delivery is well under way (and that's something to applaud!). Once the bloody show has made its debut in your underwear or on the toilet paper, chances are your baby's arrival is just a day or two away. But since labor is a process with an erratic timetable, you'll be kept in suspense until the first true contractions strike. Keep in mind, passing bloody show is different from passing the mucous plug. Though they definitely have mucous in common, bloody show is a discharge (and it's blood-tinged), while the mucous plug is more of a one-time gelatinous glob. Bloody show means it's almost show time, mucous plug means . . . maybe not so fast.

If your discharge suddenly becomes bright red (instead of blood-tinged or streaked), contact your practitioner right away.

Your Water Breaking

"I woke up in the middle of the night with a wet bed. Did I lose control of my bladder, or did my water break?"

A sniff of your sheets will probably clue you in. If the wet spot smells sort of sweet (not like urine, which has the harsher odor of ammonia), it's probably amniotic fluid your sheets are soaked in—and that's a sign that your membranes have probably ruptured (your water has broken). Another sign: You continue leaking the pale, straw-colored fluid. Another test: You can try to stem the flow of the fluid by squeezing your pelvic muscles (Kegel exercises). If the flow stops, it's urine. If it doesn't, it's amniotic fluid.

You are more likely to notice the leaking while you are lying down. It usually stops, or at least slows, when you stand up or sit down, since baby's head acts as a cork, blocking the flow temporarily. The leakage is heavier—whether you're sitting or standing—if the break in the membranes is down near the cervix than if it is higher up.

Your practitioner has probably given you a set of instructions to follow if your water breaks. If you don't remember the instructions or have any doubts about how to proceed—call, night or day.

"My water just broke, but I haven't had any contractions. When is labor going to start, and what should I do in the meantime?"

It's likely that labor's on the way—and soon. Most women whose membranes rupture before labor begins can expect to feel the first contraction within 12 hours of that first trickle, while most others can expect to feel it within 24 hours.

About 1 in 10, however, find that labor takes a little longer to get going. To prevent infection through the ruptured amniotic sac (the longer it takes for labor to get going, the greater the risk), most practitioners induce labor within 24 hours of a rupture if a mom-to-be is at or near her due date, and a few induce as early as 6 hours after. Many women who have experienced a rupture actually welcome a sooner-than-later induction, preferring it to 24 hours of wet waiting.

The first thing to do if you experience a trickle or flow of fluid from your vagina—besides grab a towel and a box of pads—is call your practitioner (unless he or she has instructed otherwise). In the meantime, keep your vaginal area as clean as possible to avoid infection: Don't have sex (not that there's much chance you'd want to right now), use a pad (not a tampon) to absorb the flow, don't try to do your own internal exam, and, as always, wipe from front to back when you use the toilet.

Rarely, when the membranes rupture before labor begins and the baby's presenting part is not yet engaged in the pelvis (more likely when the baby is breech or preterm), the umbilical cord can become "prolapsed"—it is swept into the cervix, or even down into the vagina, with the gush of amniotic fluid. If you can see a loop of umbilical cord at your vaginal opening, or think you feel something inside your vagina, call 911. For more on what to do if the cord is prolapsed, see page 568.

Darkened Amniotic Fluid

"My membranes ruptured, and the fluid isn't clear—it's greenish brown. What does this mean?"

Your amniotic fluid is probably stained with meconium, a greenish-brown substance that is actually your baby's first bowel movement. Ordinarily, meconium is passed after birth as a baby's first stool. But sometimes—such as when the fetus has been under stress in the womb, and more often when the due date has come and gone—meconium is passed before birth into the amniotic fluid.

Meconium staining alone is not a sure sign of fetal distress, but because it suggests the possibility of distress, notify your practitioner right away. He or she will likely want to get labor started (if contractions aren't already in full swing) and will monitor your baby very closely throughout labor.

Low Amniotic Fluid During Labor

"My doctor said that my amniotic fluid is low and she needs to supplement it. Should I be concerned?"

Usually, nature keeps the uterus well stocked with a self-replenishing supply of amniotic fluid. Fortunately, even when levels do run low during labor, medical science can step in and supplement that natural source with a saline solution pumped directly into the amniotic sac through a very thin and flexible catheter inserted through the cervix into the uterus. This procedure, called amnioinfusion, can significantly reduce the possibility that a surgical delivery will become necessary because of fetal distress.

Irregular Contractions

"In childbirth class we were told not to go to the hospital until the contractions were regular and 5 minutes apart. Mine are less than 5 minutes apart, but they aren't at all regular. I don't know what to do."

Just as no two women have exactly the same pregnancies, no two women have exactly the same labors. The labor often described in books and online, in childbirth education classes, and by practitioners is what is typical—close to what many expectant moms can expect. But far from every labor is true-to-textbook, with contractions regularly spaced and predictably progressive.

If you're having strong, long (20 to 60 seconds), frequent (mostly 5 to 7 minutes apart or less) contractions, even if they vary considerably in length and time elapsed between them, don't wait for them to become regular before calling your practitioner or heading for the hospital or birthing center—no matter what you've heard or read. It's possible your contractions are about as regular as they're going to get and you're well into the active phase of your labor. Either way, better to play it safe than play it by the book.

Calling Your Practitioner During Labor

"I just started getting contractions and they're coming every 3 or 4 minutes. I feel silly calling my doctor, who said we should spend the first several hours of labor at home."

Better silly than sorry. It's true that most first-time moms-to-be (whose labors are usually initially slow-going, with a gradual buildup of contractions) can safely count on spending the first several hours at home, leisurely finishing up their packing and their baby prep. But it doesn't sound like your labor's fitting that typical first-timer pattern. If your contractions have started off strong—lasting at least 45 seconds and coming more frequently than every 5 minutes—your first several hours of labor may very well be your last (and if you're not a first-timer, your labor may be on an even faster track). Chances are much of the first stage of labor has passed painlessly and your cervix has dilated significantly during that time. This means that not calling your practitioner, chancing a dramatic dash to the hospital or birthing center at the last minute—or not getting there in time—might be sillier than picking up the phone now.

So by all means call. When you do, be clear and specific about the frequency, duration, and strength of your contractions. Since your practitioner is used to judging the phase of labor in part by the sound of a woman's voice as she talks through a contraction, don't try to downplay your discomfort, put on a brave front, or keep a calm tone when you describe what you're experiencing. Let the contractions speak for themselves, as loudly as they need to. For the

Emergency Delivery If You're Alone

You'll almost certainly never need the following instructions—but just in case, keep them handy.

1. Try to remain calm. You can do this.

2. Call 911 for the emergency medical service. Ask them to contact your practitioner.

3. Find someone nearby to help, if possible (call a neighbor, coworker, or friend).

4. Start panting to keep yourself from pushing.

5. Wash your hands and then your vaginal area with soap and water or use a wipe or hand sanitizer.

6. Spread some clean towels or sheets on a bed, sofa, or the floor, and gather other towels or blankets in case baby arrives. Unlock the door so that help can get in easily when it arrives, and then lie back, propping yourself up on pillows.

7. If despite your panting the baby starts to arrive before help does, gently ease him or her out by pushing each time you feel the urge.

8. As the top of the baby's head begins to appear, pant or blow (do not push), and press gently on your perineum (the area right under where the head is emerging) to keep the head from popping out suddenly. Let the head emerge gradually—don't pull it out. If there is a loop of umbilical cord around the baby's neck, hook a finger under it and gently work it over the baby's head.

9. Next, hold baby's head gently in both hands and, if you can, press it very slightly downward (do not pull), pushing at the same time, to deliver the front shoulder. As the upper arm appears, lift the head carefully, feeling for the rear shoulder to deliver. Once the shoulders are free, the rest of your baby should slip out easily.

10. Place baby on your abdomen or, if the cord is long enough (don't tug at it), on your chest—the skin-to-skin contact will warm baby. Quickly wrap blankets or towels over the baby.

11. Wipe baby's mouth and nose with a clean towel or cloth, and run your fingers from the inside corners of baby's eyes down the outsides of the nostrils to help drain the amniotic fluid. If help hasn't arrived and the baby isn't breathing or crying, rub his or her back, keeping the head lower than the feet. If breathing still hasn't started, clear out baby's mouth some more with a clean finger and give 2 quick and extremely gentle puffs of air into his or her nose and mouth.

12. Don't try to pull the placenta out. But if it emerges on its own before help arrives, wrap it in towels, and keep it elevated above the level of the baby, if possible. There is no need to cut the cord. If help is a long way off, tie the cord with a string or shoelace about 2 to 3 minutes after delivery.

13. Keep yourself and your baby warm and comfortable until help arrives.

same reason, don't have your partner do the speaking for you—even if you're not (understandably) in a chatty mood.

If you feel you're ready but your practitioner doesn't seem to think so, ask if you can go to the hospital/birthing center or to your practitioner's office and have your progress checked. Take your bag along just in case, but be ready to turn around and go home if you've only just begun to dilate—or if nothing's going on at all.

Not Getting to the Hospital in Time

"I'm afraid I won't get to the hospital in time."

Fortunately, most of those sudden deliveries you've heard about take place on TV. In real life, deliveries (especially those of first-time moms) rarely occur without plenty of heads-up—and plenty of time to get to the hospital. But once in a really great while, a woman who hasn't felt any contractions, or has felt them only sporadically, suddenly feels an overwhelming urge to bear down. Often she mistakes it for a need to go to the bathroom (cue the "I delivered in the toilet" reenactment video).

Again, super unlikely to happen to you. Still, it's a good idea for both you and your coach to become familiar with the basics of an emergency delivery (see boxes facing page and page 402). Once that's done, sit back and relax, knowing you're prepared for something that you're far more likely to see on reality TV than really experience.

Having a Short Labor

"I always hear about women who have really short labors. How common are they?"

While they make for good stories, not all of the short labors you've heard about are as short as they seem. Often, an expectant mom who appears to have a quickie labor has actually been having painless contractions for hours, days, even weeks—contractions that have been dilating her cervix gradually. By the time she finally feels one, she's well into the final stage of labor.

That said, occasionally the cervix dilates very rapidly, accomplishing in a matter of minutes what the average cervix (particularly a first-time mom's cervix) takes hours to do. And happily, even with this abrupt, or "precipitous," kind of labor (one that takes 3 hours or less from start to finish), there is usually no risk to the baby.

If your labor seems to start with a bang—with contractions strong and close together—get to the hospital or birthing center quickly (so you and your baby can be monitored closely). Medication may be helpful in slowing contractions a bit to ease the pressure on your baby, on your own body, and on your emotional state (sometimes a mom-to-be who's having a very fast labor becomes understandably agitated, so slowing down the labor can help calm her).

Back Labor

"The pain in my lower back since my contractions began is so bad that I don't see how I'll be able to make it through labor."

What you're probably experiencing is known in the birthing business as "back labor"—and it definitely is a pain. A lot of pain. Technically, back labor occurs when the fetus is in a posterior position, with its face up and the back of its head pressing against your sacrum, or the back of your pelvis. (Ironically, this position is nicknamed "sunny-side up," though there's nothing cheerful about back labor.) It's possible, however, to experience back labor when the baby isn't in this position or to continue to experience it after the baby has flipped or been turned to a face-down position—possibly because the area has already become a focus of tension.

Emergency Delivery Tips for the Coach

At Home or the Office

1. Try to remain calm while at the same time comforting and reassuring the mom. Remember, even if you don't know the first thing about delivering a baby, a mother's body and her baby can do most of the job on their own.

2. Call 911 to dispatch emergency medical service. Ask them to call the practitioner.

3. Have the mom start panting, to keep from pushing.

4. Wash your hands and the vaginal area with soap and water (or use a wipe or hand sanitizer).

5. If there's time, place the mom on the bed or sofa (or as a last resort on a desk or table) with her buttocks slightly hanging off, her hands under her thighs to keep them elevated. If available, an ottoman or footstool can support her feet. Protect delivery surfaces, if possible, with towels or sheets. If baby's head is already appearing, place a few pillows or cushions under the mom's shoulders and head to help raise her to a semi-sitting position, which can aid delivery. If baby's head hasn't appeared yet, having the mom lie flat or on her side may slow delivery until help arrives.

6. As the top of the baby's head begins to appear, have the mom pant or blow (not push), and press gently against her perineum (the area between the vagina and the anus) to apply slight pressure to keep the head from popping out suddenly. Let the head emerge gradually—never pull on it. If there is a loop of umbilical cord around the baby's neck, hook a finger under it and gently work it over the baby's head.

7. Next, take the head gently in both hands and press it very slightly downward (do not pull), asking mom to push at the same time, so you can deliver the front shoulder. As the upper arm appears, lift the head carefully, watching for the rear shoulder to deliver. Once the shoulders are free, the rest of the baby should slip out easily.

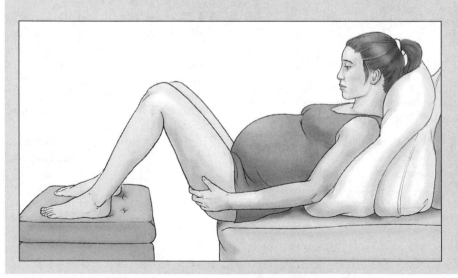

8. Place the baby on the mom's belly or, if the cord is long enough (don't tug at it), on her chest. Quickly wrap the baby in blankets, towels, or anything else that's clean.

9. Wipe baby's mouth and nose with a clean cloth and run your fingers from the inside corners of baby's eyes down the outsides of the nostrils to help drain fluid. If help hasn't arrived and the baby isn't breathing or crying, rub his or her back, keeping the head lower than the feet. If breathing still hasn't started, clear out baby's mouth some more with a clean finger, and give 2 quick and extremely gentle puffs of air into the nose and mouth.

10. Don't try to pull out the placenta. But if it emerges on its own before emergency assistance arrives, wrap it in towels, and keep it elevated above the level of the baby, if possible. There's no need to cut the cord, but you should tie it with a string or shoelace 2 to 3 minutes after birth if help hasn't arrived.

11. Keep both mom and baby warm and comfortable until help arrives.

En Route to the Hospital or Birthing Center

If you're in your car and delivery is imminent, pull over to a safe area, turning on your hazard lights. Call 911. If someone stops, ask for help contacting 911 or the local emergency medical service. If you're in a cab, ask the driver to radio or call for help.

If possible, help the mom into the back of the car. Place a coat, jacket, or blanket under her. Then, if help has not arrived, proceed as for a home delivery. As soon as the baby is born, quickly head to the nearest hospital unless the emergency dispatcher has told you help is on the way.

When you're having this kind of pain—which often doesn't let up between contractions and can become excruciating during them—the cause doesn't matter much. How to relieve it, even slightly, does. If you're opting to have an epidural, go for it (there's no need to wait, especially if you're in a lot of pain). It's possible that you might need a higher dose than usual to get full comfort from the back labor pain, so let the anesthesiologist know about it. Other options (such as narcotics) also offer pain relief. If you'd like to stay med-free, several measures may help relieve the discomfort of back labor— all are at least worth trying:

Taking the pressure off. Try changing your position. Walk around (though this may not be possible once contractions are coming fast and furious), crouch or squat, get down on all fours, lean or sit on a birthing ball, do whatever is most comfortable and least painful for you. If you feel you can't move and would prefer to be lying down, lie on your side, with your back well rounded—in a sort of fetal position.

Heat or cold. Have your coach (or doula or nurse) use warm compresses, a heating pad, ice packs, or cold compresses—whichever soothes best. Or alternate heat and cold.

Counterpressure and massage. Have your coach experiment with different ways of applying pressure to the area of greatest pain, or to adjacent areas, to find one or more that seem to help. He can try his knuckles, the heel of one hand reinforced by pressure from the other hand on top of it, a tennis ball, or a back massager, using direct pressure or a firm circular motion. Cream, oil, or powder can be applied periodically to reduce irritation.

Reflexology. For back labor, this therapy involves applying strong finger pressure just below the center of the ball of the foot.

Other alternative pain relievers. Hydrotherapy (a warm shower or jetted bath) can ease the pain somewhat. If you've had some experience with meditation, visualization, or self-hypnosis for pain, try these, too. They often work, and they certainly couldn't hurt.

Labor Induction

"My doctor wants to induce labor. But I'm not overdue yet, and I thought induction was only for overdue babies."

Sometimes Mother Nature needs a little help making a mother out of a pregnant woman. About 20 percent of pregnancies end up needing that kick in the maternity pants, and though a lot of the time induction is necessary because a baby is overdue, there are many other reasons why your practitioner might feel that nature needs a nudge, such as:

- Your membranes have ruptured and contractions have not started on their own within 24 hours (though some practitioners induce much sooner).

- Tests suggest that your uterus is no longer a healthy home for your baby because the placenta is no longer functioning optimally, amniotic fluid levels are low, or for another reason.

- Tests suggest that the baby isn't thriving and is mature enough to be delivered.

- You have a complication, such as pre-eclampsia or gestational diabetes, or a chronic or acute illness that makes it risky to continue your pregnancy.

- There's a concern that you might not make it to the hospital or birthing center on time once labor has started, either because you live a long distance away or because you've had a previous very short labor (or both).

If you're still unsure about your doctor's reasons for inducing labor, ask for a more substantial and satisfying explanation. To find out all you'll need to know about the induction process, keep reading.

"How does induction work?"

Induction, like naturally triggered labor, is a process—and sometimes a pretty long process. But unlike naturally triggered labor, your body will be getting some help with the heavy lifting if you're induced. Labor induction usually involves a number of steps (though you won't necessarily go through all of these steps):

- First, your cervix will need to be ripened (or softened) so that labor can begin. If you arrive with a ripe cervix, great—you'll probably move ahead to the next step. If your cervix is not dilated, not effaced, and not soft at all, your practitioner will likely administer a hormonal substance such as prostaglandin E in the form of a vaginal gel, insert, or tablet suppository to get things started. In this painless procedure, either a syringe is used to place the gel in the vagina close to your cervix, or your practitioner inserts the tablet or insert into the vagina near the cervix. After a few hours or longer, you'll be checked to see if your cervix is getting softer and beginning to efface and dilate. If it isn't, a second dose may be administered. In many cases, the gel or insert is enough to get contractions and labor started. If your cervix is ripe enough but contractions have not begun, the induction process continues. (Some practitioners use

Membrane Stripping

Stripping the membranes (also known as membrane sweeping) is one way your practitioner may try to jump-start labor—sometimes as part of the induction process in the hospital, sometimes during a regular prenatal visit when a mom is at or very near term. It's different from membrane rupturing, though it can lead to it. Here's what you need to know about membrane stripping:

How's it done? Your practitioner will use his or her finger to gently separate the amniotic sac (aka bag of water) from the side of your uterus near the cervix. Once the sac is separated, your body releases hormones (prostaglandins) that can eventually help get those contractions you're waiting for started. Membrane stripping could be a one-time deal, or your practitioner may ask you to come back every few days to repeat the process if the first attempt didn't get labor going. Even if your practitioner chooses to strip the membranes only once, you'll likely be asked to come back every few days to be checked for progress.

What does it feel like? Having your membranes stripped can be a little uncomfortable, though some women don't feel a thing. You might experience some crampiness for 24 hours after your membranes have been stripped (which may or may not lead to the labor contractions you're hoping for). You may also notice slight reddish, pink, or brown spotting for a few days afterward. All this is normal and nothing to worry about, though if you have severe pain or bright red bleeding, call your practitioner right away.

But . . . does it work? There is some evidence that having your membranes stripped may fast-track you to the birthing room—just maybe not so fast (it could take 3 to 5 days or more before any of those real-deal contractions start). But since it's not a slam dunk for starting labor and it's no fun for moms, many experts say it shouldn't be done routinely.

---

devices designed to ripen the cervix, such as a catheter with an inflatable balloon, graduated dilators to stretch the cervix, or even a botanical—called Laminaria japonicum—that, when inserted, gradually opens the cervix as it absorbs fluid around it and expands.)

- If the amniotic sac is still intact, your practitioner may strip the membranes (see box, above). Or he or she may artificially rupture your membranes (see page 409) to try to get labor started.

- If you're still not having regular contractions, your practitioner will slowly administer intravenous Pitocin, a synthetic form of the hormone oxytocin (which is produced naturally by the body throughout pregnancy and also plays an important role in labor), until contractions are well established. The drug misoprostol, given through the vagina, might be used as an alternative to other ripening and induction techniques.

- Your baby will be continuously monitored to assess how he or she is dealing with the stress of labor. You'll also be monitored to make sure the drug isn't overstimulating your uterus, triggering contractions that are too long or powerful. If that happens, the rate of infusion can be reduced or the process can be discontinued entirely. Once your contractions are in full swing, the oxytocin may be stopped or the dose decreased, and labor should progress just as a noninduced labor does. You can also get an epidural at this point if you'd like.

- If, after 8 to 12 hours of oxytocin administration, labor hasn't begun or progressed, your practitioner might stop the induction process to give you a chance to rest before trying again or, depending on the circumstances, the procedure may be stopped in favor of a cesarean delivery.

Eating and Drinking During Labor

"I've heard conflicting things about whether it's okay to eat and drink during labor."

Should eating be on the menu when you're in labor? That depends on who's placing the orders. Some practitioners red-light all food and drink during labor, on the theory that food in the digestive tract might be aspirated, or "breathed in," in the very, very unlikely case that emergency general anesthesia becomes necessary. These practitioners usually okay ice chips only, supplemented as needed by intravenous fluids.

Most other practitioners (and guidelines from ACOG), however, allow liquids and light solids (read: no stuffed-crust pizza) during a low-risk labor. These folks logically figure that a mom doing the hard work of labor needs both fluids and calories to stay strong and effective. Besides, they point out, the risk of aspiration (which,

again, exists only if general anesthesia is used, which it rarely is except in emergency situations) is extremely low: 7 in 10 million births. Their position has even been backed up by research, which shows that moms who are allowed to eat and drink during labor have shorter labors by an average of 90 minutes. Non-fasting moms are also less likely to need oxytocin to speed up labor, require fewer pain medications, and have babies with higher Apgar scores than moms who are forced to fast. Check with your practitioner to find out what will and won't be on the menu for you during labor.

Even if your practitioner gives you the go-ahead on eating, chances are you won't be in the market for a major meal once the contractions begin in earnest (and besides, you'll be pretty distracted). After all, labor can really spoil your appetite. Still, an occasional light, easy-to-digest snack during the early hours of labor—Popsicles, Jell-O, applesauce, cooked fruit, a banana, plain pasta, toast with jam, or clear broth are ideal choices—may help keep your energy up at a time when you need it most (you probably won't be able to, or won't want to, eat during the later parts of active labor). When deciding—with your practitioner's help—what to eat and when, also keep in mind that labor can make you feel pretty nauseous. Some laboring moms throw up, even if they haven't been eating.

Whether you can chow down or not during labor, your coach definitely can—and should (you don't want him weak from hunger when you need him most). Remind him to have a meal before you head off to the hospital or birthing center (his mind's probably on your belly, not his) and to pack a bunch of snacks to take along so he won't have to leave your side when his stomach starts growling.

Routine IV

"Is it true that I'll have to get an IV when I'm in labor—even if I'm pretty sure I don't want an epidural?"

That depends a lot on hospital policy. In some hospitals, it's routine to give all women in labor an IV, a flexible catheter placed in your vein (usually in the back of your hand or lower arm) to drip in fluids and medication. The reason is precautionary—to prevent dehydration, as well as to save a step later on in case an emergency arises that necessitates medication (there's already a line in place to administer drugs—no extra poking or prodding required). Other hospitals and practitioners omit routine IVs and instead wait until there is a clear need before hooking moms up. Check out policies in advance, and if you strongly object to having a routine IV, ask your practitioner if it can be skipped. It may be possible to hold off until the need, if any, comes up.

You'll definitely get an IV if an epidural is on the agenda. IV fluids are routinely administered before and during the placement of an epidural to reduce the chance of a drop in blood pressure, a common side effect of this pain relief route. The IV also allows for easier administration of Pitocin in case labor needs a nudge.

If you end up with a routine IV or an IV with epidural that you were hoping to avoid, you'll probably find it's not all that intrusive. The IV is only slightly uncomfortable as the needle is inserted—after that, you shouldn't even notice it (and if you do, tell your nurse). When it's hung on a movable stand, you can take it with you to the bathroom or on a stroll down the hall. If you very strongly don't want an IV but hospital policy dictates that you receive one, ask your practitioner whether a heparin lock might be an option for you. With a heparin lock, a catheter is placed in the vein, a drop of the blood-thinning medication heparin is added to prevent clotting, and the catheter is locked off. This option gives the hospital staff access to an open vein should an emergency arise but doesn't hook you up to an IV pole unnecessarily—a good compromise in certain situations.

Fetal Monitoring

"Will I have to be hooked up to a fetal monitor the whole time I'm in labor? What's the point of it anyway?"

For someone who's spent 9 months floating peacefully in a warm and comforting amniotic bath, the trip through the narrow confines of mom's pelvis will be no joyride. Your baby will be squeezed, compressed, pushed, and molded with every contraction. And though most babies sail through the birth canal without a problem, others find the stress of being squeezed, compressed, pushed, and molded too difficult, and they respond with decelerations in heart rate, rapid or slowed-down movement, or other signs of distress. A fetal monitor assesses how your baby is handling the stresses of labor by gauging the response of his or her heartbeat to contractions.

But does that assessment need to be continuous? Most experts say no, citing research showing that for low-risk moms with unmedicated deliveries, intermittent fetal heart checks using a Doppler or fetal monitor are an effective way to assess a baby's condition.

Episiotomy: No Longer a Common Cut

Chances are you've heard enough about episiotomies to know you'd rather not have one. Happily for most moms, the episiotomy—a surgical cut in a mom's perineum made to enlarge the vaginal opening just before the baby's head emerges—is no longer performed routinely at delivery. These days, in fact, midwives and most doctors rarely make the cut without a good reason, and only about 10 percent of delivering moms end up getting one.

It wasn't always that way. The episiotomy was once thought to prevent spontaneous tearing of the perineum and postpartum urinary and fecal incontinence, as well as reduce the risk in the newborn of birth trauma (from the baby's head pushing long and hard against the perineum). But it's now known that infants fare just fine without an episiotomy, and moms seem to do better without it. Skipping the procedure doesn't seem to make the average total labor any longer, and moms often experience less blood loss, less infection, and less perineal pain after delivery without an episiotomy (though you can still have blood loss and infection with a tear). What's more, research has shown that episiotomies are more likely than spontaneous tears to turn into serious third- or fourth-degree tears (those that go close to or through the rectum, sometimes causing fecal incontinence, or the inability to control bowel movements).

But while routine episiotomies are no longer recommended, there is still a place for them in certain birth scenarios. Episiotomies may be indicated when a baby is large and needs a roomier exit route, when the baby needs to be delivered rapidly, when forceps or vacuum delivery needs to be performed, or for the relief of shoulder dystocia (a shoulder gets stuck in the birth canal during delivery).

If you do need an episiotomy, you'll get an injection (if there's time) of local pain relief before the cut, though you may not need a local if you're already anesthetized from an epidural or if your perineum is thinned out and already numb from the pressure of your baby's head during crowning. Your practitioner will then take surgical scissors and make either a median (also called midline) incision (a cut made directly toward the rectum) or a mediolateral incision (which slants away from the rectum). After delivery of your baby and the placenta, the practitioner will stitch up the cut (you'll get a shot of local pain medication if you didn't before or if your epidural has worn off).

If you haven't already, discuss the episiotomy issue with your practitioner. It's very likely he or she will agree that the procedure should not be performed unless there's a good reason. Document your feelings about episiotomies in your birth plan, too, if you like. But keep in mind that, very occasionally, episiotomies do turn out to be necessary, and the final decision should be made in the delivery or birthing room—when that cute little head is crowning.

So if you fit in that category, you probably won't have to be attached to a fetal monitor for your entire labor (you almost certainly won't be if you're delivering with a midwife). If, however, you're being induced, have an epidural, or have certain risk factors (such as meconium staining), you're most likely going to be hooked up to a monitor throughout your labor.

There are three types of continuous fetal monitoring:

External monitoring. In this type of monitoring, used most frequently, 2 devices are strapped to the abdomen. One, an ultrasound transducer, picks up the fetal heartbeat. The other, a pressure-sensitive gauge, measures the intensity and duration of uterine contractions. Both are connected to a monitor, and the measurements are recorded on a digital and paper readout. When you're connected to an external monitor, you'll be able to move around in your bed or on a chair nearby, but you won't have complete freedom of movement, unless telemetry monitoring is being used (see below).

During the second (pushing) stage of labor, when contractions may come so fast and furious that it's hard to know when to push and when to hold back, the monitor can be used to accurately signal the beginning and end of each contraction. Or the monitor may be removed entirely while you're pushing, to make sure it doesn't interfere with your concentration. In this case, your baby's heart rate will be checked periodically with a Doppler.

Internal monitoring. When more accurate results are required—such as when there is reason to suspect fetal distress—an internal monitor may be used. In this type of monitoring, a tiny electrode is inserted through your vagina onto your baby's scalp, and a catheter is placed in your uterus or an external pressure gauge is strapped to your abdomen to measure the strength of your contractions. Though internal monitoring gives a slightly more accurate record of the baby's heart rate and your contractions than an external monitor, it's used only when necessary (since its use comes with a slight risk of infection). Your baby may have a small bruise or scratch where the electrode was attached, but it'll heal in a few days. You'll be more limited in your movement with an internal monitor, but you'll still be able to move from side to side.

Telemetry monitoring. Available only in some hospitals, this type of monitoring uses a transmitter on your thigh to transmit the baby's heart tones (via radio waves) to the nurse's station—allowing you to take a lap or two around the hallway while still having constant monitoring.

Be aware that with both internal and external types of monitoring, false alarms are common. The machine can start beeping loudly if the transducer has slipped out of place, if the baby has shifted position, if mom has shifted position, if the monitor isn't working right, or if contractions have suddenly picked up in intensity. Your practitioner will take all these factors and others into account before concluding that your baby really is in trouble. If the abnormal readings do continue, several other assessments can be performed (such as fetal scalp stimulation) to determine the cause of the distress. If fetal distress is confirmed, then a cesarean delivery is usually called for.

Artificial Rupture of Membranes

"I'm afraid that if my water doesn't break on its own, the doctor will have to rupture the membranes. Won't that hurt?"

Most moms-to-be actually don't feel much at all when their membranes are artificially ruptured, particularly if labor's already well underway (there are far more significant pains to cope with then). The procedure, done with an amniohook (a long, thin plastic device with a hook at the end, designed to puncture the sac), isn't likely to be any more uncomfortable than all those internal exams you'll be getting to check on your progress. Chances are, all you'll really notice is a gush of water, followed soon—at least that's the hope—by harder and faster contractions that will get your baby moving.

Artificial rupture of the membranes doesn't seem to decrease the need for Pitocin but does seem to shorten the length of labor—at least in labors that are induced—and many practitioners will turn to artificial rupture in an attempt to help move a sluggish labor along. If there's no compelling reason to rupture them (labor's moving along just fine), you and your practitioner may decide to hold off and let them rupture naturally. (Occasionally, artificial rupture may be performed to allow for another procedure, like internal monitoring.)

Once in a while, membranes stay stubbornly intact throughout delivery (the baby arrives with the bag of waters still surrounding him or her, which means it will need to be ruptured right after birth), and that's fine, too.

Vacuum Extractor

"Why would the doctor use a vacuum extractor during delivery? The idea of suctioning my baby's head out sounds like it would be painful for her and me."

Vacuum extractors can ease babies out of some pretty tight delivery spots. Don't think Hoover—the vacuum extractor is a simple plastic cup that's placed on the baby's head, and uses gentle suction to help guide her out of the birth canal (see illustration, below). The suction prevents the baby's head from moving back up the birth canal between contractions and can be used to help mom out while she is pushing during contractions. Vacuum extraction is used in about 5 percent of deliveries and offers a good alternative to both forceps (which are rarely used these days; see next question) and c-section under the right circumstances.

What are the right circumstances? Vacuum extraction might be considered when the cervix is fully dilated and the membranes have broken but a mom is just too exhausted from labor to push effectively or to keep pushing, or if she has a heart condition or very high blood pressure that might make strenuous pushing risky. The

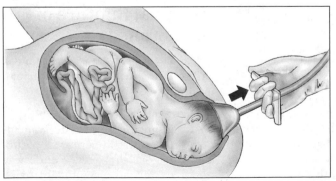

Vacuum Extractor

procedure might also be used if the baby needs to be delivered in a hurry because of possible distress (assuming the baby is in a favorable position—for example, close to crowning).

Babies born with vacuum extraction experience some swelling on the scalp, but it usually isn't serious, doesn't require treatment, and goes away within a few days. If the vacuum extractor isn't working successfully to help deliver the baby, a cesarean delivery will likely be performed.

Before turning to vacuum extraction, your practitioner may suggest (time permitting) letting you rest up for a few contractions before trying to push again (sometimes even a short break can give you the second wind you need to push your baby out effectively). A change of position (getting on all fours, squatting with a birthing bar, sitting on a birthing ball) might also push delivery along by enlisting the force of gravity to shift baby's head.

Ask your practitioner any questions you have about the possible use of vacuum extraction (or forceps, see next question), including whether you'll need an episiotomy before a vacuum delivery. The more you know, the better prepared you'll be for anything that comes your way during childbirth.

Forceps

"How likely will it be that I'll need forceps during delivery?"

Pretty unlikely these days. Forceps—long, curved tonglike devices designed to help a baby make his or her descent down the birth canal—are used in only a very small percentage of deliveries (vacuum extraction is more common; see previous question). Not because they aren't as safe as vacuum

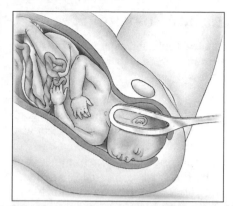

Forceps

extraction or a c-section (they are actually even safer for the baby when used correctly), but because fewer and fewer doctors have been trained in how to use them or have used them enough to feel comfortable using them. The possible reasons for using forceps are the same as those for vacuum delivery.

If forceps are used in your delivery, your cervix will have to be fully dilated, your bladder empty, and your membranes ruptured first. Then you'll be numbed with a local anesthetic (unless you already have an epidural in place). You'll also likely receive an episiotomy to enlarge the vaginal opening to allow for placement of the forceps. The curved tongs of the forceps will then be cradled one at a time around the temples of the baby's crowning head, locked into position, and used to gently deliver the baby (see illustration, above). There may be some bruising or swelling on the baby's scalp from the forceps, but it will usually go away within a few days after birth.

If an attempt at a forceps delivery is unsuccessful, you'll likely have a c-section.

Labor Positions

"I know you're not supposed to lie flat on your back during labor. But what position is best?"

There's no need to take labor lying down, and in fact, lying flat on your back is probably the least efficient way to birth your baby: first because you're not enlisting gravity's help to get your baby out, and second because there's the risk of compressing major blood vessels (and possibly interfering with blood flow to the baby) when you're on your back for an extended period of time. Expectant moms are encouraged to labor in any other position that feels comfortable and to change their position as often as they can (and want to). Getting a move on during labor, as well as varying your position often, not only eases discomfort but may also yield speedier results.

You can choose from any of the following labor and delivery positions (or variations of these):

Standing or walking. Getting vertical not only helps relieve the pain of contractions but also takes advantage of gravity, which may allow your pelvis to open and your baby to move down into your birth canal. While it's unlikely you'll be heading for the track once contractions are coming fast and furious, walking (or just standing leaning against a wall or your coach) during the early stages of labor can be an effective move.

Standing or walking

Rocking. Sure, your baby's not even born yet, but he or she will still enjoy a little rocking—as will you, especially when those contractions start coming. Slip into a chair or remain upright, and sway back and forth on your own or in the arms of your partner (or rock on a birthing ball; see facing page). The rocking motion may allow your pelvis to open and encourage your baby to descend. And again, staying upright allows you to use the force of gravity to help in the process.

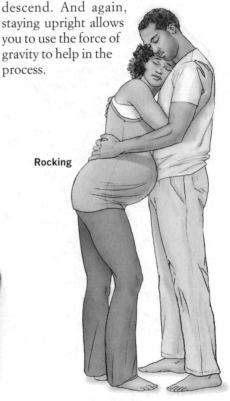

Rocking

Leaning over. Many laboring moms-to-be find it relaxing to lean forward during contractions—and it's an especially helpful position if you've got back labor. Stack a bunch of pillows on a bed or table and lean forward on them, resting your head and arms on the pillows and relaxing your body.

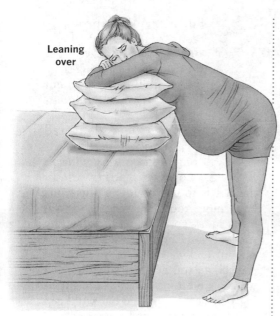

Leaning over

This position is also helpful if you want to sway or rock but don't have the energy to hold your body up.

Sitting. Whether in bed (the back of the birthing bed can be raised so you're almost sitting upright), in your partner's arms, or on a birthing ball, sitting can ease the pain of contractions and may allow gravity to help coax your baby down into your birth

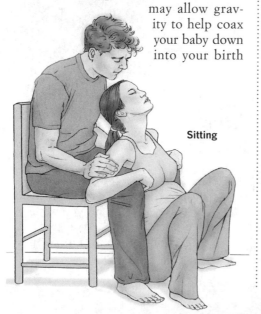

Sitting

canal. Another option, if it's available, is a birthing chair, specifically designed to support a woman in labor. A plus: Moms get to see more of the birth in this position.

On a birthing ball. Sitting on one of these large exercise balls can help open up your pelvis—and it's a lot easier than squatting for long periods. The curve of the ball gives a slight counterpressure to the perenium during labor. If you'd rather lean forward on your hands and knees (see illustration, next page), take advantage of the curve of the ball to rock back and forth (or side to side or even in gentle circles). Using the ball for support this way can help with back labor and can also take the strain off your wrists while still allowing you to labor in whatever position feels best for you.

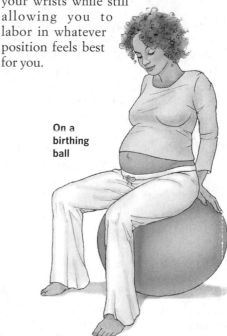

On a birthing ball

Kneeling. Got back labor? Kneeling over a birthing ball, a chair, or over your spouse's shoulders can be soothing and productive when the back of baby's head is pushing against your spine. It

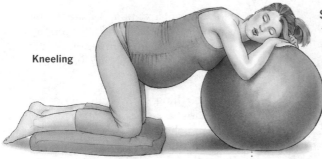

Kneeling

Squatting. You probably won't be able to stand and deliver, but once you get closer to the pushing stage of childbirth, you might want to consider squatting. There's a reason why women have delivered their babies in a squatting position for centuries: It works. Squatting allows the pelvis to open wide, giving your baby more room to move on down. You can use your partner for squatting support (you'll probably be a little wobbly, so you'll need all the support you can get), or you can use a squatting bar, which is often attached to the birthing bed (leaning on the bar will keep your legs from tiring out as you squat—ask if one will be available ahead of time if you think you might want to use it).

encourages the baby to move forward, taking that load off your back. Even if you don't have back labor, kneeling can be an effective labor and delivery position. Because it allows you to shift and transfer some of the pressure toward the lower spine while you push your baby out, kneeling seems to reduce childbirth pain even more than sitting does.

Hands and knees. Getting on all fours is another way to cope more comfortably with back labor—and to help get that puppy out faster. This position allows you to do pelvic tilts for comfort while giving your spouse or doula access to your back for massage and counterpressure. You might even consider delivering in this position (no matter what kind of labor you're having), since it opens up the pelvis and uses gravity to coax baby down. (You can also use a birthing ball in this position; see above.)

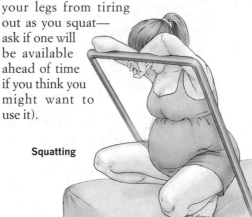

Squatting

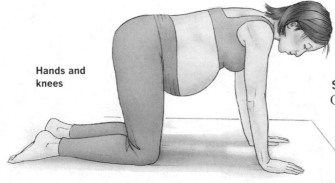

Hands and knees

Side lying. Too tired to sit? Or squat? Just need to lie down? Lying on your side (left side is best) is much better than lying on

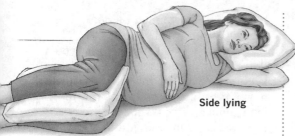

Side lying

your back, since it doesn't compress the major veins in your body. It's also a good delivery option, helping to slow a too-fast birth as well as easing the pain of some contractions.

In a tub. Even if you're not open to a water birth (or if the option isn't open to you), laboring in a tub can help ease the pain of contractions, enhance relaxation, and even help speed your progress. No tub in your birthing room? A warm shower can help relieve pain, too.

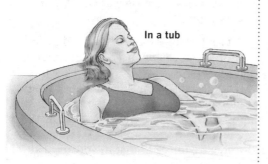

In a tub

Remember that the best labor position is the one that's best for you. And what's best in the early phases of labor might make you miserable when you're in the throes of labor, so change positions as often—or as little—as you want. If you're being continuously monitored, your positions are somewhat limited. It'll be hard to walk, for instance—but you'll have no problem squatting, rocking, sitting, getting on your hands and knees, or lying on your side. Even if you have an epidural, sitting, side lying, or rocking are all options for you.

Being Stretched by Childbirth

"I'm concerned about stretching during delivery. Will my vagina ever be the same again?"

Mother Nature definitely had moms in mind when thinking up vaginas. Their incredible elasticity and accordion-like folds allow this amazing organ to open up for childbirth (and the passage of that 7- or 8-pound baby) and then—over a period of weeks after delivery—return to close to original size. In other words, your vagina's definitely designed to take it.

The perineum is also elastic but less so than the vagina. Massage during the months before delivery (and during delivery) may help increase its elasticity and reduce stretching in a first-time mom (though it's not a must-do; see page 384). Likewise, exercising the pelvic muscles with Kegels during this period may enhance their elasticity, strengthen them, and speed their return to normal tone.

Most women find that the slight increase in vaginal roominess typically experienced postpartum is imperceptible and doesn't interfere at all with sexual enjoyment. For those who were previously too snug, that extra room can be a real plus—making sex more of a pleasure and in some cases, literally, less of a pain. Very occasionally, however, in a woman who was "just right" before (or a couple who were a perfect fit before), childbirth does stretch the vagina enough that sexual satisfaction decreases. Often, the vaginal muscles tighten up again in time. Doing Kegels faithfully and frequently helps speed that process. If 6 months after delivery you still find that your vagina's too slack for comfort, talk to your doctor about other possible treatments.

Handling the Sight of Blood

Most expectant dads—and moms—worry about how they'll handle seeing blood at delivery. But chances are you won't even notice it, never mind be bothered by it—for a couple of reasons. For one, there typically isn't very much blood to see. For another, the excitement and wonder of watching your baby arrive is likely to keep you both pretty preoccupied (that, and the efforts of birthing, of course).

If at first glance the blood does bother you (and it's really likely it won't), keep your eyes focused on your spouse's face as you coach her through those last pushes. You'll probably want to turn back to the main event for that momentous moment—at that point, blood is going to be the last thing you'll notice.

The Sight of Blood

"The sight of blood makes me feel faint. I'm not sure if I'll be able to handle watching my delivery."

Here's some good news for the squeamish. First of all, there isn't all that much blood during childbirth—not much more than when you have your period. Second, you're not really a spectator at your delivery—you'll be a very active participant, putting every ounce of your concentration and energy into pushing your baby those last few inches. Caught up in the excitement and anticipation (and, let's face it, the pain and fatigue), you're unlikely to notice, much less be unsettled by, any bleeding. If you ask friends who've given birth before, few will be able to tell you just how much blood, if any, there was at their deliveries.

If you still feel strongly that you don't want to see any blood, simply keep your eyes off the mirror at the moment of birth (and look away, too, in the unlikely event that an episiotomy is performed). Instead, just look down past your belly for a good view of your baby as he or she emerges. From this vantage point, virtually no blood will be visible. But before you decide to opt out of watching your own delivery, watch someone else's by viewing a childbirth on YouTube. You'll probably be much more awestruck than horrified.

Delaying Cord Clamping

"What's this I hear about not clamping the umbilical cord right away after the baby is born?"

It's a part of the birth that used to go pretty much unnoticed in the birthing room, at least by parents, who were too busy basking in the glow of baby's first moments—gazing into those just-opening eyes, enjoying those first cuddles, counting fingers, toes, and blessings—to realize (or care) that the doctor had already clamped the umbilical cord within just a few moments of delivery.

While midwives delivering babies in birthing centers and at home have long taken their time with umbilical cord clamping, it has traditionally been done in a flash in hospital settings—without fanfare, and certainly without delay (wham-bam-clamp-you-mom). The reason for this quick clamping? Because it was believed to reduce the risk of hemorrhaging (mom losing too much blood after delivery).

But the latest research seems to show that faster may not be better—and that delayed cord clamping not only

Wear and Tear During Delivery

When a little baby with a pretty big head tries to squeeze through a much narrower opening, there's a good chance that opening will not only be stretched out to accommodate it, but also might tear a little. In fact, it's common, given the pressure from a baby's head pushing through, to experience tears and lacerations in the perineum (the area between your vagina and your anus) and sometimes the cervix as well. As many as half of all women who deliver vaginally will experience at least a small tear during delivery (though your chances of tearing in second and subsequent labors are lower). First-degree tears (where only the skin is torn) and second-degree tears (when skin and vaginal tissue are torn) are the most common types of tears.

In most cases, a tear requires stitches (they're generally required in tears that are longer than 2 cm, or about 1 inch). After the tear is repaired, you'll likely experience tenderness at the site as it heals over the next week to 10 days. But here's the good news: Recovering from a small tear that happens naturally is a lot easier than healing after an episiotomy—a procedure that's (thankfully) rarely used these days in uncomplicated births (see box, page 408).

To reduce the possibility that you'll tear, some experts recommend perineal massage (see page 384) for a few weeks before your due date if you're a first-time mom. (If you've delivered vaginally before, you're already stretched, so do-ahead massage probably won't accomplish much.) During labor, the following can also help: warm compresses to lessen perineal discomfort, perineal massage with oils or lubricants, standing or squatting and exhaling or grunting while pushing to facilitate stretching of the perineum. During the pushing stage, your practitioner will probably use perineal support (applying gentle counterpressure to the perineum so your baby's head doesn't push out too quickly and cause an unnecessary tear) and perineal massage.

---

doesn't increase the risk of a mom hemorrhaging, but may offer real benefits to baby. A clamping delay after delivery allows the placenta to give a few more pulses of blood to the newborn, and this extra dose of blood can represent as much as 30 to 40 percent of a baby's blood volume. And pumping up that blood supply can significantly improve a baby's iron and hemoglobin levels, preventing anemia in the first 6 months of life. And how's this for a possible (if unexpected) perk: Delayed cord clamping may boost social and fine motor skills later in life.

How long a wait is long enough? That depends who you ask. Many midwives routinely wait until the cord stops pulsating, which can take several minutes, often more. The World Health Organization (WHO) already recommends waiting 1 to 3 minutes after birth to cut the umbilical cord. ACOG and the AAP recognize the benefits of delaying clamping until 60 seconds after birth, but say there's not enough evidence to recommend delaying beyond the 1-minute mark. They point to a slightly increased risk (about 2 percent) of newborn jaundice in babies whose cord clamping was delayed longer than 1 minute (due to the extra blood baby receives)—and to the fact that babies born in the U.S. are rarely iron deficient (making the extra blood inconsequential). The exception: preemies, who can

Lotus Birth

If delaying cord clamping might be beneficial—what about not cutting the cord at all? That's the theory behind the controversial practice of lotus birth: Instead of cutting the cord, parents opt to leave the umbilical cord and placenta attached to their baby until it dries out and falls off by itself—a process that can take 3 to 10 (or more) days. Advocates say this allows the baby to reap the benefit of complete blood transfer from the cord and placenta.

Problem is, there are no scientific studies on the safety of the practice, and experts haven't been reassuring. They say that without active blood circulation, the cord and placenta are essentially dead tissue that will rot (and smell). Bacteria can colonize in the placenta and potentially be a source of infection that can spread to the newborn. Which means that lotus birth most likely isn't a smart trend to embrace, and may even be downright dangerous.

Still curious? Be sure to discuss the practice with your practitioner before making the decision to try it.

definitely benefit from the extra blood and the lowered risk of anemia. Both ACOG and AAP recommend delaying cord clamping for at least a minute when a baby is born preterm.

Still, the birthing room times (and the timing of cord clamping) are changing. Despite the lack of an official thumbs-up from ACOG and AAP, many doctors (and most midwives) allow—and even encourage—a longer-than-1-minute delay in clamping at all births. Wondering what your practitioner's cord clamping practice is? Now, before the cord is delivered (along with your baby and the placenta), is the time to ask—and to specify any preferences you have in your birth plan. For healthy moms with normal pregnancies, a 2- to 3-minute delay might be just what the doctor ordered (and it won't interfere with cord blood harvesting).

ALL ABOUT:
Childbirth

After 9 months at it—graduating from queasiness and bloating to heartburn and backache—you almost certainly know what to expect when you're expecting by now. But what should you expect when you're laboring and delivering?

That's actually hard to predict (make that impossible). Like every pregnancy before it, every labor and delivery is different. Still, just as it was comforting to know what you might expect during those months of growing your baby, it'll be comforting to have a general idea of what you might have in store for you during those hours of childbirth. Even if it turns out to be nothing like you expected (with the exception of that very happy and cuddly ending).

Stage One: Labor

Phase 1: Early Labor

This phase is usually the longest phase of labor—but fortunately, it's also by far the least intense. Over a period of hours, days, or weeks (often without noticeable or bothersome contractions), or over a period of 2 to 6 hours of no-doubt-about-it contractions, your cervix will efface (thin out) and dilate (open) to between 4 to 6 cm.

Contractions in this phase usually last 30 to 45 seconds, though they can be shorter. They are mild to moderately strong, may be regular or irregular. They may start as far apart as 20 minutes, but will become progressively closer together (about 5 minutes apart by the end of early labor), though not necessarily in a consistent pattern.

What you may be feeling. During early labor, you might experience any or all (or none) of the following:

- Backache (either constant or with each contraction)

- Menstrual-like cramps

Stages and Phases of Childbirth

Childbirth progresses in 3 stages: labor, delivery of the baby, and delivery of the placenta. First up (unless a planned c-section eliminates this stage entirely) is labor, which is divided into three phases: early labor, active labor, and transitional labor. All women who deliver vaginally will experience all 3 phases of labor (though some moms may barely notice much of the first phase at all), but moms who end up requiring a cesarean delivery at some point during labor may skip one or more of those phases. Though every labor is different, the timing and intensity of contractions can help pinpoint which phase of labor you're in at any particular time, and so can some of the symptoms you're experiencing along the way. Periodic internal exams will confirm your progress. (Keep in mind that different practitioners define phases differently, which is why you'll notice a range of centimeters dilated within each phase below.)

Stage One: Labor

- **Phase 1: Early (Latent)**—Thinning (effacement) and opening (dilation) of the cervix to between 4 to 6 cm; contractions are 30 to 45 seconds long, 20 minutes apart or less (getting to about 5 minutes apart by the end of early labor).

- **Phase 2: Active**—Dilation of cervix from between 4 to 6 cm to between 7 to 8 cm; contractions are 40 to 60 seconds long, coming 3 to 4 minutes apart.

- **Phase 3: Transitional**—Dilation of cervix from between 7 to 8 cm to 10 cm (fully dilated); contractions are 60 to 90 seconds long, about 2 to 3 minutes apart.

Stage Two: Pushing and delivery of the baby

Stage Three: Delivery of the placenta

- Lower abdominal pressure

- Indigestion

- Diarrhea

- A sensation of warmth in your abdomen

- Loss of mucous plug; bloody show (blood-tinged mucus)

- Rupture of your membranes (your water breaking), though it's more likely that they'll rupture (or be ruptured) during active labor.

Emotionally, you may be all over the map—from relaxed, relieved, excited, and chatty to tense, anxious, and apprehensive. You may also be impatient while you're waiting (and waiting) for labor to get more active.

What you can do. Of course you're full of anticipation, but it's important to relax—or at least try to relax. This could take a while.

- If contractions start during the night but your water hasn't broken, try to sleep (you might not be able to later, when the contractions are coming fast and furious). If you can't sleep—what with all the adrenaline pumping—get up and do things around the house that will distract you. Bake some muffins or cook up a batch of chili or chicken breasts to add to your postpartum freezer stash, do the laundry, or log on to see if anyone else in the WhatToExpect.com community is in the same early labor boat.

- If it's daytime, go about your usual routine, as long as it doesn't take you far from home (remember to take your cell phone with you). If you're at work, you might want to head home (it's not like you're going to get anything done anyway). If you have nothing planned, find something relaxing to keep you occupied. Go for a walk, watch TV, text friends and family or keep them posted on Facebook, finish packing your bag. Feel like starting labor and delivery fresh—even if you won't end up that way when it's over? Take a shower and wash your hair.

- Alert the media. Okay, maybe not the media (yet)—but you'll definitely want to put your partner on alert if he's not with you. He probably doesn't have to rush to your side just yet if he's at work—unless he really wants to—since there's not much for him to do this early on. If you have hired a doula, issue a bulletin to her, too. And if you have older children who will need watching while you're laboring, alert the babysitter.

- Eat a light snack or meal if you're hungry (broth, toast with jam, plain pasta or rice, Jell-O or pudding, an ice pop, a banana, watermelon, or something else your practitioner has suggested)—now's the best time

---

Call Your Practitioner If . . .

Your practitioner probably told you not to call until you're in more active labor, but may have suggested that you call early on if labor begins during the day or if your membranes rupture. Definitely call immediately, however, if your membranes rupture and the amniotic fluid is murky or greenish, if you have any bright red vaginal bleeding, if you feel no fetal activity (try the test on page 315), or if there's an extremely marked slowdown or other dramatic change of fetal movement.

What You Can Do During Early Labor

If you're around during this phase, here are some ways you can help out:

- Practice timing contractions. The interval between contractions is timed from the beginning of one to the beginning of the next. Time them periodically (you'll both get frustrated if you time early contractions too often), and keep a record. When they are coming less than 10 minutes apart, time them more frequently.

- Spread the calm. Right now, your most important job is to keep your partner relaxed. And the best way to do that is to keep yourself relaxed, both inside and out. It's possible to spread stress without even realizing it, communicating it not just through words but touch and expressions (so no tensed-up foreheads, please). Doing relaxation exercises together or giving her a gentle massage may help. It's too soon, however, to begin using breathing exercises—save them for when they're needed so she doesn't burn out. For now, just breathe.

- Offer comfort, reassurance, and support. She'll need them from now on.

- Keep your sense of humor, and help her keep hers—time flies, after all, when you're having fun. It'll be easier to laugh now than when contractions are coming fast and hard (she probably won't find very much of anything funny then).

- Try distraction. Suggest activities that will help keep both your minds off her labor: playing games on the iPad, watching a silly sitcom or reality show, baking something for the postpartum freezer stash, taking short strolls.

- Keep up your own strength so you'll be able to reinforce hers. Eat periodically but empathetically (don't go wolfing down a Big Mac when she's sticking to pudding). Prepare a sandwich to take along to the hospital or birthing center, but avoid anything with a strong odor. She probably won't be in the mood to be sniffing salami or onions on your breath.

to stock up on energy foods. But don't eat heavily, and avoid hard-to-digest foods (burgers, potato chips, pizza). You may also want to skip anything acidic, such as orange juice or lemonade. And definitely drink some water—it's important to stay hydrated.

- Make yourself comfortable. If you're achy, take a warm shower or use a heating pad where it hurts. You can also take some acetaminophen (Tylenol) if your practitioner approves, but don't take aspirin or ibuprofen (Advil, Motrin).

- Time contractions (from the beginning of one to the beginning of the next) for half an hour if they seem to be getting closer than 10 minutes apart and periodically even if they don't. But try not to be a constant clock-watcher.

- Remember to pee often, even if you're not feeling the urge to. A full bladder could slow down the progress of labor.

- Use relaxation techniques if they help, but don't start breathing exercises yet or you'll burn out on them long before you really need them.

On to the Hospital or Birthing Center

Sometime near the end of the early phase or the beginning of the active phase (probably when your contractions are 5 minutes apart or less, sooner if you live far from the hospital or are likely to face traffic, or if this isn't your first baby), your practitioner will tell you to pick up your bag and get going. The going will be easier, of course, if your coach can be reached and get to you quickly (or you have a backup plan if he can't, like taking a taxi or having a friend drive you—don't try to drive yourself). It will also be a smoother ride if you've planned your route in advance, are familiar with parking, and know which entrance will get you to labor and delivery fastest. En route, get as comfortable as you can (recline the seat, if possible, bring a blanket if you have chills) but don't forget to fasten your seat belt.

Once you reach the hospital or birthing center you can probably expect something like the following (since protocols differ, your experience may be a little different):

- If you've preregistered (and it's best if you have), the admission process will be quick and easy. If you haven't preregistered, you (or better yet, your coach) will have to go through a more lengthy process, so be prepared to fill out a bunch of forms and answer a lot of questions.

- Once you've arrived at labor and delivery, a nurse will probably take you to your room (likely an LDR, or labor, delivery, and recovery room). If it's not clear you're in active labor you may be brought first to a triage (assessment) room (this is standard practice in some hospitals).

- Your nurse will take a brief history, asking (among other things) when the contractions started, how far apart they are, whether your membranes have ruptured, when and what you last ate.

- Your nurse will ask for your signature (or your spouse's) on routine consent forms.

- Your nurse will give you a hospital gown to change into and might request a urine sample. He or she will check your pulse, blood pressure, respiration, and temperature, look for leaking amniotic fluid, bleeding, or bloody show, and will listen to baby's heartbeat with a Doppler or hook you up to a fetal monitor, if necessary. He or she may also evaluate baby's position.

- Your nurse, your practitioner, or a staff doctor or midwife will examine you internally to see how dilated and effaced your cervix is. Have questions? Now's a great time to ask them. Have a birth plan? Now's a good time to hand it to the nurse so it can be added to your chart.

If at any time during the intake it's determined that you're not actually in active labor, you may be sent home (don't worry—you'll be back!) or asked to stay for a few hours before checking you again.

Phase 2: Active Labor

The active phase of labor is usually shorter than the early phase, lasting an average of 2 to 3½ hours (with, again, a wide range of normal). The contractions are more concentrated now, accomplishing more in less time, and they're also increasingly intense (in other words, painful). As they become stronger, longer (40 to 60 seconds, with a distinct peak about halfway through), and more frequent (generally 3 to 4 minutes apart, though the pattern may not be regular), the cervix dilates to 7 to 8 cm. With fewer breaks in the action, there's less opportunity to rest between contractions.

What you may be feeling. You'll likely be in the hospital or birthing center by now, and you can expect to feel all or some of the following (though you won't feel pain if you've had an epidural):

- Increasing pain and discomfort with contractions (you may not be able to talk through them now)

- Increasing backache

- Leg discomfort (aches in the legs, thighs, or butt) or heaviness

- Fatigue

- Increasing bloody show

- Rupture of your membranes (if they haven't earlier)

Emotionally, you may feel restless and find it more difficult to relax—or your concentration may become more intense and you may become completely absorbed in your labor efforts. Your confidence may begin to waver ("How will I make it through?"), along with your patience ("Will this labor never end?"), or you may feel excited and encouraged that things are really starting to happen. Whatever your feelings, they're normal—just get ready to start getting "active."

What your practitioner or nurse will be doing. During active labor, assuming all is progressing normally and safely, your birth attendants will check and monitor you as needed, but also allow you to work through your labor with your coach and other support people without interference. You can expect them to:

- Take your blood pressure

- Monitor baby with a Doppler or fetal monitor

- Time and monitor the strength of your contractions

- Evaluate bloody show

- Start an IV if you're going to want an epidural or if hospital policy dictates

- Administer an epidural (or other pain relief) if you choose to have one (the anesthesiologist will have to be called in for this)

- Possibly, rupture your membranes if they're still intact

- Jump start your labor if it's progressing very slowly by administering Pitocin

- Periodically examine you internally to check how labor is progressing and how dilated and effaced your cervix is

Don't Hyperventilate

With all the breathing going on during labor, some moms start to hyperventilate or over-breathe, causing low levels of carbon dioxide in the blood. If you feel dizzy or lightheaded, have blurred vision or a tingling and numbness of your fingers and toes, let a nurse or your doula know. You'll be given a paper bag to breathe into (or told to breathe into your cupped hands). A few inhales and exhales will get you feeling better in no time.

When Labor Slows Down

Feel like lingering over labor? Of course not—you'd like to keep labor moving. And making good progress during labor—which happens most of the time—requires three main components: strong uterine contractions that effectively dilate the cervix, a baby that is in position for an easy exit, and a pelvis that is roomy enough to permit passage of the baby. But in some cases, labor doesn't progress by the book, because the cervix takes its time dilating, the baby takes longer than expected to descend, or pushing isn't getting you (or your baby) anywhere. Contractions can also slow down after an epidural kicks in, too—but keep in mind that expectations for the progress of labor and delivery are different for those who have an epidural (first and second stage may take longer, and that's typically nothing to worry about).

To get a stalled labor back up and running, there are a number of steps your practitioner (and you) can take:

- If you're in early labor and your cervix just isn't dilating or effacing, your practitioner may suggest some activity (such as walking) or just the opposite (sleep and rest, possibly aided by relaxation techniques). This will also help rule out false labor (the contractions of false labor usually subside with activity or a nap).

- If you're not dilating or effacing as quickly as expected, your practitioner may try to rev things up by administering Pitocin (oxytocin), prostaglandin E, or another labor stimulator. He or she might even suggest a labor booster that you can take into your own hands (or your coach's): nipple stimulation.

- If you're already in the active phase of labor, but your cervix is dilating

They'll also be able to answer any questions you might have (don't be shy about asking or having your coach ask) and provide additional support as you go through labor.

What you can do. It's all about your comfort now. So:

- Don't hesitate to ask your coach for whatever you need to get and stay as comfortable as possible, whether it's a back rub to ease the ache or a damp washcloth to cool your face. Speaking up will be important. Remember, as much as he's going to want to help, he's going to have a hard time anticipating your needs, especially if this is his first time coaching labor.

- Start your breathing exercises, if you plan to use them, as soon as contractions become too strong to talk through. Didn't plan ahead and practice? Ask the nurse or doula for some simple breathing suggestions. Remember to do whatever relaxes you and makes you feel more comfortable. If the formulaic breathing exercises aren't working for you, don't feel obligated to stick with them. Or ask the nurse (or your doula) to help you redirect your breathing.

- Try to relax fully between contractions, so you can conserve energy that you'll need later. This will become increasingly difficult as they come more frequently, but it will also become increasingly important as your energy reserves are drained.

slowly (less than 1 to 1.2 cm per hour if you're having your first baby and 1.5 cm per hour if you've delivered before), or if your baby isn't moving quickly enough down the birth canal (at a rate of more than 1 cm per hour if you're a first-timer or 2 cm per hour if you're not), your practitioner may rupture your membranes and/or start (or continue) administering oxytocin. Some practitioners (especially midwives) will encourage a woman to labor longer than this before resorting to interventions—as long as baby's heart rate is good and mom doesn't have a fever.

- If you're a first-time mom, you'll probably be allowed to push for 3 hours if you haven't had an epidural and 4 hours if you have. If you're a second-timer or more, you'll probably be allowed to push for 2 hours if you haven't had an epidural and 3 hours if you have had one. If the pushing goes on too long, your practitioner will reassess your baby's position, see

how you're feeling, perhaps attempt to birth your baby using vacuum extraction or (less likely) forceps, or decide to do a cesarean delivery.

To keep the ball (and the baby) rolling throughout labor, remember to urinate periodically, because a full bladder can interfere with the baby's descent. (If you have an epidural, chances are your bladder is being emptied by a catheter.) Full bowels may do the same, so if you haven't moved your bowels in 24 hours, give it a try. You might also try to nudge a sluggish labor along by using gravity (sitting upright, squatting, standing, or walking). When it comes to giving slow pushing a push, a semi-sitting, semi-squatting, or all-fours position may help deliver results.

Most practitioners will turn to a cesarean delivery after 24 hours of active labor (sometimes sooner) if sufficient progress hasn't been made by that time. Some will wait longer, assuming both mom and baby are doing well.

- If you'd like some pain relief, now's a good time to ask for it. An epidural can be given as early as you feel you need it and as soon as an anesthesiologist can get to your room.

- Stay hydrated. With your practitioner's green light, drink clear beverages frequently to replace fluids and to keep your mouth moist. If you're hungry, and again, if you have your practitioner's okay, have a light snack (like a Jell-O or Popsicle). If your practitioner doesn't allow anything else by mouth, sucking on ice chips can be refreshing.

- Stay on the move if you can (you won't be able to get around much if you have an epidural). Walk around,

if possible, or at least change positions as needed (see page 412 for suggested labor positions). Taking a shower or soaking in a tub now can help ease your pain, if you don't have an epidural.

- Pee periodically. Because of tremendous pelvic pressure, you may not notice the need to empty your bladder, but a full bladder can prevent baby's descent and keep you from making the progress you'll definitely want to be making. No need to trek to the bathroom if you have an epidural (not that you could anyway), because you've probably been given a catheter to empty your bladder.

What You Can Do During Active Labor

Labor's getting more active, and that means you'll be getting busier supporting your laboring spouse. Here are some ways you can help her:

- Hand a copy of the birth plan to the nurse so that it can be placed in your partner's chart (if it hasn't been already). If the shift changes, make sure the new nurse is in the loop, too.

- If mom wants pain relief, let the nurse or practitioner know. Support whatever decision she makes—to continue unmedicated or to go for pain relief (even if this decision represents a change of plans).

- Take your cues from her. Whatever mom wants, mom should get. Keep in mind that what she'll want may change from moment to moment (the TV blaring one second, TV off the next). Ditto for her mood and her reaction to you. Don't take it personally if she doesn't respond to, doesn't appreciate—or is even annoyed by—your attempts to comfort her. Ease up, if that's what she seems to prefer—but be prepared to step it up 10 minutes later if she wants. Remember that your role is important, even if you sometimes feel unneeded, unwanted, or just plain in the way. She'll appreciate you in the morning (or whenever it's all over).

- Set the mood. If possible, keep the door to the room closed, the lights low, and the room quiet to promote a relaxed and restful atmosphere. Soft music may also help (unless she'd rather watch TV—remember, she's the boss right now). Continue encouraging relaxation techniques between contractions and breathing with her through the contractions—but don't push if she's not into them or if the relaxation agenda is starting to stress her out. If distractions seem to help her, turn to cards or game apps, light music, or TV. But distract her only as much as she seems to want to be distracted.

- Pump her up. Reassure her and praise her efforts (unless your verbal reassurance is making her more edgy), and avoid criticism of any kind (even the constructive type). Be her cheerleader (but keep it low-key, since she probably won't appreciate full-on exuberance). Particularly if progress is slow, suggest that she take her labor one contraction at a time, and remind her that each pain brings her closer to seeing the baby. If she finds your cheers irritating, however, just support her gently. Stick to sympathy if that's what she seems to need.

- Keep track of the contractions. If she's on a monitor, ask the practitioner or the nurse to show you how to read it. Later, when contractions are coming one on top of the other, you can announce each new contraction as it begins—the monitor may detect the tensing of the uterus before she can, and can let her know when she's having one if she can't feel them, thanks to an epidural. You can also encourage mom through those tough contractions by telling her when each peak is ending. If there is no monitor, ask a nurse to show you how to recognize the arrival and departure of contractions with your hand on her abdomen (unless she doesn't want it there).

- Massage her neck or back, or use counterpressure or any other techniques you've learned, to make her more comfortable. Let her tell you what kind of stroking or touching or massage helps. If she prefers not to be touched at all, comfort her verbally. Remember, what feels good one moment might rub her the wrong way the next, and vice versa.

- Remind her to take a bathroom break at least once an hour if she doesn't have a catheter. She might not feel the urge, but a full bladder can stand in the way of labor progress.

- Suggest a change of positions. You'll find a variety of labor positions to try starting on page 412. Or suggest a shower or a soak in the tub to help ease the pain.

- Be the ice man. Find out where the ice machine is, and keep those chips coming. If she's allowed to sip on fluids or snack on light foods, offer them periodically. Popsicles may be especially refreshing, so ask the nurse if there's a stash you can help yourself to.

- Keep her cool. Use a damp washcloth, wrung out in cold water, to help cool her body and face. Refresh it often.

- If her feet are cold, offer to get out a pair of socks and put them on her (reaching her own feet won't be easy).

- Be her voice and her ears. She has enough going on, so lighten her load. Serve as her go-between with medical personnel as much as possible. Intercept questions from them that you can answer, and ask for explanations of procedures, equipment, and use of medication, so you'll be able to tell her what's happening. For instance, now might be the time to find out if a mirror will be provided so she can view the delivery. Be her advocate if she's unhappy about a procedure or policy, but stay calm as you intervene on her behalf so she doesn't get more upset.

Phase 3: Transitional Labor

Transition is the most demanding phase of labor but, happily, typically the quickest. Suddenly, the intensity of the contractions picks up. They become very strong, 2 to 3 minutes apart, and 60 to 90 seconds long, with very intense peaks that last for most of the contraction. Some moms, particularly those who have given birth before, experience multiple peaks. You may feel as though the contractions never disappear completely and you can't completely relax between them. The final 2 to 3 cm of dilation, to a full 10 cm, will probably take place in a very short time: on average, 15 minutes to an hour, though it can also take as long as 3 hours.

What you may be feeling. You'll feel plenty when you're in transition (unless, of course, you've had an epidural), and may experience some or all of the following:

- More intense pain with contractions

- Strong pressure in the lower back and/or perineum

- Rectal pressure

- An increase in your bloody show as more capillaries in the cervix rupture

- Feeling very warm and sweaty or chilled and shaky (or you might alternate between the two)

- Crampy legs that may tremble uncontrollably

- Nausea and/or vomiting

- Drowsiness between contractions as oxygen is diverted from your brain to the site of the delivery

- A tightening sensation in your throat or chest

- Exhaustion

Emotionally, you may feel vulnerable and overwhelmed, as though you're reaching the end of your rope. In addition to frustration over not being able to push yet, you may feel discouraged, irritable, disoriented, and restless, and may have difficulty concentrating and relaxing (it might seem impossible to do either). You may also find excitement reaching a fever pitch in the midst of all the stress. Your baby's almost here!

What you can do. Hang in there. By the end of this phase, which is not far off, your cervix will be fully dilated, and it'll be time to begin pushing your baby out.

- Continue to use breathing techniques if they help. If you feel the urge to push, resist. Pant or blow instead, unless you've been instructed otherwise. Pushing against a cervix that isn't completely dilated can cause it to swell, which can delay delivery.

What You Can Do During Transitional Labor

The going's getting tough—but here's how to help your partner-in-labor keep going.

- If your laboring spouse has an epidural or other kind of pain relief, ask her if she needs another dose. Transition can be quite painful, and if her epidural is wearing off, she won't be a happy camper. If it is, let the nurses or the practitioner know. If mom's continuing unmedicated, she'll need you more now than ever (read on).

- Be there, but give her space if she seems to want it. Often, women in transition don't like being touched— but, as always, take your cues from her. Allow her to lean on you if she wants. Abdominal massage may be especially offensive now, though counterpressure applied to the small of her back may continue to provide some relief for back pain. Be prepared to back off—even from her back—as directed.

- Don't waste words. Now's not the time for small talk, and probably not for jokes, either. Offer quiet comfort, and guide her with words that are brief and direct.

- Offer lots of encouragement, unless she prefers you to keep quiet. At this moment, eye contact or touch may communicate more expressively than words.

- Breathe with her through every contraction if it seems to help her through them.

- Help her rest and relax between contractions, touching her abdomen lightly to show her when a contraction is over. Remind her to use slow, rhythmic breathing in between contractions, if she can.

- If her contractions seem to be getting closer and/or she feels the urge to push—and she hasn't been examined recently—let the nurse or practitioner know. She may be fully dilated.

- Offer her ice chips or a sip of water frequently, and mop her brow with a cool damp cloth often. If she's chilly, offer her a blanket or a pair of socks.

- Stay focused on the payoff you're both about to get. It won't be long before the pushing begins—and that anticipated bundle arrives in your arms.

Baby's Movements During Labor

You've been counting (and enjoying) baby's kicks for the last few months, attuned to your wee one's every wiggle. But what about during labor? Is your baby still kicking up those cute little feet—and will you be able to feel those movements? The answer is yes . . . and maybe. Your baby will still move around during labor—and in fact may do some impressive spins to help ease out of the birth canal—but you may not feel much of that movement at all. First, your focus (understandably) is likely to be on those contractions, making movements easy to miss. Second, if you've had an epidural, you'll be numb—which means you might not feel a thing (including those movements). But that's where fetal monitors or Dopplers come in—to track baby's heartbeat, assuring all is well. One less thing for you to have to worry about during labor!

- If you didn't have an epidural before but would like one now, ask for it.
- If you don't want anybody to touch you unnecessarily, if your coach's once comforting hands now irritate you, don't hesitate to let him know.

- Try to relax between contractions (as much as is possible) with slow, deep, rhythmic breathing.
- Keep your eye on the prize: That bundle of joy will soon be arriving in your arms.

Laboring Down

Woo-hoo—you've reached that magic 10 cm mark! You're fully dilated and it's finally time to start pushing out baby, right? Not so fast—or at least that's what your doctor or midwife will tell you if he or she practices the art of "laboring down." Laboring down allows your uterus to do most of the work of bringing baby farther down the birth canal, and it means you won't need to start pushing in earnest until baby's head is at +2 station or nearly crowning (or until you feel that tremendous urge to push)—even if you're already fully dilated. This process of waiting for baby to come down the birth canal on his or her own can take a few minutes or an hour or two, during which you'll follow only natural, gentle urges to push (or not push at all). In fact, contractions often slow down or stop during this time, giving you a break from the hard labor you've been experiencing. The benefit to laboring down? You'll get to conserve energy until it's really needed, and take a rest while your uterus does the heavy lifting. Plus, studies show that laboring down significantly decreases pushing time. Have an epidural? You can still labor down.

Stage Two: Pushing and Delivery

Up until this point, your active participation in the birth of your baby has been negligible. Though you've definitely taken most of the abuse, your cervix and uterus (and baby) have done most of the work. But that's about to change. Now that dilation is complete, it's your turn to push your baby the rest of the way through the birth canal—and out (unless you'll be laboring down, in which case you can catch a break before you begin pushing; see box, page 429). Pushing and delivery generally take between 30 minutes and an hour, but can sometimes be accomplished in 10 (or even fewer) short minutes or in 2, 3, or even more very long hours.

The contractions of the second stage are usually more regular than the contractions of transition. They are still about 60 to 90 seconds in duration but sometimes further apart (usually about 2 to 5 minutes) and possibly less painful, though sometimes they are more intense. There now should be a well-defined rest period between them, though you may still have trouble recognizing the onset of each contraction.

What you may be feeling. Common in the second stage (though you'll definitely feel the following a lot less—and you may not feel anything at all—if you've had an epidural):

- Pain with the contractions, though possibly not as much

- An overwhelming urge to push (though not every mom feels this, especially with an epidural)

- Tremendous rectal pressure (ditto)

- A burst of renewed energy (a second wind) or fatigue

- Very visible contractions, with your uterus rising noticeably with each

- An increase in bloody show

- A tingling, stretching, burning, or stinging sensation at the vaginal opening as your baby's head crowns (it's called the "ring of fire" for good reason)

- A slippery wet feeling as your baby emerges

Emotionally, you may feel relieved, exhilarated, and excited that you can now start pushing—or, if the pushing stretches on for much more than an hour, frustrated or overwhelmed. In a prolonged second stage, you may find your preoccupation is less with seeing the baby than with getting the ordeal over with (and that's perfectly understandable). Some moms can also feel inhibited or unsure when they begin pushing, especially if they don't quite get the hang of it at first. After all, birthing a baby is a natural process—but it doesn't always come naturally.

What you can do. It's time to get this baby out. So get into a pushing position (which one will depend on the bed, chair, or tub you're in, what's most comfortable and effective for you, and your practitioner's preferences). A semi-sitting or semi-squatting position is often the best because it enlists the aid of gravity in the birthing process and may offer you more pushing power. Tucking your chin to your chest when you're in this position will help you focus your pushes where they need to be. Sometimes, if the pushing isn't moving your baby down the birth canal, it may be helpful to change positions. If

What You Can Do During Pushing and Delivery

It's push time, and here's how you can help:

- Continue giving comfort and support (a whispered "I love you" can be more valuable to her during the pushing stage than anything else), but don't feel hurt if the object of your efforts doesn't seem to notice you're there. Her energies are necessarily focused elsewhere.

- Help her relax between the contractions—with soothing words, a cool cloth applied to forehead, neck, and shoulders, and, if feasible, back massage or counterpressure to help ease backache. If she's laboring down (see box, page 429), encourage her to rest up.

- Continue to supply ice chips or sips of ice water to moisten her mouth as needed—she'll be parched from pushing.

- Support her back while she's pushing, if necessary. Hold her hand, wipe her brow—or do whatever else seems to help her. If she slips out of position, gently help her back into it.

- Periodically point out her progress. As the baby begins to crown, remind her to keep an eye on the mirror so she can have visual confirmation of what she is accomplishing. When she's not looking, or if there's no mirror, give her inch-by-inch descriptions. Take her hand and touch baby's head together for renewed inspiration.

- If you're offered the opportunity to catch your baby as he or she emerges or, later, to cut the cord, don't be afraid. Both are relatively easy jobs, and you'll get step-by-step directions and backup from the attendants. You should know, however, that the cord can't be snipped like a piece of string. It's tougher than you may think.

you've been semi-sitting, for example, you might want to get up on all-fours.

Once you're ready to begin pushing, give it all you've got. The more efficiently you push and the more energy you pack into the effort, the more quickly your baby will make the trip through the birth canal. Frantic, disorganized pushing wastes energy and accomplishes little—plus it can take its toll on you. Keep these pushing pointers in mind:

- Relax your upper body and your thighs and then push as if you're having a bowel movement (the biggest one of your life). Focus your energy on your vagina and rectum, not your chest (which could result in chest pain after delivery) and not your face (straining with your face could cause bruises on your cheeks and bloodshot eyes, not to mention do nothing to help get your baby out). It may help to look down, past your bump, as you push.

- Speaking of bowel movements, since you're bearing down on the whole perineal area, anything that's in your rectum may be pushed out, too—trying to avoid this while you're pushing can slow your progress. Don't let inhibition or embarrassment break the pushing rhythm. Involuntary pooping (or peeing) is experienced by nearly everyone during delivery. No one else in the room will think twice about it, and neither should you (you probably won't even notice it). Pads will immediately whisk away anything that comes out.

- Take a few deep breaths while the contraction is building so you can gear up for pushing. As the contraction peaks, take a deep breath and then push with all your might—holding your breath if you want or exhaling as you push, whatever feels right to you. If you'd like the nurses or your coach to guide you by counting to 10 while you push, that's fine. But if you find it breaks your rhythm or isn't helpful, ask them not to. There is no magic formula when it comes to how long each push should last or how many times you should push with each contraction—the most important thing is to do what comes naturally. You may feel as many as 5 urges to bear down, with each push lasting just seconds—or you may feel the urge to bear down just twice, but with each push lasting longer. Follow those urges, and you'll deliver your baby. Actually, you'll deliver your baby even if you don't follow your urges or if you find you don't have any urges at all. Pushing doesn't come naturally for every woman, and if it doesn't for you, your practitioner, nurse, or doula can help direct your efforts, and redirect them if you lose your concentration.

- Don't become frustrated if you see the baby's head crown and then disappear again. Birthing is a 2-steps-forward, 1-step-backward proposition. Just remember, baby's moving in the right direction.

- Rest between contractions. If you're really exhausted, especially when the pushing stage drags on, your practitioner may suggest that you not push for several contractions so you can rebuild your strength.

- Stop pushing when you're instructed to (as you may be, to keep the baby's head from being born too rapidly). If you're feeling the urge to push when you are asked not to push, pant or blow instead.

- Remember to keep an eye on the mirror (if one is available) once there's something to look at. Seeing your baby's head crown (and reaching down and touching it) may give you the inspiration to push when the pushing gets tough. Besides, unless your coach or someone else is taking a video, there won't be any replays to watch.

What your practitioner and nurse will be doing. While you're pushing, the nurses and/or your practitioner will give you support and direction (and if necessary, will use their hands to apply some gentle pressure on your abdomen to help coax baby down), continue to monitor your baby's heartbeat with either a Doppler or fetal monitor, and prepare for delivery by spreading sterile drapes and arranging instruments, donning surgical garments and gloves, and sponging your perineal area with antiseptic (though midwives generally just don gloves and don't do any draping). Most practitioners will use their fingers to gently stretch the perineum (much like perennial massage described on page 384) before your baby's head emerges. Some will use lubricants or oils (like olive or mineral oil) to make your perineum slippery, enabling baby's head to glide out more easily (and avoid tears). If necessary (it's unlikely), an episiotomy will be performed, or possibly vacuum extraction, or even less likely, forceps will be used.

A Baby Is Born

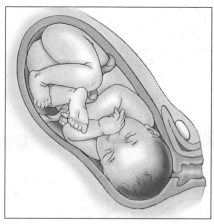

1. The cervix has thinned (effaced) somewhat but has not begun to dilate much.

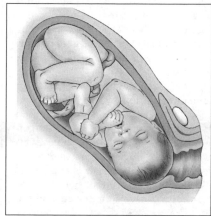

2. The cervix has fully dilated and the baby's head has begun to press into the birth canal (vagina).

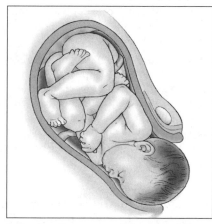

3. To allow the narrowest diameter of the baby's head to fit through the mother's pelvis, the baby usually turns sometime during labor. Here, the slightly molded head has crowned.

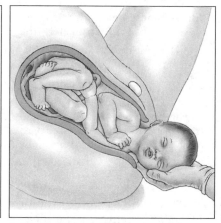

4. The head, the baby's broadest part, is out. The rest of the delivery should proceed quickly and smoothly.

Once your baby's head emerges, your practitioner will suction your baby's nose and mouth to remove excess mucus, then help ease the shoulders and torso out. You probably will have to give only one more small push to help with that—the head was the hard part, and the rest slides out pretty easily.

A First Look at Baby

After 40 or so weeks of waiting (and too many hours of laboring and delivering), there's no doubt that your just-born baby will be a sight for your sore eyes: perfectly beautiful to you in every way.

That said, 9 months of soaking in an amniotic bath, followed by compression in a contracting uterus and cramped birth canal can take a temporary toll on a newborn's appearance. Babies who were neatly plucked from their uterine homes (especially if they arrived via scheduled c-section, before labor started) will have an initial edge in the looks department—they'll be rounder and smoother. What can you expect your newborn baby to look like at first sight, besides picture perfect? Here's a realistic heads-up on some typical newborn characteristics, head to toe:

Oddly shaped head. At birth, an infant's head is, proportionately, the largest part of the body, with a circumference as large as his or her chest. As your baby grows, the rest of the body will catch up. Often, the head has molded to fit through mom's pelvis, giving it an odd, possibly pointed "cone" shape. If baby has pressed hard against your cervix before it was fully dilated, there may be a lump on that sweet noggin, too. The lump will disappear in a day or two, the molding within 2 weeks, at which point your baby's head will begin to take on that cherubic roundness.

Newborn hair. Some newborns are virtually bald or sport just a light coating of peach fuzz, some have a thick mane. But hair today will be gone, eventually. All babies lose their newborn hair (though this may happen so gradually that you don't notice), and it will be replaced by new growth, possibly of a different color and texture.

Vernix coating. Remember that cheesy coating that was keeping baby's skin protected in that amniotic bath? Premature babies have quite a lot of this coating at birth, on-time babies have just a little, and overdue babies may have none at all—except possibly in skin folds and under fingernails.

Swelling of breasts and genitals. Boy and girl parts can appear swollen at birth. Breasts of both male and female newborns can also be swollen (and sometimes even engorged, secreting a white or pink substance nicknamed "witch's milk"), thanks not to their own

Your baby will be handed to you or placed on your belly, the umbilical cord will be clamped (see page 416) and cut—either by the practitioner or by your coach—and the midwife or nurse will give baby a rub to help get his or her breathing and crying going. (If you've arranged for cord blood collection, it will be done now.) This is a great time for some caressing and skin-to-skin contact, so lift up your gown and bring baby close. In case you need a reason to do that, studies show that infants who have skin-to-skin contact with their mothers just after delivery sleep longer and are calmer hours later. Breastfeeding could be initiated now or, if need be, after the initial evaluation (see below). Here's a fun fact: If you keep your newborn skin-to-skin on your belly after birth, he or she will instinctively creep (over a period of 20 minutes to an hour or longer) toward your breast, find your nipple (bobbing hormones, but mom's. Those same hormones may also stimulate a white, sometimes blood-tinged vaginal discharge in baby girls. These effects are normal and will disappear in a week to 10 days.

Puffy eyes. Swelling around the eyes, normal for someone who's been soaking in amniotic fluid for 9 months and then squeezed through a narrow birth canal, may be exacerbated by the ointment used to protect baby's eyes from infection. Most of the puffiness will—poof!—disappear within a few days.

Eye color, TBD. Brown? Green? Blue? For most babies, it's way too early to call. Caucasian baby eyes are usually (but not always) slate blue, no matter what color they will turn later on. In babies of color, eyes are usually brown at birth, but the shade of brown may ultimately do some changing.

Skin surprises. Your baby's skin will appear pink, white, or even grayish at birth (even if it will eventually turn brown or black). That's because pigmentation doesn't show up until a few hours after birth. A variety of rashes, tiny "pimples," and whiteheads may also mar your baby's skin thanks to maternal hormones, but all are temporary. You may also notice skin dryness and cracking, caused by such a long soak in an amniotic bath and first-time exposure to air—these, too, will pass without any treatment.

Lanugo. Fine downy hair, called lanugo, may cover the shoulders, back, forehead, and temples of full-term babies. This will usually be shed by the end of the first week. Such hair can be more abundant, and will last longer, in a premature baby and may already be gone in an overdue one.

Birthmarks. A reddish blotch at the base of the skull, on the eyelid, or on the forehead, called a salmon patch, is very common, especially in Caucasian newborns. Mongolian spots—bluish-gray pigmentation of the deep skin layer that can appear on the back, buttocks, and sometimes the arms and thighs—are more common in Asians, southern Europeans, and African Americans. These markings eventually disappear, usually by age 4. Hemangiomas, elevated strawberry-colored birthmarks, vary from tiny to about quarter size or even larger. They eventually fade to a mottled pearly gray, then often disappear entirely. Coffee-with-cream colored (café au lait) spots can appear anywhere on the body—they're usually inconspicuous and don't fade.

For much more on your baby, head to toe, see *What to Expect the First Year*.

---

that cute little head while searching for it), and then latch on.

What's next for your baby? The nurses and/or a pediatrician will evaluate baby's condition, and rate it on the Apgar scale at 1 minute and 5 minutes after birth (see *What to Expect the First Year* for more), give a brisk, stimulating, and drying rubdown, possibly take baby's footprints for a keepsake, attach an identifying band to your wrist (and to baby's dad's wrist) and to your baby's ankle, administer nonirritating eye ointment to prevent infection (you can ask that the ointment be administered after you've had time to cuddle with your newborn), weigh baby, and then wrap him or her to prevent heat loss. (In some hospitals and most birthing centers, some of these procedures may be omitted—in others, many will be attended to later, so you can have more time to bond with your newborn.)

Then you'll get your baby back (assuming all is well) and you may begin breastfeeding if you haven't already and you'd like to (see Beginning Breastfeeding, page 478). Sometime after that, baby will get a more complete pediatric exam and some routine protective procedures (including a heel stick, vitamin K shot, and hepatitis B vaccine), either in your room or in the hospital nursery (dad can go along or stay with you). Once your baby's temperature is stable, he or she will get a first bath, which you (and/or dad) may be able to help give.

Stage Three: Delivery of the Placenta

The worst is over, and the best has already come. All that remains is tying up the loose ends, so to speak. During this final stage of childbirth (which generally lasts anywhere from 5 to 30 minutes or more), the placenta, which has been your baby's life support inside the womb, will be delivered. You will continue to have mild contractions approximately a minute in duration, though you may not feel them (after all, you're preoccupied with your newborn!). The squeezing of the uterus separates the placenta from the uterine wall and moves it down into the lower segment of the uterus or into the vagina so it can be expelled.

Your practitioner will help deliver the placenta by either pulling the cord gently with one hand while pressing and kneading your uterus with the other or exerting downward pressure on the top of the uterus, asking you to push at the appropriate time. You might get some Pitocin (oxytocin) via injection or in your IV to encourage uterine contractions, which will speed delivery of the placenta, help shrink the uterus back to size, and minimize bleeding. Once the placenta is out, your practitioner will examine it to make sure it's intact. If it isn't, he or she will inspect your uterus manually for placental fragments and remove any that remain. (If you'd like to keep the placenta, be sure your practitioner knows about this plan, and that both he or she and the hospital have agreed to it ahead of time. See page 362 for more.)

Now that the work of labor and delivery is done, you may feel overwhelmingly exhausted or, conversely, experience a burst of renewed energy. You are likely to be very thirsty and, especially if labor has been long (and particularly if you weren't allowed to eat), hungry. Some women experience chills in this stage, while all experience a bloody vaginal discharge (called lochia) comparable to a heavy menstrual period.

How will you feel emotionally after you've delivered your baby? Every new mom reacts a little differently, and your reaction is normal for you. Your first emotional response may be joy, but it's just as likely to be a sense of relief. You may be exhilarated and talkative, elated and excited, a little impatient at having to push out the placenta or submit to the repair of a tear or an episiotomy, or so in awe of what you're cuddling in your arms (or so beat, or a little bit of both) that you don't notice. You may feel a closeness to your spouse and an immediate bond with your new baby,

What You Can Do After Delivery

Your baby is here! While you're basking in the moment, you can also:

- Offer some well-earned words of praise to the new mom—and congratulate yourself, too, for a job well done.

- Begin bonding with your little one—with some holding and cuddling, and by doing soft singing or talking. Remember, your baby has heard your voice a lot during his or her stay in the uterus and is familiar with its sound. Hearing it now will bring comfort in this strange new environment.

- Don't forget to do some cuddling and bonding with mom, too.

- Ask for an ice pack to soothe her perineal area, if the nurse doesn't offer one.

- Ask for some juice for mom—she may be very thirsty. After she's been rehydrated, and if both of you are in the mood, break out the bubbly—champagne or sparkling cider if you brought some along.

- Snap baby's first photos or capture your amazing newborn on video.

- You'll also have the opportunity to be with your newborn for the first exam, first bath, and other routine procedures.

or (and this is just as normal) you may feel somewhat detached (who is this stranger sniffing at my breast?). No matter what your response now, you will come to love your baby intensely. These things just sometimes take time. (For more on bonding, see page 471.)

What you can do

- Do some quality snuggling, skin-to-skin. Speak up, too. Since your baby will recognize your voice, cooing, singing, or whispered words will be especially comforting (it's a strange new world, and you'll be able to help baby make some sense out of it). Under some circumstances, your baby may be kept in a heated bassinet for a while or be held by your coach while the placenta is being delivered—but not to worry, there's plenty of time for baby bonding.

- Spend some time bonding with your coach, too—and enjoying your cozy new threesome.

- Help deliver the placenta, if necessary, by pushing when directed. Some moms don't even have to push at all for the placenta to arrive. Your practitioner will let you know what to do, if anything.

- Hang in there during repair of any episiotomy or tears.

- Continue (or start) breastfeeding if baby is still with you.

- Take pride in your accomplishment—you did it, mama!

All that's left to do, then, is for your practitioner to stitch up any tear (if you're not already numbed, you'll get a local anesthetic) and clean you up. You'll likely get an ice pack to put on your perineum to minimize swelling—ask for one if it's not offered. The nurse will also help you put on a maxipad or add some thick pads under your bottom (remember, you'll be bleeding a lot). Once you're feeling up to it, you'll be transferred to a postpartum room.

Cesarean Delivery

You won't be able to participate actively at a cesarean delivery the way you would at a vaginal one, and some would consider that a definite plus. Instead of huffing, puffing, and pushing your baby into the world, you'll get to lie back and let everybody else do all the heavy lifting. In fact, your most important contribution to your baby's cesarean birth will be preparation: The more you know, the more comfortable you'll feel. Which is why it's a good idea to look this section over ahead of time, even if you're not having a planned cesarean delivery.

Thanks to regional anesthesia (like epidurals) and the liberalization of hospital regulations, most moms (and their coaches) are able to be full-on spectators at their cesarean deliveries. Because they aren't preoccupied with pushing or pain, they're often able to relax (at least to some degree) and marvel at the birth. This is what you can expect in a typical cesarean birth:

- An IV infusion will be started (if it isn't already in) to provide speedy access if additional medications or fluids are needed. Most doctors will give you antibiotics through your IV to prevent infection down the road.

- Anesthesia will be administered: either an epidural or a spinal block (both of which numb the lower part of your body but allow you to be fully awake and alert). In rare emergency situations, when a baby must be delivered immediately, a general anesthetic (which puts you to sleep) may be used.

- Your abdomen will be washed down with an antiseptic solution. A catheter (a narrow tube) will be inserted into your bladder to keep it empty and out of the surgeon's way.

- Sterile drapes will be arranged around your exposed abdomen. A screen will be put up at about shoulder level so you won't have to see the incision being made, though some hospitals have clear drapes so you can have a view of baby emerging.

- If your coach is going to attend the delivery (which he probably will be able to), he will be suited up in sterile garb. He will sit near your head so that he can give you emotional support and hold your hand, and he may have the option of viewing the actual surgery. If you've planned to have a doula with you during the delivery, she can be with you during your c-section as well.

- If yours is an emergency cesarean delivery, things may move very quickly. Try to stay calm in the face of all that activity, and don't let it worry you—that's just the way things work in a hospital sometimes.

- Once your doctor is certain that the anesthetic has taken effect, an incision

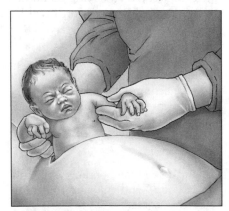

Cesarean delivery

Tying Your Tubes After Delivery

Thinking about ending your baby-making career after this delivery—and contemplating a permanent solution to birth control? Though it's far easier for dads to take this step (vasectomy, the male version of sterilization, is much less invasive), moms choosing to have their tubes tied can opt to add the procedure to their birth plans. Whether you're delivering vaginally or via c-section, having a tubal ligation right after your baby's birth definitely saves time and money and will certainly make postpartum sex (when you finally get around to it) more convenient. Not sure if you're done, done, done? See more about birth control on page 511.

If you've delivered via cesarean. Since an incision has already been made to get your baby out—and you're already numb from the anesthesia—there's little extra fuss or muss involved.

Your doctor will simply clip (or clamp) your fallopian tubes before stitching your incision back up.

If you've delivered vaginally. The doctor will make a small incision under the belly button. The benefit to doing the procedure right after delivery is that your uterus is still large, so there's easy access to your fallopian tubes. Most doctors will perform a tubal ligation right after a vaginal birth only if mom has received an epidural during labor and it's still in place.

You likely won't need any extra recovery time or experience any extra pain from the procedure—beyond what you'd experience anyway after delivery (and if you did, it would be hard to differentiate one pain from the other). You probably also won't need any additional pain medication (again, beyond what you might take for postpartum pain).

(usually a horizontal bikini cut) is made in your lower abdomen, just above the pubic hairline. You may feel a sensation of being "unzipped," but you won't feel any pain.

- A second incision (usually a low-horizontal one) is then made, this time in your uterus. The amniotic sac is opened, and, if it hasn't already ruptured, the fluid is suctioned out—you may hear a sort of gurgling or swooshing sound.

- The baby is then eased out, usually while an assistant presses on the uterus. With an epidural (though not likely with a spinal block), you will probably feel some pulling and tugging sensations, as well as some pressure. If you're eager to see your baby's

arrival and drapes are blocking the view, ask the doctor if the screen can be lowered slightly.

- Your baby's nose and mouth are then suctioned—then you'll hear the first cry, the cord will be quickly clamped and cut, and you'll be allowed a quick glimpse of your newborn. In a hospital offering a "gentle c-section," your baby may be placed on your chest and you'll be able to hold (or even breastfeed) your baby right away.

- While the baby is getting the same routine attention that a vaginally delivered infant receives, the doctor will remove the placenta.

- Now the doctor will quickly do a routine check of your reproductive organs and stitch up the incisions that

Don't Forget to Cover Baby

One of the many calls you'll have to make now (or within the next few weeks) is to your health insurance company so your baby can be added to your plan. Not insured or want to change Affordable Care Act plans? Since having a baby qualifies you for a Special Enrollment Period, you can enroll in or change Marketplace coverage now even if it's not Open Enrollment time, for 60 days after the birth of your little one. Go to healthcare.gov for more information.

were made. The uterine incision will be repaired with absorbable stitches, which do not have to be removed. The abdominal incision may be closed with either stitches (which may or may not be absorbable) or surgical staples.

■ An injection of oxytocin may be given intramuscularly or into your IV to help contract the uterus and control bleeding.

You may have some cuddling time—and even some skin-to-skin time in the delivery room, but a lot will depend on your condition and the baby's, as well as hospital rules. Many hospitals allow skin-to-skin time after a cesarean delivery as long as your baby is medically stable (just ask the nurses to hand you your baby)—and especially if "gentle cesareans" are offered. If you can't hold your baby, perhaps your spouse can. If your baby has to be whisked away to the NICU (neonatal intensive care unit) or the nursery, don't let it get you down. This is standard in some hospitals after a cesarean delivery and is more likely to indicate a precaution than a problem. And as far as bonding is concerned, later can be just as good as sooner—so not to worry if the snuggles have to wait a little while.

CHAPTER 15

Expecting Multiples

Have two (or more) passengers aboard the mother ship? Then chances are, you have at least double the joy and excitement—and at least double the questions: Will the babies be healthy? Will I be healthy? Am I more likely to have complications? Will I be able to stick with my regular practitioner, or will I have to see a specialist? How much food will I have to eat, and how much weight do I have to gain? Will there be enough room inside of me for two babies? Will I be able to carry them to term? Will I have to go on bed rest? Will giving birth be twice as hard?

Carrying one baby comes with its share of challenges and changes. Carrying more than one—well, you've probably already done the math. But not to worry. You're up for it—or at least you will be once you're armed with the information in this chapter . . . and the support of your partner and your practitioner. So sit back (comfortably, while you still can) and get ready for your amazing multiple pregnancy.

What You May Be Wondering About

Choosing a Practitioner

"We just found out we're having twins. Can I use my regular ob, or do I need to see a specialist?"

Having twins is definitely special— but it doesn't definitely require a specialist's care. Just make sure you really like your regular ob before you commit—since twin pregnancies always come with more office visits, you'll be seeing a lot of each other.

Do you like your ob but also like the idea of extra-careful care? Many general ob practices send patients who are pregnant with multiples to a specialist for periodic consultations, or refer them to a specialist later in pregnancy (or at any point if things take a turn for the complicated)—a good compromise if you'd like to combine the familiar comfort of your ob's care with the expertise of a specialist's. Moms-to-be of multiples who have any other risk factors (they're older, have a history of miscarriage, or have a chronic health condition) may want to start off with or consider switching over full-time to a maternal-fetal medicine specialist (also known as a perinatologist). Talk that possibility over with your ob if your pregnancy falls into a higher risk category. If you're carrying triplets or more, your best bet is to get your prenatal care from a perinatologist right from the beginning.

When choosing a practitioner for your multiple pregnancy (likely a physician, since most midwives don't offer care for multiple pregnancies; see box, facing page), you'll also want to factor in hospital affiliation. Ideally, you'll want to deliver at a facility with the ability to care for premature babies (one with a NICU) in case your bundles arrive early, as multiples often do.

Also ask about the doctor's policy on topics specifically related to multiple births: Will you be induced at 37 or 38 weeks as a matter of course, or will you have the option of carrying beyond that time frame if all is going well? Will a vaginal birth be possible under certain circumstances (or at least a trial of labor), or does this doctor routinely schedule moms of twins for cesarean delivery? Will you be able to deliver vaginally in a birthing room or

Fraternal or Identical?

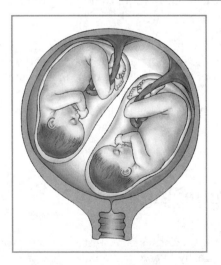 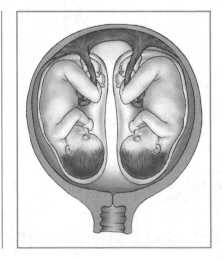

Fraternal twins (left), which result from 2 eggs being fertilized at the same time, each have their own placenta. Identical twins (right), which come from 1 fertilized egg that splits and then develops into 2 separate embryos, may share a placenta and amniotic sac or—depending on when the egg splits—may each have their own.

Midwife Care for Multiples?

Even if your regular practitioner is a midwife, it's possible that you'll be able to stick with her, at least for part of your pregnancy, as long as it stays low risk—and assuming her credentials, license, and experience allow her to care for and deliver twin pregnancies.

Unfortunately, many midwives don't meet that set of criteria, which means that while it's possible you'll find one who can care for and deliver twin pregnancies, it's more likely that you won't. While some midwives will provide prenatal care for low-risk twin pregnancies, others will care for a mom of twins only up to a certain gestational age, and others won't take a twin pregnancy on at all, due to the potential of it turning high risk. What's more, some states don't allow midwives to care for or deliver multiples—and many birthing centers won't allow twin deliveries, either.

But that doesn't mean you have to write off midwife care entirely. Midwives who have collaborative agreements with obs who can act as backups in case of complications are more likely to agree to signing up a mom of twins. And even if your care does need to be transferred to an ob or perinatologist at some point, your midwife may be able to stay involved in your pregnancy and even attend your birth.

Have your heart set on a home birth? You may have a hard time finding a midwife who will deliver twins at home, especially if you live in a rural area where an ob (and hospital) backup may be too far away.

If you do decide to use a midwife for your prenatal care, at least initially—and especially if you choose to have her (or him) deliver your babies—be sure to choose someone who has plenty of experience managing twin pregnancies.

is it routine to deliver multiples in an operating room?

For more general information about choosing a practitioner, see page 10.

Pregnancy Symptoms

"I've heard that pregnancy symptoms are way worse when when you're having multiples. Is that true?"

Twice the babies sometimes spell twice (or more) the pregnancy discomforts, but not always. Every multiple pregnancy, like every singleton pregnancy, is different. An expectant mom of one may suffer enough morning sickness for two, while a mom-to-be of multiples might sail through her pregnancy without a single queasy day. The same with other symptoms, too.

But though you shouldn't expect a double dose of morning sickness (or heartburn, or leg cramps, or varicose veins), you can't count it out. The miseries do, on average, multiply in a multiple pregnancy, and that's not surprising, given the extra weight you'll be carrying around and the extra hormones you're already generating. Among the symptoms that might be—but won't necessarily be—exponentially exacerbated when you're expecting twins or more:

- Morning sickness. Nausea and vomiting can be worse in a multiple pregnancy, thanks to—among other things—the higher levels of hormones circulating in a mom's system. Morning sickness can also start earlier and last longer. And severe nausea and vomiting (hyperemesis gravidarum,

Seeing Double—Everywhere?

If it looks like multiples are multiplying these days, it's because they are. In fact, nearly 4 percent of babies in the United States are now born in sets of 2, 3, or more, with the majority (about 95 percent) of these multiple births composed of twins. At least twice as amazing, the number of twin births has jumped more than 50 percent in recent years. Rates of higher-order multiples (triplets and more) are starting to decline, but are still up about 300 percent.

So what's up with this multiple-baby boom? While identical twins usually happen by chance, your chance of having fraternal twins (the more common type of twin) increases based on the following factors (some of which can also influence the odds of having higher-order fraternal multiples, too):

Age. The older you are, the higher your odds of having fraternal twins. Moms over the age of 35 are naturally more likely to drop more than 1 egg at ovulation (thanks to often higher levels of FSH, or follicle-stimulating hormone), upping the odds of having twins.

Fertility treatments. As techniques in assisted fertility become more sophisticated, they're less likely to produce multiples, especially higher-order multiples. Still, having any kind of fertility treatments (particularly the kind that stimulates ovulation or implants more than 1 embryo) multiplies the chances of a multiple pregnancy.

Obesity. Women who are obese when they conceive (with a BMI higher than 30) are significantly more likely to have fraternal twins than women with lower BMIs.

Size. There is some evidence that larger, taller women may be slightly more likely to conceive twins than smaller women—but the connection appears weak (meaning size doesn't matter much).

Race. Twins are slightly more common among African Americans and somewhat less common among Hispanics and Asians.

Family history. Do fraternal twins run in your family? Or are you a fraternal twin yourself? Your chances of having multiples are greater than average. And if you've already had a set of fraternal twins, you're twice as likely to have another set in a future pregnancy. Now, that's a win-win-win-win.

see page 547) is more common among moms-to-be of multiples.

- Other tummy troubles. More gastric crowding (and more gastric overloading, since moms of multiples are eating for three or more) can lead to an increase in the kinds of digestive discomforts pregnancy's known for, like heartburn, indigestion, and constipation.

- Fatigue. This is a no-brainer: The more weight you're dragging around, the more you're likely to drag. Fatigue can also increase with the extra energy an expectant mom of multiples expends (your body has to work twice as hard to grow two babies). Sleep deprivation can also wear you out (it's difficult enough to settle down with a watermelon-size belly, let alone one that's the size of two watermelons). And speaking of no-brainers, expecting twins can thicken the normal brain fog of pregnancy.

- All those other physical discomforts. Every pregnancy comes with its share of aches and pains—your twin pregnancy might just come with a little more than its share. Toting that extra baby can translate to extra backache, hip pain, pelvic twinges, pelvic (and round ligament) pain, crampiness, swollen ankles, varicose veins, you name it. Breathing for a crowd can also seem to be an extra effort, especially as your uterus full of babies gets big enough to crowd out your lungs.

- Fetal movement. Though every pregnant woman might feel at some point that she's expecting an octopus, the 8 limbs you'll be carrying will really pack a punch. Make that many punches, and kicks.

Whether your multiple pregnancy ends up doubling up on discomforts or not, one thing's for sure—it'll also gift you with twice the rewards. Not bad, for 9 months' work.

Eating Well with Multiples

"I'm committed to eating well now that I'm pregnant with triplets, but I'm not sure what that means—eating 3 times as much?"

Belly up to the buffet table, mom—feeding 4 means it's always time to chow down. While you won't literally have to quadruple your daily intake (any more than a woman expecting a single baby has to double it), you will need to do some serious eating in the months to come. Moms-to-be of multiples should cash in on an extra 150 to 300 calories a day per fetus, doctor's orders (good news if you're looking for a license to eat, not so good news if queasiness or tummy crowding has your appetite cramped). Which translates to an extra 300 to 600 calories if you're carrying twins, an extra 450 to 900 calories for triplets (if you've started out with an average prepregnancy weight). But before you take that extra allotment as a free pass to Burritoville (extra guacamole for Baby A, extra sour cream for Baby B, extra refried beans for Baby C), consider this: The quality of what you eat will be just as important as the quantity. In fact, good nutrition during a multiple pregnancy has an even greater impact on baby birthweight than it does during a singleton pregnancy.

So just how do you eat well when you're expecting more than one? Check out the Pregnancy Diet (see Chapter 4) and:

Keep it small. The bigger your belly gets, the smaller you'll want your meals to stay. Not only will grazing on 5 or 6 healthy mini meals and snacks ease your digestive overload, but it'll keep your energy up—while delivering the same nutritional bottom line as 3 squares. As space gets ever tighter, you may even want to eat even less even more often — and you'll probably want to keep some nibbles bedside in case you get hungry during the night.

Make your calories count. Pick foods that pack plenty of nutrients into small servings. Studies show that a higher-calorie diet that's also high in nutrients significantly improves your chances of having healthy full-term babies. Wasting too much of that premium space on junk food means you'll have less room for the nutritious food your crew of cuties needs.

Go for extra nutrients. Not surprisingly, your need for nutrients multiplies with each baby—which means you'll have to tack on some extra servings to your Daily Dozen (see page 90). It's usually recommended that moms of multiples get 1 extra serving of protein, 1 extra serving of calcium, and 1 extra serving of whole grains. Be sure to ask your practitioner for specific recommendations in your case.

Pump up the iron. Another nutrient you'll need to ramp up is iron, which helps your body manufacture red blood cells (you'll need lots of those for the increased blood your multiple-baby factory will be using) and helps keep you from becoming anemic, which often happens in multiple pregnancies. So eat up from the list of iron-rich foods (see page 97). Your prenatal vitamin and possibly a separate iron supplement should fill in the rest—but ask your practitioner for specifics.

Keep the water flowing. Dehydration can lead to preterm labor (something moms-to-be of multiples are already at risk for), so drink up.

For more information on eating well for multiples, check out *What to Expect: Eating Well When You're Expecting.*

Weight Gain

"I know I'm supposed to gain more weight with twins, but just how much more?"

Get ready to gain. Experts advise a normal-weight mom expecting twins to gain between 37 and 54 pounds.

Why the big spread? Because recommendations differ considerably based on your particular profile and your practitioner's recommendations. Carrying triplets? Since there are no official guidelines, you'll need to check in with your practitioner for a specific target weight gain total—which will likely exceed 50 pounds (a little less if you were overweight prepregnancy, a little more if you were underweight).

Sounds like a piece of cake, right? Or maybe two pieces of cake (or hey, maybe the whole cake). But the reality is, gaining enough weight isn't always as easy as it seems when you've got two—or more—on board. In fact, a variety of challenges you may face throughout your pregnancy can keep the numbers on the scale from climbing fast enough.

Standing between you and weight gain in the first trimester might be nausea, which can make it difficult to get food down—and then keep it down. Eating tiny amounts of comforting (and, hopefully, sometimes nutritious) food throughout the day can help get you through those probably queasy months. Aim for a pound-a-week gain through the first trimester, but if you find you can't gain that much, or have trouble gaining any at all, relax. You can have fun catching up later. Just be sure to take your prenatal vitamin and stay hydrated.

What to Gain When You're Gaining for Multiples

PREGNANCY STATUS	TOTAL WEIGHT GAIN
Normal weight with twins	37 to 54 pounds
Overweight with twins	31 to 50 pounds
Triplets	Ask your practitioner for recommendations

Use the second trimester (which will probably be your most comfortable—and the easiest for you to do some serious chowing down in) as your chance to load up on the nutrition your babies need to grow. If you didn't gain any weight during the first trimester (or if you lost weight due to severe nausea and vomiting), your practitioner may want you to gain an average of 1½ to 2 pounds per week starting now. If you've been gaining steadily through the first trimester, you can aim a little lower. Either way, that may seem like a lot of weight in a short time, and you're right—it is. But it's weight that's important to gain. Supercharge your eating plan with extra servings of protein, calcium, and whole grains. Heartburn and indigestion starting to cramp your eating style? Spread your nutrients out over those 6 (or more) mini-meals.

As you head into the home stretch (the third trimester), you'll still need to continue your steady rate of gain. By 32 weeks, your babies may be 4 pounds each, which won't leave much room in your crowded out tummy for food. Still, even though you'll be feeling plenty bulky already, your babies will have to bulk up quite a bit more—and they'll appreciate the nutrition a healthy diet provides. So focus on quality over quantity, and expect to taper down to a pound a week or less in the 8th month and just a pound or so total during the 9th. (This makes more sense when you remember that most multiple pregnancies don't make it to 40 weeks.)

Exercise

"I'm a runner, but now that I'm pregnant with twins, is it safe to keep up my workouts?"

Exercise can benefit most pregnancies, but when you're staying fit for

Multiple Timeline

Already counting down your 40 weeks? You might not have to count that many after all. A twin pregnancy is considered full term a full 2 weeks earlier, at 38 weeks—certainly reason to celebrate (2 weeks less of puffiness, heartburn . . . and waiting!). But just as most singletons fail to arrive on their due date, multiples keep their moms and dads (and practitioners) guessing, too. They might just stay put until 38 weeks (or longer)—or they might make their appearance before they've clocked in even a full 37 weeks. In fact, most do.

If your babies do end up overstaying their 38-week term, your practitioner will likely elect to induce, taking into account how they're doing and how you're doing. ACOG's recommendation that low-risk twin pregnancies be delivered by the end of the 38th week may also be factored in (and that's one significant reason why few twin pregnancies are allowed to go longer than a full 38 weeks). Be sure to have an endgame discussion with your practitioner long before the end is near, because many differ on how they typically handle the late stages of a multiple pregnancy.

three, you'll have to exercise care, too. First, check in with your practitioner. Even if exercise is green-lighted during the first and second trimesters, your practitioner will likely steer you toward more gentle options and away from any workout that puts downward pressure on your cervix (like running) or that raises your body temperature significantly (running can do that, too). Most

Extra, Extra!

Not surprisingly, extra babies come with extra precautions—and that's a good thing. With extra precautions come extra-excellent chances that your multiple babies will thrive and arrive safe, sound, and healthy.

Here are some of the extras you can expect when you're expecting twins or more:

- Extra practitioner visits. Good prenatal care is the ticket to a healthy pregnancy and a healthy baby—at least doubly so when you're expecting multiples. So expect more frequent prenatal checkups—you'll likely be seen every 2 to 3 weeks (rather than every 4) up until your 7th month and even more often after that. And those visits may get more in-depth as your pregnancy progresses. You'll get all the tests singleton moms get, but you may also get transvaginal ultrasounds to keep an eye on cervical length (to check for signs of preterm labor) as well as more nonstress tests and biophysical profiles in your third trimester (see page 380). You'll also likely be screened for gestational diabetes earlier and more often than a singleton mom would be.

- Extra pictures. Of your babies, that is. You'll get extra ultrasounds to monitor your babies and make sure their development and growth is on track. Which means extra reassurance, plus extra peeks at that precious pair (or trio)—and extra pictures for your baby book (or books!).

- Extra close attention. Your practitioner will keep an extra close eye on your health to reduce your risk of certain pregnancy complications more common in multiple pregnancies (see page 451). With all that extra attention, any problem that develops will likely be caught and treated quickly.

experts recommend that moms-to-be of multiples stay away from high-impact aerobic exercise (again, like running) after 20 weeks if any cervical shortening has been detected on ultrasound (because it increases the risk of preterm labor for them), and to stop running by 28 weeks even if there is no cervical shortening. Unfortunately, these guidelines hold true for experienced runners like you, as well.

Looking for a more appropriate fitness routine for the three of you? Good choices include swimming or pregnancy water aerobics, stretching, prenatal yoga, light weight training, and riding a stationary bicycle, all exercises that don't require you to be on your feet while you do them (though do ask your practitioner if walking is safe in your case—it is most of the time). And don't forget your Kegels (page 229), the anywhere-anytime exercises designed to strengthen your pelvic floor (which needs extra reinforcement when there are extra babies inside).

No matter what you're doing during your workout, if the exertion is causing Braxton-Hicks contractions or raising any other red flags listed on page 140, stop immediately, rest, drink some water, and call your practitioner if they don't subside within 20 minutes or so.

Mixed Feelings

"Everybody thinks it's so exciting that we're going to have twins, except us. We're scared and even disappointed. What's wrong with us?"

Multiple Connections

As a multiples mother-to-be, you're about to join a special club already filled with thousands of women just like you—women who are also expecting double the delight and, chances are, double the self doubt. Never been a joiner? Membership in this particular club does come with plenty of rewards. By talking to other moms-to-be of multiples, you'll be able to share your joy, your fears, your symptoms, your funny stories (the ones nobody else would get) with those who know just how you're feeling. You'll also be able to score reassuring advice from other expectant moms who have multiples on the way (as well as from those who've already had their multistork delivery). Join a discussion group online (check out WhatToExpect.com for a multiples message board) or ask your practitioner to hook you up with other pregnant-with-multiples moms in his or her practice and start your own group. There are also national organizations that can provide you with contact information for local clubs, including the National Organization of Mothers of Twins Clubs, nomotc.org, or you can use an online search engine to find a local multiples chapter. You can also check out online sites that cater specifically to parents of multiples, including mothersof multiples.com and twinstuff.com.

Absolutely nothing. Prenatal daydreams don't usually include two babies. You prepare yourself psychologically, as well as physically and financially, for the arrival of one baby—and when you suddenly discover you're having two instead, feelings of disappointment aren't unusual. Neither is trepidation. The impending responsibilities of caring for a single infant are plenty daunting without having them doubled.

Some expectant parents are happy to hear they're expecting multiples right from the start, but many others take some time getting used to the news. It's just as common to feel initial shock as initial joy—to feel you're being deprived of experiencing the cozy bond you'd always imagined with a single baby, but can't immediately see yourselves having with a pair. Guilt about questioning your double blessing (especially if becoming pregnant was a struggle to begin with) can compound your conflicted feelings. All of these feelings (and the others you might be experiencing) are a completely normal reaction to the news that your pregnancy and your lives are taking an unexpected turn.

So accept the fact that you're ambivalent about the dual arrivals, and don't saddle yourselves with guilt (since your feelings are normal and understandable, there's absolutely nothing to feel guilty about). Instead, use the months before delivery to get used to the idea that you'll be having twins (you will!). Talk openly and honestly to each other (the more you let your feelings out, the faster you'll work through them). Talk to anyone you know who has twins, and if you don't know any moms and dads of multiples, look to message boards. Sharing your feelings with others who've felt them, and recognizing that you're not the first expectant parents to experience them, will help you accept and, in time, become excited about this pregnancy and the two beautiful babies you'll be holding one day soon. Twins, you'll find, may be double the effort at first, but they're also double the fun down the road.

Insensitive Comments

"When I told my friend that we're having twins, she said to me, 'Better you than me.' Why would she make such a nasty comment?"

That might be the first insensitive comment you've been ambushed by during your multiples pregnancy, but it probably won't be the last. From coworkers to family members to friends to those perfect (make that not-so-perfect) strangers in the supermarket, you'll be amazed at the remarkably rude things people feel completely comfortable saying to an expectant mom of multiples.

What's up with the lack of tact? The truth is, many people don't know how to react to the news that you're carrying multiples. Sure, a simple "Congratulations!" might be in order, but most people assume that twins are special (they are) and therefore need to be recognized with a "special" comment. Curious about what it must be like to be pregnant with twins, in awe of what you'll be going through once they're born, they're clueless about the right response—so they dish out the wrong one. Their intentions are good, but their follow-through stinks.

The best way to react? Don't take it personally, and don't take it too seriously. Realize that even as your friend opened her mouth and inserted her foot, she was almost certainly trying to wish you well (and she probably has no idea that she offended you, so try not to take offense). Remember, too, that you can be the best spokeswoman for moms of twins everywhere—and you'll have lots of chances to spread the wonderful word on multiples.

"People keep asking me if twins run in my family or if I had fertility treatments. I'm not ashamed that I had IVF, but it's also not something I want to share with everyone."

A pregnant woman brings out the nosy like no one else, but a woman expecting multiples becomes everybody's business. Suddenly, your pregnancy goes public—with people you hardly know (or don't know at all) prying into your personal life (and bedroom habits) and prodding you for personal information without thinking twice. But that's just the point: These people aren't really thinking twice—or even once. They're not asking to be intrusive, they're just curious (multiples are fascinating stuff, after all), and they haven't been educated in twin etiquette. If you're open to sharing the details, then by all means, go for it ("Well, first we tried Clomid, and when that didn't work, we tried IVF, which means that my husband and I went to a fertility clinic . . ."). By the time you're halfway done with your story, the questioner will probably be bored to tears and looking for the nearest exit. Or, you can try one of these responses the next time someone asks about the conception of your twins:

- "They were a big surprise." This can be true whether you've conceived with or without fertility help.
- "Twins run in the family—now." This will shut them up while keeping them guessing.
- "We had sex twice in one night." Who hasn't at some point? Even if the last time was on your honeymoon, it's not a lie—and it'll be the end of the line for their line of questioning.
- "They were conceived with love." Well, that's a given, no matter what—and where do they go from there?

- "Why do you ask?" If they're TTC (trying to conceive) themselves, then maybe it'll open up a conversation that could help them (infertility can be a lonely road, as you probably know). If not, it could stop them in their nosy tracks.

Not in the mood for a witty retort—or to even respond at all (especially after you've been asked the same question 5 times in a single day)? There's nothing wrong with letting the questioner know that the answer is none of her business, which it isn't. "That's a personal matter" says it all.

Safety in Numbers

"We'd barely adjusted to the fact that I was pregnant when we found out I'm carrying twins. Are there any extra risks for them, or for me?"

Extra babies do come with some extra risks, but not as many as you'd think. In fact, not all twin pregnancies are classified as "high risk" (though higher-order multiples definitely fall into that category), and most expectant mothers of multiples can expect to have relatively uneventful pregnancies, at least in terms of complications. Plus, entering your twin pregnancy armed with a little knowledge about the potential risks and complications can help you avoid many, and will prepare you should you encounter any. So relax (twin pregnancies are really safe), but read up.

For the babies, the potential risks include:

Early delivery. Multiples tend to arrive earlier than singletons. More than half of twins, the majority of triplets, and practically all quadruplets are born premature. While women pregnant with a single baby deliver, on average, at

39 weeks, twin delivery, on average, occurs at 35 to 36 weeks. Triplets usually come (again, on average) at 32 weeks, and quadruplets at 30 weeks. (Keep in mind that term for twins is considered 38 weeks, not 40.) After all, as cozy as it can be for your little ones in the uterus, it can also get pretty crowded as they grow. Be sure you know the signs of preterm labor, and don't hesitate to call your practitioner right away if you're experiencing any of them (see page 559).

Low birthweight. Since many multiple pregnancies end early, the average (repeat: average) baby born of a multiple pregnancy arrives weighing 5½ pounds, which is considered low birthweight. Most 5-pounders end up doing just fine health-wise, thanks to advances in caring for these small newborns, but babies born weighing less than 3 pounds are at increased risk for health complications as newborns, as well as for long-term disabilities. Making sure your prenatal health is in top-notch condition and your diet contains plenty of nutrients (including the right amount of calories) can help get your babies to a bigger bottom line. See *What to Expect the First Year* for more on low-birthweight babies.

Twin-to-Twin Transfusion Syndrome (TTTS). This in-utero condition, which happens in about 9 to 15 percent of identical twin pregnancies in which the placenta is shared, arises when one or more placental arteries from one twin deposits blood in the placenta that returns to the other twin through a placental vein. If there aren't other common vessels present to equalize the delivery of blood to both fetuses, the result can be one baby getting too much blood and the other too little. (Fraternal twins are almost never

Pregnancy Reduction

Sometimes an ultrasound reveals that one (or more) of the fetuses in a multiple pregnancy can't survive or is so severely malformed that the chances of survival outside the womb are minimal—and worse yet, that the unhealthy fetus may be endangering your other healthy one(s). Or there are so many fetuses that there is a significant risk to the mother and all her babies. In such cases, your practitioner may recommend a pregnancy reduction. Contemplating this procedure can be agonizing—it may seem like sacrificing one baby to protect another—and may leave you plagued with guilt, confusion, and conflicted feelings. You may come to your decision of whether to proceed (or not proceed) easily, or it may be an excruciating decision-making process.

There may be no easy answers, and there are definitely no perfect options, but you'll want to do whatever you can to make peace with the decision you end up making. Review the situation with your practitioner, and seek a second opinion, or third, or fourth, until you're as confident as you can be about your choice. You can also ask your practitioner to put you in touch with someone from the bioethics staff of the hospital (if that's available). You may want to share your feelings with close friends, or you may want to keep this personal decision private. If religion plays an important role in your life, you'll probably want to look to spiritual guidance. Once you make your decision, try not to second-guess: Accept that it's the best decision you can make under the difficult circumstances. Also try not to burden yourself with guilt, no matter what you choose. Because none of this is your fault, there's no reason to feel guilty about it.

If you end up undergoing pregnancy reduction, you may expect to experience the same grief as any parent who has lost one or more babies. See page 596 for help coping.

affected because they never share a placenta.) This condition is dangerous for the babies, though not to the mom. If it's detected in your pregnancy, your practitioner will likely refer you to a perinatologist who may suggest laser therapy of the placenta (using a special device placed in the uterus) to stop the transfusion. Alternatively, although less effective, the physician may opt to use amniocentesis to drain off excess amniotic fluid every week or two, which improves blood flow in the placenta and reduces the risk of preterm labor. If you're dealing with TTTS, check out fetalhope.org for more information and resources.

Other complications. There are other fetal complications that are more likely to occur in a multiple pregnancy, but that are still uncommon. Ask your practitioner about other additional risks for your babies and how you can best modify them.

A multiple pregnancy can also impact the health of the mother-to-be:

Preeclampsia. The more babies you're carrying, the more placenta you've got on board. This added placenta (along with the added hormones that come with two babies) can lead to high blood pressure, and sometimes to preeclampsia. Preeclampsia affects 1 in 4 mothers of twins and usually is caught early, thanks to careful monitoring. For more on the condition and treatment options, see page 550.

Gestational diabetes. Expectant multiples moms are slightly more likely to have GD than singleton moms. That's probably because higher hormone levels can interfere with a mom's ability to process insulin. Diet can usually control (or even prevent) GD, but sometimes extra insulin is needed (see page 548).

Placental problems. Women pregnant with multiples are at a somewhat higher risk for complications such as placenta previa (low-lying placenta, page 554) or placental abruption (premature separation of the placenta, page 556). Fortunately, careful monitoring (which you'll be getting) can detect placenta previa long before it poses any significant risk. Placental abruption can't be detected before it happens, but because your pregnancy is being carefully watched, steps can be taken to avoid further complications if an abruption occurs.

Bed Rest

"Will I have to be on bed rest just because I'm carrying twins?"

To bed rest or not to bed rest? That is the question many moms-to-be of multiples ask, and practitioners don't always have an easy answer. That's because there really isn't an easy answer. The obstetrical jury is still out on whether bed rest helps prevent the kinds of complications sometimes associated with a multiple pregnancy (such as preterm labor and preeclampsia). And even though most research shows there's no benefit, many practitioners continue to prescribe some version of bed rest, especially under certain circumstances (for instance, if mom's cervix has shortened or she has high blood pressure, or if one or both of the babies isn't growing well). Since the risk of complications increases with each additional baby, bed rest is even more likely to be prescribed in higher-order multiple pregnancies.

Be sure to have a discussion with your practitioner early in your pregnancy about his or her philosophy on bed rest. Some practitioners prescribe it routinely for all expectant moms of multiples (often beginning between 24 and 28 weeks), while most do it on a case-by-case basis, taking a wait-and-see approach.

If you are put on bed rest, see page 573 for tips on coping with it. And keep in mind that even if you aren't sent to bed, your practitioner will probably still advise you to take it easy, cut back on (or stop) work, and stay off your feet as much as possible during the latter half of your pregnancy—so get ready to rest up anyway.

Vanishing Twin Syndrome

"I've heard of vanishing twin syndrome. What is it?"

Detecting multiple pregnancies early using ultrasound technology has many benefits, because the sooner you and your practitioner discover you've got two (or more) babies to care for, the better care you'll be able to get. But there's sometimes a downside to knowing so soon. Identifying twin pregnancies earlier than ever also reveals losses that went undetected before the days of early ultrasound.

The loss of a twin during pregnancy can occur in the first trimester (often before a mom even knows she's carrying twins) or, less commonly, later in the pregnancy. During a first-trimester loss, the tissue of the miscarried twin is usually reabsorbed by the mother's body. This phenomenon, called vanishing twin syndrome, occurs in about 20 to 30 percent of multiple pregnancies. Documentation of vanishing twin syndrome has grown significantly over the past few decades, as early ultrasounds—the only way to be sure early in pregnancy that you're carrying twins—have become routine (and are used even earlier and more often in an IVF pregnancy). Researchers report more cases of vanishing twin syndrome in women older than 30, though that may be because older mothers in general have higher rates of multiple pregnancies, especially with the use of fertility treatments.

There are rarely any symptoms when the early loss of a twin occurs, though some women experience mild cramping, bleeding, or pelvic pain, similar to a miscarriage (though none of those symptoms is a sure sign of such a loss). Decreasing—not disappearing— hormone levels (as detected by blood tests) may also indicate that one fetus has been lost.

The good news is that when vanishing twin syndrome occurs in the first trimester, a mom usually goes on to experience a normal pregnancy and delivers the single healthy baby without complication or intervention. In the much less likely case that a twin dies in the second or third trimester, the remaining baby may be at an increased risk of intrauterine growth restriction, and the mother may be at risk of pre-term labor, infection, or bleeding. The remaining baby would then be watched carefully and the rest of the pregnancy monitored for complications.

For help coping with the loss of a twin in utero, see page 599.

ALL ABOUT:
Multiple Childbirth

Every delivery day is an unforgettable one, but if you're carrying twins (or more), yours probably won't be the typical birth story you've heard from moms who've delivered just one. Not surprisingly, things can get a little more complicated when you've got two babies or more heading for the exit— and a lot more interesting.

Will your labor and delivery be twice the effort? What will be the ideal way to deliver your multiple newborns into your arms? The answers can depend on a lot of factors, such as fetal position, your health, the safety of the babies, and so on. Multiple births have more variables—and more surprises—than single births. But since you'll be getting two (or more) for the price of one labor, your multiple childbirth will be a pretty good deal no matter how it ends up playing out. And remember that whatever route your babies take from your snug womb to your even snugger embrace, the best way is the one that is the healthiest and safest for them—and for you.

Laboring With Twins or More

How will your labor differ from the labor of a mother of one? Here are a few ways:

It could be shorter. Will you have to endure double the pain to end up cuddling double the pleasure? Nope. In fact, when it comes to labor, you're likely to catch a really nice break. The labor is often shorter with multiples—which means that if you'll be delivering vaginally, it may take less time to get to the point where you can start pushing. The catch? You'll be hitting the harder part of labor sooner.

Or it could be longer. Because a multiples mom's uterus is overstretched, contractions are sometimes weaker. And weaker contractions could mean that it might take longer to become fully dilated.

It'll be watched more closely. Because your medical team will have to be twice as careful during your multiple delivery, you'll be monitored more during labor than most moms of singletons. Throughout labor (if you're delivering in a hospital—the most common scenario), you'll likely be attached to two (or more) fetal monitors so your practitioner can see how each baby is responding to your contractions. Early on, the babies' heartbeats may be monitored with external belt monitors—this could allow you to go off the monitors periodically so you can walk around or hit the whirlpool tub (if you're so inclined). In the latter stages of labor, Baby A (the one closest to the exit) may be monitored internally with a scalp electrode while Baby B is still monitored externally. This will put an end to your mobility, because you'll be tethered to a machine. If you're delivering at home with a midwife, your babies will be monitored with a Doppler more frequently.

You'll probably have an epidural (again, assuming you're delivering in a hospital). If you've had your heart set on one anyway, you'll be happy to hear that epidurals are strongly encouraged—or even required—with multiple deliveries, in case an emergency c-section becomes necessary to deliver one or all of your babies. If you'd like to avoid an epidural, talk to your practitioner ahead of time.

You'll probably deliver in an operating room. Chances are, you'll be able to labor in a comfy birthing room, but when it's time to push, you'll be wheeled into the OR. Most hospitals require this, just to be on the safe side (and in case an emergency c-section becomes necessary), so ask ahead.

Delivering Twins

Here's what you can expect when delivering your twins:

Vaginal delivery. About half of all twins born these days come into the world vaginally, but that doesn't mean the birthing experience is the same as it is for singleton moms. Once you're fully dilated, delivery of Baby A may be a cinch (3 pushes) or a protracted ordeal (3 hours). Though that latter scenario is far from a given, some research has shown that the duration of pushing is usually longer in a twin delivery than in a singleton delivery. The second twin in a vaginal delivery usually comes within 10 to 30 minutes of the first, and most multiples moms report that delivering Baby B is a snap compared with Baby A. Depending on the position of Baby B, he or she may need some help from the practitioner, who can try external or internal version (see box, page 456) to move baby into the birth canal or use vacuum extraction to speed the delivery.

Mixed delivery. In rare (very rare) cases, Baby B must be delivered by c-section after Baby A has been delivered vaginally.

Position, Position, Position

Quick . . . flip a coin. Heads (up) or tails (down)? Or maybe one (or more) of each? How multiples will end up at delivery time (and how you'll end up delivering) is anybody's guess. Here's a look at the possible ways your twins may be presenting and the likely delivery scenarios for each situation.

Vertex/vertex. This is the most cooperative position that twins can wind up in on delivery day, and they wind up in it about 40 percent of the time. If both your babies are vertex (heads down), you'll likely be able to go into labor naturally and attempt a vaginal birth. Keep in mind, however, that even perfectly positioned singletons sometimes need to be delivered by c-section. This goes double for twins. If you're hoping to have a midwife attend your delivery (or even if you'd like to deliver at home), the vertex/vertex position is the best-case scenario.

Vertex/breech. The second-best-case scenario if you're hoping for a vaginal birth for your twins is the vertex/breech setup. This means that if Baby A is head-down and well positioned for delivery, it may be possible for your practitioner to manipulate Baby B from the breech position to vertex after Baby A is born. This can be done either by applying manual pressure to your abdomen (external version) or literally reaching inside your uterus to turn Baby B (internal version). The internal version sounds much more complicated than it is—because Baby A has essentially warmed up and stretched out the birth canal already, the procedure is over with pretty quickly. (Still, an arm reaching into your uterus to pull out a baby isn't pretty without pain meds—another reason why many

doctors strongly recommend epidurals for multiples moms.) If Baby B remains stubbornly breech, your practitioner may do a breech extraction, in which your baby is pulled feet first right out the exit.

Breech/vertex or breech/breech. If Baby A is breech or if both your babies are bottoms-down, your practitioner will almost certainly recommend a c-section. Though external version is commonplace for breech singletons (and can work in the above mentioned vertex/breech multiple pregnancy), it's considered too risky in this scenario.

Baby A oblique. Who knew there were so many positions for babies to lie in? When Baby A is oblique, it means his or her head is pointed down, but toward either of your hips rather than squarely at your cervix. In a singleton pregnancy with oblique presentation, a practitioner would probably try external version to bring the baby's head where it needs to be (facing the exit), but that's risky with twins. In this case, two things can happen: An oblique presentation can correct itself as contractions progress, resulting in a vaginal birth, or more likely, your practitioner will recommend a c-section to avoid a long, drawn-out labor that may or may not lead to a vaginal birth.

Transverse/transverse. In this setup, both babies are lying horizontally across your uterus. A double transverse almost always results in a c-section.

Got triplets (or more) in there? Your babies can assume any number of these positions (and maybe even keep you guessing until right up to delivery).

See facing page for more on triplet delivery.

This is usually done only when an emergency situation has come up that puts Baby B at risk, such as placental abruption or cord prolapse. (Those all-important fetal monitors tell your doctor just how well Baby B is doing after Baby A's arrival.) A mixed delivery is definitely not fun for mom. In the moment, of course, it can be very scary, and after the babies are born, it means recovery from both a vaginal birth and a surgical one—a big double ouch. But when it's necessary, it can be a baby-saving procedure, well worth the added recovery time.

Planned cesarean delivery. Possible reasons for this plan include a previous c-section (a VBAC, or vaginal birth after cesarean, is not common practice for multiples), placenta previa or other complications, or fetal positions that make vaginal delivery unsafe. With most planned c-sections, your spouse, partner, or coach can accompany you into the OR, where you will probably be given an epidural or a spinal block. You may be surprised by how fast it all goes after you're numb: Baby A's and Baby B's birth times will be separated by anywhere from seconds to just a minute or two. Hoping to hold and breastfeed your babies as soon as possible after delivery? So-called gentle cesarean deliveries are also an option for twins, assuming all is going well. See page 438 for more.

Unplanned cesarean delivery. An unplanned c-section is the other possible way your babies might enter the world. In this case, you may walk into your usual weekly prenatal appointment and find out that you're going to meet your babies the same day. Best to be prepared, so in those later weeks of pregnancy, be sure to get your bag packed and ready to go. Reasons for a surprise cesarean delivery include conditions such as intrauterine growth restriction (where the babies run out of room to grow) or a sharp rise in your blood pressure (preeclampsia). An unplanned c-section scenario may also arise during labor if there are any signs of distress in the babies or if you labor for a very long time and don't progress at all. A uterus holding 10 or more pounds of babies may be too stretched to contract effectively, so a cesarean delivery might be the only way out.

Delivering Triplets (or More)

Wondering if your higher-order multiples are destined to take the abdominal route out? A cesarean delivery is most often scheduled for triplets and quads—not only because it's usually safest, but because c-sections are more common in high-risk deliveries (a category higher-order multiples always fall into) and because they're more common among older moms (who give birth to the majority of triplets or quads). But some doctors say that vaginal delivery can be an option if Baby A (the one nearest the "exit") is in a head-down presentation and there are no other complicating factors (such as preeclampsia in the mom or fetal distress in one or more of the babies). In some rare cases, the first baby or the first and second may be delivered vaginally, and the final baby (or babies) may require a cesarean delivery. Of course, more important than having all of your babies exit vaginally is having all of you leaving the delivery room in good condition—and any route to that outcome will be a successful one.

Multiple Recovery

Besides having your hands (and if you're nursing, your breasts) twice as busy, your recovery from a multiple delivery will be very similar to that of a singleton delivery (you can read all about it in Chapters 16 and 17). You can also expect these postpartum differences:

- **You'll be going with more flow.** Your lochia (after-delivery bleeding) may be heavier and last longer. That's because more blood was stored up in your uterus during your pregnancy and it all has to go now. See page 461 for more.

- **Afterpains may be more of a pain.** Your uterus was extra-stretched by your multiple load, so it'll take more contracting to get it back to size—and those contractions may be extra painful. See page 462 for more.

- **Your back won't catch a break.** All the extra weight you carried around weakened your abs, which means they won't be as supportive of your poor, aching back, at least not until they tighten back up. Extra-loosened ligaments pose the same painful problem. In the meantime a belly band can pick up some of the slack. See page 494 for more.

- **Your tummy will take extra time.** A belly that took one (actually, two or more) for the team—generously providing room and board for multiple babies—will take longer to return to its normal size, and that's to be expected. In its way: your still extra-enlarged uterus, the extra fluids that will need to be flushed out, the extra fat reserves your body produced for your babies, and the extra-loose skin you're in. Give it (and yourself) time. See page 504 for more.

- **Your recovery will be slower.** In general, having just run a double (or triple) baby marathon will leave you lagging for longer. Especially if you were on bed rest or otherwise restricted in activity, you'll need to slowly build up your strength and stamina.

PART 3

After the Baby Is Born

CHAPTER 16

Postpartum: The First Week

·············

Congratulations! The moment you've been awaiting for 40 (or so) weeks has finally arrived. You've put long months of pregnancy and long hours of childbirth behind you, and you're officially a mother, with a new bundle of joy in your arms instead of in your belly. But the transition from pregnancy to postpartum comes with more than just a baby—none of it is nearly as cute. It also comes with a variety of new symptoms (goodbye pregnancy aches and pains, hello postpartum ones) and a variety of new questions: Why am I sweating so much? Why am I having contractions if I've already delivered? Will I ever be able to sit again? Why do I still look 6 months pregnant? Whose breasts are these anyway? Hopefully, you'll have a chance to read up on these and many more pertinent postpartum topics in advance. Once you're on full-time mom duty, finding the time to read anything (never mind finding the time to use the toilet or take a shower) won't be easy.

What You May Be Feeling

During the first week postpartum, depending on the type of delivery you had (easy or difficult, vaginal or cesarean) you may experience all, or only some, of the following:

Physically

- Vaginal bleeding (lochia) similar to but possibly heavier than your period

- Abdominal cramps (afterpains) as your uterus contracts, especially when nursing

- Exhaustion
- Perineal discomfort, pain, numbness, if you had a vaginal delivery (especially if you had stitches)
- Some perineal discomfort if you had a c-section (especially if you labored first)
- Pain around the incision and, later, numbness in the area, if you had a c-section (especially a first one)
- Discomfort sitting and walking if you had a repair of a tear, an episiotomy, or a cesarean delivery
- Difficulty urinating for a day or two
- Constipation, and a lot of discomfort with bowel movements
- Hemorrhoids, continued from pregnancy and/or new from pushing
- All-over achiness, especially if you did a lot of pushing
- Bloodshot eyes, and/or black-and-blue marks around eyes, on cheeks, elsewhere, from pushing
- Sweating, particularly at night

- Hot flashes
- Swelling in your feet, ankles, legs, and hands, continued from pregnancy, plus possibly extra from any IV fluids
- Breast discomfort and engorgement beginning around the 3rd or 4th day postpartum
- Sore or cracked nipples, if you're breastfeeding
- Stretch marks (possibly including ones you never noticed before)

Emotionally

- Elation, blues, or swings between the two
- New mom jitters—trepidation about caring for your new baby, especially if you're a first-timer
- Excitement about starting your new life with your new baby
- A feeling of being overwhelmed by the challenges now and ahead
- Frustration, if you're having a hard time getting started breastfeeding

What You May Be Wondering About

Bleeding

"I expected some bleeding after delivery, but when I got out of bed for the first time and saw the blood running down my legs, I was a little freaked out."

Grab a pile of pads, and relax. This discharge of leftover blood, mucus, and tissue from your uterus, known as lochia, is normally as heavy as (and often heavier than) a menstrual period for the first 3 to 10 postpartum days. It may total up to 2 cups before it begins to taper off (not that you'll be measuring it), and at times it may seem pretty profuse. A sudden gush when you stand up in the first few days is normal—it's just the flow that accumulates when you've been lying down or sitting. Because blood and an occasional blood clot are the predominant ingredients of lochia during the immediate postpartum

Puff Mama, Part 2

No longer pregnant, but still plenty puffy (or maybe even more puffy)? Extra fluids accumulate during pregnancy, of course, but IV fluids during labor and delivery pump in even more. So if you had an IV, you can expect to experience additional swelling in your legs and ankles (and maybe your hands and face, too) afterward. It will take time to drain those accumulated fluids, but you can help speed up the process by circling your ankles (make 10 circles clockwise, then 10 counterclockwise), getting up and moving around as soon as you're able, and drinking lots of water to flush your system.

period, your discharge can be quite red for anywhere from 5 days to 3 weeks, gradually turning to a watery pink, then to brown, and finally to a yellowish white. Maxipads, not tampons, should be used to absorb the flow, which may continue on and off for just a couple of weeks or for as long as 6 weeks. In some moms, light bleeding continues for as long as 3 months. The flow is different for everyone.

Breastfeeding—and/or Pitocin, which is routinely ordered by some practitioners (either via IV or a shot) after delivery—may reduce the flow of lochia by encouraging uterine contractions. These postdelivery contractions (aka afterpains, see next question for more) help shrink the uterus back to its normal size more quickly while pinching off exposed blood vessels at the site where the placenta separated from the uterus.

If you're in the hospital or birthing center and you think your bleeding may

be excessive, let a nurse know. Once you're home, if you experience what seems to be abnormally heavy bleeding (see page 571), call your practitioner without delay. If you can't reach him or her, go to the ER (in the hospital where you delivered, if possible). Call your practitioner, too, if you notice no bleeding at all once you get home.

Afterpains

"I've been having crampy pains in my abdomen, especially when I'm nursing. What's that about?"

Thought you'd felt the last of those contractions? Unfortunately, they don't end immediately with delivery—and neither does the discomfort (okay, pain) they can cause. Those so-called afterpains are triggered by the contractions of the uterus as it shrinks (from about 2⅓ pounds to just a couple of ounces) and makes its normal descent back into the pelvis following delivery. You can keep track of the shrinking size of your uterus by pressing lightly below your navel. By the end of 6 weeks, you probably won't feel it at all.

Afterpains can definitely be a pain, but they do important work. Besides helping the uterus find its way back to its usual size and location, those contractions help slow normal postpartum bleeding. They're likely to be more of a pain in women whose uterine muscles are lacking in tone because of previous births or excessive stretching (as with a multiple pregnancy). Afterpains can be much more intense during nursing, when contraction-stimulating oxytocin is released (a good thing, actually, since it means your uterus is shrinking faster) and/or if you had Pitocin following delivery.

The pains should subside naturally within 4 to 7 days. In the meantime, the good news is now that you've delivered, you can turn once again to ibuprofen (Advil or Motrin) for its more potent pain relief, though acetaminophen (Tylenol) should do the trick, too. If pain relievers don't work, or if the pains persist for more than a week, see your practitioner to rule out other postpartum problems, including infection.

Perineal Pain

"I didn't have an episiotomy, and I didn't tear. Why am I so sore down there?"

You can't expect 7 or 8 pounds of baby to pass unnoticed. Even if your perineum was left neatly intact during delivery, that area has still been stretched, bruised, and generally traumatized, and discomfort, ranging from mild to not so mild, is the very normal result. The pain may be worse when you cough or sneeze, and you may even find that it hurts to sit down. You can try the same tips given in the next answer for post-tear pain.

It's also possible that in pushing your baby out, you developed hemorrhoids and, possibly, anal fissures, which can range from uncomfortable to extremely painful (see page 293). Or perhaps a vulvar or vaginal varicose vein that cropped up during pregnancy was further irritated during pushing and delivery, causing even more pain now. Fortunately, these types of varicose veins usually disappear a few weeks after delivery (and in the unlikely event that they don't disappear after a few months, your doctor can easily treat and remove them).

"I tore, and now I'm incredibly sore. Could my stitches be infected?"

Everyone who delivers vaginally (and sometimes those who have a lengthy labor before delivering via cesarean) can expect some perineal pain. But, not

---

Welcome Back, Ibuprofen

Have you been missing your old buddy, ibuprofen (Advil, Motrin) during pregnancy? Once you've delivered (and unless your practitioner has advised otherwise), it's safe to pull ibuprofen out of the medicine cabinet again and enjoy its more potent pain relief for all your postpartum discomforts. It's also breastfeeding friendly.

---

surprisingly, that pain's likely to be compounded if the perineum was torn or surgically cut (aka an episiotomy). Like any freshly repaired wound, the site of a tear or episiotomy will take time to heal, usually 7 to 10 days. Pain alone during this time, unless it is very severe, is not a sign that you've developed an infection.

What's more, infection (though possible) is really very unlikely if you've been taking good care of the area. While you're in the hospital or birthing center, a nurse will check your perineum at least once daily for any signs of infection, like inflammation. The nurse will also instruct you in postpartum perineal hygiene, which is important in preventing infection not only of the repair site but of the genital tract as well (germs can get around). For this reason, the same precautions apply for moms who delivered completely intact. Here's the self-care plan for a healthy postpartum perineum:

- Use a fresh maxipad as needed, but at least every 4 to 6 hours.

- Pour or squirt warm water (or an antiseptic solution, if one was recommended by your practitioner or nurse) over your perineum while you pee to ease burning, and after you're finished peeing to keep the area clean. Pat dry (make sure your hands are clean) with gauze pads or with the paper wipes that come with some hospital-provided pads, always from front to back. Gently does it—no rubbing.

- Keep your hands off the area until healing is complete.

Though discomfort is likely to be greater if you've had a repair (with itchiness around the stitches possibly accompanying soreness), the tips below will be soothing no matter how you delivered. To relieve perineal pain:

Ice it. To reduce swelling and bring soothing relief, use chilled witch hazel pads, an ice pack or disposable glove filled with crushed ice, a maxipad with a built-in cold pack, or compression shorts with a built-in ice pack, applied to the site every couple of hours during the first 24 hours following delivery.

Heat it. Warm compresses or warm sitz baths (a bath in which only your hips and bottom are submerged) for 20 minutes a few times a day will ease discomfort. Ask if you can add Epsom salts, witch hazel, lavender oil, or chamomile oil for extra relief.

Numb it. Use local anesthetics in the form of sprays, creams, ointments, or pads recommended by your practitioner. Taking ibuprofen (Advil, Motrin) or acetaminophen (Tylenol) may also help.

Keep off it. To keep the pressure off your sore perineum, lie on your side when possible, and avoid long periods of standing or sitting. Sitting on a pillow (especially one with an opening in the center, like a Boppy) or an inflated or memory foam donut cushion can help. You can also try tightening your buttocks before sitting down.

Keep it loose. Tight clothing can rub and irritate the area, plus slow the healing. Let your perineum breathe as much as possible (for now, favor baggy sweats over spandex leggings).

Exercise it. Kegel exercises, done as frequently as possible after delivery and right through the postpartum period, will stimulate circulation to the area, promoting healing and improving muscle tone. Don't worry if you can't feel yourself doing the Kegels, since the area initially will be numb. Feeling will return to the perineum gradually over the next few weeks—and in the meantime, the work's being done even if you can't feel it.

If your perineum becomes very red, very painful, and swollen, or if you detect an unpleasant odor, you may have developed an infection. Call your practitioner.

Delivery Bruises

"I look more like I've been in a boxing ring than in a birthing room. How come?"

Look and feel like you've taken a beating? That's normal postpartum. After all, you probably worked harder birthing your child than most boxers work in the ring, even though you were facing only a 7- or 8-pounder. Thanks to powerful contractions and strenuous pushing (especially if you were pushing with your face and chest instead of your lower body), you might be sporting a variety of unwelcome delivery souvenirs. These may include black or bloodshot eyes (cold compresses for 10 minutes several times a day may help speed healing) and bruises, ranging from tiny dots on the cheeks to larger black-and-blue marks on the face or upper chest area. You may also be bringing home soreness in your chest

When to Call Your Practitioner

Few moms feel their physical (or emotional) best after delivering a baby—that's just par for postpartum. Especially in the first 6 weeks after delivery, experiencing a variety of aches, pains, and other uncomfortable (or unpleasant) symptoms is common. Fortunately, what isn't common is having a serious complication. Still, it's smart to be in the know. That's why all brand new moms should be aware of symptoms that might point to a postpartum problem, just in case. Call your practitioner without delay if you experience any of the following:

- Bleeding that saturates more than 1 pad an hour for more than a few hours. If you can't reach your practitioner immediately, call the ER or the labor and delivery unit at the hospital you delivered at. Have the triage nurse assess you over the phone and advise you on whether or not you should come into the ER.

- Large amounts of bright red bleeding that occur 1 to 2 weeks after delivery (called delayed or secondary postpartum hemorrhage). But don't worry about light menstrual-like bleeding for up to 6 weeks (in some women as long as 3 months) or a flow that increases when you're active or during breastfeeding.

- Bleeding that has a foul odor. It should smell like your period.

- Numerous or large (lemon-size or larger) clots in the vaginal bleeding. Occasional small clots in the first few days, however, are normal.

- A complete absence of bleeding during the first few postpartum days

- Pain or discomfort, with or without swelling, in the lower abdominal area beyond the first few days after delivery

- Persistent pain in the perineal area beyond the first few days, especially if it doesn't respond to pain relievers

- After the first 24 hours, a temperature of over 100°F for more than a day

- Severe dizziness or significant light-headedness when standing up

- Nausea and vomiting

- Severe headaches that persist for more than a few minutes

- Localized pain, swelling, redness, heat, and tenderness in a breast once engorgement has subsided, which could be signs of mastitis or breast infection

- Localized swelling and/or redness, heat, and oozing at the site of a c-section incision

- After the first 24 hours, difficulty urinating, excessive pain or burning when urinating, and/or a frequent urge to urinate that yields scanty and/or dark urine. Drink plenty of water while trying to reach your practitioner.

- Sharp chest pain (not chest achiness, which is usually the result of strenuous pushing); rapid breath or heartbeat; blueness of fingertips or lips

- Localized pain, tenderness, and warmth in your calf or thigh, with or without redness, swelling, and pain when you flex your foot. Rest with your leg elevated while you try to reach your practitioner. Don't massage the leg or the tender area.

- Depression or anxiety that affects your ability to cope; feelings of anger toward your baby, particularly if those feelings are accompanied by violent urges. See page 498 for more on postpartum depression.

and/or difficulty taking a deep breath, because of strained chest muscles (hot baths, showers, or a heating pad may ease it), pain and tenderness in the area of your tailbone (heat and massage may help), and/or general all-over achiness (again, heat where it hurts may help).

Difficulty Urinating

"It's been a few hours since I gave birth, and I haven't been able to pee."

Peeing doesn't come easily for most brand new moms during the first 24 postpartum hours. Some feel no urge at all, and others feel the urge but are unable to satisfy it. Still others manage to pee, but with pain and burning. There are a host of reasons why basic bladder function often becomes too much like hard work after delivery:

- The holding capacity of the bladder increases because it suddenly has more room to expand—so your need to pee may be less frequent than it was during pregnancy.

- The bladder may have been traumatized or bruised during delivery. Temporarily paralyzed, it may not send the necessary signals of urgency even when it's full.

- Having had an epidural and/or a catheter may decrease the sensitivity of the bladder or your alertness to its signals.

- Perineal pain may cause reflex spasms in the urethra, making urination difficult. Swelling of the perineum may also stand between you and an easy pee.

- The sensitivity of the site of a tear or episiotomy repair can cause burning and/or pain with urination. Burning may be eased somewhat by standing astride the toilet while peeing so the flow comes straight down, without touching sore spots. Squirting warm water on the area while you pee can also decrease discomfort (use the squirt bottle you were probably given and shown how to use).

- You may be dehydrated, especially if you didn't do any drinking during labor, and didn't receive IV fluids.

- Any number of psychological factors may keep you from going with the flow: fear of pain, lack of privacy, embarrassment over using a bedpan or needing help at the toilet.

As difficult as peeing may be, it's essential that you empty your bladder within 6 to 8 hours after delivery (or after the removal of any catheter) to avoid a UTI, loss of muscle tone in the bladder from over-distension, and excessive bleeding (because an over-full bladder can get in the way of your uterus as it attempts the normal postpartum contractions that stanch bleeding). With those marching orders in mind, the nurse will ask you frequently after delivery if you've accomplished this important goal. You might even be asked to deposit that first postpartum pee into a container or bedpan, so your output can be measured. The nurse may palpate your bladder to make sure it's not distended. To help get things flowing:

- Be sure you're drinking plenty of fluids: What goes in is more likely to go out.

- Take a walk. Getting out of bed and going for a slow stroll as soon after delivery as you're able will help get your bladder (and bowels) moving.

- If you're uncomfortable with an audience (and who isn't?), have the nurse wait outside while you pee.

- If you have to use a bedpan, try to sit on it instead of lying on it.

- Squirt warm water over your perineal area to induce urgency. You can also try warming your perineum in a sitz bath or chilling it with an ice pack

- Turn the water on while you try. Running water in the sink really does encourage your own faucet to flow.

If all efforts fail and you haven't peed within 8 hours after delivery, your practitioner may order a catheter to empty your bladder—another good incentive to try the methods above.

After 24 hours, the problem of too little generally becomes one of too much. Most new moms usually begin urinating frequently and plentifully as the excess fluids of pregnancy are excreted. If you're still having trouble peeing, or if output is scant during the next few days, it's possible you have a UTI (see page 528).

"I can't seem to control my urine. It just leaks out."

The physical stress of childbirth can put a lot of things temporarily out of commission, including the bladder. Either it can't let go of the urine—or it lets go of it too easily, as in your drippy case. Such leakage (called urinary incontinence) occurs because of loss of muscle tone in the perineal area. Kegel exercises can help restore the tone and help you regain control over the flow of urine. See page 492 for more.

That First Bowel Movement

"I delivered 2 days ago and I haven't had a bowel movement. I've felt the urge, but I've been too afraid of opening my stitches to try."

The passing of the first postpartum bowel movement is a milestone every newly delivered mom is eager to put behind her (so to speak). And the longer it takes you to get past that milestone, the more anxious—and the more uncomfortable—you're likely to become.

Several physical factors may interfere with the return of bowel-business-as-usual after delivery. For one thing, the abdominal muscles that assist in elimination have been stretched during childbirth, making them flaccid and sometimes temporarily unable to help out. For another, the bowel itself may have taken a beating during delivery, leaving it sluggish. And of course, it may have been emptied before or during delivery (remember that prelabor diarrhea? The poop that you squeezed out during pushing?), and stayed pretty empty because you didn't eat much solid food during labor.

But it's the psychological factors that most inhibit postpartum pooping: the fear that it will hurt, split open any stitches, or make your hemorrhoids worse; the natural embarrassment over lack of privacy in the hospital or birthing center; and that pressure to "perform." In other words, it's mind over fecal matter.

Here are some steps you can take to get things moving again:

Don't worry. Nothing will keep you from moving your bowels more than worrying about moving your bowels. Don't stress about opening the stitches—you won't. Finally, don't worry if it takes a few days to get things moving—that's okay, too.

Request roughage. If you're still in the hospital or birthing center, select as many whole grains (bran cereal or muffins), beans, and fresh fruits (but not bananas) and salads from the menu as you can. If you're home, make sure you're eating regularly and well—and

Should I Stay or Should I Go?

Wondering when you'll be able to bring baby home? How long you and your baby stay in the hospital will depend on the kind of delivery you had, your condition, and your baby's condition. By federal law, you have the right to expect your insurer to pay for a 48-hour stay following a normal vaginal delivery and 96 hours following a cesarean delivery. If both you and your baby are in fine shape and you're eager to get home, you'll likely be able to go home 24 hours after your vaginal delivery and 2 to 3 days after your cesarean delivery (or earlier if your practitioner gives the early green light).

If you do opt for an early checkout, keep in mind that your baby will need an early checkup, too, just to make sure no problems crop up after discharge. The most convenient option is a home nurse visit (since you won't have to venture out to get your baby checked out). Your insurance plan may pay for a home nurse visit, and all first-time low-income moms are eligible for one through the Affordable Care Act's Maternal, Infant, and Early Childhood Home Visiting program. If a checkup at home isn't an option, make sure you take your newborn for an office visit to the pediatrician within a few days. The nurse or doctor will assess baby's weight and general condition (including a check for jaundice), as well as evaluate how feeding is going. Keeping and bringing along a feeding diary (and a wet and dirty diaper count) will help.

If you do stay the full 48 or 96 hours, take advantage of the opportunity to rest as much as possible. You'll need that energy stash for when you get home.

---

that you're getting your fill of fiber. As much as you can, stay away from bowel-clogging foods like white bread and rice.

Keep the liquids coming. Not only do you need to compensate for fluids you lost during labor and delivery, but you need to take in additional liquids to help soften stool if you're clogged up. Water's always a winner, but you may also find apple or prune juice especially effective. Hot water with lemon can also do the trick.

Get off your bottom. An inactive body encourages inactive bowels. You won't be running laps the day after delivery, but you will be able to take short strolls up and down the halls. Kegel exercises, which can be practiced in bed almost immediately after delivery, will help tone up not only the perineum but also the rectum. At home, take walks with baby.

Don't strain. Straining won't break open any stitches you have, but it can lead to or aggravate hemorrhoids. If you already have hemorrhoids, you may find relief with sitz baths, topical anesthetics, witch hazel pads, suppositories, or hot or cold compresses.

Use stool softeners. Many hospitals send new moms home with both a stool softener and a laxative, for a reason: Both can help get you going.

The first few bowel movements may be a pain to pass. But fear not. As stools soften and you become more regular, discomfort will ease and eventually end—and moving your bowels will become second nature once again.

Excessive Sweating and Hot Flashes

"I've been waking up at night soaked with sweat. Is this normal?"

It's messy, but it's normal. New moms are sweaty moms (and sometimes, moms with hot flashes), and for a couple of good reasons. For one thing, your hormone levels are dropping—reflecting the fact that you're no longer pregnant. For another, perspiration (like frequent urination) is your body's way of ridding itself of pregnancy-accumulated fluids (as well as any IV-accumulated fluids) after delivery—something you're bound to be happy about. Something you might not be happy with is how uncomfortable that perspiration might make you, and how long it might continue. Some women keep sweating up a storm for several weeks or more. If you do most of your perspiring at night, as most new moms do, covering your pillow with an absorbent towel may help you sleep better (it'll also help protect your pillow).

Don't sweat the sweat. Do make sure, though, that you're drinking enough fluids to compensate for the ones you're losing, especially if you're breastfeeding but even if you're not.

Hot flashes are common postpartum, too, also because of those hormonal changes. These is-it-hot-in-here-or-is-it-me moments may be more pronounced if you're breastfeeding and may last a few weeks or more—but while they may be a preview of menopause, they're not a sign of it.

Fever

"I've just come home from the hospital, and I'm running a fever of about 101°F. Should I call my doctor?"

Just as it was during your 9 months of pregnancy, it's always a good idea to play it safe during the first week or so after delivery—and that means keeping your practitioner in the loop when you're not feeling well. Although it's always possible that the fever you're running isn't postpartum-related, your practitioner will want to rule out a postpartum infection and treat any infection that's getting you down. While a fever can also occasionally be caused by the combination of excitement and exhaustion that's common in the early postpartum period, it typically wouldn't run as high as 101°F. A brief low-grade fever (less than 100°F) occasionally accompanies engorgement when your milk first comes in, and it's nothing to worry about.

So keep playing it safe postpartum. Report to your practitioner any fever over 100°F that lasts more than a day during the first 3 postpartum weeks or that lasts more than a few hours if it's a higher fever.

Engorged Breasts

"My milk just came in, and now my breasts are gigantic, rock hard, and so painful I can't put on a bra."

Just when you thought your breasts couldn't get any bigger, they do. That first milk delivery arrives, leaving your breasts swollen, painfully tender, throbbing, granite hard—and sometimes seriously, frighteningly gigantic. To make matters more uncomfortable and inconvenient, this engorgement (which can extend all the way to the armpits) can make nursing painful for you and, if your nipples are flattened by the swelling, frustrating for baby. The longer it takes for you and baby to hook up for your first nursing sessions, the worse the engorgement is likely to be.

Happily, though, it won't last long. Engorgement, and all its miserable effects, gradually eases once a well-coordinated milk supply-and-demand system is established, typically within days. Nipple soreness, too—which usually peaks at about the 20th feeding, if you're keeping count—generally diminishes rapidly as the nipples toughen up. And with proper care, so does the nipple cracking and bleeding some women also experience (see *What to Expect the First Year* for more).

Until nursing becomes second nature for your breasts—and completely painless for you—there are some steps you can take to relieve the discomfort and get a good milk supply going (read all about it starting on page 478).

Women who have an easy time getting started with breastfeeding (especially second-timers) may not experience very much engorgement at all. As long as baby's getting those milk deliveries, that's normal, too.

Engorgement If You're not Breastfeeding

"I'm not nursing. I've heard that drying up the milk can be painful."

Your breasts are programmed to fill with milk around the 3rd or 4th postpartum day, whether you plan to use that milk to feed your baby or not. This engorgement can be uncomfortable, even painful—but it's only temporary.

Milk is produced by your breasts only as needed. If the milk isn't used, production stops. Though sporadic leaking may continue for several days, or even weeks, severe engorgement shouldn't last more than 12 to 24 hours. During this time, ice packs, mild pain relievers, and a supportive bra may help. Avoid nipple stimulation, expressing milk, or hot showers, all of which stimulate milk production and keep that painful cycle going longer.

Where's the Breast Milk?

"It's been hours since I delivered, and nothing comes out of my breasts when I squeeze them. Is my baby boy starving?"

Not only is your baby not starving, he isn't even hungry yet. Babies aren't born with a big appetite or with immediate nutritional needs. And by the time your baby begins to hunger for a breast-full of milk (on the 3rd or 4th day postpartum), you'll undoubtedly be able to serve it up.

Which isn't to say that your breasts are currently empty. Colostrum, which provides your baby with enough nourishment for now and with important antibodies his own body can't yet produce (and also helps empty baby's digestive system of excess mucus and bowels of meconium), is definitely present in the tiny amounts necessary. A teaspoon or so per feeding is all your bundle of joy needs at this point. But until the 3rd or 4th postpartum day, when your breasts begin to swell and feel full (indicating the milk has come in), it's not that easy to express by hand. A day-old baby, eager to suckle, is better equipped to extract this premilk than you are.

If your milk doesn't come in at all by the time you've hit day 4, call your practitioner.

Bonding

"I expected to bond with my baby as soon as she was born, but I'm not feeling anything at all. Is something wrong with me?"

Moments after delivery, you're handed your long-anticipated bundle of joy, and she's more beautiful

Breast Milk Timeline

Suckling on colostrum for the first few days not only gets your newborn off to the healthiest start in life, but also gets the breastfeeding party started, stimulating production of the next stage of breast milk. Here's what'll be on tap for your baby in the coming weeks:

Colostrum. You already have this thick clearish-yellow premilk at the ready as soon as baby is born—providing your cuddly cutie with crucial antibodies and just the right kind of nourishment for the first few days of life.

Transitional milk. Next up on the breast milk menu: transitional milk, which is what's filling your breasts (and baby's tiny tummy) during engorgement. It has a whitish-orange color and contains more lactose, fat, and calories than colostrum while still providing a fair amount of those all-important immunoglobulins and proteins.

Mature milk. Mature milk—which looks like watery skim milk slightly tinged light blue—takes over from transitional milk around day 10 to 14 postpartum. Mature milk has two components to it: foremilk and hindmilk. When your little one starts to suckle, the foremilk quenches baby's thirst, but not his or her appetite. As the nursing session progresses, your breast dispenses the hindmilk, which is power-packed with the filling stuff: protein, fat, nutrients, and calories—everything your growing baby needs.

---

and more perfect than you ever dared to imagine. She looks up at you, and your eyes lock in a heady gaze, forging an instant bond. As you cradle her tiny form, breathe in her sweetness, and cover her soft face with kisses, you feel emotions you never knew you had, and they overwhelm you with their intensity. You're a mom in love.

And maybe you were dreaming— or, at least, pregnant daydreaming. Birthing-room scenes like this one are the stuff dreams—and commercials— are made of, but they don't always play out. Another possible scenario: After a long, hard labor that's left you physically and emotionally drained, a wrinkled, puffy, red-faced stranger is placed in your awkward arms, and the first thing you notice is that she doesn't quite resemble the chubby-cheeked cherub you'd been expecting. The second thing you notice is that she doesn't stop crying. The third, that you have no idea how to make her stop crying. You try to feed her, but she won't latch on. You try to socialize with her, but she's more interested in sleeping— and frankly, at this point, so are you. And you can't help wondering: Have I missed my opportunity to bond with my baby?

Absolutely, positively not. The process of bonding is different for every parent and every baby, and it doesn't come with a use-by date. Sure, some moms bond quickly with their newborns—maybe because they've had experience with infants before, their expectations are more realistic, their labors were easier, or their babies are more responsive. But other moms (plenty of them!) find that the attachment doesn't cement with superglue speed. In fact, the bonds that last a lifetime generally form gradually, over time—and you and your baby have lots of that ahead of you.

Bonding with Baby

Bonding begins with that first cuddle, but it's just the very start of your relationship with your baby. That brand new connection between you will deepen and strengthen, not just over the next weeks, but over the many years you'll be sharing as father and child.

In other words, don't expect instant results. You may get them, but no worries if you don't. Look at every moment with your newborn as a new opportunity to strengthen the bond you've been building. Every cuddle, every kiss, every bath, every gaze into those beautiful eyes, every word you speak or song you sing (remember your voice linked you together even before baby was born)—you'll be bonding. Making eye-to-eye contact and skin-to-skin contact (opening your shirt and snuggling baby against your bare chest) every chance you get will tighten the bond—while according to research, helping speed your newborn's brain development. In fact, every opportunity you take to be close to your baby increases your levels of the nurturing hormone, oxytocin, which in turn increases those feelings of closeness. Yes, the relationship may seem a little one-sided at first (until your newborn is alert enough to be responsive, you'll be doing all the smiling and cooing), but every moment of your attention is contributing to your baby's fledgling sense of wellbeing, letting your baby know he or she's secure, cared for, and loved unconditionally. The feedback you'll get once the smiles start coming will confirm that the connection with your baby was there all along.

Has your spouse been mom-monopolizing the baby and the baby care? Let her know that you'd like in. If she tends to baby hog when you're both at home (moms often do this without even realizing it), send her out—or at least, out of the room. That way, she can get some alone time—and you can get the alone-with-baby time that will quickly bring you even closer.

So give yourself that time—time to get used to being a mother (it's a major adjustment, after all) and time to get to know your newborn, who, let's face it, is also a newcomer in your life. Meet your baby's basic needs (and your own), and you'll find that love connection forming—a day (and a cuddle) at a time. And speaking of cuddles, bring them on. The more nurturing you do (especially skin-to-skin, since such snuggles release more of that nurturing hormone, oxytocin), the more like a nurturer you'll feel. Though it may not seem like it's coming naturally at first, the more time you spend cuddling, feeding, massaging, singing to, cooing to, and talking to your baby—the more time you spend skin-to-skin and face-to-face—the more natural it will start feeling, and the closer you'll become. Before you know it, you'll feel like the mom you are (really!), bound forever to your baby by the kind of love you've dreamed of.

"My baby was premature and was rushed to the NICU. The doctors say he'll be there for at least 2 weeks. Will it be too late for good bonding when he gets out?"

Not at all. Sure, having a chance to bond right after birth—to make contact, skin-to-skin, eye-to-eye—is wonderful. It's a first step in the development of a lasting parent-child connection. But it's only the first step. And this step doesn't have to take place at delivery. It can take place hours or days later in a hospital bed, or through the portholes of an isolette, or even weeks later at home.

And luckily, you'll be able to touch, talk to, and probably hold your baby even while he's in the NICU. Most hospitals not only allow parent-infant contact in the NICU, but encourage it—especially kangaroo care (holding baby skin-to-skin against your chest). Talk to the NICU staff and see how you can get close to your newborn. For more on the care of premature babies, see *What to Expect the First Year.*

Keep in mind, too, that even moms and dads who have a chance to bond in the birthing room don't necessarily feel that instant attachment (see the previous question). Love that lasts a lifetime takes time to develop—time that you and your baby will start having together soon.

Recovery from a Cesarean Delivery

"What will the recovery from my c-section delivery be like?"

Recovery from a c-section is similar to recovery from any abdominal surgery, with a delightful difference: Instead of losing a gallbladder or appendix, you gain a brand new baby.

Of course, there's another less delightful difference. In addition to recovering from surgery, you'll also be recovering from childbirth. Except for a neatly intact perineum, you'll experience all the same postpartum discomforts over the next weeks (lucky you!) that you would have had if you'd delivered vaginally: afterpains, lochia, perineal discomfort (if you went through labor before the surgery), breast engorgement, fatigue, hormonal

Give It Time

So you've been a mom for a week (with the stretch marks, postpartum pains, and bags under your eyes to prove it), and by now you may be wondering: When am I going to feel like one? When will I be able to accomplish latch-on without 20 minutes of fumbling? Or finally get the hang of burping? Or stop worrying about breaking the baby every time I pick her up? When will I be able to coo without feeling awkward? When will I figure out which cries mean what—and how to respond to any of them? How do I put on a diaper so it doesn't leak? Get the onesie over baby's head without a struggle? Shampoo that little patch of hair without dripping soap into those tender eyes? When will the job that nature just signed me up for start coming naturally?

The truth is, giving birth makes you a mother, but it doesn't necessarily make you feel like one. Only time spent on this sometimes bewildering, sometimes overwhelming, always amazing job will do that. The day-to-day (and night-to-night) of parenting is never easy, but it absolutely, positively gets easier.

So cut yourself some slack, pat yourself on the back, and give yourself time, mom. Which, by the way, you are.

changes, and excessive perspiration, to name a few.

Here's what you can expect in the recovery room:

Pain around your incision. Once the anesthesia wears off, your incision wound, like any wound, is going to hurt—though just how much depends on many factors, including your personal

Rooming-in Rules

Wondering where all the babies at your local hospital went (you know, the neatly wrapped bundles that used to be on display in the nursery, in row after row of bassinets)? They're rooming-in with their moms, most likely. Full-time rooming-in has become the standard in family-centered maternity care, and for a lot of very sound reasons. It gives new parents (often both parents, since dads are typically welcome to room-in, too) the chance to start getting to know their new arrival right from the start—to spend time snuggling skin-to-skin, to become familiar with baby's hunger cues, to start practicing those soothing techniques they'll definitely need once they arrive home. It also makes it possible for new moms to breastfeed on demand, which boosts the odds of ultimate breastfeeding success. It even reduces the amount of crying and increases the amount of sleeping newborns do (and their moms, believe it or not). Rooming-in is considered so beneficial, in fact, that even NICU families are encouraged to bunk with their babies in a hospital room for a night or two (albeit with a nurse just a call button away) before heading home.

For all those reasons and more, hospital nurseries often don't have many (if any) baby boarders at any given time these days, typically taking in only newborns in need of some extra care. Some hospitals have even shut down their nurseries entirely, sending babies needing medical attention to the NICU instead.

So do new moms have a choice when it comes to rooming-in? At many hospitals, they don't—rooming-in has become a requirement (and when it's not mandatory, it's highly suggested). And that's just fine with most moms and dads—who are often just as happy not to let their brand new little ones out of their sight. But sometimes, rooming-in moms need a break, an hour or two of uninterrupted sleep, or just a chance to rest up from childbirth and get ready for childrearing. If that sounds like you—push that button now and ask for a break. You've earned it, you deserve it, and—hopefully—you'll get it. Just make sure that if you're breastfeeding, your baby isn't given any supplementary bottles while you rest.

---

pain threshold and how many cesarean deliveries you've had (the first is usually the most uncomfortable). You will probably be given pain relief medication as needed, which may make you feel woozy or drugged. It will also allow you to get some needed sleep. No stress if you're nursing—the medication won't pass into your colostrum, and by the time your milk comes in, you probably won't need any heavy painkillers (though if you do, the small amount of medication that gets into your milk won't be unsafe for baby). If the pain continues for weeks, as it sometimes does, you can also safely rely on over-the-counter pain relief like ibuprofen (Advil or Motrin)—just ask your practitioner about dosing. (If you'd like to avoid narcotic meds from the start, discuss pain relief options with your practitioner ahead of time, and make sure that anyone administering medications is aware of your preference.)

Possible nausea, with or without vomiting. This isn't always an aftereffect of the surgery, but if it is, ask about getting an antinausea medication.

Exhaustion. You're likely to feel somewhat weak after surgery, partly due to blood loss, partly due to the anesthetic, and partly due to pain meds you might be taking. If you went through some hours of labor before the surgery, you'll feel even more beat. You might also feel emotionally spent (after all, you did just have a baby—and surgery), especially if the c-section wasn't planned.

Regular evaluations of your condition. A nurse will periodically check your vital signs (temperature, blood pressure, pulse, respiration), your urinary output and vaginal bleeding, the dressing on your incision, and the firmness and level of your uterus (as it shrinks in size and makes its way back into the pelvis).

Once you have been moved to your postpartum room, you can expect:

More checking. A nurse will continue to monitor your condition.

Removal of the urinary catheter. This will probably take place several hours after surgery. Urination may be difficult, so try the tips on page 466. If they don't work, the catheter may be reinserted until you're able to pee by yourself.

Encouragement to move. Before you're able to get out of bed, you'll be encouraged to wiggle your toes, circle your ankles, flex your feet to stretch your calf muscles, push against the end of the bed with your feet, and turn from side to side. These moves will improve circulation, especially in your legs, and prevent blood clots—plus they'll also help you get rid of all that IV-accumulated fluid faster. (But be prepared for some of them to be quite uncomfortable, at least for the first 24 hours or so.) You can also resume your Kegels right after delivery.

To get up between 8 and 24 hours after surgery. With the help of a nurse, you'll sit up first, supported by the raised head of the bed. Then, using your hands for support, you'll slide your legs over the side of the bed and dangle them for a few minutes. Then, slowly, you'll be helped to step down onto the floor, your hands still on the bed. If you feel dizzy (which is normal), sit right back down. Steady yourself for a few more minutes before taking a couple of steps, and then take them slowly—walking may be very uncomfortable. Though you may need help the first few times you get up, this difficulty getting around is temporary. In fact, you may soon find yourself more mobile than the vaginally delivered mom next door—and you'll probably have the edge when it comes to sitting.

A slow return to a normal diet. Research has shown that moms who start back on solids beginning as early as 4 to 8 hours post-op have that first bowel movement earlier and are generally ready to be released from the hospital 24 hours sooner than those kept on fluids only. Procedures may vary from hospital to hospital and from physician to physician, and your condition after the surgery may also play a part in deciding when to pull the plug on the IV and when to pull out the silverware. Keep in mind, too, that reintroduction of solids will come in stages. You'll start with fluids by mouth, moving on next to something soft and easily tolerated (like Jell-O), and on (slowly) from there (don't even think about having someone smuggle in a burger and fries yet). Once you're back on solids, don't forget to push the fluids, too—especially if you're breastfeeding.

Shoulder pain. Irritation of the diaphragm can cause a few hours of sharp shoulder pain after surgery (thanks to nerve pathways that run from the diaphragm to your shoulder, "referring" pain there) after surgery. A pain reliever may help.

Probably constipation. Since the anesthesia and the surgery (plus your limited diet and any pain meds you might be taking) may slow your bowels down, it may be a few days until you pass that first movement, and that's normal. You may also experience some painful gassiness because of the constipation. A stool softener, suppository, or other mild laxative may be prescribed to help move things along, especially if you're uncomfortable. The tips on page 467 may help, too.

Gas pain. As your digestive tract (temporarily put out of commission by surgery) begins to function again, trapped gas can cause considerable pain, especially when it presses against your incision line. The discomfort may be worse when you laugh, cough, or sneeze. Ask the nurse or doctor to suggest some possible remedies. A suppository may help release the gas. Taking a hallway stroll can also help, as can lying on your side or on your back, your knees drawn up, taking deep breaths while holding your incision. Holding a pillow against the incision site when you change positions or poop (and, after discharge, when you ride in a car) can help, too. Need more help? A belly band (like the one you may have used during pregnancy) can help support the belly and protect your incision.

Swelling. Thought the days of swelling were over now that you're postpartum? They will be—eventually. But in the first week after a c-section, many moms notice increased swelling, particularly in their feet and legs. Some of this swelling comes from leftover pregnancy fluids, some comes from all the IV fluids that were pumped in during surgery. Compounding post-op puffiness is the fact that you're not moving around much, which makes it harder for your body to rid itself of the fluid. Flush it out by drinking lots of water, getting moving as much as possible (without overdoing it), and when you're in bed, keeping your legs elevated.

To spend time with your baby. You'll be encouraged to cuddle and feed your baby as soon as possible (see box, page 486). And yes, you can even lift your baby. Hospital regulations and your condition permitting, you'll probably be rooming-in—and of course, having your partner or another family member or friend bunking with you, too, will be a big help. If you don't have that help on board, don't hesitate to call the nurse, who can lend a hand.

Removal of stitches. If your stitches or staples aren't self-absorbing, they will be removed about 4 or 5 days after delivery. The procedure isn't very painful, although you may have some discomfort. When the dressing is off, take a good look at the incision with the nurse or doctor. Once your incision is truly healing (no scabbing or open skin—usually 10 to 14 days after surgery), you can put a silicone scar sheet on it (you can pick up a package of them at your local pharmacy) to help minimize the scar's appearance. Ask how soon you can expect the area to heal, which changes will be normal, and which might require medical attention.

You'll likely be able to go home about 2 to 4 days postpartum. But you'll still have to take it easy, and you'll continue to need lots of help while you recover.

Coming Home with Baby

"In the hospital, a nurse was always a call button away when I needed help with the baby. Now that I'm home with him, I'm clueless how to care for him—and I'm feeling overwhelmed."

Being There

The very best way to start off your new life as a father is at home with your new family. So if it's possible and financially feasible, consider taking off as much time as you can right after delivery—through the FMLA, which allows for 12 weeks of unpaid leave for mothers and fathers (see page 200) or the policy at your company, or by taking a chunk of vacation time. If that's impossible (or not your preference), consider working part-time for a few weeks or doing some work from home.

If none of these possibilities are practical, maximize the time you do have off from work. Make sure you're home as much as you can be, and learn to say no to overtime, early or late meetings, and business trips that can be put off or passed off. Especially in the postpartum period, when your partner is still recovering from labor and delivery, try to do more than your share of household chores and baby care whenever you're home. Keep in mind that no matter how physically or emotionally stressful your work is, there is no more demanding job than caring for a newborn.

Make bonding with your new baby a priority, but don't forget to devote some time to nurturing the new mom in your life as well. Pamper her when you're home, and let her know you're thinking of her when you're at work. Call her often to offer support (and so she can unload as much as she needs to), and surprise her with flowers or with takeout from a favorite restaurant.

It's true that babies aren't born with how-to's written on their cute, dimply bottoms (wouldn't that be convenient?). Fortunately, they do typically come home from the hospital with instructions from the staff about feeding, bathing, and changing diapers. Already lost those? Or maybe they ended up smeared with mustardy poop the first time you tried to change baby's diaper while trying to read the instructions for changing his diaper? Not to worry; there's lots of help out there as you tackle your new job as a new parent (including *What to Expect the First Year*). Plus, you've probably already scheduled the first visit to the pediatrician, where you'll be armed with even more information—not to mention answers to the dozens of questions you've managed to accumulate (that is, if you remember to write them down and bring them along). Or maybe your health insurance plan entitles you to a visit from a home nurse, who can troubleshoot problems you're having and offer some hands-on help.

Of course, it takes more than know-how to make a parenting expert out of a new parent. It takes patience, perseverance, and practice, practice, practice. Luckily, your baby won't judge as you learn. He won't care if you put his diaper on backward or you forget to wash behind his ears at bath time. What's more, he won't be shy about giving you feedback. He'll let you know when he's hungry or tired or uncomfortably wet (though at first you may have trouble telling which complaint is which). Best of all, since your baby's never had another mom (or dad) to compare you with, you definitely stack up really well in his book. In fact, you're the best he's ever had.

Still suffering from a crumbling of confidence? What might help most—

besides the passing of time and the accumulation of experience—is to know that you're in good company. All parents (even those seasoned pros you doubtless eye with envy) feel in over their heads in those early weeks, especially when postpartum exhaustion—teamed with nightly sleep deprivation and the recovery from childbirth—is taking its toll, body and soul. So cut yourself plenty of slack, and give yourself plenty of time to adjust and to get with the parenting program. Pretty soon (sooner than you think), the everyday challenges of baby care won't be so challenging anymore. In fact, they'll come so naturally, you'll be able to do them in your sleep (and will often feel as though you are). You'll be diapering, feeding, burping, and soothing with the best of them—with one arm tied behind your back (or at least, one arm folding laundry, catching up on social media, reading a book, spooning cereal into your mouth, or otherwise multitasking). You'll be a mom. And moms, in case you haven't heard, can do anything.

ALL ABOUT:
Beginning Breastfeeding

There's nothing more natural than nursing a baby, right? Well, not always, at least not right away. Babies are born to breastfeed, but they're not necessarily born knowing how to breastfeed. Ditto for moms. The breasts are standard issue and fill with milk pretty much automatically, but knowing how to position them effectively in baby's mouth, well, that's a learned art.

Truth is, while breastfeeding is a natural process, it's a natural process that doesn't necessarily come naturally—or quickly—to all moms and babies. Sometimes there are physical factors that foil those first few attempts, at other times it's just a simple lack of experience on the part of both participants. But whatever might be keeping your baby and your breasts apart, it likely won't be long before they're in perfect sync. Some of the most mutually satisfying breast-baby relationships begin with several days—or even weeks—of fumbling, bungled efforts, and tears on both sides.

Reading up on breastfeeding (or even taking a class) ahead of baby's arrival can help speed that mutual adjustment. But there's no substitute for learning on the job, baby at the breast. The following basics are meant to get you started on that job, but you'll find much more detailed help—including strategies for overcoming just about every breastfeeding bump you might encounter along the way—in *What to Expect the First Year*.

Getting Started Breastfeeding

Here's how you can get off to a good breastfeeding start:

Start early. Babies are extra alert in the first hour after birth, which makes this a perfect time for early bonding and early breastfeeding. So let your practitioner know that you'd like to begin breastfeeding right after delivery (even if it's a cesarean delivery), assuming baby doesn't need any immediate medical attention.

Enlist help. Ask if a lactation consultant (LC) or a nurse who is knowledgeable about breastfeeding can observe your technique, provide hands-on instruction, and redirect if you and your baby aren't on target. If you leave the hospital or birthing center before getting the help you need—or if you need help once you're home—find an outside LC or home nurse who can evaluate your technique and give you pointers. Contact your local La Leche League chapter (search for it on llli.org) or the International Lactation Consultant Association (ILCA) at ilca.org for an LC in your area. Some pediatricians have licensed LCs (or very experienced nurses) on staff as well—ask if your baby's doctor does.

Keep your baby bottle-free. Even if you're planning to introduce a bottle at some point in your baby's breastfeeding future, hold off for now—and make sure hospital staff does, too, unless supplementary feedings are medically necessary. Bottle feedings of glucose water or formula can sabotage early breastfeeding efforts by satisfying your newborn's tender appetite and urge to suck. And since an artificial nipple yields results with less effort, you may find your baby

---

Bottle Baby

Chose the bottle? Getting started bottle-feeding is usually a lot easier than getting started breastfeeding (especially because formula and bottles actually come with instructions, unlike breasts). But there's still plenty to learn, and you can read all about it in *What to Expect the First Year*.

---

reluctant to tackle your harder-to-work nipples after a few encounters with a bottle. Worse still, if baby's getting that sucking satisfaction elsewhere, your breasts won't be stimulated to produce enough milk—and a vicious cycle can begin, one that interferes with establishment of a good demand-and-supply system. Once you get home, stay bottle-free (even if you'll ultimately be supplementing) until breastfeeding is well established, usually at 2 to 3 weeks.

Feed around the clock. Aim for a feeding every 2 to 3 hours, timed from the beginning of one to the beginning of the next—for a total of 8 to 12 feeds per

---

Eating When You're Feeding

Milk production burns 500 calories a day, which means that you'll get to eat an extra 500 calories a day (up from your prepregnancy numbers— not your pregnancy allotment) to meet that need. As baby gets bigger and hungrier, you may have to add even more calories—that is, until solids are added to the menu and the demand for breast milk gradually decreases. You'll also need an extra serving of calcium, for a total of 5.

For more details on what to eat and what not to eat (and drink) when you're breastfeeding—plus all the breastfeeding know-how you'll need to know— see *What to Expect the First Year*. For a complete look at the Breastfeeding Diet, see *What to Expect: Eating Well When You're Expecting*.

Feeding Time

Remember how you timed your contractions—counting from the beginning of one to the beginning of the next? Good—because you'll be timing breastfeeding sessions the same way. These sessions won't be nearly as close together as contractions were, but they will last a whole lot longer, leaving you less time between feeds than you might have expected.

Still, as time-consuming as breastfeeding can be at first, it's important not to put a time limit on it. A newborn nursing session lasts an average of 30 minutes, but some sweet slowpokes can linger for as long as 45 minutes. Don't put a time limit on how long baby spends at each breast, either, because you're worried about your nipples getting sore. Sore nipples result from improper positioning of baby on the breast, and have little to do with the length of the feeding. Instead, let your baby be your guide (as you'll soon discover, your just-born newborn is wise beyond his or her days in many ways—feeding is one of those). He or she will likely tell you when it's time to switch sides (by slowing down or stopping suckling) and when it's time to call it quits on the session entirely (by conking out). The exception? If baby nods off after just a few minutes of suckling, it's time for a wake-up call (some sleepyheads would rather snooze than suckle).

Once your milk comes in (and engorgement levels off), you'll want to make sure that at least one breast is "emptied" (it'll go from feeling full to feeling soft) at each feeding. Thoroughly draining one side before moving on to the next will ensure that your little nurser gets not only the thirst-quenching foremilk that a breast dispenses at the beginning of a feed, but the high-calorie hindmilk that comes at the end. So don't pull the plug arbitrarily mid-feed. Once baby is finished with the first breast, you can offer the second, but don't push it. Just remember to start the next feeding on the breast that wasn't drained at the last session.

So sleepy yourself, you're having trouble remembering which side is up next? Use a reminder—a notation in your breastfeeding journal or app, a small scrunchie looped around your bra strap, or a nursing bracelet on your wrist—to remind you which breast is on deck for the next feed.

And speaking of keeping track, it's a good idea to keep a running tab of baby's feeds (when they begin and end) as well as of wet and soiled diapers your newborn produces. While that might sound a bit obsessive, it'll help give you a good sense of how breastfeeding is going, and also make it possible for you to report back to baby's doctor at the next checkup. Along with good weight gain, adequate output (at least 6 wet diapers—with urine that's clear, not dark—and at least 5 bowel movements over each 24-hour period) is one of the best indications of good intake—and a sign that your breasts and baby are right on target.

---

day. Not only will this round-the-clock schedule keep your baby happy (newborns love to suck even when they're not hungry), but it will stimulate your breasts, minimize engorgement, and boost production. Have a sleepyhead on your hands? If it's been more than 2 to 3 hours since the last feed, it's time for a wake-up call. Unswaddle your baby or lay him or her on your bare chest (the scent of your breast may be enough to wake your little one).

No Breasts, No Problem

It's a biological fact: There are three things that moms can do that dads can't. You can't be pregnant, you can't give birth (some would consider that a definite plus), and you can't breastfeed. But here's another fact: Those natural physical limitations don't have to send you to the sidelines. You can share in nearly all the excitement, joy, anticipation, and, let's face it, stress of your spouse's pregnancy, labor, and delivery—from the first kick to the last push—as an active, supportive participant. And though you'll never be able to put your baby to the breast (at least not with the kind of results baby's looking for), you can share in the feeding process:

Be your baby's backup feeder. Once breastfeeding is established, there's more than one way to feed a baby. And though you can't breastfeed, you can be the one to give supplementary bottles of expressed milk or formula (if those will be on baby's menu). Not only will being the supplementary feeder give mom a break (whether in the middle of the night or in the middle of dinner), it will give you extra opportunities for closeness with your baby. Make the most of the moment—instead of propping the bottle up to the baby's mouth, strike a nursing position, with your baby snuggled close and the bottle where that breast would be. Opening up your shirt, which allows for cuddly skin-to-skin contact, will enhance the experience for both of you. No supplementary bottles on the menu? You can still do skin-to-skin, every chance you get.

Share the night shift. Sharing in the joys of feeding also means sharing in those early weeks of sleepless nights. Even if you're not giving supplementary bottles, there's plenty you can do for Team Feed. You can be the one to pick baby up, do any necessary diaper changing, deliver baby to mom for feedings, and return baby to the crib or bassinet once the feed is finished. Not only will you be connecting more with baby by participating in nighttime feeds (building both lifelong bonds and lifetime memories), but you'll also be letting mom get some much-needed rest.

Double down on other duties. Breastfeeding is the only baby-care activity limited to moms. Dads can bathe, diaper, and rock with the best of moms—and yes, even better than them—given the chance to step up and step in.

Get calm, mom. Tension not only inhibits letdown (how your breasts dispense milk once it's on tap), but it can generate stress in your baby (infants are extremely sensitive to mom's moods)—and a stressed-out baby can't nurse effectively. So try to start out each feed as relaxed as possible. Do some relaxation exercises before you begin, or tune in to some soft, soothing music. Getting comfortable will also help you get your calm on, so use a nursing pillow (or a regular pillow) to position baby so breastfeeding's not a strain or a pain. Bring on baby's calm before feeds, too, by doing some gentle rocking and quiet, soothing skin-to-skin.

Breastfeeding 101

Proper positioning is essential to a good latch, and to prevent nipple soreness and other breastfeeding problems. Start by placing baby on his or

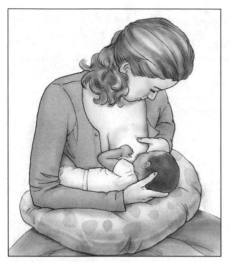

Crossover hold

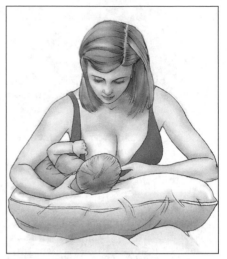

Football hold

her side, facing your nipple. Make sure baby's whole body is facing your breasts—with his or her ear, shoulder, and hip in a straight line. In other words, make sure baby's little boy or girl parts are facing (parallel to) the breast you're not feeding from. You don't want your baby's head turned to the side—it should be straight in line with his or her body. (Imagine how difficult it would be for you to drink and swallow while turning your head to the side.) Use a nursing pillow (or a regular pillow) to bring baby up to a height that will make maneuvering your little one to the breast easier.

You can try any of these positions, experimenting to find the ones that feel most comfortable for you:

Crossover hold. Hold your baby's head with the hand opposite to the breast you'll be nursing from (if nursing on the right breast, hold your baby with your left hand). Rest your wrist between your baby's shoulder blades, your thumb behind one ear, your other fingers behind the other ear. Using your other hand, cup your breast, placing your thumb above your nipple and areola

at the spot where your baby's nose will touch your breast. Your index finger should be at the spot where your baby's chin will touch the breast. Lightly compress your breast so your nipple points slightly toward your baby's nose. You are now ready to have baby latch on.

Football hold. This position, also called the clutch hold, is especially useful if you've had a c-section and want to avoid placing your baby against your abdomen, or if your breasts are large or if your baby is small or premature. Position your baby at your side, facing you, with baby's legs under your arm (your right arm if you're nursing on the right breast). Support your baby's head with your right hand and cup your breast as you would for the crossover hold.

Cradle hold. Position your baby so that sweet little head rests in the bend of your elbow and you're using the rest of your arm to support baby's body. Using your free hand, cup your breast as you would for the crossover hold.

Laid-back position ("biological nurturing"). Lean back on a bed or couch,

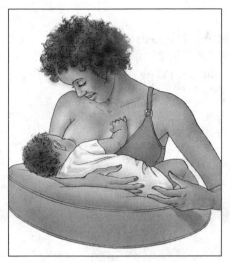

Cradle hold

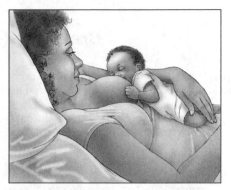

Laid-back position

well supported by pillows, so that when you put your baby tummy-to-tummy onto your body, head near your breast, gravity will keep him or her molded to you. Your baby can rest on you in any direction, as long as his or her whole front is against yours and he or she can reach your breast. Your baby can naturally latch on in this position, or you can help by directing the nipple toward his or her mouth—but otherwise you don't have to do much in the laid-back position besides lie back and enjoy.

Side-lying position. In this position, both you and your baby lie on your sides, tummy to tummy. Use your hand on the side you're not lying on to cup your breast if you need to. This position is a good choice when you're feeding in the middle of the night.

Now that baby's in position, you can latch him or her onto your breast using the following tips:

- Gently tickle your baby's lips with your nipple until his or her mouth is opened very wide, like a yawn. Some LCs suggest aiming your nipple toward your baby's nose and then directing it down to the upper lip to

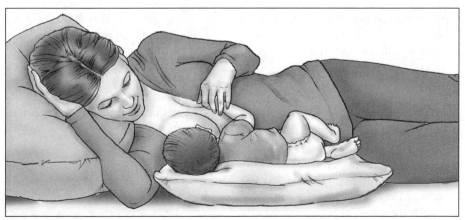

Side-lying position

Breastfeeding Multiples

Breastfeeding, like just about every aspect of caring for newborn multiples, seems as though it will be at least twice as challenging. However, once you've fallen into the rhythm of nursing your multiples (and you will!), you'll find that it's not only possible but doubly (or even triply) rewarding—and convenient. To successfully nurse twins and more, you should:

Eat up. Doing so much feeding will mean you'll also have to do more eating. To fuel your multiples milk machine, you'll need 400 to 500 calories above your prepregnancy needs for each baby you are nursing (you may need to increase your caloric intake as the babies grow bigger and hungrier or decrease it if you supplement nursing with formula and/or solids, or if

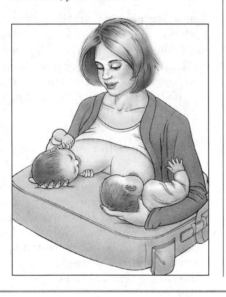 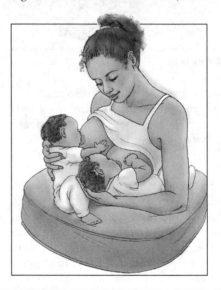

get baby to open his or her mouth very wide. This prevents the lower lip from getting tucked in during nursing. If your baby turns his or her head away, gently stroke the cheek on the side nearest you. The rooting reflex will make baby turn his or her head toward your breast.

- Once that little mouth is opened wide, move your baby closer. Do not move your breast toward your baby. Many latching-on problems occur because mom is hunched over baby, trying to shove breast

into mouth. Instead, keep your back straight and bring your baby to your breast. Remember, too, not to stuff your nipple into an unwilling mouth—instead, let your baby take the initiative. It might take a couple of attempts before your baby opens his or her mouth wide enough to latch on properly.

- Be sure baby latches on to both the nipple and the areola that surrounds it. Sucking on just the nipple won't compress the milk glands and can cause soreness and cracking.

you have considerable fat reserves you would like to burn). You'll also need an extra calcium serving for that extra baby (for a total of 6, though you can also tap into a calcium supplement to help you reach that goal). See box, page 479, for more.

Pump it up. If your babies are in the NICU and are still too small to breast-feed, consider pumping; see box, page 487.

Nurse two at a time. You've got two breasts and two (or more) mouths to feed—so why not nurse them together, tandem style? An obvious—and big—advantage of tandem-nursing is that you don't spend all day and night nursing (first Baby A, now Baby B, and back to Baby A, and so on). To nurse two at the same time, position both babies on the pillow first, and then latch them on (or ask someone to hand the babies to you one at a time, especially while you're still getting used to the juggling act). Using a nursing pillow designed for twins will make positioning much easier. You can position both babies in the football (or clutch) hold, using nursing pillows to support their heads, or you can combine the cradle hold and the football hold, again using the pillow for support and experimenting until both you and your babies are comfortable.

If tandem nursing doesn't appeal to you, don't do it. You can bottle-feed one (using either pumped milk or formula, if you're supplementing) while nursing the other (and then switch off), or nurse one baby after the other.

Got three (or more) babies to feed? Breastfeeding triplets (and even quads) is possible, too. Nurse two at a time, and then nurse the third baby afterward, remembering to switch off which baby gets solo suckling time. For more information on breastfeeding higher-order multiples, check out raisingmultiples .org.

Treat each diner differently. Even identical twins have different personalities, appetites, and nursing patterns. So try to tune in to the needs of each. And keep extra-careful records to make sure each baby is well fed at each feeding.

Give both breasts a workout. Switch breasts for each baby at each feeding so both breasts are stimulated equally.

- Once baby is properly latched on, check to see if your breast is blocking your baby's nose. If it is, lightly depress the breast with your finger. Elevating baby slightly may also help provide a little breathing room. But as you maneuver, be sure not to loosen baby's grip on the areola.

- Not sure if baby's suckling? Check those sweet cheeks—you should see a strong, steady, rhythmic motion. That means your little feeder is getting fed—successfully suckling and swallowing.

Now that the feed has started, how long should it last? See the box on page 480.

If your baby has finished suckling but is still holding on to the breast, pulling it out abruptly can cause injury to your nipple. Instead, break the suction first by depressing the breast or by putting your finger into the corner of the baby's mouth to let in some air.

Breastfeeding After a Cesarean Delivery

Eager to get your baby to breast, even though you've had a c-section? How soon you can get baby to latch on and get busy depends on how you're feeling and how baby's doing. More and more hospitals are allowing skin-to-skin (and breast nuzzling) time right after delivery, baby's condition permitting. And the most progressive hospitals are giving new moms the opportunity to breastfeed right after their c-section—while they're still in the operating room. Of course you'll have a hard time moving (you just had major surgery after all), so be sure to enlist your partner, a nurse, your doula, or an LC to help you get propped up (or shifted to your side) and in position, ready for baby to be handed to you.

You'll probably find breastfeeding after a c-section uncomfortable at first (at least once your pain meds wear off). Your best bet will be to find a position that puts the least amount of pressure on your incision. Do this by placing a regular or breastfeeding pillow on your lap under the baby, or by lying on your side, or by using the football hold (page 482), again supported by a pillow, to nurse. A belly band can also take some of the pressure off your incision, helping make breastfeeding a little more comfortable. Some positions will be more comfortable than others, so be sure to find the best one for you.

If you're groggy from general anesthesia or your baby needs immediate care in the nursery, this first nursing session may have to wait. If after 12 hours you still haven't been able to get together with your baby, ask about using a pump to express colostrum and get lactation started.

A few more things to keep in mind: First, since you've been pumped up with a lot of fluids thanks to your IV, your baby will have a little more "water weight" on him or her. Your little one will get rid of those fluids by peeing a lot and appearing to lose a lot of weight (more than a typical vaginal birth baby). Be sure that normal weight loss isn't used as a reason to give a supplementary bottle (unless it has been prescribed as medically necessary), since that could hurt your chances of early breastfeeding success (see page 479). Second, some moms who have had a cesarean delivery find that their milk comes in a little later than expected, probably due to the extra stress of surgery. You can keep your milk supply on track by cuddling skin-to-skin with your baby often and getting those first nursing sessions started as soon as possible. Be sure you've documented your wishes in your birth plan and that you've got advocates on your side (your partner, an LC, a doula, the pediatrician) helping you be reunited with your baby as soon as possible. Finally, you'll be given pain meds (often narcotics) after your delivery—don't hesitate to take them if you need them (and want them). Being in intense pain can unnecessarily interfere with your breastfeeding efforts. As long as you use them only short-term and at a safe dose (take only one tablet every 6 to 8 hours maximum, and watch for excessive drowsiness in baby), they're safe for your little one and compatible with breastfeeding.

If you've been given antibiotics after your c-section, be aware that it might increase your newborn's chances of getting thrush. Taking a probiotic can help reduce that risk.

Breastfeeding the NICU Baby

B reast is best for babies of every size—including the tiniest ones. In fact, preemies and babies who are small for gestational age or have other medical problems at birth do much better on breast milk, even if they're not ready to tackle a breast. So don't give up on breastfeeding. Talk to your baby's neonatologist and the nurse in charge to see how you can best feed your very little one—and feed him or her the very best—while in the NICU. And then, if you can, get pumping (a double electric is best, and if you can rent a hospital grade pump, better still). If baby isn't ready for latching on yet, your pumped milk may be given to your baby via tube feeding or bottle. Even if that's not possible at first, you can pump milk to store until baby's ready for it—and to keep your supply pumped up until baby's ready to feed from you directly. Can't produce enough breast milk or can't pump at all? Ask the hospital about the possibility of donor milk, often used to supplement preemies. For much more on feeding preemies (as well as much more on preemie care), see *What to Expect the First Year.*

Postpartum: The First 6 Weeks

B y now you're probably either settling into your new life as a fledgling mom or figuring out how to juggle new baby care with the demands of older children. Almost certainly, much of your daily—and nightly—attention is focused on that recently arrived little bundle. Babies, after all, don't take care of themselves. But that doesn't mean you should neglect your own care (yes, you need care, too, especially while you're still in recovery mode).

Though most of your questions and concerns are likely to be baby-related right now, you're sure to have some that are a little more mommycentric, too, from the state of your emotions ("Will I ever stop crying during those silly insurance commercials?") to the state of your sexual union ("Will I ever want to do 'it' again?") to the state of your waist ("Will I ever be able to wear jeans that zip?"). The answers: yes, yes, and yes—just give it time.

What You May Be Feeling

The first 6 weeks postpartum are considered a "recovery" period. Even if you sailed through your pregnancy and had the easiest labor and delivery on record (and especially if you didn't), your body has still been stretched and stressed to the max—and it needs a chance to regroup. Every new mom, like every expectant one, is different—so all will make that recovery at a different rate, with a different collection of postpartum symptoms. Depending on the type of delivery you had, how much help you have at home, and a variety of other individual factors, you may experience all, or only some, of the following:

Physically

- Continued lochia, first dark red, then pink, turning brownish, then yellowish white

- Fatigue, of course

- Some continuing pain and numbness in the perineum, if you had a vaginal delivery (especially if you had stitches) or labored before having a cesarean delivery

- Diminishing incision pain, continuing numbness, if you had a c-section

- Gradual easing of constipation and, hopefully, hemorrhoids

- Gradual slimming of your belly as excess fluids are flushed out and your uterus shrinks and recedes into the pelvis

- Gradual weight loss

- Gradual decrease in swelling

- Breast discomfort and nipple soreness until breastfeeding is well established

- Backache (from weakened abdominal muscles and from carrying baby)

- Joint pain (from joints still loosened from pregnancy)

- Achiness in arms and neck (from carrying and feeding baby)

- Continued excessive sweating

- Continued hot flashes

- Hair loss

Emotionally

- Elation, moodiness, or swings between them

- A sense of being overwhelmed, a growing feeling of confidence, or swings between the two

- Little interest in sex or, less commonly, stepped-up desire

Expect the Unexpected Postpartum

Like pregnancy, the postpartum period can deliver a bundle of unexpected symptoms. For one, phantom kicks—occasionally feeling your baby kicking from the inside when (clearly) your baby is living on the outside. Or diaper rash (on you, not baby)—from wearing pads for so long (you can switch brands, use witch hazel pads, or even borrow baby's diaper rash cream). Postpartum hives, which can erupt days, weeks, or even months after delivery—even among moms who have never had an allergic reaction in their lives. These hives seem to be associated either with breastfeeding hormones or a postpartum immune reaction (ask your doctor for a treatment plan, which will probably include a breastfeeding-safe antihistamine). Another unexpected symptom that can affect breastfeeding moms postpartum: a fleeting feeling of sadness every time baby starts to suckle (see box, page 506, for more on this syndrome).

Stumbled on another symptom you didn't expect now that you're no longer expecting? Check out this and the previous chapter, and if you still can't figure out the trigger, check with your practitioner.

What You Can Expect at Your Postpartum Checkup

Your practitioner will probably schedule you for a checkup 4 to 6 weeks postpartum. (If you had a cesarean delivery, you may be asked to come in at about 2 to 3 weeks postpartum to have your incision looked at.) During your postpartum visit, you can expect the following to be checked, though the exact rundown of the visit will vary:

- Blood pressure

- Weight, which may be down by about 17 to 20 pounds

- Your uterus, to see if it has returned to prepregnant shape, size, and location

- Your cervix, which will be on its way back to its prepregnant state but will still be somewhat engorged

- Your vagina, which will have contracted and regained much of its muscle tone

- Any tear or episiotomy repair site

- Your incision site, if you had a cesarean delivery

- Your breasts, to check for lumps, redness, tenderness, cracked nipples, or any abnormal discharge

- Hemorrhoids or varicose veins, if you have either

- Your emotional state (screening for PPD)

- Questions or problems you want to discuss—have a list ready

At this visit, your practitioner will also discuss with you the method of birth control you're planning to use. See page 511 for birth control options.

What You May Be Wondering About

Exhaustion

"I knew I'd be tired after giving birth, but I haven't gotten any sleep in weeks, and I'm so beyond exhausted, it's not funny."

No one's laughing—especially none of the other sleep-deprived new parents out there. And no one's really wondering why you're so exhausted, either. After all, you're juggling endless feeding (especially if you're breastfeeding), burping, changing, rocking, and pacing. You're trying to tackle the mountain of laundry that seems to grow larger and more daunting each day and the pile of thank-you notes that never seem to get written. You're shopping (out of diapers—again?), and you're schlepping (who knew how much baby stuff you'd need to lug just to pick up milk at the supermarket?). And you're doing it all on an average of about 3 hours of sleep (if you're lucky) a night, with a body that's still recovering from childbirth. In other words, you have multiple good reasons why you're feeling like Our Lady of Perpetual Exhaustion.

Is there a cure for this maternal fatigue syndrome? Not really—at least not until baby starts sleeping through the night. But in the meantime, there are many ways of regaining some of your get-up-and-go—or at least enough so you can keep getting up and going:

Get some help. Hire help if you can afford to (a postpartum doula might be just the ticket). If you can't, now's a good time to let family and friends lend their helping hands. Enlist them to take baby out for a stroll while you grab a power nap or suggest that they pick up your groceries.

Share the load. Parenting—when there are two parents around—is a two-person job. Even if your partner-in-parenting is holding down a 9 to 5, he should share the baby load when he's home. Ditto the cleaning, laundry, cooking, and shopping. Together, divide and conquer the responsibilities, then write down who's on for what and when, so there's no confusion. (If you're a single parent or your partner is deployed, lean on a close friend or family member to help out.)

Don't sweat the small stuff. The only small stuff that matters right now is your baby. Everything else should take a distant backseat until you're feeling more energetic. So let the dust bunnies breed where they may (even if it's on top of those still-blank thank-you notes). And while you're ignoring those thank-you notes, buy some time by sending out a bulk email with baby's picture attached.

Find deliverance. Whether it's the hot meal you never have time to cook, or the baby nail clippers you forgot to buy, or the diapers you're forever running out of, there's an app for everything you need delivered to your door (except for a nap), so load up your phone and get busy.

Sleep when the baby sleeps. Yes, you've heard it before, and probably snorted at the thought. After all, baby's naptime is the only time you can tackle the 300 other things that never seem to get done. But stop snorting and start snoring. Lie down for even 15 minutes during one of the baby's daytime naps, and you'll feel better able to handle the crying when it starts again.

Feed your baby, feed yourself. Sure, you're busy feeding baby—but don't forget to feed yourself, too. Just as you did when you were expecting, fight fatigue by grazing on mini meals that combine protein and complex carbs to serve up long-term energy. Keep your fridge, your glove compartment, and your diaper bag stocked with grab-and-go snacks so you're never running on empty. While sugar and caffeine (that giant cupcake and that 5-shot latte, taken in quick succession) may seem the obvious solution for the energy challenged, remember this: Though they may give you the boost you crave in the short term, they'll quickly lead to an energy crash and burn. And don't just eat—drink plenty of water, too, because dehydration can lead to exhaustion.

If you're really beat, check with your practitioner to rule out any other physical cause (such as postpartum thyroiditis; see box, page 501). If you're feeling a little down, take steps to boost your mood (see page 495), because baby blues are tied to fatigue as well. If all else checks out and it's Diagnosis: New Mommy, rest assured (that is, when you can rest at all) that your zombie days are numbered. You will live to sleep again.

Hair Loss

"My hair seems to be falling out suddenly. Am I going bald?"

You're not going bald—you're just going back to normal. Ordinarily, the average head sheds 100 hairs a day (just not all at once, so you don't usually notice the shedding), and those hairs are being continually replaced. During pregnancy, however, hormonal changes keep those hairs from falling out, which means your head hangs on to them. But all good things must come to an end, including your reprieve on hair fall. All those hairs that were slated to go during pregnancy will be shed sometime after delivery, usually in the first 6 months postpartum—and often in unsettling clumps. Some women who are breastfeeding exclusively find that hair fall doesn't begin in earnest until they wean their baby or supplement with formula or solids. You'll take comfort knowing that by the time your baby is ready to blow out the candles on that 1st birthday cake (and probably has a full head of hair of his or her own), your hair should be back to normal-for-you.

To keep your hair healthy, continue taking your prenatal supplement (or switch to a supplement designed for breastfeeding moms if you're nursing), eat well, and treat your mane humanely. That means shampooing only when necessary (as if you had time for any extra shampoos now), using a wide-toothed comb or detangling brush if you have to untangle, not frying your hair with curling or flat irons (as if you have the time to style it, anyway), and using soft scrunchies or gentle clips to put up your mom-do.

Talk to your practitioner if your hair loss seems really excessive, since that can be a symptom of postpartum thyroiditis (see box, page 501).

By the way, if you also had a reprieve from waxing and shaving during pregnancy—because hair stopped growing on your legs, under your arms, and other places you typically keep groomed—that party may be over. Unfortunately, hair will probably resume its growth in the places you'd prefer it didn't. However, if you had a fuzzy belly or extra facial hair throughout your pregnancy, you'll likely be shedding that soon, thankfully.

Postpartum Urinary Incontinence

"I gave birth nearly 2 months ago and I'm still peeing when I cough or laugh. Am I ever going to stop leaking?"

So your new-mom bladder is letting you—and your panties—down? It's completely normal to involuntarily leak a little urine in the months (yes, months) after delivery, usually while laughing, sneezing, coughing, or performing any strenuous activity—and it's pretty common (more than a third of moms spring a postpartum leak). That's because pregnancy, labor, and delivery weaken the muscles around the bladder and pelvis, making it harder for you to control the flow of urine. Plus, as your uterus shrinks in the weeks after delivery, it sits directly on the bladder, compressing it and making it more difficult to stem the tide. Hormonal changes after pregnancy can also batter your bladder.

It can take between 3 and 6 months, or even longer, to regain complete bladder control. Until then, use panty liners, maxipads, or bladder control pads to absorb the leak (depending on how much you're leaking). You can also take these steps to help regain control faster:

Keep up your Kegels. Thought you were finished with your Kegels now

Help for Leaks That Won't Let Up

Tried every do-it-yourself trick for dealing with postpartum urinary or fecal incontinence—including Kegeling until you're blue in the face—but still left with a leak? Don't let embarrassment keep you from talking to your practitioner. He or she might suggest biofeedback (see page 82), other treatments (such as physical therapy), or in a particularly tough case, eventual surgery. Fortunately, leaks usually resolve themselves without that kind of intervention.

that your baby's delivered? You'll actually need them more than ever to speed your recovery. Among other perks: Continuing those pelvic-floor–strengthening exercises will help you regain bladder control now and preserve it later on in life.

Start losing it. Extra pounds gained during pregnancy are still applying pressure to your bladder. Once you've reached the 6-week mark, start shedding weight sensibly to take that pressure off.

Train your bladder to behave. Pee every 30 minutes—before you have the urge—and then try to extend the time between pees, going (without going) a few more minutes each day.

Stay regular. Try to avoid constipation, so full bowels don't put pressure on your bladder.

Drink up. It might seem that cutting back on fluids would cut down on the leaking, but dehydration makes you vulnerable to UTIs. An infected bladder is

more likely to leak, and a leaking bladder is more likely to become infected. When reaching for the fluids, however, consider limiting caffeine, since too much can irritate the urinary tract.

Tired of pulling out pads to absorb all those leaks, or not crazy about graduating to the bladder leak variety? Another option once you've completely finished your postpartum healing (check with your practitioner first): a bladder-support product—a specially designed tampon-like product that's inserted vaginally to gently lift and support the urethra to prevent leaks (don't use real tampons). Leak won't let up? See box, this page.

Fecal Incontinence

"I've been passing gas involuntarily lately and even leaking some feces, which is gross. What can I do about it?"

As a new mother, you definitely expected to be cleaning up after your baby—but you probably didn't count on cleaning up after yourself. Yet some newly delivered moms do add fecal incontinence and the involuntary passing of gas to that long list of unpleasant postpartum symptoms. That's because during labor and childbirth, the muscles and nerves in the pelvic area are stretched and sometimes damaged, which can make it difficult for you to control how and when waste (and wind) leaves your body. In most cases, the problem takes care of itself as the muscles and nerves recover, usually within a few weeks.

Until then, skip hard-to-digest foods (nothing fried, no beans, no cabbage), and avoid overeating or eating on the run (the more air you gulp, the more you are likely to pass it as gas). Keeping up with your Kegels can also help tighten up those slack muscles as well as the ones that control urine (which also may be leaking these days). Check in with your practitioner about it, too. If fecal leaking continues, you may want to ask for a referral to a physical therapist for pelvic floor therapy.

Postpartum Backache

"I thought all my back pain would go away after delivery, but it hasn't. Why?"

Welcome back, backache. If you're like nearly half of all newly delivered moms, your old not-so-friendly pal from pregnancy has returned for an unwelcome visit. Some of the pain still has the same cause—hormonally loosened ligaments that haven't yet tightened up. It may take time, and several weeks of soreness, before these ligaments regain their strength. Ditto for the stretched-out and weakened abdominal muscles that altered your posture during pregnancy, putting strain on your back. And of course, now that you've got a baby around, there's another reason for that pain in your back: all the lifting, bending, rocking, feeding, and toting you're doing. Especially as that cute little load you're carrying around gets bigger and heavier, your back will be up against growing stress and strain. One thing that you can't blame your backache on: an epidural. Research shows that lingering back pain beyond the first postpartum days isn't related to having had an epidural.

While time heals most things, including those postpartum aches and pains, there are other ways to get your back back on track:

- Tone that tummy. Ease into some undemanding exercises to strengthen the muscles that support your back (see page 520 for more).

- Get support. Use a belly binder, belt, band, or compression shorts to help support your abdominal muscles, easing back pain.

- Mend when you bend. And lift. Give your back a break by bending properly: Spread your feet apart to give yourself a wide base of support, bend at your knees (not your waist), tighten your core as you lift (or lower), lift using your leg muscles, and hold the object as close to your body as you can. If an object is too heavy or awkward, don't lift it.

- Get off your feet. Sure, you're running (and rocking) all the time, but whenever you don't have to, take a seat. When you have to stand, place one foot on a low stool to take some pressure off your back.

- Put your feet up. Who deserves to put their feet up more than you? Plus, elevating your feet slightly when sitting—and baby feeding—will ease the strain on your back.

- Don't be a slouch on the couch. When feeding your baby, don't slump over (as tempting as that might be, given your state of exhaustion). Your back will thank you if it's well supported.

- Watch your posture. Listen to your mom, Mom—and stand up straight, even when you're swaying from side to side. Slouched shoulders result in an aching back. As your baby gets bigger, avoid resting that growing weight on one hip, which will throw your back off further, plus lead to hip pain.

- Wear your baby. Instead of always holding your baby, wear him or her in a sling or wrap. Not only will it be soothing to baby (and you), but it'll be a relief to your achy back and arms.

- Pull a switch. Many moms play favorites with their arms, always carrying (or bottle-feeding) baby in the left arm or the right. Instead, alternate arms so they each get a workout (and you don't get a lopsided ache).

■ Rub it. Can't spare the time and change for the professional massage your muscles are aching for? Ask your spouse to step in and rub.

■ Turn up the heat. A heating pad can spell relief from back pain and muscle aches. Apply it often, especially during those marathon feeding sessions. Ask your practitioner (or the baby's pediatrician) whether it's okay to use topical creams or heat patches if you're breastfeeding. You'll probably get the green light, but it's good to ask, just to be on the safe side.

As your body adjusts to toting a baby all the time, you'll probably find that pain in your back (and arms, and hips, and neck) diminishing, and you may even find yourself sporting some new baby biceps. In the meantime, here's something else that might help ease your aches by easing your load: Unload that diaper bag. Lug around only what you absolutely need, which is plenty heavy anyway.

Baby Blues

"I was sure I'd be over the moon once my baby was born. But I'm feeling down instead. What's going on?"

How can something so happy make you feel so sad? That's what an estimated 60 to 80 percent of new moms end up asking themselves soon after childbirth, thanks to so-called baby blues. Baby blues appear seemingly out of the blue—usually 3 to 5 days after delivery, but sometimes a little earlier or a little later—bringing on unexpected sadness and irritability, bouts of crying, restlessness, and anxiety. Unexpected

FOR FATHERS

Your Baby Blues

Becoming a dad was the happiest moment of your life—and holding your bundle of joy fills you with more joy than you even knew was possible. So why are you so emotionally spent? After all that buildup, all the planning and preparation and dreaming and drama and anticipation and exhilaration, your child has been born, and you feel not only run down (that's the sleep deprivation talking) but also a tiny bit let down. Welcome to the Postpartum Club, when you suddenly realize why the word "baby" is so often followed by the word "blues." Not every new parent experiences the so-called baby blues (about 10 percent of new dads do), but you can pretty predictably expect a potent cocktail of emotions in both of you (fortunately, it's likely only one of you will experience down feelings at a time). Be ready. And be strong. You'll need the patience of a saint, the endurance of a triathlete, and a sense of humor (big time) to work through this period of adjustment. Adapt the tips for her baby blues (on these pages) to your needs during this rough patch. If those don't help, and baby blues progress to depression, talk to your doctor about getting the help you need so you can start enjoying life with your new baby.

because—well, for one thing, isn't having a baby supposed to make you over the moon, not down in the dumps?

It's actually easy to understand why you're feeling this way if you step back for a moment and take an objective look at what's been going on in your life, your body, and your psyche, including any or all of the following: rapid changes in hormone levels (which drop precipitously after child-birth) and a draining delivery followed by an exhausting homecoming, all compounded by the round-the-clock demands of newborn care, sleep deprivation, possible feelings of new mommy self-doubt, breastfeeding stumbling blocks (sore nipples, painful engorgement), unhappiness over your looks (the bags under your eyes, the pooch around your belly, the fact that there are more dimples on your thighs than on your baby's), and stress from inevitably shifting relationship dynamics. With such an overwhelming laundry list of challenges to confront (and don't even get you started on the laundry that's on that list), it's no wonder you're feeling down.

The baby blues will likely fade over the next couple of weeks as you adjust to your new life and start getting a little more rest—or, more realistically, begin functioning more effectively on less rest. In the meantime, try the following tips to help lift yourself out of that postpartum slump:

Lower the bar. Feeling overwhelmed and underprepared in your role as a newbie mom? It may help to remember that you won't be for long. After just a few weeks on the job, you're likely to feel much more comfortable in those mom shoes. In the meantime, lower your expectations for yourself—and for your baby. Then lower them some more. Make this your mommy (or daddy) mantra, even after you've become a parenting pro: There's no such thing as a perfect parent. Expecting too much means you'll be letting yourself down—and bringing your mood down, too. Instead, just do the best you can (which at this point may not be as well as you'd like, but that's okay).

Don't go it alone. Nothing is more depressing than being left alone with a crying newborn, that mountain of spit-up-stained laundry, a leaning tower of dirty dishes, and the promise (make that guarantee) of another sleep-deprived night ahead. So if it's feasible, ask for more help—from your partner, your mother, your sister, your friends.

Dress yourself. Yes, you're busy dressing (and diapering) your baby—but have you forgotten to dress yourself? It sounds trite, but it's surprisingly true. Spending a little time making yourself look good will actually help you feel good—even if baby's the only one seeing you all day. So hit the shower and maybe even the blow-dryer before your spouse hits the commuter train in the morning, trade in the stained sweats for a clean pair, and consider applying a little makeup (and a lot of concealer).

Wear your baby. Babywearing can boost your mood and baby's (babies who are worn more cry less, and that's a happy fact). See box, facing page.

Leave home. It's amazing what a change of scenery can do for your state of mind—especially when the scenery doesn't include the cluttered mess that was once your home. So try to get out of the house with baby at least once a day: Take a walk, stroll the mall, grab a coffee with friends. Anything that will keep you from hosting another (understandable) self-pity party.

Treat yourself. Next time you have 30 minutes to yourself, grab it. Take a nap, a long shower, a mini-mani, or a chance to catch up on social media or a guilty pleasure celebrity gossip site. Occasionally, make yourself a priority. You deserve it.

Get moving. Exercise boosts those feel-good endorphins, giving you an all-natural (and surprisingly lasting) high. So join a postpartum exercise class (look for one that includes babies in the fun), work out to a post-pregnancy

Wearing Away the Baby Blues

There's no doubt it's the ultimate in hands-free baby care, allowing you to soothe your baby, rock your baby, even eventually feed your baby without lifting a finger—leaving your hands and arms available for just about anything else you have to get done. But can babywearing (wearing your little one in a sling or carrier) also wear away the baby blues in new moms (and dads)? Or even help ease postpartum depression?

Some say yes—and for several reasons:

- Wearing your baby close to you (like skin-to-skin contact) increases your levels of oxytocin, one of the body's happiest hormones. Also known as the "bonding hormone," oxytocin not only helps cement your emotional connection to your baby, but relieves stress and eases postpartum aches—both of which can bring a new mama down. In fact, low levels of oxytocin have been linked to postpartum depression, as well as postpartum anxiety disorders. Pumping up the oxytocin by wearing your baby may actually boost your mood.

- Wearing your baby makes your baby happier. Babies who are worn more cry less and sleep and feed better—and what could make a new parent happier (and more confident) than that?

- Wearing your baby leaves your arms and legs free—free to eat a meal, catch up on work, get the laundry done, and yes, even do your hair (your hair!). All of which can make you feel better.

- Wearing your baby lets you get out more. There's no easier way to take a walk, do the marketing, have lunch with a friend. Plus, a baby who's worn isn't easily touched by prying (possibly germy) strangers—an added perk.

Of course, if babywearing isn't for you—you just don't feel comfortable doing it—don't feel obligated. Remember, every mom is different—and what feels right for you is almost always what's best for you. Keep in mind, too, that while babywearing may be very therapeutic for new moms battling the baby blues or even mild depression or anxiety, it may not be the answer for every mom, and it's likely not enough to treat more serious postpartum depression.

exercise DVD or a YouTube video, step out for some exercises that tone with the help of a stroller full of baby, or just simply step out for a walk.

Be a happy snacker. Too often, new moms are too busy filling their babies' tummies to worry about filling their own. A mistake, since low blood sugar sends not only energy levels plummeting but moods, too. To keep yourself on a more even keel, physically and emotionally, stash sustaining, healthy, easy-to-munch snacks within quick reach. Tempted to reach for a chocolate bar instead? Go ahead and reach—especially if chocolate really makes you happy—just remember sugar-induced blood sugar highs have a way of crashing quickly. (Opt for dark chocolate when you can, since it's much lower in sugar and is believed to have mood-boosting properties.)

Cry—and laugh. If you need a good cry, go for it. But when you're finished, watch something silly on TV or online and laugh. Try laughing, too, at all the mishaps you're likely having—you know, the diaper blowout, the breasts that leaked in line at the market, the spit-up that spewed only after you realized you had left home without wipes. You know what they say: Laughter is the best medicine. Plus, a good sense of humor is a parent's best friend.

Still blue, no matter what you do? Keep on reminding yourself that you'll outgrow the baby blues within a week or two—most moms do—and you'll be enjoying the best of times, most of the time, in no time.

But also remember that there's a big—and very significant—difference between baby blues and postpartum depression. If the baby blues just don't fade, or appear later than expected, if feelings of sadness persist (lasting more than 2 weeks) or get worse, and/or if you start to feel very anxious, you may be suffering from postpartum depression.

"I don't have any sign of baby blues—but my partner seems really down. Could he have baby blues?"

Does your partner seem to be down while you're flying high? Studies show that a new dad is far more likely to experience baby blues when the new mom in his life escapes them (and conversely, he's unlikely to be down when she is—perhaps nature's way of ensuring that both parents don't slump at the same time). Hormonal changes (dads experience those, too, postpartum) may be a trigger when dad gets the blues, as may all the inevitable life changes that come with a new baby. Either way, it's important that he not keep his feelings under wraps, something a new dad may feel compelled to do to avoid dumping on his spouse. Encourage him to talk them out—and to see the box, page 495.

Postpartum Depression

"I felt so happy after we brought our baby home. But in the last couple of weeks, I've started feeling really down. Sad, hopeless even. Should I write it off as baby blues?"

Though "baby blues" and "postpartum depression" are often used interchangeably to describe new mom moodiness, they're actually two very different conditions. The far more common baby blues appear and fade quickly. True postpartum depression (PPD) is much less prevalent (affecting about 15 percent of new moms) and much more enduring (lasting anywhere from a few weeks to a year or even more). It may have roots in pregnancy depression, it may begin at delivery, or (more often) it may not start until a month or two after baby's born. Sometimes PPD comes far later—it doesn't begin until a new mom gets her first postpartum period or until she weans her nursing baby (possibly because of fluctuating hormones). More susceptible to PPD are women who've had it before, have a history of depression or severe PMS, spent a lot of time feeling down or depressed during pregnancy, had a complicated pregnancy or delivery, or have a premature or sick baby. Women who have had a miscarriage or stillbirth are more susceptible to postpartum depression (and anxiety) with a subsequent healthy delivery, often because they can't shake the feeling that something will go wrong again.

The symptoms of PPD are similar to those of baby blues, though much more pronounced. They include crying and irritability, sleep problems (not being able to sleep or wanting to sleep the day away), eating problems (having no appetite or wanting to do nothing but eat), persistent feelings of sadness,

Keep an Eye on Her Mood

Baby blues are one thing (they're normal and self-limiting), but true postpartum depression (PPD) is another. It's a serious medical condition that requires prompt, professional treatment. The same goes for other postpartum mood disorders, including postpartum anxiety disorder, postpartum OCD, post-partum PTSD, and postpartum psychosis. If the mom in your life still seems truly overwhelmed, sad, angry, anxious, or hopeless several weeks after the baby comes home, isn't sleeping or is sleeping all the time, won't leave the house or let anyone come over to visit, isn't eating or isn't otherwise functioning normally—as normally as can be expected given her demanding new mom life—sit down with her and tell her you're worried about her wellbeing. Focus on the behaviors you've seen—crying constantly, raging for no apparent reason, refusing to leave the house or answer the phone, being uncharacteristically anxious, jittery, or stressed, not interacting well with the baby—and encourage her to share her feelings with you. Reassure her that whatever she's going through is in no way her fault—it's not because she's weak or a bad mother. And remind her that you are and will be there to support her every step of the way. Emotional support from a partner is an essential component in the recovery from PPD.

But don't stop there. Encourage her to talk to her practitioner about it and, as needed, to get a referral to a psychotherapist or psychologist. Don't leave it up to her if she says no—make the calls yourself. She may not recognize the signs of depression. Be sure you know the signs (see facing page), and understand that she may not experience all of the symptoms (postpartum depression and anxiety are not one-size-fits-all illnesses). Make sure she gets the treatment she needs to feel better, and be as supportive as you can of the treatment plan that's proposed. If one treatment method doesn't work (and it won't necessarily, at least at first), encourage her to be open to others—and not to give up. PPD is treatable, but finding the right treatment sometimes takes time.

And though much of your focus will understandably be on your partner as you try to help her get better, realize that—for now—she may not be up to much, or (in a severe case of PPD) any of the baby care. Step in to provide the nurturing your newborn needs, and if you can't provide it all because of your work schedule, try to find a friend or family member (or baby nurse, if you can afford one) to fill in as needed. Keep in mind that it's normal for you to feel frustrated or disappointed that your partner isn't over the moon happy in her new role with your new baby—so don't fault yourself for feeling that way. Find ways to give yourself a break, too, and remember there are other dads who know exactly what you're going through. Check out the support pages for dad on postpartum.net.

Be aware, too, that dads can also suffer from PPD. Your own hormones are in flux postpartum, too, and it's natural for the combination of the new baby, the stress of the past 9 months, and the new sense of responsibility to take their toll. In fact, 1 in 4 dads experience paternal postnatal depression (PPND), a dad's version of PPD. You may feel left out, or you may feel overwhelmed by everything that's expected of you. If you suspect you have PPND, talk to your partner or a trusted friend or family member about it, and don't hesitate to seek professional treatment—for the health and wellbeing of both you and your baby.

Getting Help for PPD

No new mother should have to suffer from PPD. Sadly, too many do, either because they believe it's normal and inevitable after delivery (it isn't) or because they're ashamed to ask for help (they shouldn't be). PPD can keep a new mom from nurturing her little one, which could lead to slower development (babies of depressed moms are less vocal, less active, make fewer facial expressions, and are more anxious, passive, and withdrawn).

Luckily, there is more and more awareness about PPD and the need for new moms who are suffering from it to get the help and treatment they need. Most hospitals send new moms home with educational materials about PPD so that they (and just as important, their partners and other family members) will be more likely to spot the symptoms early and seek treatment. Practitioners are becoming better informed, too—learning how to look for risk factors during pregnancy that might predispose a woman to PPD, to screen routinely for the illness postpartum, and to treat it quickly, safely, and successfully.

Pediatricians—who have many more opportunities to interact with new moms than obs or midwives do—are often the first line of defense when it comes to spotting PPD. The AAP recommends that pediatricians screen for PPD at 1-, 2-, and 4-month visits by asking new moms to complete a short checklist called the Edinburgh Postnatal Depression Scale—basically 10 questions designed to reveal whether a new mother is struggling with PPD.

PPD is one of the most treatable forms of depression. So if it strikes you, don't suffer with it any longer than you have to. Speak up—and get the help you need now. For more help, contact Postpartum Support International at 800-944-4PPD (4773) or postpartum.net.

---

emptiness, hopelessness, and helplessness, an inability (or lack of desire) to take care of yourself or your newborn, social withdrawal, excessive worry, aversion to your newborn, feeling all alone, and memory loss.

If you haven't already tried the tips for getting the baby blues to fade (see page 496), do try them now. Some of them may be helpful in easing PPD, too. But if moderate symptoms continue for more than 2 weeks without any noticeable improvement, or if you're having more serious symptoms for more than a few days, chances are your PPD won't go away without professional attention. Don't wait to see if it does (and don't delay at all if you're having symptoms that might result in harm to yourself or your baby). And don't be put off by reassurances that such feelings are normal postpartum—they're not. Call your practitioner and be up front about how you're feeling. Ask for a referral to a therapist who has a clinical background in the treatment of PPD, and make an appointment promptly. Therapy, the first line of defense, can help you feel better fast, and if your therapist thinks medications will help, too, there are several antidepressants that are safe even if you're breastfeeding (though it can take time to figure out the right meds at the right dose). Bright light therapy can also be effective in reducing symptoms of PPD by causing a positive biochemical change in your brain that can cheer you up. Other CAM therapies, healthy

Thyroiditis Got You Down?

Nearly all new mothers feel run-down and tired. Most have trouble losing weight. Many feel blue at least some of the time, and just about all experience hair loss. It may not be a pretty picture, but for the majority of moms, it's a completely normal one in postpartum—and one that gradually begins to look better as the weeks pass. For the estimated 7 to 8 percent of women who suffer from postpartum thyroiditis (PPT), however, this picture may not improve with time. And, because the symptoms of PPT are so similar to those weathered by most new moms, the condition may go undiagnosed and untreated.

PPT may start anywhere from 1 to 4 months after delivery with a brief episode of hyperthyroidism (too much thyroid hormone). This period of excess thyroid hormone circulating in the bloodstream may last 2 to 8 weeks. During this hyperthyroid period, a new mom may be tired, irritable, and nervous, feel very overheated, and experience increased sweating and insomnia—all of which are common in the immediate postpartum period anyway, making an easy diagnosis more elusive. That's okay, because treatment isn't usually needed for this phase.

In about 25 percent of women with PPT, this hyperthyroid period will be followed by one of hypothyroidism (too little thyroid hormone) that often lasts about 2 to 6 months. With hypothyroidism, fatigue continues, along with depression (longer lasting and often more severe than typical baby blues), muscle aches, excessive hair loss, dry skin, cold intolerance, poor memory, and an inability to lose weight. Again, so close to typical new mom symptoms that they may be easy to write off as postpartum-as-usual.

Some new moms with PPT experience only hyperthyroidism, while others have only hypothyroidism, which begins 2 to 6 months after delivery.

If your postpartum symptoms seem to be more pronounced and persistent than you would have expected, and especially if they are interfering with your ability to function and enjoy your baby, check with your practitioner. A blood test can easily determine whether PPT is the cause of your symptoms. Be sure to mention any personal history of thyroid problems or a family history (especially on your mom's side of the family, since there is a very strong genetic link).

Most women recover from PPT within a year after delivery. In the meantime, treatment with supplementary thyroid hormone can help them feel much better much faster. About 25 percent of women who have the condition, however, remain hypothyroid, requiring lifetime treatment (which is as easy as taking a pill every day and having a yearly blood test). Even in those who recover spontaneously, thyroiditis is likely to recur during or after subsequent pregnancies. For this reason, it makes sense for women who have had PPT to have a yearly thyroid screening and, if they are planning another pregnancy, to be screened in the preconception period and during pregnancy (because an untreated thyroid condition can interfere with conception and cause problems during pregnancy).

eating, and exercise can also help minimize symptoms, as can babywearing (see box, page 497). Since postpartum thyroiditis can trigger depression (see box above), your practitioner may also want to check your thyroid levels. The

Beyond Postpartum Depression

New moms often have ups and downs, occasional moments of feeling overwhelmed and stressed, even anxious—and most do more than their share of unnecessary worrying. For the most part, that's the adjustment talking—and the sleep deprivation. And it's to be expected.

But sometimes, it's not as easy as that—or as normal. Postpartum mood disorders are distinctly different from typical new mom mood swings—and they come in many forms, sometimes accompanying PPD or appearing instead of it. All the following postpartum mood disorders need prompt diagnosis and treatment. If you notice any symptoms of these conditions, don't delay in getting the help you need:

Postpartum anxiety disorder. Some new moms, instead of (or in addition to) feeling depressed postpartum, feel extremely anxious or fearful, sometimes experiencing panic attacks that include rapid heartbeat and breathing, hot or cold flashes, chest pain, nausea, insomnia, dizziness, and shaking. Women with a history of anxiety or panic attacks (during pregnancy or before) are more likely to experience these symptoms postpartum.

Postpartum anxiety affects about 10 percent of new moms, and about half of those who have PPD will also experience postpartum anxiety. A mom with postpartum anxiety may feel a constant sense of dread—as if something is about to go terribly wrong. Or she'll worry constantly about her baby's health and development, her ability to parent well, and how she's going to balance parenting and the rest of her responsibilities at work and home. These worries aren't the normal new mom worries (they're more extreme) and are typically not based on any real problem or threat. For instance, a mom suffering from postpartum anxiety may be fearful that her baby is alarmingly sick or in pain every time he or she cries. Or that she might fall asleep while holding her baby and drop him or her. Or have a pervasive, nagging fear that her baby has died or that she's left her baby in the hot car or that someone is going to break into the house and kidnap her sleeping baby. Sometimes a new mom suffering from postpartum anxiety may feel restless and jittery all the time—even though she's exhausted. Postpartum anxiety, like PPD, requires prompt treatment by a qualified therapist. Such treatment may include therapy (talk or cognitive behavioral therapy), learning techniques such as meditation, relaxation exercises, and mindfulness training, and, if necessary, medication.

Postpartum obsessive-compulsive disorder (PPOCD). About 30 percent of women suffering from PPD also exhibit signs of postpartum obsessive-compulsive disorder (PPOCD), though PPOCD can also occur by itself. Symptoms of PPOCD include obsessive-compulsive behaviors, such as waking up every 15 minutes to make sure the baby is still breathing, developing an obsessive order for doing ordinary

same tips that are used to deal with pregnancy depression (see page 44) apply to PPD as well.

Whichever treatment (or combination of treatments) you and your therapist decide is right for you—and even if it takes time to figure out the best treatment in your case—the most important first step is the one you're taking: acknowledging that you're tasks (like tapping on the light switch 3 times before turning it on) and worrying that straying from the order will cause her baby harm, furious housecleaning, or having obsessive thoughts about harming her newborn (such as throwing the baby out the window or dropping him or her down the stairs). Women suffering from PPOCD are horrified by their gruesome and violent thoughts, though they won't act on them (only those suffering from postpartum psychosis might; see below). Still, they can be so afraid of losing control and following through with these impulses that they may end up neglecting their babies. Like PPD, treatment for PPOCD includes a combination of therapy and antidepressants. If you're having obsessive thoughts and/or behaviors, be sure to get help by telling your practitioner about your symptoms.

Postpartum psychosis. Much more rare and much more serious than PPD is postpartum psychosis. Its symptoms include loss of reality, hallucinations, and/or delusions. If you're experiencing suicidal, violent, or aggressive feelings, are hearing voices or seeing things, or have other signs of psychosis, call your doctor and go to the emergency room immediately. Don't underplay what you're feeling, and don't be put off by reassurances that such feelings are normal postpartum—they're not. To be sure you don't act out any dangerous feelings if you're alone while you're waiting for help, try to get a neighbor, relative, or friend to stay with you or put your baby in a safe place (such as the crib). You can also call 911 or the National Suicide Prevention Hotline at 1-800-273-8255.

(If you're a dad noticing symptoms of postpartum psychosis in your spouse, get her help immediately—and in the meantime, don't leave her alone with the baby for even a moment.)

Postpartum Post Traumatic Stress Disorder (P-PTSD). The safe delivery of a healthy baby should be a moment to remember with joy. But for the estimated 9 percent of new moms who suffer from P-PTSD, childbirth becomes a source of pain and anxiety. Triggered by a traumatic event during labor, delivery, or postpartum (such as an umbilical cord prolapse, shoulder dystocia, a severe tear, hemorrhage, or an emergency c-section) or by a perceived trauma (feelings of being powerless or not having adequate support during childbirth), P-PTSD can leave a new mom with flashbacks and nightmares that vividly replay (and possibly magnify) the traumatic birth. Or she may feel detached from her baby and others, have difficulty sleeping, anxiety and panic attacks, an exaggerated startle response, and disturbing, intrusive thoughts. Women with a history of depression, anxiety, or prior trauma (a sexual assault, for instance, or a terrible car accident) are at higher risk of developing P-PTSD. P-PTSD is temporary and treatable—usually with therapy—so if you're experiencing any of the symptoms of the condition, don't wait to seek professional help. Without treatment, new moms suffering from P-PTSD are less likely to get routine postpartum care, less likely to breastfeed, and more likely to have challenges bonding with and caring for their newborns.

depressed and seeking help. Without the right treatment, PPD can prevent you from bonding with, caring for, and enjoying your baby. It can also have a devastating effect on your baby's emotional, social, and physical development (see box, facing page), on the other relationships in your life, and on your own health and wellbeing.

Losing Weight Postpartum

"I knew I wouldn't be ready for my skinny jeans right after delivery, but I still look 6 months pregnant 2 weeks later."

Loved your pregnancy bump, but not such a fan now that you're no longer pregnant? Though childbirth produces more rapid weight loss than any fad diet (an average of 12 pounds overnight), most new moms don't find it rapid enough. Particularly once they catch a glimpse of their still pregnant-looking postpartum profiles in the mirror.

The fact is, no one comes out of the delivery room looking all that much slimmer than when they went in. Part of the reason for that protruding postpartum belly is your still-enlarged uterus, which will be reduced to prepregnancy size and relocated to its previous pelvic position by the end of 6 weeks, shrinking your girth in the process. Another reason for your belly bloat might be leftover fluids, which should be getting flushed out soon. And then there are those stretched-out abdominal muscles and skin, which will likely take some effort to tone up—plus a few extra fat stores that helped nurture your baby during pregnancy (and are still nurturing baby if you're breastfeeding).

As hard as it might be to put it out of your mind, don't even think about the shape your body's in during the first 6 weeks, especially if you're breastfeeding. This is a recovery period, during which ample nutrition is important for your energy, mood, resistance to infection, and general wellbeing.

Sticking to a healthy postpartum diet should start you on the way to slow, steady weight loss for now. If, after 6 weeks, you aren't losing any weight, you can start cutting back sensibly on calories. If you're breastfeeding, don't go overboard. Eating too few calories can reduce milk production, and burning fat too quickly can release toxins into the blood, which can end up in your breast milk. If you're not breastfeeding, you can aim to lose weight somewhat faster once you've passed the 6-week mark, but stick to diets that are well balanced and provide enough calories to fuel the energy every new mom needs.

Some women find that the extra pounds melt off while they're breastfeeding, while others are bummed to find the scale doesn't budge. If the latter turns out to be the case with you, don't worry—you'll be able to shed any remaining weight once you've weaned your baby.

How quickly you return to your prepregnant weight will also depend on how many pounds you put on during pregnancy. If you didn't gain much more than 25 to 35 pounds, you'll likely be able to pack away those maternity jeans in a few months, without strenuous dieting. If you gained 35 or more pounds, you may find it takes more effort and more time—anywhere from 10 months to 2 years—to return to prepregnancy weight and your skinny jeans.

Either way, give yourself a break—and give yourself some time. Remember, it took you 9 months to gain that pregnancy weight, and it may take at least that long to take it off.

C-Section Recovery, Continued

"It's been a week since my c-section. What can I expect now?"

While you've definitely come a long way since you were wheeled into recovery, like every new mom, you're still in recovery mode. And like every mom who's had a c-section, you're recovering not only from pregnancy and childbirth, but from surgery. You'll recover faster if you follow your doctor's instructions both for post-op and for all those things new moms aren't known for in general (getting enough rest and not overdoing it come to mind). In the meantime you can expect:

Progressive improvement in pain. Most of the pain should dissipate by the end of the first 6 weeks (though some moms experience occasional pain and other twinges much longer, even months later). Your scar will be sore and sensitive for the first few weeks, but it should improve steadily. Occasional sensations of pulling or twitching and other brief pains around the incision site are a normal part of healing and eventually subside. Itchiness around and on the scar (another normal—if extra annoying—part of the healing process) may follow. If it does, ask your practitioner to recommend an anti-itch ointment that you can apply. The numbness surrounding the scar will last longer, possibly several months. Lumpiness in the scar tissue will probably diminish, and the scar may turn pink or purple before it finally fades.

Narcotics during the first 2 weeks after birth are considered okay in safe doses if you feel you need them, but acetaminophen (Tylenol) or ibuprofen (Advil) should do the trick after the first week, so try to wean yourself off any pain meds as quickly as you're able, particularly if you're breastfeeding. If pain at the incision site gets worse, or if the area around the incision turns an angry red, or if a brown, gray, green, or yellow discharge oozes from the wound, call your doctor. The incision may have become infected. (A small amount of clear fluid discharge is usually normal, but report it to your doctor anyway.)

You may find that wearing a belly band or other type of postpartum support system can help minimize pain while giving support to your healing incision and shrinking abdomen.

A 4-week wait (at least) for sex. The guidelines are pretty much the same as they are for those who've delivered vaginally (yes, even though your baby didn't exit vaginally), though how well your incision is healing may also be factored into how long you'll need (and want) to wait. See page 507 for more on resuming sex.

To get moving. Ease your way back to exercise with a 5-minute walk a few times a week starting as soon as you feel up to it, building up to low-impact workouts after the first 5 to 6 weeks. Once you reenter the world of workouts, do it gradually, building up as your stamina does—but also try for consistency (if you're looking for results, occasional workouts won't cut it). As you're working your way back to your old exercise routine, concentrate on exercises that tighten the abs (see page 520), but be sure to start off slow. Expect it to take several months at least before you're able to work out the way you did pre-baby. And remember, Kegels are still important even if you delivered with your perineum intact, because pregnancy took its toll on those pelvic floor muscles, even if childbirth didn't.

Breast Infection

"I've got a lot of pain and redness in one of my breasts and I'm running a fever. Do I have an infection?"

Sounds like mama has mastitis—a breast infection that can happen anytime during lactation but is most common between the 2nd and 6th week postpartum. What causes it? Often a combination of germs entering the milk ducts through a crack in the nipple,

Feeling Down with Let-Down

There's nothing more joyful than putting your baby to breast—that rush of oxytocin, the feel-good hormone, as it courses through your veins, filling your baby with nourishment and you with blissful, peaceful pleasure.

But what if that's not what you feel at all each time baby latches on? What if you feel—instead of that expected happiness and serenity—a fleeting moment of sadness, agitation, dread, guilt, anger, or resentment? Feelings that pass quickly but leave you unsettled, wondering what could be triggering such an unexpected response to breastfeeding?

It's little known and discussed, but a small percentage of breastfeeding moms suffer from Dysphoric Milk Ejection Reflex (D-MER)—a rare condition in which the milk let-down reflex itself brings on a range of negative emotions. The emotions begin immediately before the milk lets down and last anywhere from 30 seconds to a few minutes.

Experts say D-MER isn't psychological (it's not an aversion to breastfeeding, and it's not related to postpartum depression), rather it's a physiological hormonal response, related to the sudden decrease in the brain chemical dopamine (responsible for mood stabilizing and happy thoughts) immediately before milk let-down.

So what can you do if you're experiencing D-MER? First, know that the condition will pass—gradually improving and eventually disappearing (likely by the time baby's 6 months old). Second, remember that those negative emotions don't represent your true feelings—they're just a momentary hormonal response. Moms with D-MER (unlike moms with PPD) feel fine throughout the rest of the day. Understanding what is happening, and reminding yourself that it's very temporary, can help you cope with D-MER. It may also help to keep track of those surges of negative feelings to see whether there's a pattern of intensity to them (maybe they come on more strongly when you're dehydrated or extra tired) and whether there are proactive steps you can take to ease them. Third, ask your practitioner if there are any therapies (such as breastfeeding-safe herbal remedies, acupuncture, or dietary changes) that might help. Exercise can boost dopamine levels naturally, which means that taking a walk with baby before feeds may give you a lift during let-down. Finally, reach out to your social media mom network to see if you can find other moms who have experienced the symptoms of D-MER. As always, knowing that you're not alone in what you're feeling can be incredibly reassuring.

failure to drain breasts at each nursing, and lowered resistance in mom due to stress and fatigue.

The most common symptoms of mastitis are severe soreness or pain, hardness, redness, heat, and swelling of the breast over the affected duct, plus flulike symptoms—chills and a fever of about 101°F to 102°F—though occasionally the only symptoms are fever and fatigue. If you develop such symptoms, contact your doctor right away. Prompt medical treatment is necessary and may include bed rest, antibiotics, pain relievers, increased fluid intake, and heat applications. You should begin to feel drastically better within 36 to 48 hours after beginning the antibiotics. If you don't, let your practitioner know. He or she may need to prescribe a different type of antibiotic. Finish up the entire prescription unless you're advised not to (or prescribed a different one). Taking probiotics during the course of antibiotics (though not at the same time of day) will help prevent yeast infection and thrush.

Continue to breastfeed during treatment. The antibiotics prescribed for the infection will be safe during breastfeeding, and draining the breast will help prevent clogged milk ducts. Breastfeed on the infected breast if you can handle the pain, and express whatever baby doesn't finish. If the pain is so bad that you can't nurse from the affected breast at all, see if pumping to drain it is tolerable.

Delay in treating mastitis or discontinuing treatment too soon could lead to the development of a breast abscess, the symptoms of which include excruciating, throbbing pain, localized swelling, tenderness, and heat in the area of the abscess, and temperature swings between 100°F and 103°F. Treatment includes antibiotics and, frequently, surgical drainage under local anesthesia. Breastfeeding on that breast may be able to be continued (depending on the location of the abscess), but in many cases it won't be possible. But you can keep nursing with the other breast until you wean your baby.

Resuming Sex

"I've heard a lot of different answers to this question—but when can we start having sex again?"

That's at least partly up to you, though you'll also want to include your practitioner in the decision (probably not in the heat of the moment). Couples are typically advised to pick up where they left off sex-wise whenever the woman feels physically ready—usually around 4 weeks postpartum, though some practitioners give the green light to sex as early as 2 weeks postpartum,

and others still follow the old 6-week rule routinely. In certain circumstances (for instance, if healing has been slow or you had an infection), your practitioner may recommend waiting longer. If your practitioner still has you in a holding pattern, but you think you're ready to move forward, ask if there's a reason why you shouldn't, and if there isn't, whether you can get busy earlier. If it turns out there is a reason, hold off and wait for clearance. Keep in mind that time will fly when you're caring for a newborn. In the meantime, assuming you're in the mood, satisfy each other with lovemaking that doesn't involve penetration.

"My midwife told us we can start having sex, but I'm afraid it's going to hurt. Plus, to be honest, I'm really not in the mood."

Doing "it" isn't topping your to-do list these days—or, more likely, isn't even making the top 20? No surprise there (or down there). Most women lose that loving feeling during the postpartum period—and beyond—for a variety of reasons. First, as you already suspect, postpartum sex can be more pain than pleasure—especially if you delivered vaginally, but, surprisingly, even if you labored and then had a c-section. After all, your vagina has just been stretched to its earthly limits, and possibly torn or surgically cut and sutured to boot—leaving you too sore to sit, never mind contemplate sex. Adding to the pain potential no matter which exit your baby took: Low levels of estrogen cause the vaginal tissue to remain thin, and thin is not in as far as vaginas are concerned. And, your natural lubrications haven't turned on yet, making you feel uncomfortably dry where you'd rather be moist—especially if you're breastfeeding (breastfeeding hormones can keep you dry longer).

Postpartum Sex?

So, maybe you're experiencing the longest sexual dry spell you've had since freshman year—and you're pretty sure you're exhibiting the symptoms of dreaded DSB (deadly semen backup). You're as ready for action as you've ever been—but action may not be in your partner's plans right now. And you get that. After all, she's recovering from a significant shock to her system—not just the birthing, but the 9 months preceding. She's been through the wringer physically—and you feel for her, even if you don't literally feel her pain. You probably even hesitate to bring up sex. The doctor or midwife may have already said that sex is technically okay to start up again—but understandably, your partner (and her body) may have a different timetable in mind (as in, sex is tabled until she changes her mind). And she will, eventually.

Once she does agree to give postpartum sex a try—and even if she's just as eager as you (or even more eager) to resume where you last left off—proceed very slowly and extremely gently. Ask her what feels good, what hurts, what you can do to help. Keep in mind that you'll need to serve up lots of tender foreplay appetizers before you even consider laying into the main course, both to get her in the mood and help her get her juices going (she'll be dry due to hormonal changes, so extra lubrication will be helpful, too). Don't

be surprised if you get an accidental eyeful of milk right in the middle of the action (milk happens, especially early on). Share a laugh, and get back to business.

Or maybe the issue with getting back into the sack isn't with her, but with you? Perhaps you're hesitant to hitch a ride on the sex bandwagon because being a new parent is making you feel incredibly happy but distinctly unsexy? Many brand new dads find both the spirit and the flesh somewhat less willing after delivery (although there's nothing abnormal about those who don't) for many very understandable reasons: fatigue, fear that baby will wake up and cut you off at first base (or when you're trying to steal second), unease about having sex so nearby your newborn (particularly if he or she is sharing your room), concern that you may hurt your spouse by having sex before her body is completely healed, and, finally, a general physical and mental preoccupation with your newborn, which sensibly concentrates your energies and interests where they are most needed at this stage of your lives. Your feelings may also be influenced by the temporary increase in estrogen and drop in testosterone that many new fathers experience, because it's testosterone—in both women and men—that fuels libido. That's probably nature's way of helping you nurture—and

But your libido has other problems to contend with postpartum besides the physical ones: your understandable preoccupation with a very little and very needy person, who is given to waking up with a full diaper and an empty tummy at the least opportune times.

Not to mention a number of other very effective mood killers (the pungent smell of day-old spit-up on your sheets, the pile of dirty baby clothes at the foot of your bed, the baby massage oil on your nightstand where there used to be couples massage oil, the fact that you nature's way of keeping sex off your mind when there's a new baby in the house. (Though keep in mind, being in the mood for sex doesn't make you less of a nurturer.)

Remember, as with all matters sexual, there is a wide range of normal. For some couples, desire precedes even the practitioner's go-ahead. For others, 6 months can pass before sex makes a postpartum comeback. Some moms find their libidos lacking until they stop breastfeeding, but that doesn't mean they can't enjoy the closeness of lovemaking.

While you're waiting for your libidos (yours, hers, or both) to make their inevitable return (and they will!), make sure you're paying your partner plenty of the attention she's undoubtedly in need of. Even if she's not in the mood for love—she's definitely in the mood to hear that you love her (and think she's beautiful and sexy). It can't hurt, either, to try some romantic moves to get you both back into the mood—as challenging as that might be to accomplish when you've got a newborn in the house. Light some scented candles once baby's finally asleep to mask that pervasive aroma of dirty diapers. Offer her a sensuous-but-no-strings-attached massage. Bring on the cuddles while you're both collapsed on the coach. Who knows—you might both feel that libido return sooner than you'd think.

can't remember when you had your last shower). It's no wonder sex isn't on the schedule, or even on your mind.

Will you ever live to make love again? Absolutely. Like everything else in your new and often overwhelming life, it'll just take time and patience—from your partner, too, who may already be ready for this dry spell to end (or not; see box, facing page). So wait until you're feeling ready, or help yourself get ready with the following tips:

Lubricate. Using K-Y, Astroglide, or another lubricant until your own natural secretions return can reduce pain and, ideally, increase pleasure. Buy them in economy sizes, so you'll be more likely to use them liberally—on both of you.

Loosen up. Speaking of lubrication, drinking a small glass of wine can also help you unwind—and keep you from tensing up and experiencing pain during sex (just make sure you sip it right after a feeding if you're nursing). Another great way to loosen up is massage, so request one before closing the deal.

Warm up. Your partner may be as eager as he's ever been to get down to business. But though he's not likely to need much—if any—foreplay, you definitely do. So ask for it. And then ask for some more. The greater the effort he puts into warming you up (time permitting before baby wakes up again), the better the main event will be for both of you.

Tell it like it is. You know what hurts and what feels good, but your partner doesn't unless you provide him with clearly marked route guidance ("Turn left . . . no, right . . . no, down . . . up just a smidge—there, perfect!"). So speak up when you'd like things to heat up.

Position properly. Experiment and find a position that puts less pressure on any tender areas and gives you control over the depth of penetration (this is one time when deeper will definitely not be better). Woman-on-top (if you have the energy) or side-to-side positions are both great postpartum picks for those reasons. Whoever's in charge of the strides, make sure they're performed at a comfortably slow speed.

Pump it up. No, not that kind of pumping. Pump blood and restore muscle tone to your vagina by doing the exercise you're probably sick of hearing about (but should keep doing anyway): Kegels. Do them day and night (and don't forget to do them when you're doing "it," too, since that squeeze can please you both).

Find alternative means of gratification. If you're not having fun yet through intercourse, seek sexual satisfaction through (gentle for you) mutual masturbation or oral sex (ditto). Or if you're both too pooped to pop, find pleasure and intimacy in just being together. There's absolutely nothing wrong (and everything right) about lying in bed together and cuddling.

Bottom line on your postpartum bottom line: Even if sex does hurt a bit the first time (and second and third time), don't write it off—or give it up. It won't be long (though it may seem that way) before the pleasure will be all yours—and your partner's—again.

One more step before you resume sex: Make sure you're all squared away with birth control; see facing page.

Breastfeeding as Birth Control?

"I've heard that breastfeeding keeps you from getting pregnant. Is that true?"

Breastfeeding is a form of birth control . . . just not the most reliable one. So unless you don't mind becoming pregnant again soon, it's best not to bet on lactation for contraception—or at least, not to put all your contraceptive eggs in the breastfeeding basket.

It's true that, on average, women who breastfeed resume normal cycles later than those who don't—a sign that, on average, they're not fertile as fast. In moms who aren't nursing, periods usually kick in again between 6 and 12 weeks after delivery, while in nursing moms the average is between 4 and 6 months. As usual, however, averages don't tell the whole story. Nursing moms have been known to begin their periods as early as 6 weeks or as late as 18 months after giving birth.

Though there's no way to predict where you'll fall on that first period timetable, several variables can offer clues: for example, frequency of nursing (more than 3 times a day seems to suppress ovulation better), duration of nursing (the longer you continue, the longer the delay in ovulation), and whether you're breastfeeding exclusively or supplementing (giving baby formula or solids can interfere with the ovulation-suppressing effect). Which means that while it's far from a sure thing, the odds are pretty good that you won't get pregnant again right away if you're exclusively breastfeeding, feeding frequently, and haven't gotten your period yet.

So why worry about using birth control, at least until you get that first postpartum period? Because the timetable for first postpartum ovulation is as unpredictable as the timetable for first postpartum period. Some women have a sterile first period—that is, they don't ovulate during that initial cycle. Others ovulate before having a period, which means they could conceivably go from pregnancy to pregnancy without ever unpacking the tampons. Since you don't know which will come first, the period or the egg, contraception makes sense if you're hoping to plan your next pregnancy.

Think you might already be pregnant again? See page 27 for information on back-to-back pregnancies.

Birth Control Options

"I'm definitely not ready to have another baby yet. What are my options for birth control?"

Okay, maybe sex isn't the first thing on your minds these days—and these sleep-deprived nights. Maybe it's the last thing on your mind most of the time. Yet there will come a night (or a Sunday afternoon when baby's napping) when you'll get the urge to sweep the pacifiers and burping cloths off the bed and sweep each other off your feet—when lust will return to your life, and passion will pick up where it left off (approximately) pre-baby.

So be prepared. If you'd like to avoid back-to-back pregnancies, you'll need to use some form of birth control as soon as you begin having sex again. And because you never know when the urge might strike, it's good to have that birth control in hand (or by your bed) well in advance.

Unless you're a gambling twosome, counting on breastfeeding to provide birth control is dicey (see previous question). In other words, you'll want to consider a more reliable form of birth control—and there are plenty to choose from, even if you're a breastfeeding mom. There might even be some new options on the market since the last time you picked a birth control method (or ones that better fit your needs now).

Before you decide on which form of contraception is best for you, read up on all the following methods, and discuss them with your partner and your practitioner. Each of the methods has its benefits and drawbacks, depending on your medical and gynecological history, your lifestyle, whether you want to become pregnant again in the future (and how certain you want to be about avoiding pregnancy in the meantime), your practitioner's recommendation, and your feelings and your partner's. All of these methods are effective when used correctly and consistently, though some offer more reliable results than others:

Oral contraception. Available in most states by prescription only (a few states allow over-the-counter sales), oral contraception (OC or "the Pill") is among the most effective nonpermanent methods of birth control, with a success rate of about 99.5 percent (most failures are due to a user's missing a day or taking pills in the wrong order). Another plus: It allows for spontaneity in sex.

There are two basic types of oral contraception: combination pills (which contain both estrogen and progestin) and progestin-only pills (mini-pills). Both work by preventing ovulation and by thickening cervical mucus to keep sperm from reaching an egg, should one be released. They also prevent a fertilized egg from implanting in the uterus. The combination pills are slightly more effective in preventing pregnancy than the minis. For maximum effectiveness, the mini-pills must be taken at the same time every day (combination pills have a slightly longer window).

Some women experience side effects from OC (which vary, depending on the pill), most commonly: fluid retention, weight changes, nausea, breast tenderness, an increase or decrease in sex drive, hair loss, and menstrual irregularities. After the first few cycles of pill use, side effects often diminish or disappear completely. In general, today's oral contraceptives trigger fewer side effects than OC did years ago.

Some versions of the Pill (Yasmin, Cyclessa) deliver constant levels of estrogen and a new type of progestin (these are called monophasic pills) or use three different levels of estrogen and progestin (called triphasic) to reduce bloating and PMS. Another option that may be especially appealing to women who aren't fond of their monthly flow is Seasonale. It comes in a package with 84 hormone pills and 7 inactive pills; women take the hormones for 12 weeks straight before taking a break for their period (which then comes only 4 times a year). Some women, however, experience more breakthrough bleeding with Seasonale than with monthly pills. Most doctors agree that it's safe to take any monophasic pill continually—by skipping the inactive pills—to avoid having a monthly period altogether.

Women who are over age 35 and heavy smokers may be at increased risk of serious side effects (such as blood clots, heart attack, or stroke) from OC. The Pill may also be unsuitable for women with certain medical conditions, including a history of blood clots, diabetes, hypertension, and certain types of cancer. And OC sometimes is less effective in overweight or obese women.

On the plus side, OC appears to protect against a whole host of conditions, including ovarian and uterine cancer. Other benefits experienced by some women who take OC are diminished PMS, very regular periods, and (with certain varieties) clearer skin. There is some controversy about whether OC affects your breast cancer risk, so talk to your doctor about any concerns you may have, especially if there's a family history of premenopausal breast cancer.

If you're planning to have another baby, fertility may take longer to return if you're using OC than if you're using a barrier contraceptive. Ideally, you should switch to a barrier method (see page 515) about 3 months before the time you plan to start TTC (trying to conceive). About 80 percent of women ovulate within the first 3 months after stopping the Pill, 95 percent within a year.

If you decide to try OC (or go back to it), your doctor will help you determine which type and which dose is best for you, based on whether you're breastfeeding (oral contraception containing estrogen is not recommended during breastfeeding, so nursing moms are limited to a progestin-only pill, aka the mini-pill), as well as on your menstrual cycle, weight, age, and medical history. Making sure the Pill works the way it's supposed to is up to you—so take it as prescribed. If you miss even one pill, or if you have diarrhea or vomiting (which can interfere with absorption of OC by your body), use backup protection (such as a condom) until your next period. See your doctor every 6 months to 1 year for monitoring of your health, report any problems or signs of complications that show up between visits, and be sure to inform anyone prescribing medication of any kind that you are on oral contraception (some herbs and medications, such as antibiotics, interact adversely with OC, making it less effective).

The Pill doesn't protect against STDs, so use a condom, too, if there's a chance of contracting an STD from your partner. OC increases the need for B_6, B_{12}, C, riboflavin, zinc, and folic acid (it reduces the need for other nutrients), so continue taking your prenatal (or a breastfeeding supplement) while on the Pill.

Injection. Hormonal injection, such as Depo-Provera, is a highly effective method of birth control (with a success rate of 99.7 percent) that stops ovulation and thickens cervical mucus to keep sperm and egg from meeting. The shot, given in the arm or buttock, is effective for 3 months. Depo-Provera is a progestin-only injection, so it is safe for breastfeeding mothers.

As with oral contraception, side effects of hormonal injections can include irregular periods, weight gain, and bloating. For some women, periods become fewer and lighter, and many women will have no periods while using Depo-Provera. Other women might experience longer and heavier periods. And, like OC, the shot is not for every woman, depending on her specific health and medical condition, and it doesn't protect against STDs.

The greatest advantage to the shot is that it prevents pregnancy for 12 weeks, and this can be compelling for someone who doesn't like to have to think about birth control or who often forgets to take a pill or insert a diaphragm. It also protects against endometrial and ovarian cancers. But there are disadvantages, too: having to return to your practitioner every 12 weeks for another shot, the fact that the effects of the shot can't be immediately reversed (if you suddenly want to TTC), and that it may take up to a year for fertility to return after you stop Depo-Provera.

Patch. The Ortho Evra patch, a matchbox-size adhesive patch, delivers the same hormones as the combination pill but in patch form. Unlike OC, the patch maintains a steady state of hormonal levels because it continuously delivers hormones through the skin. The patch is worn for 1 week at a time and is replaced on the same day of the week for 3 consecutive weeks (you can use an app or an alarm on your phone as a reminder). The 4th week is "patch free," during which you'll get your period. The patch can be changed any time of the day. If you forget to change the patch and leave it on beyond the 7 days, the hormones are still effective for an additional 2 days.

Most women choose to wear the patch on the abdomen or bottom. It can also be worn on the upper torso (excluding the breasts), the back, or the upper outer arm. Since the patch isn't affected by moisture, humidity, temperature, or activity, it can be worn in any weather, when showering or working out, even in a sauna or hot tub.

Like other hormonal contraceptives, the patch is highly effective (about 99.5 percent). It may be less effective in overweight or obese women. Side effects are similar to those of OC, but there may be a greater risk of blood clots with the patch. It does not protect against STDs.

Ring. The NuvaRing is a small (about the size of a silver dollar), transparent, flexible plastic ring that can flatten like a rubber band, be inserted into the vagina, and left in place for 21 days. Once inserted, the ring releases a steady flow of low doses of estrogen and progestin. The exact positioning of the ring inside the vagina isn't a key to effectiveness because it's not a barrier method of birth control. You can easily insert the ring yourself once a month (you won't feel it once it's inserted, and neither will your partner during sex). Once you remove it (again, easily), you'll get your period. Then 1 week after the last one was removed, you'll insert a new ring, even if your period hasn't stopped yet. If you're likely to have trouble remembering the monthly insertion, a calendar reminder or app can keep you on track. Studies show that the level of cycle control with the NuvaRing is better than that with OC, which means there's little breakthrough bleeding. Because the hormones are the same as those used in the combination pills, side effects are generally the same, and those women who are advised not to use OC are also advised not to use contraceptive rings. The ring is also not for breastfeeding mothers. It has a success rate of about

99 percent, and is a good choice for obese women. The NuvaRing does not protect against STDs.

Implant. The under-the-skin progestin implant has been shown to be a safe and effective method of birth control (with a success rate of about 99.9 percent), though the method may be less effective in obese women. Nexplanon is a single flexible plastic rod about the size of a matchstick that is implanted under the skin of the upper arm. It releases a low, steady dose of progestin to thicken cervical mucus and thin the lining of the uterus, as well as stop ovulation. The implant is safe during breastfeeding, and it can prevent pregnancy for up to 3 years. The most common side effect is irregular bleeding—especially in the first 6 to 12 months of use. Most women find their periods become fewer and lighter (though some have longer, heavier periods), and some women stop having periods completely. Serious problems with Nexplanon are rare. It does not protect against STDs.

IUD (Intrauterine device). The IUD is the most widely used reversible birth control method for women in the world, but not so in the U.S., where only 11 percent of women using contraception opt for it. Which is surprising, since today's IUDs are considered among the safest methods of birth control—and are as effective as sterilization (over 99 percent). They're also the most convenient, and, for most women, trouble free—definitely worth considering.

An IUD is a small plastic device that is inserted into a woman's uterus by her gyn provider, and can be left in place (effectively preventing pregnancy) for a number of years, depending on the type of IUD. There are two types of IUDs. The ParaGard copper IUD releases copper in the uterus to immobilize sperm, and also prevents implantation. This long-lasting IUD can be left in for 10 years (talk about set it and forget it!). The Mirena IUD releases progestin into the uterine walls, thickening cervical mucus and blocking sperm, while also preventing implantation. It lasts for 5 years—still a pretty good chunk of protected time.

The major advantage of an IUD is that it offers the ultimate in convenience. Once it is inserted (which, by the way, can happen any time you'd like, including right after your vaginal or cesarean delivery, or at your 6-week postpartum checkup), it needs absolutely no maintenance, except to check regularly (monthly is a good idea) for the string attached to it. This allows for a completely spontaneous sex life—with no pausing to find and insert a diaphragm or put on a condom, or remembering to take a daily pill. Another plus: The IUD does not interfere with breastfeeding, and the hormones in the Mirena are safe for a breastfeeding baby.

You can increase the already excellent protection from pregnancy provided by the IUD if you use condoms and/or spermicides for the first 2 or 3 months after insertion (when most failures, which are rare to begin with, occur).

The IUD should not be used by a woman who has untreated gonorrhea or chlamydia. It should also not be used by a woman with active pelvic inflammatory disease (PID), known or suspected uterine or cervical malignancy or premalignancy, or abnormalities of the uterus or an unusually small uterus. Ask your doctor about the safety of an IUD if you (or your partner) have an STD. An allergy or suspected allergy to copper rules out the use of a copper IUD.

Possible complications include cramping (which can be mild to moderate) during insertion (and, rarely, for a few hours or even days following), uterine perforation (extremely rare), accidental expulsion (it might go unnoticed and leave you unprotected), and tubal or pelvic infections (also rare). Having an IUD in place does not increase the risk of an ectopic pregnancy. Some women may experience spotting between periods during the first few months after insertion. The first few periods may also last longer and be heavier. It's also not unusual for a woman to continue having heavier and longer periods while using an IUD, though the progestin-releasing Mirena may lessen the amount of bleeding (most women find their periods get lighter or disappear completely with the Mirena). Keep in mind that IUDs don't protect against STDs.

Diaphragm. The diaphragm is a barrier method of birth control—a dome-shaped rubber cap that's placed over the cervix before sex to block the entry of sperm. It's 94 percent effective when used properly (meaning, it's the right size, it's inserted properly, and it doesn't slip) along with a spermicidal gel, meant to inactivate any sperm that might slip past the barrier. Aside from possible increases in urinary tract infections and an occasional allergic reaction triggered by either the spermicide or the rubber, the diaphragm is safe. In fact, used with a spermicide, it appears to reduce the risk of pelvic infections that can lead to infertility (though it doesn't protect against STDs). It in no way affects breastfeeding.

With the diaphragm, size absolutely matters. It must be prescribed and fitted by a medical professional—and refitted after every delivery, since pregnancy and childbirth change the size and the shape of the cervix. As for the spontaneity factor, the diaphragm doesn't exactly get high marks—you have to stop to insert it (or insert it before things get

started), then check to make sure it's properly inserted before each sex session (unless you'll be having an encore sexual performance within a few hours, in which case you just need to add more spermicide). The diaphragm then has to be left in place for at least 6 to 8 hours after sex (but no longer than 24 hours in a row). Some experts suggest it's probably prudent to remove it within 12 to 18 hours, and some recommend women insert their diaphragms as part of their bedtime routines so they don't forget or neglect to use it in a moment of passion (though again, it can't be kept in place for more than 24 hours at a time). Either way, there's a lot of keeping track and clock-watching. And there's maintenance involved, too—cleaning the diaphragm after use, storing it properly in its case (not loose in the bottom of your purse or in your jeans pocket), and checking it regularly for holes by holding it up to a light.

Cervical cap. The cervical cap is similar to the diaphragm in many ways. It must be fitted by a medical professional, must be used with a spermicide, and does its job by acting as a barrier to sperm. Its success at preventing pregnancy is lower than the diaphragm's (approximately 60 to 75 percent), but it does offer a couple of advantages. Shaped like a large thimble, the pliable rubber cap has a firm rim that fits snugly around the cervix, making it only about half the size of the diaphragm. A convenience plus: Instead of the 24-hour outside limit recommended for the diaphragm, the cap can be left in place for 48 hours (though an unpleasant odor can develop when it's left in that long).

The FemCap, another type of cervical cap (with a success rate of 85 percent), is a silicone dome shaped like a sailor's hat. It comes in three sizes and fits over the cervix with a brim that seals against the vaginal walls and has a groove that stores the spermicide and traps the sperm. It also has a removal strap.

Vaginal sponge. The Today sponge, which covers the cervix and blocks sperm from entering the uterus while also continuously releasing a spermicide that keeps sperm from moving, is made of plastic foam. It is soft, round, and about 2 inches in diameter with a nylon loop attached to the bottom for removal. The upsides to the sponge: It doesn't require a visit to the doctor or a prescription, is relatively easy to use, provides continuous protection for a full 24 hours after insertion, and has no effect on breastfeeding. On the downside, it's somewhat less effective than the diaphragm (about 80 percent), can increase the risk of yeast infections, and can be uncomfortable to insert. It should not be left in longer than recommended, and you'll need to check carefully to make sure the whole sponge is removed intact (a piece left behind could cause odor and infection). The sponge also can't be reused, so you'll have to stay stocked up.

Condom. Also called a rubber, a condom (as you probably know) is essentially a penis cover designed to trap sperm when they're ejaculated so they can't gain access into the vagina. It's made of latex or natural skin (from the intestines of a sheep)—and if used consistently and correctly, it's a pretty effective birth control method (with a success rate of 98 percent). The condom is totally harmless—that is, unless one or both partners has an allergic reaction to the latex material or the spermicide (if latex is an issue, opt for the natural skin). It has the advantage of being easily available and portable (for on-the-fly activities), and of reducing the risk of transmitting STDs, such as gonorrhea,

chlamydia, and HIV (the latex variety is better at preventing transmission of HIV), as well as the Zika virus. Because it in no way interferes with breastfeeding and because it clearly doesn't require postpartum refitting (as does the diaphragm), it is an ideal "transitional" method. Some couples find that condoms get in the way of spontaneous fun—especially because you have to wait until erection to put it on—and some find it decreases sensitivity and/or causes vaginal irritation (with more potential for irritation postpartum). Other couples don't mind condoms a bit, and may even find a way to make putting it on part of foreplay.

To increase effectiveness, you shouldn't linger long after sex when you're using a condom—the penis should be withdrawn before the erection is totally lost and while the condom is held on, to avoid leakage of semen. The use of a lubricating cream (or a lubricated condom) will help slip the covered penis in more comfortably during those dry postpartum and breastfeeding months. But choose your lube with care: Don't use oil-based lubricants or Vaseline, because they can damage a latex condom (always check the instructions on the package before using an oil-based lubricant).

Thought condoms kept only guys covered? There's one for you, too. The female condom is a thin, lubricated polyurethane pouch that lines the vagina and is held in place by a closed inner ring near the cervix and an outer open ring at the opening of the vagina. A female condom is inserted into the vagina up to 8 hours before intercourse and is removed right after. The downsides to the female condom: It is more expensive than the male condom, may prevent full sensation, and is clearly noticeable once in place. Plus, it's yet another birth control method that depends on a woman's compliance, unlike the male condom, which at least shares the load. And it's a little less effective than the male condom (about 95 percent). But like the male condom, it prevents STDs.

Spermicide foams, creams, jellies, suppositories, and contraceptive films. Used alone, these antisperm agents are only so-so effective (approximately 72 to 94 percent) at preventing pregnancy. They are available without a prescription, but can be messy and inconvenient. They can be inserted up to 1 hour before intercourse.

Emergency contraception. The emergency contraception pill (ECP) is the only method of birth control that can be used after unprotected sex (or as backup when your contraceptive method has failed, as with a broken condom, slipped diaphragm, or missed pills) but before a pregnancy is established. ECP is sold over-the-counter as Plan B One-Step, Take Action, Next Choice One Dose, and My Way. Ella, another ECP, is available with a prescription. ECPs reduce a woman's risk of pregnancy by 75 percent when taken within 72 hours of unprotected sex. The sooner ECPs are taken after unprotected sex, the more effective they are. (Your doctor might also recommend using ordinary birth control pills as emergency contraception, but check to confirm the dose you should use.) Emergency contraception pills will not work if you're already pregnant. Important distinction: ECP is not a so-called abortion pill, like RU486. ECPs work primarily by temporarily stopping ovulation. ECPs are not recommended for use during the first 6 weeks postpartum because their high estrogen content can increase the risk of blood clots and are not recommended while breastfeeding.

Sterilization. Sterilization is frequently the choice of couples who feel that their families are complete, don't have a problem with closing (and locking) the door to conception, and are eager to dispense with contraception altogether (and who's not eager for that?). It's increasingly safe (with no known long-term health effects) and virtually foolproof. The occasional failure can be attributed to a slip-up in surgery or, in the case of vasectomy, not using alternative birth control until all viable sperm have been ejaculated. Though sterilization is sometimes reversible, it should be considered permanent.

A vasectomy (the tying or cutting of the vasa deferentia, the tubes that transport sperm from testicles to penis) is an easy, in-office procedure done with local anesthesia, and it carries far fewer risks than female sterilization. It doesn't (as some men fear) affect the ability to achieve erection or ejaculate—all that's missing is the sperm (not the semen). Research has also shown that there is no increased risk of prostate cancer for men with vasectomies.

Tubal ligation is a procedure done on women under regional or epidural anesthesia (right after delivery if you want; see page 439) in which a small incision is made in the abdomen (near the belly button or bikini line) and the fallopian tubes are cut, tied, or blocked. It does require some downtime, usually 2 days to a week (sometimes more) of only light activity for most women—which you're going to be adhering to anyway if you just delivered.

Another permanent birth control option for women is called Essure. An alternative to tubal ligation, this type of sterilization doesn't require an abdominal incision (as tubal ligation does). A soft, flexible microinsert is placed into each fallopian tube via a catheter (tube) inserted through the cervix. Over the course of 3 months, new tissue grows in the fallopian tube (inside the insert), blocking the tubes completely. A backup method of birth control must be used until the doctor can confirm through testing that your tubes are effectively blocked (usually after 3 months). Sounds pretty perfect, but this method isn't without controversy. The FDA is investigating reports that the procedure may cause pain, bloating, and heavy bleeding.

Fertility awareness. Couples who prefer not to use contraception at all can opt for the fertility awareness method (FAM), aka natural family planning. This approach relies on becoming aware of a number of body signs or symptoms to determine the time of ovulation. If done perfectly correctly, the FAM approach can be just as successful at avoiding pregnancy as some other birth control methods (in the 90 percent effectiveness range).

So what makes for perfect practice of fertility awareness? The more factors a couple takes into consideration, the better the success rate—and there's a long list of factors, including cervical mucus changes (the mucus is clear, copious, thin, has an egg-white consistency, and can be pulled into a long string at ovulation), basal body temperature changes (the baseline temperature, measured first thing in the morning, drops slightly just before ovulation, reaches its lowest point at ovulation, and then immediately rises to a high point before returning to the baseline for the rest of the cycle), and cervical changes (the normally firm cervix becomes a little softer, and it's also slightly higher and more open than normal during ovulation). Ovulation predictor kits can also help to pinpoint ovulation (though using them every month to prevent pregnancy can get pretty pricey). Saliva tests for ovulation can also help some women predict when ovulation is about to happen and are more cost effective. Once you're armed with all the ovulation information you need, the key will be avoiding sex from the first sign that you're about to ovulate until 3 days after. Need more ovulation information? See *What To Expect Before You're Expecting*.

ALL ABOUT:
Getting Back into Shape

It's one thing to look 6 months pregnant when, in fact, you are 6 months pregnant . . . and another to look it when you've already delivered. Yet most new moms can expect to leave the birthing room with a little bundle in their arms—and a sizable one still around their middles.

How soon after you become a new mother will you stop looking like a mother-to-be? Genes will play a role in how quickly you'll slip back into your skinny jeans, as will your metabolism, how much weight you gained during pregnancy, and, of course, your postpartum eating habits. But there's no getting around it: Getting back into shape (and out of those baggy sweats) will definitely take getting back into the exercise habit.

"Who needs exercise?" you may wonder. "I haven't stopped moving since I got home from the hospital. Doesn't that count?" Unfortunately,

Workout Rules for the First 6 Weeks

- Wear a supportive bra and comfortable clothing (nothing that rubs on tender spots, traps moisture, or doesn't allow breathing room).

- Try to divide your exercise schedule into 2 or 3 brief sessions rather than doing a single long session a day (this tones muscles better and will be easier on your recovering body—plus you're more likely to be able to fit it in and keep it up).

- Start each session with the exercise you find least strenuous.

- Do exercises slowly, and don't do a rapid series of repetitions. Instead, rest briefly between movements (the muscle buildup occurs then, not while you are in motion).

- Avoid jerky, bouncy, erratic motions during the first 6 weeks postpartum, while your ligaments are still loose. Also avoid knee-to-chest exercises, full sit-ups, and double leg lifts during this period.

- Keep a water bottle next to you during your workouts, and sip often.

- Take it slowly and sensibly. "No pain, no gain" wasn't a motto created with new moms in mind. Don't do more than recommended, even if you feel you can, and stop before you feel tired (that is, more tired than being a new mom has already made you). If you overdo it, you probably won't feel it until the next day, by which time you may be so exhausted and achy that you won't be able to exercise at all. Plus, pushing yourself can actually slow your postpartum recovery.

- Don't let taking care of your baby stop you from taking care of yourself. Your baby will love lying on your chest as you go through your floor routine.

not that much. Exhausting as it is caring for a newborn, that kind of activity won't tighten up the perineal and abdominal muscles that have been stretched and left saggy by pregnancy and childbirth—only a regular workout program will. And the right kind of postpartum exercise will do more than tone you up. It will help keep baby-toting backaches at bay, promote healing and recovery from labor and delivery, help pregnancy-loosened joints tighten up, and improve circulation. Kegel exercises, which target the perineal muscles, will help you avoid stress and urinary incontinence and postpartum sexual problems. Finally, exercise can make you happier. As exercise-released endorphins circulate in your system, boosting your mood and your ability to cope, you'll find yourself much better equipped to handle the stresses of new parenthood, and even beat back baby blues. In fact, research shows that moms who resume exercising within 6 weeks of delivery feel better about themselves—and just plain feel better.

Don't even think about starting off with a bang, however, even if you feel surprisingly well and mega-motivated. Instead, ease your recovering body slowly and steadily back into workout mode with the following basic exercises. Supplement these with an online or DVD postpartum workout, take a class for new moms, or just make daily strolls (or Strollercize) with baby a part of your daily routine.

First Weeks After Delivery

Eager to get that prebaby body back? Then you'll be happy to hear that it's time to step up to the exercise ladder. But before you take that step, make sure the pair of vertical muscles that form your abdominal wall have not separated during pregnancy. If they have, you'll have to close them up before the workouts start heating up (see box, facing page). Once the separation has closed, or if you've never had one, you can work up to the following exercises. At first, do these exercises in bed, then move on to a well-cushioned floor, or an exercise or yoga mat:

Pelvic Tilt. Lie on your back, knees bent, soles flat on the floor. Support your head and shoulders with pillows, and rest your arms flat at your sides. Take a breath. Then exhale as you press the small of your back against the floor for 10 seconds. Then relax. Repeat 3 or 4 times to start, increasing gradually to 12, and then 24.

Pelvic Tilt

Leg Slides. Lie on your back, knees bent, soles flat on the floor. Support your head and shoulders with pillows, and rest your arms flat at your sides. Slowly extend both legs until they are flat on the floor. Slide your right foot, flat on the floor, back toward your buttocks, inhaling as you go. Keep the small of your back against the floor. Exhale as you slide your leg back down. Repeat with your left foot. Start with 3 or 4 slides per side, and increase gradually until you can do a dozen or more comfortably. After 3 weeks, move to a modified leg lift (lifting one leg at a time slightly off the floor and lowering it again very slowly), if it is comfortable.

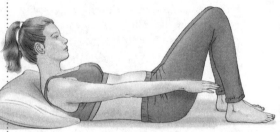

Head/Shoulder Lift

Head/Shoulder Lift. Lie on your back, knees bent, soles flat on the floor. Support your head and shoulders with pillows, and rest your arms flat at your sides. Take a deep, relaxing breath, then raise your head very slightly and stretch your arms out, exhaling as you do. Lower your head slowly and inhale. Raise your head a little more each day, gradually working up to lifting your shoulders slightly off the floor. Don't try full sit-ups during the first 6 weeks—and then only if you have always had very good abdominal muscle tone. Check first, too, for an abdominal separation (see box, facing page).

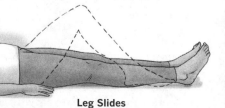

Leg Slides

Close the Gap

Don't look now, but there might be a hole in the middle of your belly (and it's not your navel). A very common pregnancy condition known in obstetrical circles as diastasis (up to half of moms experience it), it's a gap in your abdominal muscles that can develop as the abdomen expands. It can take a month or two after delivery for this gap to close, and you'll have to wait until it does before you start those crunches and other abdominal exercises, or you'll risk an injury. To determine if you have a separation, examine yourself this way: Lie on your back, knees bent, soles flat on the floor. Support your head and shoulders with pillows, and rest your arms flat at your sides. Raise your head slightly with your arms extended forward, then feel for a soft lump above your navel. Such a lump indicates a separation.

If you do have a separation, you may be able to help correct it more quickly with this exercise: Lie on your back, knees bent, soles flat on the floor. Support your head and shoulders with pillows, rest your arms flat at your sides, and inhale. Cross your hands over your abdomen, using your fingers to draw the sides of your abdominal muscles together as you breathe out, pulling your belly button inward toward the spine while raising your head slowly. Exhale as you lower your head slowly. Repeat 3 or 4 times, twice a day.

After Your Postpartum Checkup

Now, with your practitioner's go-ahead, you can gradually graduate to a more active workout program that includes power walking, running, biking, swimming, water workouts, aerobics, yoga, Pilates, weight training, or similar routines. Or sign up for a postpartum exercise class. But don't try to do too much too soon. As always, let your body be your guide.

PART 4

Staying Healthy When You're Expecting

CHAPTER 18

If You Get Sick

S o you were probably expecting to experience at least a few of the less pleasant pregnancy symptoms during your 9 months of expecting (a little morning sickness, a few leg cramps, some heartburn and fatigue), but maybe you weren't expecting to come down with a nasty cold or an ugly (and itchy) infection. The truth is, pregnant women can get sick with the best of them—actually, even better than the best of them, since the normal suppression of the immune system (so mom's body doesn't reject her baby as "foreign") makes expectant moms easier targets for germs of every variety. What's more, being sick for two can make you at least twice as uncomfortable—especially since so many of the remedies you're used to reaching for may need to stay behind medicine cabinet doors for now.

Prevention is, of course, the best way to avoid getting sick in the first place and to keep that healthy glow of pregnancy going strong. But when it fails (as when a coworker brings a stomach bug to the office, your nephew's wet kisses are sweet but saturated with cold germs, or you pick up some bacteria with those fresh-picked blueberries), quick treatment, in most cases under the supervision of your practitioner, can help you feel better fast.

What You May Be Wondering About

The Common Cold

"I'm sneezing and coughing, and my head is killing me. What can I take that won't affect my baby?"

C ommon colds are even more common when you're pregnant, because your normal immune system is suppressed. The good news is that you're the only one those nasty bugs will be bugging. Your baby can't catch your cold or be affected by it in any way. The not-so-good news: The medications and supplements that you might be used to reaching for to find relief (or to prevent a cold), including ibuprofen, extra doses of vitamin C and zinc, and herbals (like echinacea), are usually off limits when you're expecting (see page 538 for information on taking medications during pregnancy). So before you pick the shelves of your local drugstore clean, pick up the phone and call your practitioner to find out which over-the-counter remedies are considered safe in pregnancy, as well as which will work best in your case. (If you've already taken a few doses of a medication that isn't recommended for pregnancy use, don't worry. But do check with your practitioner for extra reassurance.)

Even if your standard cold remedy is shelved for now, you don't have to suffer with a runny nose and hacking cough. Some of the most effective cold remedies don't come in a bottle and are also the safest for both you and your baby. These tips can help nip a cold in the bud, before it blossoms into a nasty case of sinusitis or another secondary infection, while helping you feel better faster. At the very first sneeze or tickle in the throat:

- Rest, if you need it. Taking a cold to bed doesn't necessarily shorten its duration, but if your body is begging for rest, be sure to listen—especially now that it's begging for two. On the other hand, if you feel up to it (and you're not running a fever or coughing), light to moderate exercise can actually help you feel better faster.

- Feed your cold, and your baby. Eat as well as you can, given how crummy you feel and how little appetite you probably have. Especially seek vitamin-C-rich foods, like citrus and melon.

- Flood your cold with fluids. A runny nose can cost your body fluids you and your baby need. Warm fluids (like ginger tea or chicken broth) will be particularly soothing for your scratchy throat.

- Stay up even when you're lying down. Elevating your head with a couple of pillows will make it easier for you to breathe through a stuffy nose. Nasal strips (which gently pull your nasal passages open, making breathing easier) may help, too. Or try decongesting with a vapor rub, like Vicks.

- Stay moist. Keeping your nasal passages moist will ease congestion, so run a humidifier, especially at night, and use saline nasal spray (it's drug free, so you can use it as often as needed) or saline rinses (but steer clear of neti pots, since they're more apt to spread germs).

- Soothe with salt water. Gargling with warm salt water (¼ teaspoon of salt to 8 ounces of warm water) can ease a sore or scratchy throat, wash away postnasal drip, and help control a cough.

- Calm a dry cough the sweet way. A couple of teaspoons of honey can actually suppress the kind of dry cough that often comes with and after a cold as effectively as an OTC cough syrup. Honey's too sweet straight up? Mix it with hot water and lemon.

Colds don't typically come with a fever, but if your temperature rises to over 100°F, bring it down promptly with acetaminophen (Tylenol) and call your practitioner (see page 527 for more on fever). Also call if your cold is severe enough to interfere with eating or sleeping, if you're coughing up greenish or yellowish mucus, if you have a cough with chest pain or wheezing, if your sinuses are throbbing (see the next question), or if symptoms last more than 10 to 14 days. It's possible that your cold has progressed to a secondary infection and that prescribed medication may be needed.

Sinusitis

"I've had a bad cold for more than 10 days. Now my forehead and cheeks are starting to really hurt. What should I do?"

Sounds as if your nasty cold may have evolved into an even nastier case of sinusitis—an inflammation of the tissues lining your sinuses. In addition to a lingering or worsening stuffy nose, signs of sinusitis often include pain and tenderness in the forehead and/or one or both cheeks (beneath the eye), achiness around the teeth, and possibly a temporary loss of the sense of smell. The pain of sinusitis usually worsens when you bend over or shake your head. Fever sometimes accompanies these symptoms, but not always.

Sinusitis following a cold is fairly common, but it is far more common among pregnant women. That's because pregnancy hormones tend to swell mucous membranes (including those in and leading to the sinuses), trapping air and mucus behind the narrowed sinus openings, and causing blockages that allow germs to build up and multiply in the sinuses. These germs tend to linger longer there, because immune cells, which destroy invading germs, have difficulty reaching the sinuses' deep recesses. As a result, the symptoms can persist for weeks (or longer, becoming chronic).

Most sinus infections are caused by viruses (sometimes they're caused by allergies), but about 10 percent of the time bacteria get the blame. If your sinus infection is caused by bacteria (often the case when your sinus symptoms are lingering for longer than 10 days or if they're severe and accompanied by fever), your practitioner will prescribe a pregnancy-safe antibiotic to clear it up. If your sinusitis is caused by a virus, antibiotics won't be helpful, so treatment will focus on easing symptoms with pain relievers, nasal steroids, and nasal rinses (some practitioners will okay limited use of certain decongestants after the first trimester; see page 540).

Flu Season

"I usually get a flu shot in the fall, but now I'm wondering if I should skip it this year. Is it safe during pregnancy?"

A flu shot is definitely your best line of defense during flu season. Not only is it safe to receive while you're pregnant, it's considered a very smart move. In fact, the CDC recommends that all moms-to-be get the flu shot. That's because the flu can be much more severe when you're expecting, and is more likely to lead to serious complications requiring hospitalization. And since the CDC puts pregnant women at the top of the priority list (along with the elderly and children between the ages of 6 months and 5 years), moms-to-be can waddle to the front of the flu-shot line, even if the vaccine is in short supply. Talk to your practitioner about getting a flu shot—many ob practices offer it to pregnant patients. You can also stop by a flu shot clinic at your local pharmacy or supermarket.

The flu vaccine offers the most protection if it's given before or early in each flu season (preferably by October). It's never 100 percent effective, because it protects only against the flu viruses that are expected to cause the most problems in a particular year. Still, it greatly increases the chance that you will escape the season flu-free (and H1N1-free, too). And even when it doesn't prevent the flu, the vaccine usually reduces the severity of symptoms—which is extra important when you're expecting, since flu can hit pregnant women especially hard. Side effects occur infrequently and are generally mild.

Flu Shot for Two

Getting a flu shot protects you when you're expecting, but did you know that its benefits carry over to your soon-to-be newborn as well? Researchers have found that babies born to moms who were given the flu shot during the last trimester of pregnancy appear to be protected against the virus until they're old enough to get their own shot, at 6 months. Of course, if you're in the first or second trimester when flu season begins, don't wait to get your shot—you'll need to be protected throughout flu season.

In case you were wondering, you'll have to stick with the needle when it comes to your seasonal flu vaccine, since the nasal spray vaccine (FluMist, which is made from live flu virus), is not approved for or given to pregnant women.

If you suspect you might have the flu (symptoms include fever, achiness, headache, sore throat, and cough), call your doctor right away so that you can be treated (and so that the flu doesn't progress to pneumonia). Treatment may include an antiviral medication (like Tamiflu) along with steps aimed at reducing fever (see next question) and other symptoms.

Fever

"I'm running a little fever. What should I do?"

While a low-grade fever (one that's under 100°F) usually isn't something to worry about when you're expecting, it's also something you shouldn't ignore. So take steps to bring

it down promptly, but also keep an eye on the thermometer to make sure the numbers don't start rising.

If your fever reaches 100°F call your practitioner the same day or the next morning if it's the middle of the night. If it climbs to 101°F call right away, even if it's the middle of the night. That's because not only could a fever that goes higher than that be harmful to your developing baby, but the cause of the fever (for instance, an infection that requires treatment) might be harmful even if the fever isn't. While you're waiting to speak to your practitioner, take acetaminophen (Tylenol) to start reducing the fever. Taking a tepid bath or shower, drinking cool beverages, and keeping clothing and covers light will also help bring your temperature down. Aspirin or ibuprofen (Advil or Motrin) should not be taken at any time during pregnancy unless they've been specifically recommended by your practitioner.

Strep Throat

"My preschooler came down with strep throat. If I catch it, is there a risk to the baby?"

If there's one thing kids are good at sharing, it's their germs. And the more kids you have at home (particularly of the daycare-attending or school-going variety), the greater your chances of coming down with colds and other infections while you're expecting.

So step up preventive measures (see box, page 531). But if you do suspect that you've succumbed to strep, call your practitioner, who will likely run a throat culture. Strep infection won't hurt the baby, as long as it is treated promptly with the right type of antibiotic—one that's effective and pregnancy safe. Don't take medication that was prescribed for your child or someone else in the family.

Urinary Tract Infection

"I'm afraid I have a urinary tract infection."

Your poor battered bladder, which spends months on end being pummeled by your growing uterus and its adorable occupant, is the perfect breeding ground for less welcome visitors: bacteria. Those little bugs (which usually live quietly in your skin and in your feces) have an easier-than-usual time entering your urinary tract when you're expecting, thanks to the flood of muscle-relaxing hormones. Once there, bacteria make themselves at home and make you miserable—multiplying fast in areas where compression from your expanding uterus (the same compression that has you getting up to pee several times a night) has allowed urine to pool or flow slowly. In fact, urinary tract infections (UTIs) are so common in pregnancy that at least 5 percent of pregnant women can expect to develop at least one, and those who have already had one have a 1 in 3 chance of an encore. In some women, a UTI is "silent" (without symptoms) and diagnosed only after a routine urine culture. In others, symptoms can range from mild to quite uncomfortable (an urge to urinate frequently, pain or a burning sensation when urine—sometimes only a drop or two—is passed, pressure or sharp pain in the lower abdominal area). The urine may also be foul smelling and cloudy.

Diagnosing a UTI is as simple as dipping a stick into a urine sample at your practitioner's office—the stick will react to red or white blood cells in the sample, both of which can indicate an infection. The urine will then be sent off to the lab for further analysis. Treating a UTI is simple, too. Your practitioner will prescribe a course of pregnancy-safe antibiotics specifically targeting the type of bacteria the lab finds in your urine.

Of course, prevention is always the best strategy—but especially when you're expecting. Here are some steps you can take to prevent a UTI—you can also use them, in conjunction with your prescribed treatment, to help speed your recovery from an infection:

- Drink plenty of fluids, especially water, which can help flush out any bacteria. Cranberry juice may also be beneficial, possibly because the tannins it contains keep bacteria from sticking to urinary tract walls. Avoid coffee and tea (even decaffeinated), which may increase irritation.

- Wash your vaginal area well and empty your bladder just before and after sex.

- Every time you urinate, take the time to empty your bladder thoroughly. Leaning forward on the toilet will help accomplish this. It sometimes also helps to "double void": After you pee, wait 5 minutes, then try to pee again. And don't put off the urge when you have it, since regularly holding it in increases susceptibility to infection.

- To give your perineal area breathing room, wear cotton-crotch underwear and panty hose, avoid wearing tight pants or leggings, don't wear panty hose or tights under pants, and sleep without panties or pajama bottoms on if possible (and comfortable).

- Keep your vaginal and perineal areas meticulously clean and irritation-free. Wipe front to back after using the toilet to keep fecal bacteria from entering your vagina or urethra. Wash daily (showers are better than baths), and avoid bubble bath and perfumed products: powders, shower gels, soaps, sprays, detergents, and toilet paper.

- Ask your practitioner about taking probiotics to help restore the balance of beneficial bacteria.

UTIs in the lower part of the urinary tract are no fun, but a more serious potential risk is that bacteria from an untreated UTI will travel up to your kidneys. Kidney infections that aren't treated can be quite dangerous and may lead to premature labor, low birthweight, and other complications. The symptoms are the same as those of UTIs but are frequently accompanied by fever (often as high as 103°F), chills, blood in the urine, backache (in the midback on one or both sides), nausea, and vomiting. If you experience these symptoms, notify your practitioner immediately so you can be treated promptly.

Yeast Infection

"I think I have a yeast infection. Should I go get some of the cream I usually use, or do I need to see the doctor?"

Pregnancy is never a time for self-diagnosis or treatment—not even when it comes to something as seemingly simple as a yeast infection. Even if you've had yeast infections a hundred times before, even if you know the symptoms backward and forward (a yellowish, greenish, or thick and cheesy discharge that has a foul odor, accompanied by burning, itching, redness, or soreness), even if you've treated yourself successfully with over-the-counter preparations in the past—this time around, call your practitioner.

What kind of treatment you'll get will depend on what kind of infection you have, something only lab tests can determine. If it does turn out to be a yeast infection, which is very common

Bacterial Vaginosis

Bacterial vaginosis (BV) is the most common vaginal condition in women of childbearing age, affecting more than three-quarters of all women and up to 16 percent of pregnant women. BV, which occurs when certain types of bacteria normally found in the vagina begin to multiply in large numbers, is often accompanied by an abnormal gray or white vaginal discharge with a strong fishlike odor, pain, itching, or burning (though some women with BV report no signs or symptoms at all). Experts are not exactly sure what causes the normal balance of bacteria in the vagina to be disrupted, though some risk factors have been identified, including having multiple sex partners, douching, or having an IUD.

Why should you be concerned about something that's so common? It's because during pregnancy, BV is associated with a slight increase in complications—premature rupture of the membranes, for instance, or amniotic fluid infection—which may lead to premature labor. It may also be linked to a slight risk of miscarriage and low birthweight. Though it's unclear whether treating symptomatic BV with antibiotics during pregnancy decreases the risk of complications, most practitioners will treat anyway.

Be sure to mention any symptoms you may have to your practitioner so you can get the right diagnosis . . . and if necessary, the right treatment.

in pregnancy, your practitioner may prescribe vaginal suppositories, gels, ointments, or creams. The oral anti-yeast agent fluconazole (Diflucan) may be prescribed if necessary, but only in low doses and for no longer than 2 days because of the possible increased risk of miscarriage at higher doses.

Unfortunately, medication may banish a yeast infection only temporarily—the infection often returns off and on until after delivery and may require repeated treatment. You may be able to speed your recovery and prevent reinfection by staying as clean and dry as you can: Always wipe front to back, rinse your vaginal area thoroughly after soaping in the shower or bath (showers are preferable), skip perfumed soaps and bubble baths (and anything else irritating), wear cotton underwear, avoid tight pants or leggings (especially those that aren't cotton), and let the area breathe as much as possible (sleep without underwear if you can).

Eating yogurt containing live probiotic cultures may help keep those yeast bugs at bay. You can also ask your practitioner about taking an effective probiotic supplement. Some chronic yeast infection sufferers find that cutting down on foods yeast feeds on, like sugar and baked goods made with refined flour, helps as well. Do not douche, because it upsets the normal balance of bacteria in the vagina (which may be linked to BV; see box, page 529) and exposes you to harmful phthalates (good reasons never to douche, whether you're pregnant or not). You also don't need feminine vaginal wipes, but if you can't live without that "fresh feeling," choose wipes that are chemical- and alcohol-free, as well as pH safe, since changing the pH of your natural juices could increase the risk of infection.

Stomach Bugs

"I've got a stomach bug, and I can't keep anything down. Will this hurt my baby?"

Just when you thought it was safe to come out of the bathroom, you're back with a bug (goodbye morning sickness, hello stomach virus). And if you're still in your first trimester when the bug hits, it could be hard to differentiate the symptoms from those of morning sickness (unless you're bugged by diarrhea, too).

Luckily, having a stomach bug won't hurt your little one, just your stomach. But that doesn't mean it shouldn't be treated. And whether your tummy is turning from hormones, a virus, or egg salad that sat on the lunch cart too long, the treatment is the same: Get the rest your body's aching for and focus on fluids, especially if you're losing them through vomiting or diarrhea. They're much more important in the short term than solids.

If you're not urinating frequently enough or your urine is dark (it should be straw-colored), you may be dehydrated. Fluid needs to be your best buddy now: Try taking frequent small sips of water, diluted juice (white grape is easiest on the tummy), clear broth, weak tea, or hot water with lemon. If you can't manage to sip, suck on ice chips or an ice pop. Follow your stomach's lead when it comes to adding solids—and when you do, keep it bland, simple, and fat-free (dry toast, applesauce, bananas). And don't forget that ginger's good for what ails any sick stomach. Take it in tea or in flat ginger ale (best if there's actually ginger in it) or another ginger beverage, or suck or chew on some ginger candies. Getting your vitamin insurance is an especially good idea now, so try to take your prenatal when it's least likely to come back

Staying Well When You're Expecting

In pregnancy, when you need to stay well for two, the proverbial ounce of prevention is worth far more than a pound of cure. The following suggestions will increase your chances of staying well when you're expecting (and when you're not):

Keep your resistance up. Eat the best diet possible, get enough sleep and exercise, and don't run yourself down by running yourself ragged. Reducing stress in your life as much as you can also helps keep your immune system in tip-top shape.

Avoid sick people like the plague. As best as you can, try to stay away from anyone who has a cold, flu, stomach virus, or anything else noticeably contagious. Keep your distance from coughers on the bus, avoid hugging a friend who's complaining of a sore throat, and evade the handshake of a colleague with a runny nose (handshakes spread germs, not just greetings). Also avoid crowded or cramped indoor spaces when you can.

Wash your hands. Hands are the major spreader of infections, so wash them often and thoroughly with soap and warm water (about 20 seconds does the trick), particularly after exposure to someone you know is sick and after spending time in public places or riding on public transit. Hand washing is especially important before eating. Keep a hand sanitizer or hand sanitizing wipes in your glove compartment, in your desk drawer, and in your handbag or briefcase so you can wash up when there's no sink in sight.

Don't share the germs. At home, try to limit germ-spreading contact with sick kids or a sick spouse as much as possible. Avoiding finishing up their sandwich scraps and drinking from their cups. And while every sick child needs a dose of kiss-and-hug therapy from mom now and then, be sure to wash your hands and face (or wipe them down with hand sanitizer) after those comforting cuddles. Wash up with soap and water or wipe down with hand sanitizer, too, after touching germy sheets, towels, and used tissues, especially before touching your own eyes, nose, and mouth. See that little patients wash their hands frequently, also, and try to get them to cough and sneeze into their elbows instead of their hands (a good tip for adults, too). Use disinfectant spray or wipes on phones, tablets, keyboards, remotes, and other surfaces they handle.

If your own child or a child you care for or regularly spend time with develops a rash of any kind, avoid close contact and call your doctor as soon as you can unless you already know that you are immune to chicken pox, fifth disease, and measles.

Be pet smart. Keep pets in good health, updating their immunizations as necessary. And be sure to wash your hands after handling pet food or bowls (they sometimes harbor bacteria). If you have a cat, take the precautions to avoid toxoplasmosis (page 73).

Look out for ticks and mosquitoes. Avoid areas where Lyme disease or the Zika or West Nile virus are prevalent, or be sure to protect yourself adequately (see page 537 and the box on page 536).

To each their own. Maintain a no-sharing policy when it comes to toothbrushes and other personal items (and don't let those toothbrushes mingle bristle-to-bristle). Use disposable cups for rinsing in the bathroom.

Eat safe. To avoid food-borne illnesses, practice safe food preparation and storage habits (see page 117).

up (a powder may go and stay down easier). Don't worry, however, if you just can't handle your prenatal for a few days or so—no harm done.

If you can't get anything down, talk to your practitioner. Dehydration is a problem for anyone suffering with a stomach bug, but it's especially problematic if you're pregnant. You might be advised to take some rehydration fluid (like Pedialyte, which also comes in a soothing freezable form) or electrolyte water. Coconut water may be helpful, too. If you can't keep even that down, your doctor might want you to come in for IV fluids. Also call in if you're running a fever with those tummy troubles (see page 527).

Check with your practitioner before you open up your medicine cabinet looking for relief. Antacids like Tums and Rolaids are considered safe to take during pregnancy, and some practitioners may okay gas relievers, but ask first. Your practitioner may also okay certain antidiarrheal medicines, but probably only after your first trimester is safely behind you.

And sick tummies, take heart: Most stomach bugs clear up by themselves within a day or so.

CMV

"I'm a preschool teacher, and we've had an outbreak of CMV at our school. Is this something I should worry about catching during pregnancy?"

Fortunately, it's not likely that you can pick up CMV from one of your students and pass it on to your baby. That's because most adults were infected with CMV during childhood. If you're among that majority or if you've had CMV as an adult—and as someone who spends a lot of time with little ones, that's definitely possible—you

can't catch it now (though the CMV could be "reactivated"). Even if you do come down with a new CMV infection during pregnancy, the risks to your baby are low. Though half of expectant moms infected with CMV give birth to infected infants, only a small percentage of them show ill effects. The risks are lower still in a baby whose mom had a reactivated infection during pregnancy.

Still, because there is the potential for serious birth defects with CMV infection, it's smart to play it as safe as possible. Unless you know for sure that you're immune to CMV because you've had the infection before or because you were tested preconception, your best defense is a good offense (as it would be with any viral infection you're trying to avoid). As someone who works with little ones (and their germs), you probably know the hygiene drill. Be especially meticulous in practicing standard protocol for preventing the spread of any type of infection, such as washing your hands often and carefully, especially after changing diapers or helping children out at the potty—and of course, resist nibbling on leftovers.

Though CMV often comes and goes without any obvious symptoms, it's occasionally marked by fever, fatigue, swollen glands, and sore throat. If you notice any of these symptoms, check with your doctor. No matter if these symptoms signal CMV or another illness (such as flu or strep throat), you'll need some sort of treatment.

Fifth Disease

"I was told that a disease I had never even heard of before—fifth disease—could cause problems in pregnancy."

Fifth disease, caused by the parvovirus B19 (not to be confused with the parvovirus that affects dogs and cats), is the 5th of a group of 6 diseases that cause fever and rash in children. But unlike its sister diseases (such as measles and chicken pox, the ones that get all the attention), fifth disease isn't widely known because its symptoms are mild and can go unnoticed—or may even be totally absent. Fever is present in only 15 to 30 percent of cases. For the first few days, the rash gives the cheeks the appearance of having been slapped, then spreads in a lacy pattern to trunk, buttocks, and thighs, recurring on and off (usually in response to heat from the sun or a warm bath) for 1 to 3 weeks. It can be confused with the rash of other childhood illnesses or even a sun- or windburn. Adults don't typically show the "slapped cheek" rash.

Concentrated exposure from caring for a child sick with fifth disease or from teaching at a school where it is epidemic somewhat increases that very small risk of contracting the illness. But half of all women of childbearing age had fifth disease during childhood and are already immune, so infection, happily, isn't common among pregnant women. In the unlikely event that a mom-to-be catches fifth disease and her fetus does become infected, the virus can disrupt the developing baby's ability to produce red blood cells, leading to a form of anemia or other complications. If testing reveals you've contracted fifth disease, your practitioner will follow you for signs of fetal anemia with weekly ultrasounds for 8 to 10 weeks. If the baby is infected during the first half of pregnancy, the risk of miscarriage increases.

Again, the odds that fifth disease will affect you, your pregnancy, or your baby are very remote. Still, as always, it makes sense to take the appropriate steps to avoid any infection while you're expecting (see box, page 531).

Chicken Pox (Varicella)

"My toddler was exposed to chicken pox at her childcare center. If she comes down with it, could the baby I'm now carrying be hurt?"

Not likely. Well insulated from the rest of the world, your baby can't catch chicken pox from a third party—only from you. Which means you would have to catch it first, something that's unlikely. First of all, your child probably won't catch it and bring it home if she was immunized with the varicella vaccine (it's recommended that all tots get their first dose of the varicella vaccine at age 1 year—hopefully yours did). Second of all, it's very likely you had the infection as a child (85 to 95 percent of the U.S. adult population has had it) or had the vaccine, and are already immune. Ask your parents or check your health records to find out whether you have had chicken pox or received the vaccine (which became available in 1995). If you can't find out for sure, ask your practitioner to run a test now to see if you are immune.

Though the chances of your becoming infected are slim if you aren't immune, an injection of varicella-zoster immune globulin (VZIG) within 96 hours of a documented personal exposure (in other words, direct contact with someone who has been diagnosed with chicken pox) may be recommended. It isn't clear whether or not this will protect the baby if you do end up with chicken pox anyway, but it should minimize complications for you—a significant plus, since this mild childhood disease can be quite severe in adults. If you should be hit with a severe case, you may be given an antiviral drug to further reduce the risk of complications.

Measles, Mumps, and Rubella

Chances are good that you're already immune to measles, mumps, and rubella. That's because you (like most women of reproductive age) probably received the MMR vaccine, which protects against all 3 diseases, when you were a child—or less likely, that you had the diseases and can't catch them again. But with rising lapses in vaccination rates resulting in new outbreaks of these potentially dangerous diseases, you might be wondering if there's any risk to your pregnancy or your baby. Here's what you need to know:

Measles. In the very unlikely scenario that you're directly exposed to someone with measles and are certain you're not immune, your doctor may administer gamma globulin (antibodies) during the incubation period—between exposure and the start of symptoms—to decrease the severity of the illness should you come down with it. Measles does not appear to cause birth defects, though it may be linked to an increased risk of miscarriage or premature labor. If you were to contract measles near your due date, there is a risk that your newborn might catch the infection from you.

Mumps. It's not that easy to get mumps these days. It isn't highly contagious through casual contact, and only a few hundred Americans contract mumps each year, thanks to routine childhood immunization. However, because the disease appears to trigger uterine contractions and is associated with an increased risk of miscarriage in the first trimester or preterm labor later, pregnant women who aren't immune should be alert for early symptoms of mumps (possibly vague pain, fever, and loss of appetite, followed by the salivary glands becoming swollen, then ear pain and pain while chewing or with acidic or sour food or drink). Notify your practitioner of such symptoms immediately, because prompt treatment can reduce the chance of problems.

If you become infected during the first half of your pregnancy, the chances are very low (around 2 percent) that your baby could develop a condition called congenital varicella syndrome, which can cause some birth defects. If you come down with chicken pox later in your pregnancy, there's almost zero danger to the baby. The exception is if you get chicken pox just before (within a week of) giving birth or just after delivery. In that extremely unlikely scenario, there's a small chance your newborn will arrive infected and would develop the characteristic rash within a week or so. To prevent neonatal infection, your baby would be given an infusion of chicken pox antibodies immediately after delivery (or as soon as it becomes apparent that you've been infected postpartum).

Shingles, or herpes zoster, which is a reactivation of the chicken pox virus in someone who had the disease earlier (and happens only rarely in pregnant women), does not appear to be harmful to a fetus, probably because the mom—and so her baby—already has antibodies to the virus.

If you are not immune and escape infection this time, ask your doctor about getting immunized after delivery, to protect any future pregnancies. Immunization with the 2 doses taken between 4 and 8 weeks apart should be finished at least a month before any new conception.

Rubella. Because rubella can be very dangerous during pregnancy, your practitioner will perform a simple test—a rubella antibody titer—that measures the level of antibodies to the virus in your blood at the first prenatal visit to be absolutely certain you're immune. In the unlikely event you turn out not to be immune (or if the antibody levels in your blood are low, meaning that your immunity is waning), there's still no reason to worry. Happily, the CDC considers rubella to be eradicated in the U.S., making it nearly impossible for you to catch it here (and for the virus to be harmful you'd actually have to come down with the illness). The symptoms, which show up 2 or 3 weeks after exposure, are usually mild (malaise, slight fever, and swollen glands, followed by a slight rash a day or so later) and may sometimes pass unnoticed. If you did come down with rubella during pregnancy (and, again, the odds are extremely remote), whether your baby would be at risk would depend on when you contracted it. During the 1st month of pregnancy, the chance of a baby developing a serious birth defect is pretty high. By the 3rd month, the risk is significantly lower. After that, the risk is lower still.

Don't remember if you were ever vaccinated with the MMR, or if you ever had measles, mumps, or rubella? Check your medical records (or with your parents, who would most likely know whether they chose to opt out of routine vaccines like the MMR). If you're definitely not immune (or if titers show your immunity is low), you won't receive the MMR (or a booster) during pregnancy. Though there has never been a problem reported among babies of women who were inadvertently vaccinated before they knew they were pregnant, experts advise not taking the theoretical risk. But you can be vaccinated with the MMR (or if your titers are low for only one of the diseases, with just that individual vaccine) right after delivery. This will not only help protect your little one until he or she is fully immunized, but will protect your future pregnancies as well.

Hepatitis A

"I just heard about a recall of packaged fruit because of possible hepatitis A contamination—after I had already bought and eaten some. If I get hepatitis A, could it affect my pregnancy?"

Hepatitis A infection is rare these days in the U.S. (it's more prevalent in countries with poor sanitation) and is usually passed along through the fecal-oral route (by ingesting something that has been contaminated with the feces of an infected person). Most infections result from close personal contact, but the virus can also be spread by an infected food worker—likely the reason the food you purchased was recalled (and another good case for safe hygiene practices while cooking and preparing food). The infection is often mild, with no noticeable symptoms (especially in young children). Older children and adults typically experience muscle aches, headache, abdominal discomfort, loss of appetite, fever, and malaise, and in some cases jaundice (a yellowing of the skin and eyes). In rare cases the symptoms become severe enough to require hospitalization. Symptoms usually last no longer than 2 months, and those infected with hepatitis A recover completely (usually without any treatment needed) and end up immune to the infection for the future. (You're also immune if you were ever vaccinated against hep A.)

Protecting Against Zika Virus

Zika virus is an infection spread by mosquitoes (and in some cases through sex). Though it isn't normally risky for the general population, usually causing mild symptoms (or sometimes no noticeable symptoms at all), the virus has been linked both to miscarriage and serious birth defects—such as microcephaly (a small head) and brain damage—in babies of moms infected during pregnancy. If you live in or must travel to a region where Zika is prevalent (the CDC recommends that you don't travel to these areas), protect yourself against mosquito bites (see box, page 269). If your partner has traveled to a Zika-affected region, the CDC advises that you abstain from sex or use a condom during sex for the rest of your pregnancy. If you do become infected with the Zika virus during pregnancy (or if you think you might have been infected with it), you'll get a blood test and ultrasound and your pregnancy will be monitored more closely. For the latest information, visit cdc.gov/zika.

Happily, the infection is rarely passed on to a fetus or newborn. That's because the antibodies your body produces after exposure pass right away through the placenta, completely protecting the baby from the infection. So even if you did catch it, it's unlikely to affect your pregnancy. Still, your practitioner may suggest you get a shot of immunoglobulins within 2 weeks of exposure, just to be on the extra-safe side (the shot itself is safe, too).

If you are planning to travel to an area with high rates of infection, or if you have hepatitis B or C, ask your physician about immunization against hepatitis A, which can be given during pregnancy.

Hepatitis B

"I'm a carrier of hepatitis B and just found out that I'm pregnant. Will my being a carrier hurt my baby?"

Knowing that you're a carrier for hepatitis B is the first step in making sure your condition won't hurt your baby. Luckily it's unlikely the infection will be passed on to your baby while in utero. But because this liver infection can be passed on to baby during delivery, prompt steps will be taken at your baby's birth to make sure that doesn't happen. Your newborn will be treated within 12 hours with both hepatitis B immune globulin (HBIG) and the hepatitis B vaccine (which is routine at birth anyway). This treatment can almost always prevent the infection from developing. Your baby will also be vaccinated at 1 or 2 months and then again at 6 months (this, too, is routine for all babies), and may be tested at 12 to 15 months to be sure the therapy has been effective.

Hepatitis C

"Should I be worried about hepatitis C during pregnancy?"

Because hep C is usually transmitted via blood (for instance, through past transfusions or illegal drug injections), unless you've had a transfusion or are in a high-risk category, it's unlikely you'd be infected. Hepatitis C can be transmitted from infected mother to child during delivery, with a transmission rate of about 4 to 7 percent. The infection, if diagnosed, can potentially be treated, but not during pregnancy.

Lyme Disease

"I live in an area that's high risk for Lyme disease. Do I need to take any extra precautions now that I'm pregnant?"

As you probably already know, Lyme disease is most common among those who spend time in wooded areas where deer ticks hide out—but those ticks can occasionally hitch a ride into the suburbs and city, too, via greenery brought in from the country.

The best way to protect yourself is by taking preventive measures. If you are out in woodsy or grassy areas, or if you are handling greenery grown in such areas, wear long pants, tucked into boots or socks, and long sleeves, and use an insect repellent effective for deer ticks (such as one containing DEET) on exposed skin and treat clothing with permethrin. When you return home, check your skin carefully for ticks (if you can't easily see certain parts of your body now that you're pregnant, have your partner or someone else screen those areas of skin). If you find a tick, remove it right away by pulling straight up on it with tweezers (removing a tick within 24 hours almost entirely eliminates the possibility of infection). There is no need to save the tick for testing.

If you find a tick and notice the characteristic blotchy, bull's eye rash at the bite site, see your doctor—a blood test may be able to determine whether you are infected. Early symptoms of Lyme may include fatigue, headache, stiff neck, fever and chills, generalized achiness, and swollen glands near the site of the bite. Later symptoms may include arthritis-like pain and memory loss.

Fortunately, studies have shown that prompt treatment with antibiotics completely protects a baby whose mother is infected with Lyme—and keeps mom from becoming seriously ill.

Bell's Palsy

"I woke up this morning with pain behind my ear, and my tongue felt numb. When I looked in the mirror, the whole side of my face looked droopy. What's going on?"

It sounds like you may have Bell's palsy, a temporary condition caused by damage to the facial nerve, resulting in weakness or paralysis on one side of the face. Though it's quite uncommon in general, Bell's palsy strikes pregnant women 3 times more often than it does women who are not pregnant, and occurs most often in the third trimester or early postpartum. Its onset is sudden, and most people with the condition wake up without warning to find their face drooping.

The cause of this temporary facial paralysis is unknown, though experts suspect that certain viral or bacterial infections may cause swelling and inflammation of the facial nerve, triggering the condition. Other symptoms sometimes accompanying the paralysis include pain behind the ear or in the back of the head, dizziness, drooling (because of the weak muscles), dry mouth, inability to blink, impaired sense of taste, tongue numbness, and even impaired speaking.

The good news is that Bell's palsy will not spread beyond your face and won't get worse. More good news: Most cases completely resolve within 3 weeks to 3 months without treatment (though for some it can take as long as 6 months to go away completely). And the best news of all: The condition poses no threat to your pregnancy or your baby and needs no treatment. But since the signs of a stroke (which is slightly more common during pregnancy even in young and healthy women) can mimic those of Bell's palsy, it's critical that you call your practitioner right away if you notice a sudden onset of a facial droop.

ALL ABOUT:
Medications During Pregnancy

What do just about all prescription and over-the-counter medications have in common? Check out the fine print on those labels and package inserts and you'll see: Virtually all warn pregnant women against using them without a doctor's advice. Still, if you're like the average expectant mom, you'll wind up taking at least one prescription drug during your pregnancy and even more over-the-counter medications. How will you know which are safe and which aren't?

Fortunately, only a few drugs are definitively known to be harmful during pregnancy, and many drugs can be used safely. Still, no drug—prescription or over-the-counter, traditional or herbal—is 100 percent safe for 100 percent of the people, 100 percent of the time. And when you're pregnant, there's the health and wellbeing of two people, one very small and vulnerable, to consider every time you take a drug. Weighing the potential risks of taking a medication against the potential benefits it will provide is always wise—but it's smarter still when you're pregnant. Likewise, involving your practitioner in the decision of whether or not to take a drug is a good idea in general, but when you're pregnant, it's essential.

So, just like the labels say: Always ask first. Before you take any medication while you're expecting—even if you've popped it routinely in the past-without thinking twice—check with your practitioner about whether it's safe now.

Common Medications

Here's the lowdown on some of the more common medications you might consider taking during pregnancy. Even if a medication on this list is believed to be safe, be sure to ask your practitioner before taking it for the first time during pregnancy.

Tylenol. Acetaminophen is usually given the green light for short-term use during pregnancy, but be sure to ask your practitioner for the proper dosage.

Aspirin. Aspirin is generally not recommended—especially during the third trimester, since it increases the risk for complications before and during delivery, such as excessive bleeding, as well as problems in the newborn. Some studies suggest that very low dosages of aspirin may help to prevent preeclampsia in certain circumstances, but only

---

Keeping Current

The many lists of safe, possibly safe, possibly unsafe, and definitely unsafe drugs and medication during pregnancy change all the time, especially as new medications are introduced, others change from being prescription-only to over-the-counter, and still others are being studied to determine their safety during pregnancy. To stay current on what is or isn't safe, always ask your practitioner first. You can also turn to the U.S. Food and Drug Administration (fda.gov), the March of Dimes Resource Center at (888) MODIMES (663-4637) or marchofdimes.org, or safefetus.com to check on the safety of a certain medication during pregnancy.

your practitioner will be able to tell you whether it should be prescribed in your case. Other studies suggest that low-dose aspirin, in combination with the blood-thinning medication heparin, may reduce the incidence of recurrent miscarriage in some women with a condition known as antiphospholipid antibody syndrome. Again, only your practitioner can tell you whether it would be advisable in your case.

Advil or Motrin. Ibuprofen generally shouldn't be used in pregnancy, especially during the first and third trimesters, when it can have the same blood-thinning effects as aspirin. Use it only if it's specifically recommended by a physician who knows you are pregnant.

Aleve. Naproxen, a nonsteroidal anti-inflammatory drug (NSAID), is not recommended for use in pregnancy at all.

Nasal sprays. For relief from a stuffy nose, most steroid-containing nasal sprays are fine to use. Check with your practitioner for a preferred brand and dosing. Saline sprays are always safe to use, as are nasal strips. When it comes to nonsteroidal nasal decongestant sprays containing oxymetazoline (like Afrin), steer clear unless you have a clear okay from your prenatal practitioner. Many practitioners will not give the green light to these sprays at all, and others will advise only limited use (1 or 2 days at a time) after the first trimester.

Antacids. Heartburn that won't quit (you'll have plenty of that) often responds to Tums or Rolaids—plus you'll get a dose of calcium to boot. Maalox and Mylanta are also usually given the green light. For all these choices, be sure to check with your practitioner for the right dosage.

Gas aids. Many practitioners will okay gas aids, such as Gas-X or Mylicon, for

---

Get Smart About Antibiotics

Antibiotics can be a lifesaver, literally, when used against potentially dangerous bacterial infections—but they can also be overused or used the wrong way, leading to antibiotic-resistant infections. Here are some smart facts about antibiotics:

- Antibiotics are prescribed for bacterial infections. They don't work (and shouldn't be used) on viral infections, like colds or the flu.

- There are many antibiotics that are safe for pregnancy use, so don't hesitate to take them if your practitioner prescribes them for a bacterial infection (like a UTI).

- Take your antibiotics exactly as your practitioner tells you. Don't skip doses, and always finish the entire course of antibiotics unless instructed not to do so.

- Discard any leftover medications, and never save antibiotics for the next time you become sick.

- Only take antibiotics prescribed for you, by a doctor who knows you're pregnant.

- When taking antibiotics, consider taking a probiotic supplement to replenish beneficial bacteria. Try to space out the doses—probiotics shouldn't be taken within a couple of hours of antibiotics.

---

the occasional relief of pregnancy bloat, but check first.

Antihistamines. Not all antihistamines are safe during pregnancy, but several will probably get the green light from your practitioner. Benadryl (generic name: diphenhydramine) is the antihistamine most commonly recommended

Medication and Lactation

Wondering whether you can open the medicine cabinet more often (and with less worry) when you're breastfeeding than when you were expecting? The good news is that most medications—both over-the-counter and prescription—are compatible with breastfeeding and safe for baby. Even when a certain drug must be shelved during lactation, there's often a safe substitute—which means you probably won't have to give up breastfeeding if you must take a medication. Also remember: While it's true that what goes into your body usually does make its way into your milk supply, the amount that ultimately ends up in your baby's meals is a tiny fraction of what ends up in you.

Most drugs, in typical doses, appear to have no effect on a nursing baby at all. These include common medications such as:

- Acetaminophen (Tylenol)

- Ibuprofen (Advil, Motrin)

- Antacids (Maalox, Mylanta, Tums)

- Laxatives (Metamucil, Colace)

- Antihistamines (such as Claritin; Benadryl is also safe but may cause drowsiness in a baby)

- Decongestants (Afrin, Allegra, and so on)

- Bronchodilators (Albuterol)

- Most antibiotics

- Most anti-yeast/fungal medications (Lotrimin, Mycelex, Diflucan, Monistat)

- Corticosteroids (Prednisone)

- Thyroid drugs (Synthroid)

- Most antidepressants

during pregnancy. Claritin (loratadine) is also considered safe by most experts, but check with your practitioner, because not all will give it the okay, particularly in the first trimester. Some practitioners allow the use of chlorpheniramine (Chlor-Trimeton) and triprolidine on a limited basis, but most advise choosing a better alternative, so be sure to ask before reaching for those.

Decongestants. Most practitioners say to stay clear of decongestants containing phenylephrine and pseudoephedrine (such as Sudafed, Claritin-D, and DayQuil). Some will okay very limited use after the first trimester (for example, once or twice daily for no more than a day or so), since more frequent use can reduce blood flow to the placenta. Don't take decongestants without asking your practitioner first, but don't worry if

you've already taken them—just let your practitioner know. Vicks VapoRub is safe to use as directed.

Antibiotics. If your doctor has prescribed antibiotics for you during pregnancy, it's because the risk posed by the infection you're fighting is greater than any risk of taking the medication (and many are considered completely safe). You'll likely be put on antibiotics that fall into the penicillin or erythromycin families. Certain antibiotics are not recommended (such as tetracyclines, often used to treat acne), so be sure that any doctor prescribing antibiotics knows that you're pregnant.

Cough medicines. Expectorants such as Mucinex, and cough suppressants such as Robitussin or Vicks 44, as well as most cough drops, are considered safe

- Most sedatives
- Most medications for chronic conditions (such as for asthma, heart conditions, high blood pressure, diabetes, and so on)

A few classes of medications can be significantly harmful for the breastfeeding mom's milk supply and her baby. Drugs like some beta-blockers, epilepsy and seizure drugs, cancer drugs, lithium, ergots (used to treat migraines), and lipid-lowering drugs should be shelved when you're breastfeeding.

The research jury is still out on other medications (certain classes of antihistamines, for instance, or certain types of antidepressants). And other medications are safe, but only if they are used sparingly and temporarily (such as narcotics for pain after a cesarean delivery). Be sure to check with your practitioner or your baby's pediatrician for the most up-to-date info on what's safe and what isn't. You can also check out the National Library of Medicine's Drug and Lactation database (LactMed) at toxnet.nlm.nih.gov (click on LactMed), the Infant Risk Center at infantrisk .com, or MotherRisk at motherrisk.org for more information on which medications are safe and which aren't when you're breastfeeding.

In some cases, a less-safe medication can safely be discontinued while a mom is breastfeeding, and in others, it's possible to find a safer substitute. When medication that isn't compatible with breastfeeding is needed short-term, nursing can be stopped temporarily, with breasts pumped to keep up supply but milk tossed (pump and dump). Or dosing can be timed for just after nursing or before baby's longest sleep.

The bottom line on medication and lactation: Make sure you get the green light from your practitioner or baby's pediatrician on any medication you take or are thinking about taking while you're breastfeeding, as well as any herbal remedy or supplement.

during pregnancy, but ask your practitioner about dosing.

Sleep aids. Unisom, Tylenol PM, Sominex, Nytol, Ambien, and Lunesta are generally considered safe during pregnancy, and they are okayed by many practitioners for occasional use. Always check with your practitioner before taking these or any sleep aids.

Antidiarrheals. Most antidiarrheals aren't recommended for use during pregnancy (both Kaopectate and Pepto-Bismol contain salicylates—an active ingredient that is considered off-limits when you're expecting), though Imodium usually gets the green light after the first trimester.

Anti-nausea. Unisom Sleep Tabs (which contain the antihistamine doxylamine), taken in combination with vitamin B_6, decrease the symptoms of morning sickness but get dosing instructions from your practitioner. The downside of taking this remedy during the day: sleepiness. Diclegis, a time-released formula that combines those same ingredients and is available by prescription, may cause less drowsiness and is considered completely safe.

Topical antibiotics. Small amounts of topical antibiotics when needed for a cut or other injury, such as bacitracin or Neosporin, are safe during pregnancy.

Topical steroids. Small amounts of topical hydrocortisones (such as Cortaid) are safe during pregnancy. Use sparingly on rashes or bug bites when necessary.

Antidepressants. Though the research on the effects of antidepressants on pregnancy and on the fetus is ever-changing,

Making the Most of Your Meds

If you rely on oral medications to control a chronic condition, you may have to do a little adjusting now that you're expecting. For instance, if morning sickness has you down, taking your meds right before going to bed—so that they can build up in your system before the morning upchucking begins—may keep you from losing most of the dose through vomiting. If you must take a medication on an empty stomach (especially first thing in the morning) yet find it impossible to do because of nausea, ask your practitioner about using an anti-nausea medication that comes in suppository form (like Phenergan) before taking your medication.

Something else that you'll have to keep in mind—and that your team of doctors will have to keep an eye on: Some medications are metabolized differently during pregnancy, so the dosage you're used to isn't necessarily the right dosage now that you're expecting. If you're not sure whether your dosing is correct now that you're pregnant or if you think it might need to be adjusted because you have gained a lot of weight—or if you just have a hunch you're getting too much medicine or not enough—check with your doctors.

it does appear that there are several meds that are safe to use, others that should be completely avoided, and still others that can be considered on a case-by-case basis, their use weighed against the risk of untreated (or undertreated) depression. See page 45 for more.

If You Need Medication During Pregnancy

Has your practitioner recommended or prescribed a medication for you? Here are some steps you can take to help ensure that you're medicating safely for two:

- Lower risks and boost benefits. While weighing the risks and benefits of taking a medication with your practitioner, see if you can tip the scales even further in your favor and your baby's by boosting benefits (like taking a cold medication at night, when it will help you sleep) or reduce the risks (perhaps taking the medication for the shortest possible time, at the lowest effective dose).

- Ask and tell. Always clear a medication that's been prescribed by a different health care provider (say, an antibiotic for an ear infection prescribed by the ENT or an antidepressant prescribed by your internist or therapist) with your ob practitioner.

- Watch out for multitasking medications. Many OTC meds combine several active ingredients for multi-symptom relief, and one or more of these may not be pregnancy safe. For instance, an acetaminophen-based pain reliever might be combined with a sleep aid or a decongestant, or in some cases, even a cough suppressant. So check the active ingredients list to make sure the product you're choosing contains only the ingredient (or ingredients) your practitioner has cleared.

- Ask your practitioner ahead of time about side effects to look out for and which you should report, if any.

PART 5

The Complicated Pregnancy

CHAPTER 19

Managing Complications

....

I f you've been diagnosed with a complication or suspect you may be having one, you'll find information about symptoms and treatments in this chapter. If you've had a problem-free pregnancy so far—and there's no reason to believe it will be anything but smooth sailing throughout—this need-to-know chapter is not for you. In fact, you don't need to know any of it. While information is definitely empowering when you need it, reading about all the things that could go wrong when they're not going wrong (and aren't likely to go wrong) is only going to stress you out—and for no good reason. Skip it, and save yourself some unneeded worry.

Pregnancy Complications

The following pregnancy complications, though more common than some, are still unlikely to be experienced by the average mom-to-be. So read this section only if you've been diagnosed with a complication or you're experiencing symptoms that might indicate one. If you are diagnosed with a complication, use the information about the condition in this section as a general overview—so you have an idea of what you're dealing with—but expect to receive more specific (and possibly different) advice from your practitioner. That's, of course, the advice you should follow.

Subchorionic Bleed

What is it? A subchorionic bleed (also called a subchorionic hematoma) is the accumulation of blood between the uterine lining and the chorion (the outer fetal membrane, next to the uterus) or under the placenta itself, often (but not always) causing noticeable spotting or bleeding.

Bleeding During Pregnancy

Thankfully, most bleeding or spotting during pregnancy doesn't mean anything is wrong with your baby or your pregnancy. But sometimes, bleeding indicates something more serious—a problem with the placenta, for instance, a threatened miscarriage, or rarely, an ectopic pregnancy. Which is why you should report any spotting or bleeding you notice to your practitioner.

During the first trimester, call if you notice:

- Light, pink to dark red spotting. It's usually nothing to worry about, but check in anyway. It could be the result of implantation, irritation of the cervix after sex or a pelvic exam, a minor vaginal infection, or something else innocuous (see page 143).

- Light to heavy bright red spotting. Often, this type of spotting doesn't mean something is wrong, but you should definitely check in with your practitioner. Light to heavy red spotting could indicate a subchorionic bleed (facing page) or a threatened miscarriage (page 546).

- Spotting (pink, red, or brown) accompanied by cramping—call right away. Though such symptoms may not mean anything worrisome is happening, it's important to get checked out right away, since such symptoms could sometimes indicate a threatened miscarriage (page 546) or an inevitable miscarriage (page 582). Your practitioner will want to check to see if the cervix is opened or closed, and will likely use ultrasound to check for a fetal heartbeat.

- Heavy bleeding and cramping—call right away. Some women bleed heavily during the first trimester—even accompanied by cramping—and their pregnancies proceed normally. But about half of all women who have bleeding and cramping in the first trimester end up experiencing a miscarriage. For more information on early miscarriage, see page 582.

- Bleeding and very sharp pain in the lower abdomen with tenderness, shoulder pain, and/or rectal pressure—call right away (or dial 911). These symptoms could indicate an ectopic pregnancy (see page 588) that has ruptured or is about to.

In the second trimester, call if you notice:

- Spotting (light bleeding) or heavy bleeding (in the second or third trimester). Call your practitioner right away, since bleeding in the last 2 trimesters could be caused by placenta previa (page 554), placental abruption (page 556), a tear in the uterine lining, or (if it's after week 20) premature labor (page 559)—all of which need to be checked out and treated (if possible) as soon as possible. While spotting or bleeding during the second or third trimesters is not a definitive sign that there is something serious going on, it's a good idea to have it evaluated, just to be on the safe side.

- Heavy bleeding with blood clots, accompanied by cramping. In the second trimester, these symptoms unfortunately usually mean a late miscarriage is inevitable. See page 589 for more on late miscarriage.

The vast majority of women who have a subchorionic bleed go on to have perfectly healthy pregnancies. But because (in rare cases) bleeds or clots that occur under the placenta can cause problems if they get too large, all subchorionic bleeds are monitored.

How common is it? Of those women who experience first-trimester bleeding, 20 percent of them are diagnosed with a subchorionic bleed as the cause.

What are the signs and symptoms? Spotting or bleeding, often beginning in the first trimester, may be a sign. But many subchorionic bleeds are detected during a routine ultrasound, without there being any noticeable signs or symptoms.

What can you and your practitioner do? If you have spotting or bleeding, call your practitioner. An ultrasound may be ordered to see whether there is a subchorionic bleed, how large it is, and where it's located.

Threatened Miscarriage

What is it? A threatened miscarriage is a condition that suggests a miscarriage might take place. There is usually (but not always) some vaginal bleeding,

---

You'll Want to Know . . .

Occasional cramping in your lower abdomen early in pregnancy is probably the result of implantation, normally increased blood flow, or ligaments stretching as the uterus grows, not a sign of an ectopic pregnancy. For more on ectopic pregnancy, see page 588.

You'll Want to Know . . .

Roughly half of all expectant women who are diagnosed with a threatened miscarriage go on to have a perfectly healthy pregnancy and baby.

---

and sometimes abdominal cramps, but the cervix remains closed and the fetal heartbeat can be seen on ultrasound.

How common is it? About 1 of every 4 pregnant women has some bleeding during the first few months.

What are the signs and symptoms? Symptoms of a threatened miscarriage include:

- Abdominal cramps with or without vaginal bleeding during the first 20 weeks of pregnancy, with a cervix that remains closed

- Vaginal bleeding during the first 20 weeks of pregnancy without cramps, with a cervix that remains closed

What can you and your practitioner do? The first thing your practitioner will do if you have bleeding and/or cramping is a pelvic exam to check whether the cervix is opened or closed, and to gauge the amount of bleeding. You'll also likely get an ultrasound to check for the baby's heartbeat.

Your practitioner may also test your blood hCG level over a period of days to be sure the levels are rising, indicating the pregnancy is continuing. A blood test might also be used to check your progesterone levels.

Depending on the results of these tests, your practitioner may prescribe bed rest (plus pelvic rest, see page 576), and may, depending on your particular

Wait and See

Sometimes it's too early to see a fetal heartbeat or visualize the fetal sac on ultrasound, even in a healthy pregnancy. Dates could be off or the ultrasound equipment not sophisticated enough. If your cervix is still closed, you are spotting only lightly, and the ultrasound isn't definitive, a repeat ultrasound will be performed in a week or so to let you know what's really going on. Your hCG levels will also be followed. It's important to stay realistic but also to stay positive, as well as hold off on any action until the pregnancy has proved to be unviable.

circumstance, recommend you take supplemental progesterone to help sustain the pregnancy.

If an exam shows that your cervix is opened, or if there is no fetal heartbeat on ultrasound, a miscarriage is unfortunately considered inevitable. For more information on miscarriage, see Chapter 20.

Hyperemesis Gravidarum

What is it? Hyperemesis gravidarum (HG) is the medical term for severe pregnancy nausea and vomiting that is continuous and debilitating (not to be confused with typical morning sickness, even a pretty bad case). HG begins early in the first trimester (with a diagnosis usually coming about 9 weeks into pregnancy) and usually starts to lift between weeks 12 and 16. Most cases fully resolve by week 20, but in some women, the condition can continue throughout pregnancy.

Left untreated, HG can lead to weight loss (usually about 10 pounds or 5 percent of prepregnancy body weight), malnutrition, and dehydration. Treatment of severe HG often requires hospitalization—mostly for the administration of IV fluids and antinausea drugs, which can effectively safeguard your wellbeing and your baby's.

How common is it? HG occurs in about 1 to 2 percent of all pregnancies. It is more common in first-time moms, in young moms, in obese moms, and in moms carrying multiples. Extreme emotional stress (not your run-of-the-mill, everyday stress) may also increase your risk, as might endocrine imbalances (high thyroid levels) and vitamin B or other nutrient deficiencies. And if you had HG in a previous pregnancy, you're somewhat more likely to encounter it with subsequent pregnancies.

What are the signs and symptoms? The symptoms of HG include:

- Very frequent and severe nausea and vomiting (in other words, vomiting all day, every day)

- The inability to keep any food or even liquid down

- Signs of dehydration, such as infrequent urination or dark, scant urine

- Weight loss of more than 5 percent

- Blood in the vomit

What can you and your practitioner do? Diclegis (a combination of vitamin B_6 and doxylamine, the antihistamine found in Unisom SleepTabs) is often prescribed for tough morning sickness cases. You can combine the medication with some of the natural remedies used to fight morning sickness, including ginger, acupuncture, and acupressure wristbands (see page 137). Some experts suggest that magnesium

You'll Want to Know . . .

As miserable as hyperemesis gravidarum makes you feel, it's very unlikely to affect your baby. Most studies show no health or developmental differences between infants of moms who experience HG and those who don't.

supplements (oral or spray form) or even Epsom salt baths may help ease symptoms, so ask your practitioner about these options, too. But if you're vomiting continually and/or losing significant amounts of weight, your practitioner will assess your need for bed rest, IV fluids, and/or hospitalization, as well as some sort of antiemetic (antinausea) drug (such as Phenergan, Reglan, or scopolamine), if Diclegis alone hasn't worked. Once you're able to keep food down again, it may help to tweak your diet to eliminate fatty and spicy foods, which are more likely to cause nausea, as well as to avoid any smells or tastes that tend to set you off. In addition, try to graze on many small high-carb and high-protein meals throughout the day, and be sure your fluid intake is adequate. Keeping an eye on your urinary output is the best way to assess whether you're dehydrated—dark, scant urine is a sign you're not getting, or keeping down, enough fluids.

One thing to remember is that you're not alone—even if you think the typical pregnant woman who complains about her morning sickness can't relate. For support from moms who have been there, done that, and gotten through it (and given birth to healthy babies), check out the HER Foundation at hel-pher.org.

Gestational Diabetes

What is it? Gestational diabetes (GD)—a form of diabetes that appears only during pregnancy—occurs when the body becomes more resistant to insulin (the hormone that lets the body turn blood sugar into energy) and is less able to regulate the increased blood sugar of pregnancy effectively. Since GD usually begins between weeks 24 and 28 of pregnancy, a glucose screening test is routine at around 28 weeks. If you came into pregnancy obese, however, GD may show up earlier (or you may have undiagnosed Type 2 diabetes), which is why your practitioner may recommend screening earlier and more often. GD almost always goes away after delivery, but if you've had it, you'll be checked postpartum to make sure it's gone.

Diabetes, both the kind that begins in pregnancy and the kind that started before conception, is not harmful to either a mom or her baby if it is well controlled. But if excessive sugar is allowed to circulate in a mother's blood and then enter the fetal circulation through the placenta, the potential problems for both mother and baby are serious. Women who have uncontrolled GD are more likely to have a too-large baby, which can complicate delivery. They are also at risk for developing preeclampsia (see page 550) and stillbirth. Uncontrolled diabetes could also lead to potential problems for the baby after birth, such as jaundice, breathing difficulties, and low blood sugar levels. Later in life, he or she may be at an increased risk for obesity and Type 2 diabetes. Research also suggests that early uncontrolled GD (before 26 weeks) in a mom is associated with a greater chance of autism in her child. But it's important to remember: Those potential negative effects don't apply to moms who get the help they need to keep their blood sugar under control.

How common is it? GD is fairly common, affecting around 7 to 9 percent of expectant moms. Because it's more common among obese women, rates of GD are rising along with rising obesity rates in the U.S. Older moms-to-be are more likely to develop GD, as are women with a family history of diabetes or GD. Native Americans, Hispanic Americans, and African Americans are also at somewhat greater risk for GD.

What are the signs and symptoms? Most women with GD have no symptoms, though a few may experience:

- Unusual thirst

- Frequent urination in large amounts

- Fatigue (which may be difficult to differentiate from pregnancy fatigue)

- Sugar in the urine (detected at a routine practitioner visit)

What can you and your practitioner do? Around your 28th week (earlier if you're overweight or obese or have other risk factors), you'll be given a glucose screening test (see page 294) and, if necessary, a more elaborate 3-hour glucose tolerance test. If these tests show you have GD, your practitioner will likely put you on a special diet (similar to the Pregnancy Diet), suggest you exercise regularly, and recommend you keep your weight gain within recommended limits to keep your GD under control. You may also need to check your blood glucose levels at home. If diet and exercise alone aren't enough to control your blood sugar level (they usually are), you may need supplementary insulin. The insulin can be given in shots, or metformin (or less often,

glyburide) might be used as an alternative treatment for GD. Fortunately, virtually all of the potential risks associated with GD can be eliminated through the careful control of blood sugar levels achieved by good self-care and medical care.

Can it be prevented? Many of the same steps that can be taken to control GD can also help prevent it in the first place. Conceiving at an ideal weight lowers risk, as can gaining the right amount of weight during pregnancy. So, too, can good dietary habits (eating plenty of fruits and vegetables, lean protein, beans, and whole grains, limiting sugar, refined grains, and white potatoes, and making sure you're getting enough folic acid) and regular exercise (research shows that obese women who exercise cut their risk of developing GD by half).

Having GD during pregnancy does put you at greater risk of developing Type 2 diabetes after pregnancy. But keeping your diet healthy, staying at or getting to a normal weight, and, even more important, continuing to exercise after baby is born (and beyond) significantly cuts that risk. So does breastfeeding your baby. Experts say that breastfeeding improves glucose metabolism and insulin sensitivity, cutting the risk of developing diabetes down the road by half—and the longer you breastfeed, the lower your risk becomes.

You'll Want to Know . . .

If your GD is well controlled and your pregnancy carefully monitored, it's very likely your pregnancy will progress normally and your baby will be born healthy.

Preeclampsia

What is it? Preeclampsia is a disorder that generally develops late in pregnancy (after week 20) and is characterized by a sudden onset of high blood pressure, often (but not always) protein in the urine, and possibly other signs and symptoms. There may be excessive swelling (especially of the hands and face) with preeclampsia, but a diagnosis of the condition won't be made on the basis of swelling alone (swelling in pregnancy is usually completely normal). Pregnancy-induced hypertension involves only an increase in blood pressure, and is not the same as preeclampsia.

While it's unclear exactly what causes preeclampsia (see box, facing page), experts believe that it occurs when blood vessels in the placenta don't develop properly—they're narrower than normal—limiting the amount of blood that flows through them. These changes in blood flow to the placenta lead to high blood pressure and excessive swelling in the mom. And because the placenta doesn't function properly, it isn't as able to eliminate waste products fast enough, so those waste products build up in the blood, causing certain proteins that should stay in the bloodstream to leak into the urine. All this damage to the walls of these blood vessels can also result in changes in blood clotting, which in turn can lead to a host of other problems.

If preeclampsia goes untreated, it could progress to eclampsia, a much more serious condition involving seizures (see page 563). Unmanaged preeclampsia can also cause a number of other pregnancy complications, such as premature delivery or intrauterine growth restriction.

How common is it? About 8 to 10 percent of pregnant women are diagnosed with preeclampsia, with the risk higher for women carrying multiple fetuses, women over 40, obese women, and women with high blood pressure, diabetes, or gestational diabetes. Preeclampsia is more common in first pregnancies, and if you're diagnosed with preeclampsia in one of your pregnancies, you have a 1 in 3 chance of developing the condition in future pregnancies. That risk is higher if you're diagnosed with preeclampsia in your first pregnancy or if you develop preeclampsia early in any pregnancy.

What are the signs and symptoms? Symptoms of preeclampsia can include any or all of the following:

- A rise in blood pressure (to 140/90 or more in a woman who has never had high blood pressure before)

- Protein in the urine

- Severe headaches that aren't relieved by acetaminophen (Tylenol)

- Pain in the upper abdomen

- Blurred or double vision

- Rapid heartbeat

- Scant and/or dark urine

- Abnormal kidney function

- Exaggerated reflex reactions

- Severe swelling of hands and face

- Severe swelling of the ankles that doesn't go away

- Sudden excessive weight gain unrelated to eating

What can you and your practitioner do? Regular prenatal care is the best way to catch preeclampsia in its early stages (your practitioner might be tipped off by a rise in your blood pressure, or any of the symptoms listed above). Being alert to any such symptoms (and alerting your practitioner if you notice them)

The Reasons Behind Preeclampsia

No one knows for sure what causes preeclampsia, though there are a number of theories:

- A genetic link. Researchers hypothesize that the genetic makeup of the fetus could be one of the factors that predisposes a pregnancy to preeclampsia. So, if your mother or your partner's mother had preeclampsia during their pregnancies with either of you, you are somewhat more likely to have preeclampsia during your pregnancies. But the baby's genes are not the only ones in play. Something in the mom-to-be's genetic makeup can also predispose her to preeclampsia, say experts.

- A blood vessel defect. It has been suggested that this defect causes the blood vessels in some women to constrict during pregnancy instead of widen (as usually happens). As a result of this vessel defect, researchers theorize, there is a drop in the blood supply to organs like the kidney and liver, leading to preeclampsia. The fact that women who experience preeclampsia during pregnancy are at an increased risk later in life of having some sort of cardiovascular condition also seems to indicate that the condition may be the result of a predisposition to high blood pressure.

- Gum disease. Pregnant women with severe gum disease are more than twice as likely to have preeclampsia than women with healthy gums. Experts theorize that the infection causing the periodontal disease may travel to the placenta or produce chemicals that can cause preeclampsia. Still, it is not known if periodontal disease causes preeclampsia or if it is just associated with it.

- An immune response to a foreign intruder: the baby. This theory suggests that the woman's body becomes "allergic" to the baby and placenta. This "allergy" causes a reaction in the mother's body that can damage her blood and blood vessels. The more similar the father's and mother's genetic markers are to each other, the more likely this immune response will occur.

also helps, particularly if you had a history of hypertension before pregnancy, developed it during this pregnancy, or if you have diabetes or gestational diabetes.

In 75 percent of cases, preeclampsia is mild. However, even a mild case can progress to severe preeclampsia or eclampsia very quickly if it's not diagnosed and treated promptly. In severe preeclampsia, blood pressure is consistently much higher and can lead to organ damage and other more serious complications if not properly managed.

If you have a mild case, your doctor will probably recommend regular blood and urine tests (assessing platelet counts, liver enzymes, kidney function, urinary protein levels) to check if the condition is progressing, a daily kick count in the third trimester (recommended anyway; see page 315), blood pressure monitoring, changes to your diet (including eating more protein, fruits, veggies, low-fat dairy, and healthy fats, and less salt, as well as drinking enough water). Some form of bed rest may also be prescribed, as well as an early delivery (as close to 37 weeks as possible).

> ## You'll Want to Know . . .
>
> Fortunately, in women who are receiving regular medical care, preeclampsia is almost invariably caught early on and managed successfully. With appropriate and prompt medical care, a woman with preeclampsia near term has virtually the same excellent chance of having a positive pregnancy outcome as a woman with normal blood pressure.

In a more severe case, you'll most likely be treated in the hospital with careful fetal monitoring (including nonstress tests and ultrasounds to check for fetal wellbeing and growth), medication to lower your blood pressure, magnesium sulfate (an electrolyte with antiseizure properties that may help prevent progression to eclampsia), and early delivery—often once you've reached 34 weeks of pregnancy if your condition is stable. If it becomes unstable, the doctor may give you corticosteroids to speed your baby's lung maturity and deliver him or her right away, regardless of gestational age.

Keep in mind that while preeclampsia can be kept in check, the only way to absolutely cure the condition is by delivering your baby. The good news is that 97 percent of women with preeclampsia recover completely, with a speedy return to normal blood pressure, after delivery. That said, women with a history of preeclampsia have a higher risk of stroke, blood clots, and heart attack later in life, so be sure you continue to practice healthy habits— eating well, exercising, not smoking, and so on—and get good medical care and follow-up after your baby is born.

Can it be prevented? Research has suggested that for women at risk for preeclampsia, aspirin or other anticlotting drugs during pregnancy may reduce the risk. This has led to the recommendation that women who have a higher risk of preeclampsia, but don't have signs or symptoms, be prescribed a low-dose aspirin daily (81 milligrams per day) after the 12th week of pregnancy.

Coming into pregnancy at a healthy weight may lower the risk of preeclampsia. Some research has also suggested that good nutrition—including adequate intakes of vitamins and minerals (especially magnesium)—may reduce risk, as may regular exercise and proper dental care. One unexpected (and yummy) way to help prevent preeclampsia: regularly eating dark chocolate during the second half of pregnancy.

HELLP Syndrome

What is it? Like preeclampsia, HELLP syndrome is a serious pregnancy complication related to blood pressure. It can occur by itself or in conjunction with preeclampsia, almost always in the last trimester. The acronym stands for H (hemolysis, in which red blood cells are destroyed too soon, causing a low red-cell count), EL (elevated liver enzymes, which indicates that the liver is functioning poorly and is unable to process toxins in the body efficiently), and LP (low platelet count, which makes it difficult for the blood to form clots).

When HELLP develops, it can threaten both a mother's life and that of her baby. Women who don't get the diagnosis and aren't treated quickly run about a 1 in 4 chance of suffering serious complications, primarily in the form of extensive liver damage or stroke.

How common is it? About 50,000 moms-to-be in the U.S. develop HELLP each year, with the risk higher in women who have preeclampsia or eclampsia (about 10 to 20 percent of these women also develop HELLP) or have had HELLP in a previous pregnancy.

What are the signs and symptoms? The symptoms of HELLP are very vague, consisting of (in the third trimester):

- Nausea

- Vomiting

- Headaches

- General malaise

- Pain and tenderness in the right upper abdomen or chest

- Viral-type illness symptoms

Blood tests reveal a low platelet count, elevated liver enzymes, and hemolysis (the breakdown of red blood cells). Liver function rapidly deteriorates in women with HELLP, so treatment is critical.

What can you and your practitioner do? The only effective treatment for HELLP syndrome is delivery of your baby, so the best thing you can do is be aware of the symptoms of the condition (especially if you already have or are at risk for preeclampsia) and call your practitioner immediately if you develop any. If you have HELLP, you might also be given steroids (to treat the condition and help mature the baby's lungs) and magnesium sulfate (to prevent seizures).

Can it be prevented? Because a woman who has had HELLP in a previous pregnancy is at increased risk of having it again, close monitoring is necessary in any subsequent pregnancy. Taking the same steps to prevent and treat preeclampsia (see facing page) may help prevent a recurrence of HELLP.

Intrauterine Growth Restriction

What is it? Intrauterine growth restriction (IUGR) is a term used when a baby is smaller than normal during pregnancy. A diagnosis of IUGR is given if your baby's weight is below the 10th percentile for gestational age based on ultrasound measurements. IUGR can occur if the health of the placenta or its blood supply is impaired or if the mother's nutrition, health, or lifestyle prevents the healthy growth of her fetus.

Babies who have IUGR often have a low weight at birth—called small for gestational age (or SGA). But not all babies who are SGA had IUGR. Some are healthy babies who are just born smaller than average because they're genetically destined to be.

There are two types of IUGR: symmetrical IUGR, in which all parts of the baby's body are proportionally small, and asymmetrical IUGR, when the baby has a normal size head and brain but the rest of the body is small.

How common is it? IUGR occurs in about 10 percent of all pregnancies. It's more common in first pregnancies, in fifth and subsequent ones, in women who are under age 17 or over age 35, in those who had a previous low-birthweight baby, and in those who have placental problems or uterine

You'll Want to Know . . .

More than 90 percent of babies who are born small for gestational age do fine, catching up with their bigger birth buddies in the first couple of years of life.

You'll Want to Know . . .

A mom who has already had a low-birthweight baby has only a modestly increased risk of having another one—and, to her advantage, statistics show that each subsequent baby is actually likely to be a bit heavier than the preceding one. If you had an IUGR baby the first time around, controlling all the possible contributing factors can reduce the risk this time.

abnormalities. Carrying multiples is also a risk factor, but that's often simply the result of crowded conditions (it's hard to fit more than one 7-pounder in a single womb).

What are the signs and symptoms? Surprisingly, carrying small is not usually a tip-off to IUGR. In fact, there are rarely any obvious outward signs that the baby isn't growing in utero as he or she should be. Instead, IUGR is usually detected during a routine prenatal exam when the practitioner measures the fundal height—the distance from your pubic bone to the top of your uterus—and finds that it's measuring too small for the baby's gestational age, or through an ultrasound, which can detect a baby whose growth is slower than expected for his or her gestational age.

What can you and your practitioner do? One of the best predictors of a baby's good health is birthweight, so having IUGR can lead to some health problems in a newborn, including having difficulty maintaining a normal body temperature or fighting infection. That's why it's so important to diagnose and begin treating the problem as early

as possible during pregnancy to boost baby's chances of a healthy bottom line at birth. A variety of approaches may be tried, depending on the suspected cause, including bed rest, IV feedings if necessary, and medications to improve placental blood flow or to correct a diagnosed problem that may be contributing to the IUGR. If the uterine environment is poor and can't be improved, and the fetal lungs are mature, prompt delivery—which allows baby to start living under healthier conditions—is usually the best way to go.

Can it be prevented? Optimum nutrition, good prenatal care, and the right weight gain for mom can all greatly improve the chances that a baby will grow, develop, and thrive as he or she should—as can eliminating lifestyle factors that can contribute to IUGR (such as mom's smoking, drinking, or using recreational drugs), treating an eating disorder, minimizing physical and excessive psychological stress (such as from depression), and controlling chronic hypertension. Happily, even when prevention and treatment are unsuccessful (or impossible) and a baby is born smaller than normal, the chances that he or she will do well are increasingly good, thanks to the many advances in neonatal (newborn) care.

Placenta Previa

What is it? The definition of placenta previa is a placenta that partially or completely covers the opening of the cervix. In early pregnancy, a low-lying placenta is common, but as pregnancy progresses and the uterus grows, the placenta usually moves upward and away from the cervix. If it doesn't move up and partially covers or touches the cervix, it's called partial previa. If it completely covers the cervix, it's called total or complete previa. Either can physically block your baby's passage into the birth canal, making a vaginal delivery impossible. It can also trigger bleeding late in pregnancy and at delivery. The closer to the cervix the placenta is located, the greater the possibility of bleeding.

How common is it? Placenta previa occurs in 1 out of every 200 deliveries. It is more likely to occur in women over the age of 30 than in women under the age of 20, and it is also more common in women who have had at least one other pregnancy or any kind of uterine surgery (such as a previous c-section or a D&C that's performed after a miscarriage). Carrying multiple fetuses also increases the risks, as does smoking during pregnancy.

What are the signs and symptoms? Placenta previa is most often discovered not on the basis of symptoms but during a routine second-trimester ultrasound. Sometimes the condition announces itself in the third trimester (occasionally earlier) with bright red bleeding. Typically, bleeding is the only symptom. There's usually no pain involved.

What can you and your practitioner do? If you have no bleeding, and no signs of the more complicated placental condition placenta accreta (see page 565), nothing needs to be done until the third trimester, by which point most early cases of placenta previa have corrected themselves. Even later on, there is no treatment necessary if you've been diagnosed with previa but aren't experiencing any bleeding (you'll just need to be alert to any bleeding or to signs of premature labor, which is more common with placenta previa). If you're experiencing bleeding related to a diagnosed previa, your practitioner will likely put you on pelvic rest (no sex), advise you to

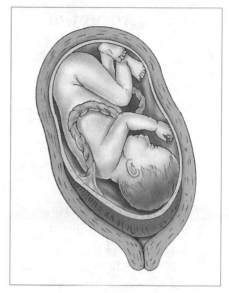

Placenta previa

take it easy and avoid strenuous activities or exercise, and monitor you closely. If preterm labor seems imminent, you may receive steroid shots to mature your baby's lungs more rapidly. Even if the condition hasn't presented your pregnancy with any problems at all (you haven't had any bleeding and you've carried to term), your baby will still be delivered via c-section.

You'll Want to Know . . .

Placenta previa is considered to be the most common cause of bleeding in the latter part of pregnancy. Most previas are found early and managed well, with the baby delivered successfully by c-section. About 75 percent of cases are delivered by scheduled c-section before labor starts.

Placental Abruption

What is it? Placental abruption is the early separation of the placenta from the uterine wall during pregnancy, rather than after delivery. If the separation is slight, there is usually little danger to the mother or baby as long as treatment is prompt and proper precautions are taken. If the abruption is more severe, however, the risk to the baby is considerably higher. That's because a placenta's complete detachment from the uterine wall means the baby is no longer getting oxygen or nourishment.

How common is it? It occurs in less than 1 percent of pregnancies, almost always in the second half of the pregnancy and most often in the third trimester. Placental abruption can happen to anyone, but it occurs more commonly in women who have had a previous abruption or have a predisposition to clotting, as well as in those who are carrying multiples, have GD, or have preeclampsia or other high blood pressure conditions of pregnancy. It's also more common in women who smoke or use cocaine. A short umbilical cord or trauma caused by an accident is occasionally the cause of an abruption.

What are the signs and symptoms? The symptoms of placental abruption depend on the severity of the detachment, but will usually include:

- Bleeding (light to heavy, with or without clots)

- Abdominal cramping or achiness

- Uterine tenderness

- Pain in the back or abdomen

What can you and your practitioner do? Let your practitioner know immediately if you have abdominal pain accompanied by bleeding in the second half of your pregnancy. Along with those symptoms, testing for fetal distress (nonstress and stress tests; see page 380) may be helpful in making the diagnosis and deciding on the management strategy, as can ultrasound (though only about 25 percent of abruptions can actually be seen on ultrasound).

If it's been determined that your placenta has separated slightly from the uterine wall but has not completely detached, and if your baby's vital signs stay regular, you'll probably be monitored closely and told to take it easy. If the bleeding continues, you may need to be hospitalized for continuous monitoring and IV fluids. Your practitioner may also administer steroids to speed up your baby's lung maturation in case you need to deliver early. If the bleeding remains manageable and the baby doesn't show any signs of distress, a vaginal delivery may be possible. But if the abruption is significant or if it continues to progress, the only way to treat it is to deliver the baby, usually by c-section.

Chorioamnionitis

What is it? Chorioamnionitis is a bacterial infection of the amniotic membranes and fluid that surround and protect your baby. It's caused by common bacteria such as E. coli or by group B strep (routinely tested for at about week 36). Infection is believed to be a major cause of preterm premature rupture of the membranes (PPROM) as well as of premature delivery.

How common is it? Chorioamnionitis occurs in 1 to 2 percent of pregnancies. Women who experience PPROM are at increased risk for chorioamnionitis because bacteria from the vagina can seep into the amniotic sac after it has ruptured. Women who've had the infection during their first pregnancy are more likely to have it again in a subsequent pregnancy.

What are the signs and symptoms? Diagnosis of chorioamnionitis is complicated by the fact that no simple test can confirm the presence of infection. The symptoms of chorioamnionitis can include:

- Fever

- Tender, painful uterus

- Increased heart rate in both you and your baby

- Leaking, foul-smelling amniotic fluid (if membranes have already ruptured)

- Unpleasant-smelling vaginal discharge (if membranes are intact)

- Increased white blood cell count (a sign the body is fighting an infection)

What can you and your practitioner do? Be sure to call your practitioner if you notice any leaking of amniotic fluid, no matter how small, or if you notice a foul-smelling discharge or any other of the symptoms listed above. If you are diagnosed with chorioamnionitis, you will likely be prescribed antibiotics and delivered immediately. You and your baby will also be given antibiotics after delivery to make sure no further infections develop.

Oligohydramnios

What is it? Oligohydramnios is a condition in which there is not enough amniotic fluid surrounding and cushioning the baby. It usually develops in the latter part of the third trimester, though it could show up earlier in pregnancy. Though the majority of women diagnosed with oligohydramnios will have a completely normal pregnancy, there is a slight risk of umbilical cord constriction if there's too little fluid for your baby to float around in. The condition may result from a puncture in the amniotic sac after amniocentesis or a spontaneous fluid leak at any time during pregnancy (one so small, you wouldn't necessarily notice it). A low level of amniotic fluid can also suggest a problem in the baby, such as poor fetal growth or a kidney or urinary tract condition (the baby normally excretes urine into the surrounding amniotic fluid, so when that process isn't working as it should, a first indicator is low amniotic fluid).

How common is it? Four percent of pregnant women are diagnosed with oligohydramnios, but the rate rises to 12 percent in pregnancies that are post-term (those that have reached 42 weeks).

What are the signs and symptoms? There are no symptoms, but signs that would point to the condition are a uterus that measures smaller than it should and a decreased amount of amniotic fluid, detected via ultrasound. There might also be a noticeable decrease of fetal activity and sudden drops in the fetal heart rate in some cases.

What can you and your practitioner do? If you're diagnosed with oligohydramnios, you'll need to get a lot of rest and drink plenty of water. The amount of amniotic fluid will be closely monitored. If at any point oligohydramnios endangers the wellbeing of your baby, your practitioner may opt for a prompt delivery. If the low level of fluid is the result of a problem with the baby's urinary tract, fetal surgery to correct it may be an option.

Hydramnios

What is it? Too much amniotic fluid surrounding the fetus causes the condition known as hydramnios (also called polyhydramnios). Most cases of hydramnios are mild and transient, simply the result of a temporary change in the normal balance of the amniotic fluid production, with any extra fluid likely to be reabsorbed without any treatment.

But when fluid accumulation is severe (which is rare), it may signal a problem with the baby, such as a central nervous system or gastrointestinal (or other congenital) defect, or an inability to swallow (normally, babies swallow amniotic fluid). Consistently high levels of amniotic fluid somewhat increase the risk for preterm premature rupture of the membranes, preterm labor, placental abruption, breech presentation, or umbilical cord prolapse.

How common is it? Hydramnios occurs in about 1 percent of all pregnancies. It is more likely to occur when there are multiple fetuses or when there are fetal abnormalities, and can be related to poorly controlled diabetes or gestational diabetes in the mother.

What are the signs and symptoms? More often than not, there are no symptoms at all with hydramnios, though some women may notice:

- Difficulty feeling fetal movements (because there's too much of a cushion from the extra fluid)

- Discomfort in the abdomen or chest (because the larger-than-normal uterus presses on the abdominal organs and chest wall)

Hydramnios is usually detected during an ultrasound that measures amniotic fluid or at a prenatal exam, when your fundal height—the distance from your pubic bone to the top of your uterus—measures larger than normal (though this finding on a physical exam will be followed up with an ultrasound for confirmation).

What can you and your practitioner do? Unless the fluid accumulation is fairly severe, there's absolutely nothing you need to do except to keep your appointments with your practitioner, who will continue to monitor your condition with ultrasounds (perhaps even weekly). If the accumulation is more severe, your practitioner may suggest you undergo a procedure called therapeutic amniocentesis, during which fluid is withdrawn from the amniotic sac to reduce the level.

Preterm Premature Rupture of the Membranes (PPROM)

What is it? PPROM refers to the rupture of the membranes (or "bag of waters") that cradle the fetus in the uterus, before 37 weeks (in other words, before term). The major risk of PPROM is a premature birth. Other risks include infection of the amniotic fluid and prolapse or compression of the umbilical cord. Rupture of the membranes that

---

You'll Want to Know . . .

With prompt and appropriate diagnosis and management of PPROM, both mom and baby should be fine, though if the birth is premature, there may be a long stay in the NICU for baby.

takes place before labor starts but after 37 weeks, is covered on page 378.

How common is it? Preterm premature rupture of membranes occurs in 3 percent of pregnancies. Women most at risk are those who smoke during pregnancy, have certain STDs, have chronic vaginal bleeding or placental abruption, have had PPROM previously, have bacterial vaginosis (BV), or are carrying multiples.

What are the signs and symptoms? The symptoms are leaking or gushing of fluid from the vagina. The way to tell whether you're leaking amniotic fluid and not urine is by taking the sniff test: If it smells like ammonia, it's probably urine. If it has a somewhat sweet smell, it's probably amniotic fluid (unless it's infected, in which case the fluid will be foul smelling). If you have any doubts about what you're leaking, call your practitioner to be on the safe side.

What can you and your practitioner do? If your membranes have ruptured after 34 weeks, you'll likely be induced and your baby delivered. If it's too soon for your baby to be delivered safely, you'll probably be put on in-hospital bed rest and given antibiotics to ward off infection, as well as steroids to mature your baby's lungs as quickly as possible for a safer early delivery.

Rarely, the break in the membranes heals and the leakage of amniotic fluid stops on its own. If that happens, you'll be allowed to go home and resume your normal routine while remaining alert to signs of further leakage.

Preterm Labor/Delivery

What is it? Labor that begins after week 20 but before the end of week 37 of pregnancy is considered to be preterm labor.

You'll Want to Know . . .

A baby born prematurely will likely need to spend time in a NICU (neonatal intensive care unit) for the first few days or weeks (or, in some cases, months) of life. Though prematurity has been linked to slow growth and developmental delays, most babies who arrive early and at a healthy (for a preemie) birthweight catch up and have no lasting problems at all. Thanks to advances in medical care, your chances of bringing home a normal, healthy infant after a premature birth are very good.

How common is it? Preterm labor and preterm birth are fairly common. About 12 percent of babies are born preterm in the U.S.

While no one knows for sure what causes premature labor, experts point to a number of factors that increase risk (see page 32 for a list of risk factors). Keep in mind that having one or more of these risk factors doesn't mean you'll necessarily go into preterm labor—and having no risk factors doesn't mean that you won't. In fact, at least half of the women who go into preterm labor have no known risk factor.

What are the signs and symptoms? Signs of premature labor can include all or some of the following:

- Menstrual-like cramps

- Regular contractions that intensify and become more frequent even if you change positions

- Back pressure

- Unusual pressure in your pelvis

Predicting Preterm Labor

Even among women who are at high risk for preterm labor, most will carry to term. One way to predict preterm labor is to examine cervical or vaginal secretions for a substance known as fetal fibronectin (fFN). Studies show that some women who test positive for fFN stand a good chance of going into preterm labor within 1 to 2 weeks after the test. The test, however, is better at predicting which women are not at risk for going into preterm labor (by detecting no fFN) than predicting which women are at risk. When fFN is detected, steps should be taken to reduce the chances of preterm labor. The test is now widely available, but is usually reserved for high-risk women only. If you aren't considered high risk for preterm birth, you don't need to be tested.

Another screening test is one for cervical length. Via ultrasound before 30 weeks, the length of your cervix is measured to see if there are any signs that the cervix is shortening or opening. A short cervix puts you at an increased risk of preterm labor, especially if it began shortening early in pregnancy.

Though not yet widely available, there is also a blood test that may be able to help predict preterm labor (ask your practitioner about it).

- Bloody vaginal discharge

- Rupture of membranes

- Changes in the cervix (thinning, opening, or shortening) as measured by ultrasound

What can you and your practitioner do? Because each day a baby remains in the womb improves the chances of both survival and good health, holding off delivery as long as possible will be the primary goal. Unfortunately, however, there often isn't much that can be done to stop early labor. The measures that were once routinely recommended (bed rest, hydration, monitoring for uterine activity) don't seem to work to stop or prevent contractions, though many doctors still prescribe them. Progesterone supplementation should be used in women with a prior spontaneous preterm delivery or those who have a short cervix and are not carrying multiples. Antibiotics (if a GBS culture is positive; see page 359) or tocolytics (that can temporarily halt contractions and give your practitioner time to administer steroids to help your baby's lungs mature more quickly, should a preterm birth become inevitable or necessary) may also be given. If at any point your practitioner determines that the risk to you or your baby from continuing the pregnancy outweighs the risk of preterm birth, no attempt will be made to postpone delivery.

Can it be prevented? Not all preterm births can be avoided, since not all are caused by preventable risk factors. However, all the following measures may reduce the risk of preterm delivery (while boosting your chances of having the healthiest pregnancy possible):

- Taking folic acid or a prenatal supplement for a year before pregnancy

- Spacing pregnancies at least 18 months apart, if possible

- Reaching an ideal weight before conception

- Getting good dental care before pregnancy

- Getting early prenatal care

- Eating well

- Receiving a weekly progesterone shot starting at 16 weeks of pregnancy and continuing through week 36 if you've delivered early before (but not if you're carrying multiples)

- Getting tested for and, if necessary, treated for any infections such as BV and UTIs during pregnancy

- Sticking to any limitations on activity (on the job, for instance, or, if needed, bed rest) prescribed by your practitioner

- Avoiding smoking, drinking, cocaine, and other drugs not prescribed by your doctor

The good news is that 80 percent of women who go into preterm labor will deliver at (or safely close to) term.

Pelvic Girdle Pain (PGP) or Symphysis Pubis Dysfunction (SPD)

What is it? Pelvic Girdle Pain, or PGP (also sometimes called symphysis pubis dysfunction, or SPD) is pain in the pelvic area and joints of the pelvis. It often happens because the ligaments that normally keep your pelvic bone aligned become overrelaxed and stretchy sooner than they should (as delivery nears, things are supposed to start loosening up significantly). This, in turn, can make the pelvic joints unstable, causing mild to severe pain. The pain may also result when a pelvic joint becomes stiff and stops moving normally, causing irritation in the other joints.

How common is it? The incidence of diagnosed PGP is about 1 in 300 pregnancies. However, some experts believe that up to 25 percent of all pregnant women experience PGP—but most of those cases aren't diagnosed.

What are the signs and symptoms? The most common symptom is a wrenching pain (as though your pelvis is coming apart) and difficulty walking. Typically, the pain is focused on the pubic area, but in some women it radiates to the upper thighs and perineum. The pain can worsen when you're walking and doing any weight-bearing activity, particularly one that involves lifting one leg, such as when you're climbing up stairs, getting dressed, getting in and out of a car, even turning over in bed. In very rare cases, the joint may gape apart, causing more serious pain in your pelvis, groin, hips, and buttocks.

What can you and your practitioner do? Avoid aggravating the condition by limiting weight-bearing positions and minimizing as best you can any activity that involves lifting or separating your legs—even walking, if it's very uncomfortable (some practitioners will even recommend modified bed rest so the pain doesn't worsen). Try stabilizing those floppy ligaments by wearing a pelvic support belt or band that corsets the bones back into place. Support shorts with built-in ice packs can help with both stabilizing joints and minimizing pain. Kegels and pelvic tilts can help to strengthen the muscles of the pelvis. Physical therapy may be especially helpful, so ask your practitioner for a referral. You can also ask about acupuncture and chiropractic therapies, as well as safe pain relievers.

Very rarely, PGP can make a vaginal delivery impossible and your practitioner may opt for a c-section instead. Even more rarely, PGP can worsen after delivery, requiring surgery. But for most moms, once baby is born and production of ligament-relaxing hormones stop, ligaments return to normal.

Cord Knots and Tangles

What is it? Once in a while, the umbilical cord becomes knotted, tangled, or wrapped around a fetus, often at the neck (when it is known as a nuchal cord). Some knots form during delivery, while others form during pregnancy when the baby moves around. As long as the knot remains loose, it's not likely to cause any problems at all. But if the knot becomes tight, it could interfere with the circulation of blood from the placenta to the baby and cause oxygen deprivation. Such an event happens only rarely, but when it does, it is most likely to occur during baby's descent through the birth canal.

How common is it? True umbilical cord knots occur in about 1 in every 100 pregnancies, but only in 1 in 2,000 deliveries will a knot be tight enough to present problems for the baby. The more common nuchal cords occur in as many as a quarter of all pregnancies but are usually harmless, very rarely posing any risk to the baby. Babies with long cords and those who are large-for-gestational age are at greater risk for developing true knots.

Researchers speculate that nutritional deficiencies that affect the structure and protective barrier of the cord, or other risk factors, such as carrying multiples, having hydramnios, or smoking or drug use may make a woman more prone to having a pregnancy with a serious cord knot.

What are the signs and symptoms? The most common sign of a cord knot is decreased fetal activity after week 37. If the knot occurs during labor (which is when knots are most often detected), a fetal monitor will detect an abnormal heart rate.

What can you and your practitioner do? You can keep a general eye on how your baby is doing, especially later in pregnancy, by doing regular kick counts and calling your practitioner if you notice any pronounced decrease in fetal activity. If a loose knot tightens during delivery, your practitioner will be able to detect the drop in your baby's heart rate, and will make the appropriate decisions to ensure your baby's safe entry into the world. Immediate delivery, usually via c-section, is often the best approach.

Two-Vessel Cord

What is it? In a normal umbilical cord, there are 3 blood vessels—1 vein (which brings nutrients and oxygen to the baby) and 2 arteries (which transport waste from the baby back to the placenta and the mother's blood). But in some cases, the umbilical cord contains only 2 blood vessels—1 vein and 1 artery.

How common is it? About 1 percent of singleton and 5 percent of multiple pregnancies will have a 2-vessel cord. The condition is more common among Caucasians, moms over age 40, and moms with diabetes. It's also more common in multiple pregnancies. Female fetuses are more often affected than males.

What are the signs and symptoms? There are no signs or symptoms with this condition—it's typically detected during a routine anatomy scan ultrasound.

What can you and your practitioner do? If you've been found to have a 2-vessel cord, your pregnancy will be monitored more closely, since the condition comes with a small increased risk of poor fetal growth and occasionally is linked to a malformation. In the absence of any other abnormalities, however, a 2-vessel cord doesn't impact the pregnancy. The baby is most likely to be born completely healthy.

Uncommon Pregnancy Complications

The following complications of pregnancy are, for the most part, rare. The average pregnant woman is extremely unlikely to encounter any of them. So, again (and this deserves repeating), read this section only if you need to—and even then, read just what applies to you. If any of these complications are diagnosed during your pregnancy, use the information here to learn about the condition and its typical treatment (as well as how to prevent it in future pregnancies), but realize that your practitioner's protocol for treating you may be different.

Eclampsia

What is it? Eclampsia is the result of uncontrolled or unresolved preeclampsia (see page 550). Depending on when in pregnancy a woman becomes eclamptic, her baby may be at risk of being born prematurely since immediate delivery is often the only treatment. Although eclampsia is life-threatening for the mother, maternal deaths from it are quite rare in the U.S. With optimum treatment and careful follow-up, the majority of women with eclampsia return to normal health after delivery.

How common is it? Eclampsia is much less common than preeclampsia and occurs in only 1 out of every 2,000 to 3,000 pregnancies, typically among women who have not been receiving regular prenatal care.

What are the signs and symptoms? Eclampsia is always preceded by preeclampsia. Seizures—usually close to or during delivery—are the most characteristic symptom of eclampsia. Seizures can also occur postpartum, usually within the first 48 hours.

What can you and your practitioner do? If you start to seize, you'll be given oxygen and drugs to stop the seizures and your labor will be induced or a c-section performed when you're stable. The majority of moms with eclampsia rapidly return to normal after delivery, though careful followup is necessary to be certain blood pressure doesn't stay up and seizures don't continue.

Can it be prevented? Regular prenatal care will help ensure that symptoms of preeclampsia will be picked up early. If you are diagnosed with preeclampsia, your practitioner will keep a close eye on you (and your blood pressure) to make sure your condition doesn't progress to eclampsia. Taking steps to try to prevent preeclampsia can also help avoid eclampsia.

Cholestasis

What is it? Cholestasis of pregnancy is a condition in which the normal flow of bile in the gallbladder is slowed (as a result of pregnancy hormones), causing the buildup of bile acids in the liver, which in turn can spill into the bloodstream. Cholestasis is most likely to occur in the last trimester, when hormones are at their peak. Happily,

You'll Want to Know . . .

Very few women receiving regular prenatal care ever progress from the manageable preeclampsia to the more serious eclampsia.

cholestasis usually goes away after delivery.

Cholestasis may increase the risks for fetal distress, preterm birth, or still-birth, which is why early diagnosis and treatment are crucial.

How common is it? Cholestasis affects 1 to 2 pregnancies in 1,000. It's more common in moms carrying multiples, those who have previous liver damage, and those whose mother or sister had cholestasis.

What are the signs and symptoms? Most often, the only symptom noticed is severe itching, particularly on the hands and feet, usually late in pregnancy. This itching shouldn't be confused with itching from dry, stretching skin (which is very common and completely normal during pregnancy).

What can you and your practitioner do? The goals of treating cholestasis of pregnancy are to relieve the itching and prevent pregnancy complications. Itching can be treated with topical anti-itch medications, lotions, or corticosteroids. Medication is sometimes used to help decrease the concentration of bile acids. If cholestasis is endangering the wellbeing of the mother or fetus, an early delivery may be necessary.

Deep Venous Thrombosis

What is it? Deep venous thrombosis, or DVT, is the development of a blood clot in a deep vein. These clots show up most commonly in the lower extremities, particularly the thigh. Women are more susceptible to clots during pregnancy and delivery, and particularly in the postpartum period. This happens because nature, wisely worried about too much bleeding at childbirth, tends to increase the blood's clotting ability—occasionally too much. Another factor that can contribute is the enlarged uterus, which makes it difficult for blood in the lower body to return to the heart. If untreated, a DVT can result in the clot moving to the lungs and becoming life threatening.

How common is it? DVT occurs in 1 in every 500 to 2,000 pregnancies, including the postpartum period. DVT is more common if you are older, over-weight, sedentary, a smoker, have a family or personal history of clots, or have hypertension, diabetes, or a variety of other conditions, including vascular diseases. Prolonged bed rest with little activity can also put you at higher risk of DVT, as can long plane rides.

What are the signs and symptoms? The most common symptoms of a deep vein thrombosis include:

- A heavy or painful feeling in the leg

- Tenderness in the calf or thigh

- Slight to severe swelling

- Distension of the superficial veins

- Calf pain on flexing the foot (turning the toes up toward the chin)

If the blood clot has moved to the lungs (a pulmonary embolus), there may be:

- Chest pain

- Shortness of breath

- Coughing with frothy, bloodstained sputum

- Rapid heartbeat and breathing rate

- Blueness of lips and fingertips

- Fever

What can you and your practitioner do? If you've been diagnosed with DVT or any kind of blood clot in previous

Cancer in Pregnancy

Sometimes, life can take a joyful turn and a challenging one, all at once—as when pregnancy and cancer happen at the same time. Whether you were already dealing with cancer when you found you were pregnant, or received a cancer diagnosis after discovering you were pregnant, there will be plenty of information to gather and choices to make in conjunction with both your prenatal team and your oncology team.

Treatment for cancer during pregnancy is a delicate balancing act between providing the best care for mom and limiting possible risk to her baby. The type of treatment you'll get will depend on many factors: how far along in pregnancy you are, the type of cancer, the stage of the cancer, and, of course, your wishes. The decisions you may face weighing your own wellbeing against your baby's may be emotionally wrenching, and you'll need plenty of support in making them.

While surgery may be performed if it's needed, doctors usually delay any other treatment (such as chemotherapy) until the second or third trimesters, when it's safer. Any treatment that might be harmful to the baby (for instance, radiation) will probably be postponed until after delivery. When cancer is diagnosed later in pregnancy, doctors may wait until after the baby is born to begin treatment, or they may consider inducing labor early. The reassuring news is that women diagnosed during pregnancy respond just as well to cancer treatment as women who are not pregnant, all other factors being equal.

For more help, contact the National Cancer Institute at cancer.gov, as well as hopefortwo.org, a support network for expectant moms with cancer.

---

pregnancies, let your practitioner know. In addition, if you notice swelling and pain in just one leg at any time during your pregnancy, call your practitioner right away. Don't massage the swelling.

Ultrasound may be used to diagnose a blood clot in the leg, and either a special scan (ventilation-perfusion) or CT study can diagnosis a clot in the lung. If it turns out that you do have a clot, you might be treated with heparin to thin your blood and prevent further clotting (though the heparin may need to be discontinued as you near term, to prevent you from bleeding excessively during delivery). Your clotting ability will be monitored along the way.

Can it be prevented? You can prevent clots by keeping your blood flowing—getting enough exercise and avoiding long periods of sitting will help you do this. If you have to fly, get up and move around every hour or two and do ankle roll exercises while you sit. Take stretching breaks frequently during long car rides, too. Staying well hydrated can also help prevent a blood clot. If you're at high risk, you can also wear support hose to prevent clots from developing in your legs. If you've been put on bed rest, take steps to reduce your risk (see page 577 for suggestions).

Placenta Accreta

What is it? Placenta accreta is an abnormally firm attachment of the placenta to the uterine wall. Depending on how deeply the placental cells invade, the condition may be called placenta

When Home Birth Isn't Best

You might have started your pregnancy low risk and had your heart set on a home birth, but when certain complications arise, it's wise to rethink your plans and opt for a hospital birth (or one at a birthing center attached to a hospital). Here are some circumstances when plans for a home birth might need to be changed:

- If you develop any of the pregnancy complications listed in this chapter (other than hyperemesis gravidarum or subchorionic bleed, if those have resolved)

- If you're pregnant with multiples

- If your baby is breech

- If you go into preterm labor

- If your baby has fetal distress

It's also not considered safe to plan for a home birth if you've had a prior cesarean delivery. Though some midwives will attend home VBACs (vaginal births after cesarean), experts agree that the risks far outweigh the benefits.

percreta or placenta increta. Placenta accreta increases the risk of heavy bleeding or hemorrhaging during delivery of the placenta.

How common is it? Only 1 out of 2,500 pregnancies will have an attachment abnormality. Placenta accreta is by far the most common of these, accounting for 75 percent of cases. In placenta accreta, the placenta digs deeply into the uterine wall, but does not pierce the uterine muscles. Your risk of placenta

accreta increases if you have placenta previa and have had one or more cesarean deliveries in the past. In placenta increta, which accounts for 15 percent of cases, the placenta pierces the uterine muscles. In placenta percreta, which accounts for the final 10 percent, the placenta not only burrows into the uterine wall and its muscles, but also pierces the outer part of the wall and may even attach itself to other nearby organs.

What are the signs and symptoms? There are usually no symptoms. The condition is usually diagnosed via color Doppler ultrasound or may be noticed only during delivery when the placenta doesn't detach (as it normally would) from the uterine wall after the baby is born.

What can you and your practitioner do? Unfortunately, there is little you can do. In most cases, the placenta must be removed surgically after delivery to stop the bleeding. When the bleeding cannot be controlled by tying off the exposed blood vessels, removal of the entire uterus may be necessary.

Vasa Previa

What is it? Vasa previa is a condition in which some of the fetal blood vessels that connect the baby to the mother run outside the umbilical cord and along the membrane over the cervix. When labor begins, the contractions and opening of the cervix can cause the vessels to rupture, possibly causing harm to the baby. If the condition is diagnosed before labor, a c-section will be scheduled and the baby will be born healthy nearly 100 percent of the time.

How common is it? Vasa previa is rare, affecting 1 in 5,200 pregnancies. Women who also have placenta previa, a history of uterine surgery (including c-section) or D&C, or a multiple pregnancy are at greater risk. Women who became pregnant through IVF are also at slightly higher risk.

What are the signs and symptoms? There are usually no signs of this condition.

What can you and your practitioner do? Diagnostic testing, such as with ultrasound or, better yet, a color Doppler ultrasound during the second trimester, can detect vasa previa. Women who are diagnosed with the condition will deliver their babies via c-section, usually before 37 weeks, to make sure labor doesn't begin on its own. Researchers are studying whether vasa previa can be treated using laser therapy to seal off the abnormally positioned vessels. You can read more about vasa previa at vasaprevia.com.

Childbirth and Postpartum Complications

Many of the following conditions can't be anticipated before labor and delivery—and there's no need to read up on them (and start worrying) ahead of time, since they're very unlikely to occur during or after your childbirth. They are included here so that in the unlikely event you experience one, you can learn about it after the fact, or in some cases, learn how you can prevent it from happening in your next labor and delivery.

Fetal Distress

What is it? Fetal distress is a term used to describe what occurs when a baby's oxygen supply is compromised in the uterus, either before or during labor. The distress may be caused by a number of factors, such as preeclampsia, uncontrolled diabetes, placental abruption, too little or too much amniotic fluid, umbilical cord compression, prolapse, or entanglement, or intrauterine growth restriction. It can also occur when the mother has been in a position for an extended period of time (such as flat on her back) that puts pressure on major blood vessels, depriving the baby of oxygen. Sustained oxygen deprivation and/or decreased heart rate can be serious for the baby and must be corrected as quickly as possible—usually with immediate delivery (most often by c-section, unless a vaginal birth is imminent).

How common is it? The exact incidence of fetal distress is uncertain (especially because some cases are only temporary), but estimates range from 1 in every 25 births to 1 in every 100 births.

What are the signs and symptoms? Babies who are doing well in utero have strong, stable heartbeats and respond to stimuli with appropriate movements. Babies in distress experience a decrease in heart rate, a change in their pattern of movement (or even no movement at all), and/or pass their first stool, called meconium, while still in the uterus. The only way you might suspect your baby is in distress is because of a noticeable slowdown of movement (after 28 weeks) or if your water broke and it was stained with meconium. The only way to know for sure is with a fetal monitor, nonstress test, or a biophysical profile ultrasound.

What can you and your practitioner do? If you think your baby might be in distress because you've noticed a change in fetal activity (it seems to have slowed down significantly, stopped, or otherwise has you concerned), call your practitioner immediately. Call your practitioner, too, if your water breaks and you notice it's meconium stained (see page 398). Once you are in your practitioner's office or in the hospital (or in labor), you'll be put on a fetal monitor to see whether your baby is indeed showing signs of distress. You may be given oxygen and IV fluids to help better oxygenate your blood and return your baby's heart rate to normal. If the reason your baby's in distress is that you've been on your back for a prolonged period of time, turning onto your left side to take pressure off your major blood vessels may also do the trick. If these techniques don't work, the best treatment is a quick delivery. The same steps will be taken if you didn't notice any symptoms but your baby was seen to be in distress during a routine checkup or nonstress test.

Cord Prolapse

What is it? A cord prolapse occurs during labor when the umbilical cord slips through the cervix and into the birth canal before the baby does. If the cord becomes compressed during delivery (as when your baby's head is pushing against a prolapsed cord), the baby's oxygen supply is compromised.

How common is it? Fortunately, cord prolapse is not common, occurring in 1 out of every 300 births. Certain pregnancy complications increase the risk of prolapse. These include hydramnios, breech delivery or any position in which the baby's head does not cover the cervix, a baby who's small for gestational age, and premature delivery. It can also occur during delivery of a second twin. Prolapse is a potential risk with PPROM or even near term if your water breaks before your baby's head has begun to "engage," or settle into the birth canal.

What are the signs and symptoms? If the cord slips down into the vagina, you may actually be able to feel it or even see it. If the cord is compressed by the baby's head, the baby will show signs of fetal distress.

What can you and your practitioner do? There's really no way to know in advance if your baby's cord is going to prolapse. If you suspect that your baby's umbilical cord has prolapsed and you are not in the hospital yet, get on your hands and knees with your head down and pelvis up to take pressure off the cord. Call 911 or have someone rush you to the hospital (on the way to the hospital, lie down on the backseat, with your bottom elevated). If you are already in the hospital when the cord prolapses, your practitioner may ask you to move quickly into a different position, one in which it will be easier to disengage the baby's head and take pressure off the umbilical cord. Delivery of your baby will need to be very quick, most likely by c-section. Quick delivery will usually prevent any of the problems (such as lack of oxygen) that may occur with a prolapsed cord that becomes compressed.

Shoulder Dystocia

What is it? Shoulder dystocia is a complication of labor and delivery in which one or both of the baby's shoulders become stuck behind the mother's pelvic bone as the baby descends into the birth canal.

How common is it? Size is what matters most when it comes to shoulder dystocia, which occurs most frequently in very large babies. In fact, statistics show that fewer than 1 percent of babies weighing 6 pounds have shoulder dystocia, while the rate is considerably higher in babies weighing more than 9 pounds. For that reason, mothers who have uncontrolled diabetes (gestational diabetes or diabetes developed before pregnancy) are more likely to encounter this complication during delivery. The chances also rise if your pregnancy has gone past 40 weeks (since babies who arrive late are likely to be on the larger size) or if you've previously delivered a baby with shoulder dystocia. Still, many cases of shoulder dystocia occur during labors without any of these risk factors.

What are the signs and symptoms? Delivery stalls after the head emerges and before the shoulders are out. This can occur unexpectedly in a labor that has progressed normally up to that point.

What can you and your practitioner do? A variety of approaches may be used to deliver the baby whose shoulder is lodged in the pelvis, such as changing the mother's position by sharply pressing her thighs against her belly, applying pressure on her abdomen right above the pubic bone, or trying to turn the baby's shoulder while it is still inside. If the mom is mobile (for instance, hasn't had an epidural), rotating to an all-fours position might help. In some cases (such as when the estimated weight of the baby is over 9.9 pounds and the mom is diabetic, if the baby is estimated to weigh over 11 pounds in any pregnancy, or there was a shoulder dystocia in a prior pregnancy), the doctor might recommend a scheduled c-section to avoid the potential for vaginal delivery complications, including shoulder dystocia.

Can it be prevented? Keeping your weight gain within the recommended range may lower the chances of having a baby too big to easily maneuver through the birth canal, as can carefully controlling diabetes or GD.

Serious Perineal Tears

What is it? The pressure of your baby's large head pushing through the delicate tissues of your cervix and vagina can cause tears and lacerations in your perineum, the area between your vagina and your anus.

First-degree tears (when only the skin is torn) and second-degree tears (when skin and vaginal muscle are torn) are common. But severe tears—those that get close to the rectum and involve the vaginal skin, tissues, and muscles of the anal sphincter (third degree) or those that actually cut into the rectum (fourth degree)—cause pain and increase not only your postpartum recovery time, but your risk of incontinence, as well as other pelvic floor problems. Tears can also occur in the cervix.

How common is it? Anyone having a vaginal delivery is at risk for a tear, and as many as half of moms will have at least a small tear. Third- and fourth-degree tears are much less common.

What are the signs and symptoms? Bleeding is the immediate symptom. After the tear is repaired, you may also experience pain and tenderness at the site as it heals.

What can you and your practitioner do? Generally, all lacerations that are longer than 2 cm (about 1 inch) or that continue to bleed are stitched. A local anesthetic may be given first, if one wasn't administered during delivery or if you didn't have an epidural.

If you end up tearing or having an episiotomy, sitz baths, ice packs, witch hazel, anesthetic sprays, and simply exposing the area to air can help it heal more quickly and with less pain (see page 463).

Can it be prevented? Perineal massage and Kegel exercises (see pages 384 and 229), done during the month or so before your due date, may help make the perineal area more supple and better able to stretch over your baby's head as he or she emerges (though perineal massage before labor will only be helpful if you're a first-timer). Warm compresses on the perineum and perineal massage during labor may help avoid tearing. Allowing the delivery to slow down and be controlled (pushing only when you feel the urge, not on a specific timetable) will give your perineum more time to stretch so it'll be less likely to tear. Some practitioners suggest that delivering on all fours makes it less likely you'll tear, while squatting or lying flat on your back slightly increases the chances of tearing.

Uterine Rupture

What is it? A uterine rupture occurs when a weakened spot on your uterine wall—almost always the site of a previous uterine surgery, such as a c-section or fibroid removal—tears due to the strain put on it during labor and delivery. A uterine rupture can result in uncontrolled bleeding into your abdomen or, rarely, lead to part of the placenta or baby entering your abdomen.

How common is it? Fortunately, ruptures are rare in women who've never had a previous cesarean delivery or uterine surgery. Even women who labor after a previous c-section (have a VBAC) have only a 1 in 100 chance of rupture (and the risk is far lower when

a woman undergoes a repeat c-section without labor). Women at greatest risk of uterine rupture are those attempting a VBAC who have been induced with prostaglandins—which is why VBACs are generally not done if the mom needs to be induced. Abnormalities related to the placenta (such as placental abruption or placenta accreta, or to the baby's position (such as a fetus lying crosswise) can also increase the risk of uterine rupture. Uterine rupture is more common in women who have already had 6 or more babies or have a very distended uterus (because of multiple fetuses or excess amniotic fluid).

What are the signs and symptoms? Searing abdominal pain (a sensation that something is "ripping") followed by diffuse pain and tenderness in the abdomen during labor (even in moms with epidurals) are the most common signs of uterine rupture. Most typically, the fetal monitor will show a significant drop in the baby's heart rate. The mother may develop signs of low blood volume, such as an increased heart rate, low blood pressure, dizziness, shortness of breath, or loss of consciousness.

What can you and your practitioner do? If you have had a previous c-section or uterine surgery in which the uterine wall was cut through completely and you'd like to attempt a vaginal birth, discuss with your practitioner whether you're a good candidate for VBAC (see page 357). Not being induced makes the extremely low risk of uterine rupture during VBAC even lower. If you do end up with a uterine rupture, an immediate c-section is necessary, followed by repair of the uterus. You may also be given antibiotics to prevent infection.

Can it be prevented? For women with increased risk (such as a previous c-section), fetal monitoring during labor can alert your practitioner to an impending or occurring rupture. Women who are trying for a VBAC delivery should not be induced except in certain circumstances—discuss with your ob.

Uterine Inversion

What is it? Uterine inversion is a rare complication of childbirth that occurs when part of the uterine wall collapses and turns inside out (in effect, like a sock being pulled inside out), sometimes even protruding through the cervix and into the vagina. The full range of problems that can cause uterine inversion is not fully understood, but in many cases it includes the incomplete separation of the placenta from the uterine wall—the placenta then pulls the uterus with it when it emerges from the birth canal. Uterine inversion, when unnoticed and/ or untreated, can result in hemorrhage and shock. But that's a remote possibility, since the condition is unlikely to go unnoticed and untreated.

How common is it? Uterine inversion is very rare—reported rates vary from 1 in 2,000 births to 1 in 50,000. You are at greatest risk for a uterine inversion if you've had an inversion during a previous delivery. Other factors that slightly increase the very remote risk include an extended labor (lasting more than 24 hours), several previous vaginal deliveries, or use of drugs like magnesium sulfate (given to halt preterm labor). The uterus also may be more likely to invert if it is overly relaxed or if the umbilical cord is short and is pulled too hard during delivery.

What are the signs and symptoms? Symptoms of uterine inversion include:

- Abdominal pain
- Excessive bleeding
- Signs of shock

- In a complete inversion, the uterus will be visible in the vagina

What can you and your practitioner do? Know your risk factors and tell your practitioner if you've had a uterine inversion in the past. If you do have one, your practitioner will try to push your uterus back up where it belongs, and then give you Pitocin (oxytocin) to encourage any floppy muscles to contract. In rare cases, where this does not work, surgery to reposition the uterus is an option. In either case, you might need a blood transfusion to make up for blood loss. Antibiotics may be given to prevent infection.

Can it be prevented? Because a woman who has had an inversion is at an increased risk for another, let your practitioner know if you've had one in the past.

Postpartum Hemorrhage

What is it? Bleeding after delivery, called lochia, is normal. But sometimes the uterus doesn't contract as it should after birth, leading to postpartum hemorrhage—excessive or uncontrolled bleeding from the site where the placenta was attached or from unrepaired vaginal or cervical lacerations. Hemorrhage can occur up to a week or two after delivery when fragments of the placenta are retained in, or adhere to, the uterus. Infection can also cause postpartum hemorrhage, right after delivery or weeks later.

How common is it? Postpartum hemorrhage occurs in 2 to 4 percent of deliveries. Excessive bleeding may be more likely to occur in these circumstances:

- The uterus is too relaxed and doesn't contract due to a long, exhausting labor.

- The uterus is overdistended because of multiple births, a large baby, or excess amniotic fluid.

- There was a traumatic delivery.

- Bits of the placenta were retained (unnoticed by the practitioner) after delivery.

- The placenta is oddly shaped or separates prematurely.

- Fibroids prevent symmetrical contraction of the uterus.

- The mother is very weak at the time of delivery (due to anemia, preeclampsia, or extreme fatigue, for example).

- The mother has been taking medication or supplements that interfere with blood clotting (such as aspirin, ibuprofen, ginkgo biloba, or large doses of vitamin E).

- There is an undiagnosed genetic bleeding disorder in the mother (which is very rare).

What are the signs and symptoms? The symptoms of postpartum hemorrhage include:

- Bleeding that soaks through more than 1 pad an hour for several hours in a row

- Heavy, bright red bleeding for more than just a few days

- Passing very large clots (lemon size or larger); smaller clots are normal

- Pain or swelling in the lower abdominal area beyond the first few days after delivery

The loss of large amounts of blood can make a woman feel faint, breathless, or dizzy, or cause her heart to speed up.

What can you and your practitioner do? You should expect bleeding following delivery, but alert your practitioner immediately if you notice abnormally heavy bleeding or any of the other symptoms listed above during the first postpartum week. If the bleeding is severe enough to be categorized as hemorrhage, you may need IV fluids or possibly even a blood transfusion.

Can it be prevented? After the placenta is delivered, your practitioner will examine it to make certain that it's complete—that no part of it might have remained in your uterus (which could lead to excessive bleeding or infection). He or she will probably give you Pitocin (oxytocin) or other medication and may massage your uterus to encourage it to contract to minimize bleeding. Breastfeeding (if you will be nursing) as soon as possible will also help your uterus contract, minimizing bleeding. Avoiding any supplement or medication that may interfere with blood clotting will also reduce the possibility of excessive postpartum bleeding.

Postpartum Infection

What is it? The vast majority of new moms recover from delivery without any problems at all, but childbirth can occasionally leave you open to infection. That's because it can leave you with a variety of open wounds—in your uterus (where the placenta was attached), in your cervix, vagina, or perineum (especially if you tore or had an episiotomy, even if it was repaired), or at the site of a c-section incision. Postpartum infections can also occur in your bladder or kidney if you were catheterized. A fragment of the placenta inadvertently left behind in the uterus can lead to infection, too. But the most common postpartum infection is endometritis, an infection of the lining of the uterus (the endometrium).

While some infections can be dangerous, especially if they go undetected or untreated, most often infections simply make your postpartum recovery slower and more difficult, and they take time and energy away from your most important priority: getting to know your baby. For that reason alone, it's important to get help for any suspected infection as quickly as possible.

How common is it? As many as 8 percent of deliveries result in an infection. Women who had a cesarean delivery or those who had premature rupture of the membranes are at greater risk.

What are the signs and symptoms? Symptoms of postpartum infection vary, depending on where the infection is, but there's almost always:

- Fever

- Pain or tenderness in the infected area

- Foul-smelling discharge (from the vagina in the case of a uterine infection, or from a wound)

- Chills

What can you and your practitioner do? Call your practitioner if you're running a postpartum fever of 100°F for more than a day; call right away if the fever is higher or if you notice any of the other symptoms above. If you have an infection, you'll probably receive a prescription for antibiotics (one that's breastfeeding-friendly if you're nursing). Take it as prescribed for the entire course, even if you begin to feel better. Taking probiotics when you're on the course of antibiotics (though spaced at least 2 hours apart) may prevent associated diarrhea, vaginal yeast infection, or thrush (in you or your baby, if you're breastfeeding). You should also try to get plenty of rest and drink lots of fluids.

Can it be prevented? Meticulous wound care and cleanliness after delivery can definitely help prevent infection (wash your hands before touching the perineal area, wipe from front to back, and use only maxipads—not tampons—for postpartum bleeding).

ALL ABOUT:
If You're Put on Bed Rest

Bed rest (a still-popular catchall phrase for a pregnancy prescription that's increasingly known as "activity restriction") can mean different things to different practitioners—and to the patients they prescribe it for. Maybe it's just getting off your feet every couple of hours, maybe it's that plus handing over the vacuum to your partner and turning in your gym membership for a while, maybe it's staying in bed for at least half the day, every day—and maybe it's a hospital stay for the last few weeks (or months) of your pregnancy. No matter what form it takes (or what it's called) it's estimated that bed rest is still being prescribed in about 20 percent of pregnancies in the U.S. That number may be waning, but probably not as quickly as many practitioners, many pregnant patients, and even ACOG would like.

So has this time-honored prescription for many problem pregnancies timed out? Probably not. There are still a number of reasons why a practitioner might recommend a restriction of activities, but probably the simplest rationale is that practitioners often have no other treatment options open when trying to prevent complications like preterm birth—and yet, they feel compelled to "do something."

Certain moms-to-be are more likely to wind up on some kind of bed rest, including those who are over 35 (because they're generally more at risk of pregnancy complications), as well as those who are carrying multiples, have a history of miscarriage due to cervical insufficiency, who have pregnancy bleeding (such as in a threatened miscarriage), have particular pregnancy complications such as preeclampsia, have certain chronic conditions, or have threatened preterm labor.

What Kind of Rest?

If you've been put on bed rest, it's likely your marching (or in this case, no-marching) orders came with a list of very specific can-dos and definitely don't-dos. That's because bed rest comes in a variety of packages. Here's the basic lowdown on each type of bed rest. Be sure to talk over the options with your practitioner if you're being put on any form of bed rest—to make sure it's not stricter than it needs to be.

Scheduled resting (or activity restriction). In the hopes of preventing full bed rest later, some practitioners ask moms-to-be with certain risk factors (such as multiples or a previous preterm delivery) to rest for a prescribed amount of time every day. The recommendation may be to sit with your feet up or lie down for 2 hours at the end of every workday or rest for an hour, lying down on your side (left preferably, but either side is fine), for every 4 hours that you're awake. Some practitioners may ask you to simply shorten your workday in your third trimester and restrict activities such as exercise, stair-climbing, and walking or standing for extended lengths of time.

Modified bed rest. With modified bed rest, you're generally prohibited from working in the office (though working from the comfort of home is probably okay), driving, and doing household chores (now, that's something to celebrate!). Sitting up (possibly with your feet up) is probably fine, as is standing just long enough to make yourself a sandwich or take a shower. You may even be granted one outing per week, as long as it doesn't involve a long walk or any stairs. You'll also be able to go to your monthly (or even weekly, if necessary) practitioner appointment. Moms-to-be on modified bed rest may split their day between the couch or recliner and the bed, but going up or down stairs will be kept to a minimum. Light physical therapy may be prescribed.

Strict bed rest. This usually means you need to be horizontal all day except for bathroom trips and a brief shower (using a shower chair if possible). If there are stairs in your house, you're going to have to pick a floor and stay there. (Some women will be allowed to make a round-trip between floors once a day, for others it might be just once a week.) Strict bed rest means no kitchen privileges, so unless you'll have someone around to serve up meals and snacks, you'll need a minifridge or cooler by your bed. Light physical therapy may also be prescribed at home.

Hospital bed rest. Some moms-to-be require constant monitoring, which means hospital admission. And just by the nature of being in the hospital,

Before You Head to Bed

Been sent to bed? Check this list before you crawl under the covers.

- Check in with your health insurance company. Let your health plan know you've been put on bed rest (and submit the right medical forms from your practitioner if necessary). Ask what home care, if any, will be covered. Ask, too, if you might be covered for physical therapy, medical supply rental, or even massage. You can also inquire about your coverage in case your baby is born prematurely.

- File for disability insurance. Bed rest can have enormous financial impact on a family that's about to expand (another reason to be sure it's truly necessary as prescribed). If you won't be able to work, speak to someone in the HR department (if there is one) at your workplace to see if you qualify for short term disability coverage (you should, though you and your practitioner will have to document the reasons why)—and whether your bed rest "time off" from work will cut into your FMLA coverage (see page 200), if you are entitled to any.

- Explore work-at-home options. If your job and your employer are flexible, you may be able to continue working at least part-time while on bed rest. Or if your job doesn't allow this, perhaps you can look into opportunities that do.

- Load up your phone. Make sure you've updated your contact info with numbers you may need while you're stuck in bed (your practitioner, the pharmacy, the hospital, neighbors and friends who can help you in a hurry).

- Create online or app accounts for restaurant delivery, grocery and drugstore delivery, online concierge services, dog walker services, laundry services, and so on, and let the deliveries begin—finances permitting.

- Hire help, if possible. Or enlist help from family, friends, and neighbors who have offered. You'll need a hand with light cleaning, errands, babysitting (if you have other children at home), carpooling (if you have older kids who need to get to school, activities, and play dates), meal prep, and laundry. If your friends and neighbors have offered to help, suggest they use online tools to keep things organized, such as lotsahelpinghands.com, carecalendar.org, or mealbaby.com.

- Give people who you'll want visiting access to your keys (or leave a key with a neighbor, the apartment manager, or doorman) so you don't have to get out of bed each time the doorbell rings. If possible, arrange to have a neighbor accept deliveries.

- Purchase or borrow a mini fridge that can be placed next to your bed (or couch) and stocked with drinks, cut up veggies, cheese, yogurt, and other snacks that need to stay chilled. Or consider a cooler lined with ice packs and restocked daily.

- Set up a charging station for your laptop, phone, tablet, and anything else that'll need to be recharged. All the wires should be within easy reach.

you'll be spending a lot more time in bed. However, given concerns about prolonged inactivity, if you're prescribed hospitalization, you may also be prescribed light physical therapy during your stay—a good thing, since it'll keep your muscles working in a way that's safe for you and your baby. If you've been admitted to the hospital because preterm labor has already begun, you'll likely need constant monitoring as well as IV meds. Your bed may even be positioned at a slight angle (feet higher than head) so that gravity can help keep your baby (or babies) growing in your womb for as long as possible.

Pelvic rest. Yes . . . this means exactly what it sounds like: no sex. But what "no sex" means is up for interpretation, so be sure to ask exactly what it means in your circumstance. It might mean nothing inserted into the vagina (no penis, fingers, dildos, vibrators, and so on), it might mean no oral or anal sex either, or it might just mean no orgasm for you. You might be put on pelvic rest if you've been bleeding (such as with a threatened miscarriage in the first trimester or later in pregnancy because of placenta previa), or because you have a history of preterm delivery, or if you're having premature contractions in this pregnancy, or because you have cervical insufficiency.

The Downsides of Resting

Staying off your feet (whether it's being sent to bed, your sofa, or the hospital) for weeks or even months definitely can take a physical toll. Prolonged inactivity can lead to hip and back pain, muscle loss (which can make it harder to bounce back once you deliver), skin irritation (aka bed sores), bone loss, and even blood clots in the legs. It may also aggravate many of the normal symptoms of pregnancy, such as heartburn, constipation, and leg swelling, as well as increase your risk for GD, since your body isn't breaking down glucose at its usual rate. Bed rest may decrease your appetite, which might keep you from

eating enough to nourish your baby (or babies). On the flip side, endless hours in bed can invite mindless eating—especially if you're out of your mind with boredom—and that can lead to excess weight gain, especially since you're not burning calories through regular activity and exercise.

But there can be a psychological cost to bed rest, too. Prolonged inactivity is linked to pregnancy depression and anxiety, especially if you're stuck indoors, cut off from activities that typically keep your mind and body busy, deprived of social interaction, exercise (and the natural-high hormones it releases), sex (ditto), the stimulation of work, even exposure to sunlight (which boosts mood and regulates sleep). There's a loss, too, of the "normal" pregnancy experience (the one where everyone around you becomes extra-attentive, solicitous, respectful—where that bump makes you feel extra-special wherever you go). The emotional impact (like the physical impact) may linger after delivery, and is associated with a higher risk of postpartum depression and anxiety disorders.

Staying Up When You're Lying Down

The thought of lying in bed or lounging around the house with the TV remote may sound pretty appealing—until it's prescribed in the form of bed rest. Bed rest, unfortunately, is no pajama party. Once reality sets in, taking it easy can suddenly seem like hard work. That's why it's important not to lose sight of the big picture (healthy pregnancy, healthy baby) and to remind yourself that your practitioner probably has good reason for keeping you off your feet—or at least off your regularly scheduled high-activity lifestyle.

Once you find out from your practitioner exactly which activities are allowed (and which aren't), use these tips to minimize some of the side effects.

Physically. You may be surprised at the things you can still do when you're being asked to do less. A few suggestions:

- Move what you can. Your practitioner may allow—and in fact prescribe—some low-impact exercise (walks, light weights for your upper body, resistance bands for your lower body) to minimize muscle loss and maintain your strength.

- Stretch what you can. As much as you can under your practitioner's guidelines, stretch your legs, circle your ankles, and flex your feet to help prevent blood clots and keep your muscles strong. Raise and lower your arms, do shoulder rolls, do chest expansions (lace your fingers behind your back and open your chest), and so on to keep up your strength in your upper body. And don't forget those Kegels, which you can do even if you're sent to bed.

- Monitor what you eat. A significant dip in a mom's appetite can lead to weight loss for her and a lower birthweight for her baby—so if you find yours slacking, fight back by grazing on nutritious snacks. Of course, if you find yourself eating too much (out of boredom or depression), excessive weight gain might also become an issue—so keep an eye on nonstop nibbling, and make sure you have healthy snacks handy.

- Stay hydrated. It's easy to remember to drink water when you're active (say, after a run), but it's hard to work up a thirst in bed. Getting enough fluids helps minimize swelling and constipation, which are both compounded by moving less.

- Keep comfortable. If you are confined to bed for most or part of the day, maximize blood flow to your uterus by lying on your side, not your back, and change sides every hour or so to lessen body aches and prevent bed sores. Put a pillow under your head, a body pillow under your belly and between your knees, and perhaps a pillow behind you (a regular one or a specially designed one for propping), if that helps you to balance. Staying propped up in bed (especially after eating) also helps ease heartburn.

Mentally. Living with limitations on your activity can be hard to handle—especially if you're normally a very active person. Sometimes keeping yourself busy can provide a welcome distraction. Try to:

- Stay connected. Of course, you'll want to stay in touch with family and friends via phone, text messaging, videochatting, and social media—if only so you can vent to those who love you most. But you may find the most empathy and support from those who are also sitting out pregnancy—your fellow bed-resters. You can find them on WhatToExpect.com (and don't forget to go app happy with the What To Expect app). Or check out the box on page 581 for a list of other online resources for women going through high-risk pregnancies.

- Structure the day. Try to establish a routine—even if the highlight is a short (approved) walk down the block and a shower.

- Work from home. If your job allows it, go for it. But first, get clearance from your practitioner so you're clear what your limits are (for instance, on how much stress you can be under).

Handling Bed Rest

Having her activity restricted is clearly no picnic for your partner (especially if she's actually banished to bed)—and it's certainly no vacation for you, either. In fact, you'll be working overtime trying to keep up with the household chores and errands that you may have previously shared—adding a variety of new job descriptions to your previously existing ones, from executive assistant to butler, chef (and water bottle filler), chauffeur, housekeeper, pillow fluffer, amateur (or make that "pop") psychologist, and verbal punching bag (a girl's got to vent), all juggled with your regular job. Have other children at home? Their care and feeding will be your job, too, for the most part. Her bed rest will be exhausting for you, for sure, but if you keep your eyes on the prize (a healthy mom and a healthy baby), you'll soldier through this rough patch. Here are some ways to help you (and your partner) handle the ups and downs of being put on bed rest:

Set up a steady stream of visitors. Sure, she only has eyes for you—but after many long, boring days of staying home (or mostly home), your spouse may crave a change of pace, and a change of faces. So work with your friends and family to put together a rotating schedule of visitors who will hang out with your honey. It'll be good for her, and you'll get the break you need (and deserve).

Bring on the entertainment. You'd be bored silly (or cranky), too, if you were stuck at home. Stock up on games, choose a TV series to download and binge watch together, and learn the best takeout places in the neighborhood (then order from them online). Surprise her with a mix of her favorite music.

Exercise together. She might only be able to walk around the block, but with you by her side, that walk will be a lot more fun. She's been allowed to use light weights for some upper body moves? Grab your weights and do some chest flies while she does her light bicep curls. Encourage her to bicycle her legs (if that's allowed) or do foot flexes while you do some spinning on the stationary bike next to her. Do sit-ups in bed next to her while she's doing her neck rolls.

Ask her "in" for a date. She may not be able to get out to a dinner and a movie, but you can bring the date night home (or to the hospital room). Dress up (even if it's just your best pj's), put on some dinner music, bring out the candles and the nice dishes, and have her favorite restaurant deliver (or cook her favorite meal). It may not have the same ambience she remembers from your nights out, but it'll be a welcome respite from the daily waiting game.

Treat her. If it's in your price range, or is covered by insurance, bring in a massage therapist for a prenatal rub down

- Prepare for baby. Register for your layette, order the gear, and scout for a doula, a lactation consultant, a pediatrician, even childcare options—all online.

- Create a baby playlist. Start playing the songs now, and your little one will likely be soothed by them later. Plus, music may soothe you when you need it the most (like now, when you're feeling a little savage-beast-like).

(just make sure it's cleared by her practitioner). See if a local nail salon will agree to a house call and (finances permitting) book her a mani-pedi. If that's out of your financial league or not up her alley, give her a back rub, do facials together at home (find an online recipe for one that's made from ingredients you probably have at home, like oatmeal or avocado), or offer to paint the toes she can no longer reach.

Talk her up. Just about every expectant mom could use an extra boost for her confidence, but mamas-on-bed-rest can benefit from even more sweet talking. Yes, you always think she's beautiful and sexy, even when she hasn't washed her hair in days or put on makeup in weeks, but does she know you think that? Let her know . . . as often as you can.

Lend your shoulder and your ear. Sometimes, she'll need to vent, and most times, you'll be on the receiving end of her frustrations. For best results (and because she deserves it), respond with patience, understanding, and empathy. Talk her up (or talk her down when she's feeling on the ledge)—remind her she's beautiful, strong, and your own personal hero, and that this too shall pass (leaving you both with a cuddly prize package for her efforts)—but also let her unload as much as she needs to. As you attend to her emotional needs, however, try not to ignore your own entirely. Be sure to take a break yourself now and then (that's what the rotating schedule of visitors is for) and lean on your buddies for support, too. Being on bed rest is hard—but so is being the care provider for someone on bed rest.

Watch her mood. Being stuck on bed rest is linked to an increased risk of pregnancy depression and anxiety disorder. Be alert to the signs (see page 174) and if you notice them, take the steps necessary to get her the help she needs. Be alert, too, to the signs of postpartum depression (see page 498), since pregnancy bed rest increases that risk as well. Is your mood worrying you? Depression can hit expectant and new dads, too. Check in with your doctor and make sure you get the help you need.

Help her bounce back. Think that after all that rest, she'll be ready to run new-baby marathons when it's over? Actually, the opposite will be true. The longer she has spent on restricted activity, the more deconditioned she'll become—and the less energy and stamina she'll have. Which means she'll actually be more tired than the average new mom, not more refreshed, and that she'll likely need more help during her postpartum recovery, not less. Give her that help, as well as the time she needs to get back her strength—but remember that both of you can expect to feel pretty drained for a while, thanks to your new parent positions.

■ Stream some shows. Two words: binge watch.

■ Get crafty. Knit, crochet, scrapbook, or quilt (if you don't know how, turn to a YouTube tutorial or a crafty friend).

You'll keep busy while creating keepsakes for your little one.

■ Organize. Clean up your laptop and your phone once and for all, catch up on software and app updates, upload photos into a digital frame. Create a baby announcement list, and design your e-card or paper birth announcement. Make sure you have all the addresses (or email addresses) ready to roll. You can even print out address labels in advance, if you're pretty sure you won't want to handwrite them. Order stamps while you're at it.

- Socialize. Throw a pajama party—order in pizza or have your friends bring over a potluck. And if you can't go out for your baby shower, ask your friends to throw it at your house.

- Primp and polish. Try not to fall into the "nobody's going to see me anyway" trap. Looking good makes you feel good, whether anyone sees you or not. So brush your hair, put on makeup, slather your tummy in yummy-smelling lotion (your skin might be itchy and dry anyway), treat yourself to a DIY facial or mani. If you can afford it, consider having a mobile hairstylist or manicurist make a house call. (Drop the hint to your friends that this would make a great shower gift.)

- Start a journal. Now's a great time to begin recording your thoughts in an online journal or in the *What to Expect Pregnancy Journal and Organizer.* Or consider writing a few letters to your baby, to preserve pregnancy moments you can share with your child years later. Have some feelings about bed rest you'd like to vent? You can journal those, too.

- Be a mommy-to-be blogger. Always wanted to write? Now's your chance.

- Keep your eyes on the prize. Frame one of your ultrasound pictures, and keep it by your side or put it on your phone or tablet as your wallpaper—so when the going gets tough, you can remind yourself that you have the best reason in the world not to go anywhere at all.

Bed Rest and the Rest of Your Family

Wondering how bed rest will affect the rest of your family, from your partner to other children (including your furry ones)? It will probably affect them in more ways than you'd imagine:

Your partner. When you're sent to bed, your partner may be sent to work—overtime. Depending on your restrictions, he may become responsible for most of the household cleaning and laundry, errands, grocery shopping, and meal prep—all in addition to his regular job. Sex might be taken off the table, too, so try to be gentle and patient with each other as you both power through this dry spell. And though you're probably aching for company after long days alone, encourage your partner to go out with friends occasionally—it'll do him good (and that will do you both good).

Have other children? He'll clearly have even more on his hands (and in his arms . . . and on his back . . . and in his backseat). Since he's shouldering the load, try to be especially respectful of his parenting style and techniques, which might be different from yours.

Your children. If you already have other children—especially age-appropriately clingy little ones who just want to be picked up and carted around on mom's hip—activity restriction can be an added challenge. You'll probably be looking at fewer tickle-fests and hide-and-seek marathons—and more tea parties, books, puzzles, coloring, and board (okay, bored) games. You can also spend time together looking at pictures

Moms Helping Moms

Every pregnancy comes with some challenges, but a pregnancy that's high risk (or one that's been complicated) can come with a whole lot more. Facing those challenges is always easier when you've got company—other moms who know exactly what you're going through because they're going through it, too (or have already gone through it themselves). You're likely to find that support online— check out WhatToExpect.com, sidelines.org, betterbedrest.org, and keepemcookin.com.

of your older child as a baby, helping him or her acclimate to the idea of the newborn soon to arrive. Try not to pin the blame for your bed rest on the baby-to-be, however, since that could set the stage for sibling rivalry. Instead say the doctor's orders were to rest so that the baby can grow strong and healthy. If at all possible, have someone else take your toddler for a run around outside every day, since burning off some of that energy may facilitate quieter playtime with you.

Feeling guilty about not "being there" for your older ones? That's understandable (guilt sort of comes with the mom territory), but try to let it go. Remember, your little ones cherish every mama moment, even those spent snuggling in bed together.

Your pets. For some dogs and most cats, it doesn't get better than lying in bed or on the sofa with mommy all day. But for the frisky few who need interactive playtime, mom's activity restriction can cramp their style. Ditto those who need long walks. Of course your partner can take over the pet care (and if necessary, you can try to find a dog walker), but if your fur baby is extra mommy-dependent, you'll also have to do some extra reassuring (and petting).

When the Rest Is Over

It might seem counterintuitive, but the more you rest, the more tired you can become—and that's definitely true when you've been on bed rest for any length of time. Even the littlest efforts can seem monumental when you've lost muscle tone and strength and when decreased aerobic capacity can leave you out of breath just climbing a few stairs. Add labor, delivery, and recovery to that debilitating equation, along with normal new parent sleep deprivation, and you can expect to drag physically, even more than the average mom (who's plenty tired herself).

So keep your expectations realistic after delivery. Cut yourself some postpartum slack, factoring in all your body has been through and what it's still going through now. Plan on building back up to your former fitness level slowly but surely. Start off gradually, modifying the postpartum exercises on page 520 if even those are difficult, and then building up as your stamina (and muscle mass) increases. Walking, yoga, and swimming are good activities to get back into the game. With consistent effort on your part and help from your practitioner, family, and friends, don't worry. You'll get there!

Pregnancy Loss

P regnancy is supposed to be the happiest of times, filled with excitement, anticipation, and pink-and-blue daydreams about life with your baby-to-be. And usually, it is all of those things, but not always. Sometimes a pregnancy ends unexpectedly and tragically. Even if you only saw your baby on ultrasound, you bonded with your son or your daughter each day he or she was growing inside of you. And having those dreams and hopes of a future shattered is understandably heartbreaking. If you've experienced the loss of a pregnancy or if you've had a stillborn baby, you know firsthand that the depth of your pain can be beyond words. This chapter is dedicated to helping you and your partner understand what happened, handle the pain, and cope with one of life's most difficult losses.

Types of Pregnancy Loss

Early Miscarriage

What is it? A miscarriage is the loss of an embryo or fetus before it is able to live outside the uterus, resulting in the unplanned end of a pregnancy. When such a loss happens in the first trimester, as it does 80 percent of the time, it's called an early miscarriage. (A miscarriage that occurs between the end of the first trimester and week 20 is considered a late miscarriage; see page 589.)

An early pregnancy loss is often related to a chromosomal or other genetic defect in the embryo, but it can also be caused by hormonal and other factors. Most often, the cause can't be identified. Miscarriage is not caused by exercise, sex, working hard, lifting heavy objects, a sudden scare, emotional stress, a fall, or a minor blow to the abdomen, and it isn't triggered by even the most severe morning sickness.

How common is it? Early miscarriage is far more common than most women realize. Though it's hard to know for sure, researchers have estimated that over 40 percent of conceptions end in miscarriages. But since well over half of

You'll Want to Know . . .

Happily, the vast majority of women who experience a miscarriage go on to have a perfectly normal and healthy pregnancy in the future.

miscarriages occur so early that a woman doesn't even know she's pregnant yet, they often go unnoticed, passing for a normal or sometimes heavier period. See the box on page 584 for more on the different types of early miscarriage.

Signs and symptoms. The symptoms of a miscarriage can include some or all of the following:

- Cramping or pain (sometimes severe) in the center of the lower abdomen or back

- Heavy vaginal bleeding (possibly with clots and/or tissue) similar to a period

- Light staining continuing for more than 3 days

- A sudden pronounced decrease in or loss of the usual signs of early pregnancy, such as breast tenderness and nausea (not the normal, gradual diminishing as the first trimester comes to a close)

- A cervix that appears open (dilated) when examined by the practitioner

- No embryo visible on ultrasound (the sac is empty)

- No heartbeat detected on ultrasound

What can you and your practitioner do? If your practitioner finds that your cervix is dilated and/or no fetal heartbeat is detected on ultrasound (and your dates are correct), it means that you are having a miscarriage or have already had one. Sadly, nothing can be done to prevent the loss at this stage.

If you're in a lot of pain from the cramping, your practitioner may recommend or prescribe a pain reliever. Don't hesitate to ask for relief from the pain if you need it.

Many miscarriages are complete, meaning all the contents of the uterus are expelled from the vagina (that's why there is often so much bleeding). But sometimes—especially the later in the first trimester you are—a miscarriage isn't complete, and parts of the pregnancy remain in the uterus (known as an incomplete miscarriage; see box, page 585). Or a heartbeat isn't detected on ultrasound, which means the embryo or fetus has died, but no bleeding has occurred yet (this is

Are You Spotting?

Seeing red (or pink or brown) on your panties or toilet paper is definitely scary when you're expecting. But not all spotting or bleeding means you're miscarrying or losing your baby. Some women spot on and off for their entire pregnancies. Read about the many reasons for spotting that aren't related to miscarriage on page 143.

Sometimes spotting, heavy bleeding, and/or cramping indicate a threatened miscarriage. That, too, doesn't mean you're definitely losing your baby. See page 546 for more on threatened miscarriage.

If you're not sure when to call your practitioner for spotting or bleeding, see the box on page 545. If you've experienced or are experiencing a loss, this chapter can help you cope.

Types of Early Miscarriage

I f you're experiencing an early pregnancy loss, the sadness you're feeling is the same no matter the cause or the official medical name. Still, it's helpful to know about the different types of miscarriage so you're familiar with the terms your practitioner might be using.

Chemical pregnancy. A chemical pregnancy occurs when an egg is fertilized but fails to develop successfully or implant fully in the uterus. A woman may miss her period and suspect she is pregnant—she may even have a positive pregnancy test because her body has produced some low (but detectable) levels of the pregnancy hormone hCG. But in a chemical pregnancy, there will be no gestational sac or placenta, and the pregnancy ends in what seems like a period. Experts estimate that up to 70 percent of all conceptions are chemical, and many women who experience one don't even realize they've conceived.

Often, a very early positive pregnancy test and then a late period (a few days to a week late) are the only signs of a chemical pregnancy.

Blighted ovum. A blighted ovum (or anembryonic pregnancy) refers to a fertilized egg that attaches to the wall of the uterus and begins to develop a placenta (which produces hCG), but then fails to develop into an embryo. What is left behind is an empty gestational sac (which can be seen on an ultrasound). Experts believe that up to half of all early miscarriages are blighted ovums. Most blighted ovum miscarriages occur very early in the first trimester. Some even occur before a woman realizes she's conceived, and end in what seems like a late period. Others are only noticed during a routine early ultrasound, when (after weeks 5 or 6) a gestational sac is visible but there is no embryo inside it.

called a missed miscarriage). In either of those cases, your uterus will eventually be—or need to be—emptied so that you can recover and your normal menstrual cycle can resume (and you can try to get pregnant again, if you choose to). There are several ways that this can happen:

- Expectant management. You and your practitioner may choose to let nature take its course and wait until the pregnancy is naturally expelled. Waiting out a missed or incomplete miscarriage can take anywhere from a few days to, in some cases, 3 to 4 weeks.

- Medication. Medication—usually a misoprostol pill taken orally, or vaginally as a suppository—can prompt

your body to expel the fetal tissue and placenta, and can be used in a missed or incomplete miscarriage, as well as a blighted ovum—a fertilized egg that implants but doesn't develop (see box, above). Just how long this takes varies, but typically, it's only a matter of days at the most before the miscarriage is completely expelled (though bleeding can continue for a few days longer). Side effects of the medication can include nausea, vomiting, cramping, and diarrhea.

- Surgery. Another option is to undergo a minor surgical procedure called dilation and vacuum curettage (D&C). During this procedure, the doctor gently dilates your cervix and removes (by suction) the fetal tissue and placenta

Missed miscarriage. A missed miscarriage is when the embryo or fetus dies but isn't expelled, at least not right away. Often there are no signs initially (no bleeding, for instance), and in some cases the placenta continues to produce hormones, which makes your body think you're still pregnant. A missed miscarriage is usually discovered during a routine first trimester ultrasound when there is no heartbeat detected, or later on in the first trimester when the heartbeat can't be heard with Doppler. The fact that there are no warning signs—you come to your appointment expecting to see or hear the heartbeat and there isn't one—can make the realization all the more painful. Some women notice the loss of all existing pregnancy symptoms (though that in and of itself doesn't mean that the pregnancy is lost), and less commonly, experience a brownish discharge.

Complete miscarriage. A complete miscarriage is when all the pregnancy tissue (embryo and placenta) passes from the uterus through the vagina.

The woman experiences bleeding and cramping, and the miscarriage completely empties the uterus without any medical intervention. On examination, the practitioner finds that the cervix has reclosed, and there is no sign of a pregnancy sac in the uterus on ultrasound. The earlier the miscarriage occurs (usually those earlier than 12 weeks), the more likely it is to be a complete one.

Incomplete miscarriage. An incomplete miscarriage is when the embryo or fetus is no longer viable and passes through the vagina via bleeding along with some of the tissue from the placenta, but some pregnancy tissue stays inside the uterus. With an incomplete miscarriage, a woman continues to cramp and bleed (sometimes heavily) and her cervix remains dilated. Because there is some remaining placental tissue in the uterus, it continues to produce hCG, which is detectable in blood tests and doesn't fall as expected. The remaining tissue in the uterus is also still visible on an ultrasound.

from your uterus. Bleeding following the procedure usually lasts no more than a week. Though side effects are rare, there is a slight risk of infection following a D&C.

How should you and your practitioner decide which route to take? Some factors you both can take into account include:

- How far along the miscarriage is. If bleeding and cramping are already heavy, the miscarriage is probably already well under way. In that case, allowing it to progress naturally may be preferable to a D&C. But if there is no bleeding yet (as in a missed miscarriage), misoprostol or a D&C might be better alternatives.

- How far along the pregnancy is. The farther along the pregnancy is, the more fetal tissue there will be, and the more likely a D&C will be necessary to empty your uterus completely.

- Your emotional and physical state. Waiting for a natural miscarriage to occur after an embryo or fetus has died in utero can be psychologically debilitating. It's likely that you won't be able to begin coming to terms with—and grieving for—your loss while the pregnancy is still inside you. Completing the process faster will also allow you to resume your menstrual cycles soon, and when and if the time is right, to try to conceive again.

Age and Miscarriage

More and more older moms are getting pregnant and having healthy babies at the time in their lives that's right for them and their partners—who are often older, too. But on average, with increasing age comes an increased risk of miscarriage. That's because the older eggs of older moms (and possibly their older partner's sperm) are more likely to contain a genetic defect that results in an embryo that isn't viable—that is, one that can't survive. These embryos are most often miscarried. So while a 20-year-old's odds of losing a pregnancy are 10 to 15 percent, a 35-year-old has a 20 percent chance of miscarrying, a 40-year-old has a 40 percent chance, and a 45-year-old's risk of pregnancy loss is over 80 percent.

When a woman conceives through advanced reproductive techniques like IVF (which women over 40 are more likely to do), the risks of miscarriage can be lowered (though not eliminated) through preimplantation screening, which stacks the odds of a healthy pregnancy by implanting only those embryos that appear healthy and viable.

- Risks and benefits. Because a D&C is invasive, it carries a slightly higher (though still very low) risk of infection. The benefit of having the miscarriage complete sooner, however, may greatly outweigh that small risk for some women. With a naturally occurring miscarriage, there is also the risk that it won't completely empty the uterus, in which case a D&C may be necessary to finish what nature has started.

- Evaluation of the miscarriage. When a D&C is performed, evaluating the cause of the miscarriage through an examination of the fetal tissue will be easier. If this isn't your first miscarriage, genetic testing can be performed on the tissue as well, which can help predict the likelihood of recurrence, as well as provide some measure of closure.

If you miscarry naturally and feel able (physically and emotionally, and both might be extremely difficult) to save the expelled pregnancy, you can do this in a sterile cup or small storage container, so that it can be tested later.

No matter what course is taken, and whether the ordeal is over sooner or later, the loss will likely be difficult for you. See page 592 for help in coping.

Molar Pregnancy

What is it? A molar pregnancy starts when an egg is fertilized, but instead of a normal pregnancy resulting, the placenta develops into an abnormal mass of cysts (also called a hydatidiform mole), and there is no accompanying fetus. In some cases, identifiable—but not viable—embryonic or fetal tissue is present. This is called a partial molar pregnancy.

The cause of a molar pregnancy is an abnormality during fertilization, in which 2 sets of chromosomes from the father become mixed in with either 1 set of chromosomes from the mother (partial mole)—or none of her chromosomes at all (complete mole). Most molar pregnancies are discovered within weeks of conception.

How common is it? Molar pregnancies are relatively rare, occurring in only 1 out of 1,000 pregnancies. Women under the age of 20 or over the age of

Choriocarcinoma

Choriocarcinoma is an extremely rare pregnancy-related cancer (occurring in only 1 out of every 40,000 pregnancies) that grows from the cells of the placenta. This malignancy most often occurs after a molar pregnancy, miscarriage, abortion, or ectopic pregnancy, when any left-behind placental tissues continue to grow despite the absence of a fetus. Only 15 percent of choriocarcinomas occur after a normal pregnancy.

The condition is usually diagnosed when there has been intermittent bleeding following a miscarriage, a pregnancy, or the removal of a molar pregnancy, as well as abnormal tissue discharge, elevated hCG levels that do not return to normal after a pregnancy has ended, a tumor in the vagina, uterus, or lungs, and/or abdominal pain.

If you are diagnosed, the news is very reassuring. While any type of cancer carries with it some risk, choriocarcinoma responds extremely well to chemotherapy and radiation treatments and has a cure rate of more than 90 percent. Hysterectomy is almost never necessary because of this type of tumor's excellent response to chemotherapy drugs.

And happily, with early diagnosis and treatment of choriocarcinoma, fertility is unaffected, though it's usually recommended that trying for another pregnancy be postponed for 1 year after treatment for choriocarcinoma is complete and there is no remaining evidence of disease.

35, as well as women who have had multiple miscarriages, are at a slightly increased risk for a molar pregnancy.

What are the signs and symptoms? A molar pregnancy seems like a normal pregnancy in the beginning, but then the expectant mother may notice:

- Dark brown to bright red vaginal bleeding during the first trimester

You'll Want to Know . . .

Having had a molar pregnancy doesn't put you at much higher risk for having another one. In fact, only 1 to 2 percent of women who have had a molar pregnancy go on to experience a second.

- Severe nausea and vomiting
- Sometimes, uncomfortable cramping

The practitioner may notice other signs, including:

- High blood pressure
- A uterus that is larger than expected
- A uterus that is doughy (rather than firm)
- An absence of embryonic or fetal tissue, or presence of tissue that isn't viable (as seen on ultrasound)
- Excessive levels of thyroid hormone in the mother's system

What can you and your practitioner do? If an ultrasound shows you do have a molar pregnancy, the abnormal tissue must be removed via a D&C (remember, even if there is embryonic or fetal tissue, it's not viable—that is, it can't develop into a baby). Followup is crucial to make sure it doesn't develop into a malignancy, like choriocarcinoma (see box, page 587), though luckily, the chances of this happening in a treated molar pregnancy are very low.

Ectopic Pregnancy

What is it? An ectopic pregnancy (also known as a tubal pregnancy) is a nonviable pregnancy that implants outside the uterus, most commonly in a fallopian tube, usually because something (such as scarring in the fallopian tube) obstructs or slows the movement of the fertilized egg into the uterus. An ectopic pregnancy can also occur in the cervix, on the ovary, or in the abdomen. Unfortunately, there is no way for an ectopic pregnancy to continue normally.

Ultrasound can detect an ectopic pregnancy, often as early as 5 weeks. But without early diagnosis and treatment of an ectopic pregnancy, the fertilized egg might continue to grow in the fallopian tube, leading to a rupture of the tube. If the tube bursts, its ability in the future to carry a fertilized egg to the uterus is destroyed, and if the rupture is not cared for, it can result

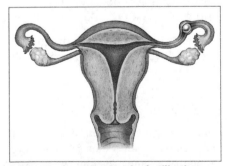

In an ectopic pregnancy, the fertilized egg implants in an area other than the uterus. Here, the egg has implanted in the fallopian tube.

> ## You'll Want to Know . . .
>
> More than half of the women who are treated for ectopic pregnancies conceive and have a normal pregnancy within a year.

in severe, even life-threatening, internal bleeding and shock for the mother. Luckily, quick treatment (usually surgery or medication) can help avoid such a rupture and removes most of the risk for the mother while greatly improving the chances of preserving her fertility.

How common is it? About 2 percent of all pregnancies are ectopic. Women at risk of having an ectopic pregnancy include those with a history of endometriosis, pelvic inflammatory disease, a prior ectopic pregnancy or tubal surgery, and women who smoke, have an STD, or conceived while using progesterone-only birth control pills. An IUD doesn't increase the risk of an ectopic pregnancy, but when pregnancies occur with an IUD, they are more commonly ectopic.

What are the signs and symptoms? Like many miscarriages, abnormal bleeding is an early sign. But with an ectopic pregnancy, there will sharp, crampy pain with tenderness, usually in the lower abdomen (it often begins as a dull ache that progresses to spasms and cramps) as well. Pain may worsen on straining of bowels, coughing, or moving. If the fallopian tube ruptures, there will be heavy bleeding inside the abdomen and you may experience:

■ Severe sharp abdominal pain

If You've Had an Early Pregnancy Loss

Though it can be hard for parents to accept it at the time, when an early pregnancy loss occurs, it's usually because the condition of the embryo or fetus wasn't compatible with life. Early miscarriage is generally a natural selection process in which an abnormal embryo or fetus (defective because of genetic abnormality, poor implantation in the uterus, maternal infection, random accident, or other, unknown reasons) is lost because it is incapable of survival.

That said, losing a baby, even at the earliest stages of life—even when the loss was inevitable from the start—can be traumatic. So allow yourself to grieve as much as you need to—it's a necessary part of the healing process. But also remember that there's no one way you should feel, since everyone experiences this kind of grief differently. You may feel far sadder than you might have expected to, or you may feel ready to move on far sooner than you thought you might, or you may feel all over the map emotionally. Grieve and heal your way, in your own time. Sharing your feelings with your partner will be essential, and finding support from others (especially those who have also experienced a pregnancy loss) may be enormously helpful, too. But again, do what feels right to you. Just try not to let guilt compound your pain—miscarriage is not your fault.

For more on coping with your loss, see page 592. For help for fathers coping with such a loss, see the box on page 600.

- Rectal pressure

- Shoulder pain (due to blood accumulating under the diaphragm)

- Heavier vaginal bleeding

- Lightheadedness, fainting, and shock

What can you and your practitioner do? If it is determined that you have an ectopic pregnancy (usually diagnosed through ultrasound and blood tests), there is, unfortunately, no way to save the pregnancy. You'll most likely have to undergo surgery (laparoscopically) to remove the tubal pregnancy or be given drugs (methotrexate), which will end the abnormally occurring pregnancy. In some rare cases, it can be determined that the ectopic pregnancy is no longer developing and can be expected to disappear over time on its own, which would also eliminate the need for surgery.

Because residual material from a pregnancy left in the tube could damage it, a follow-up test of hCG levels is performed to be sure the entire tubal pregnancy was removed or has been reabsorbed.

Late Miscarriage

What is it? The loss of a baby between the end of the first trimester and the 20th week is called a late miscarriage. Though the medical term is "miscarriage," and though the baby is still considered pre-viable (unable to live outside the womb), the loss can feel more palpable because the pregnancy felt more palpable—especially if you've watched your belly swell, felt the first kicks, and wondered at those beautiful little features developing before your eyes on ultrasound. For help coping with this kind of devastating loss, see page 594.

You'll Want to Know . . .

When the cause of a late miscarriage can be determined, it may be possible to prevent a repeat of the tragedy. If a previously undiagnosed cervical insufficiency (an incompetent cervix) was responsible, future miscarriages can be prevented by cerclage early in pregnancy, before the cervix begins to dilate (see page 34). If chronic disease, such as diabetes, hypertension, or obesity is responsible, the condition can be brought under control prior to any future pregnancy. An abnormally shaped uterus or one that is distorted by the growth of fibroids, polyps, or a septum (a piece of tissue that divides all or part of the uterine cavity in two) in some instances can be corrected by surgery. The presence of antibodies that trigger placental inflammation and/or clotting may be treated with low-dose aspirin and heparin injections in a subsequent pregnancy. Some causes of late miscarriage, such as acute infection, are very unlikely to recur.

How common is it? Late miscarriages occur in about 6 in 1,000 pregnancies. A late miscarriage is usually related to the mother's health (a chronic condition such as antiphospholipid antibody syndrome or, rarely, poorly controlled diabetes), the condition of her uterus, cervical insufficiency (see page 34), an untreated bacterial infection, or problems of the placenta. Sometimes a late miscarriage is due to chromosomal or other genetic abnormalities in the fetus.

What are the signs and symptoms? The signs and symptoms of a late miscarriage include:

- Heavy bleeding (possibly including blood clots), accompanied by strong cramping and abdominal pain

- A dilated cervix (found during examination)

- No fetal heartbeat detected on ultrasound or with Doppler

- A complete cessation of baby's movements (if the mother has already begun feeling movement consistently)

What can you and your practitioner do? If you're experiencing the type of heavy bleeding and painful cramping that signal a miscarriage, there's usually nothing, unfortunately, that can be done to stop the inevitable. The miscarriage may be complete, or your practitioner may need to perform a D&C to remove any remnants of the pregnancy. If the miscarriage hasn't begun on its own, yet it's clear during a routine office visit or on ultrasound that there is no fetal heartbeat, your practitioner might bring you into the hospital to induce labor using misoprostol or for a procedure similar to a D&C called a D&E—dilation and evacuation—in which surgical methods are used to deliver the fetus and placenta. A D&E is considered safer than induction because of decreased risk of infection and bleeding, but talk to your practitioner about the relative risks and benefits of both options. If induction is chosen, depending on how far along in the pregnancy you are, you may have the opportunity to hold your baby, and doing so may help in the grieving process (see page 595 for more).

A late miscarriage will be emotionally painful and it is also likely to be physically painful, so be sure to ask for medication if you need it.

Lactation Suppression When a Baby Dies

When you've suffered the loss of a baby, the last thing you need is another reminder of what would have been. Sadly, nature can deliver that reminder when the end of pregnancy (even when it has ended tragically) automatically signals the beginning of lactation, and your breasts fill with the milk that was intended to feed your baby. That will be emotionally painful, of course, but breast engorgement will also make it physically painful. Ice packs, mild pain relievers, and a supportive bra can help minimize the physical discomfort you'll feel. Avoiding hot showers, nipple stimulation, and expressing milk from your breasts will help stop further milk production. The engorgement will pass within a few days.

Stillbirth

What is it? The loss of the baby in utero anytime after the 20th week is called a stillbirth. Most stillbirths occur before labor begins, though a small number of stillbirths occur during labor and delivery. After so many months of becoming attached to your baby, preparing for your baby, and feeling and seeing your baby's kicks, the pain of a stillbirth is profoundly heartbreaking.

How common is it? Stillbirth occurs in about 1 in 160 pregnancies. The reasons babies die in utero range from birth defects (about 15 percent of stillborn babies have one or more birth defects) to poor fetal growth (which accounts for about 35 percent of stillborn babies), placental problems like placental abruption (which account for about 20 percent of stillbirths), knots in the umbilical cord (2 percent), chronic health conditions in the mother like diabetes, hypertension, or obesity (about 10 percent), and maternal or fetal infections (around 10 percent of the time). Severe trauma (for instance, from a serious car accident or lack of oxygen during a difficult delivery) can also be the cause of a stillbirth.

What are the signs and symptoms? The pregnant woman may suspect that something is wrong if fetal movement suddenly stops. An ultrasound will confirm that there is no fetal heartbeat. During labor, the lack of a heartbeat could be detected by the fetal monitor or Doppler.

What can you and your practitioner do? Even if your baby's movements have stopped—leading you to fear the worst—there is no way to prepare for the news that your baby has died in your uterus. You are likely to be in a fog of disbelief and grief after being told your baby's heartbeat can't be located. It may be difficult or even impossible for you to carry on with any semblance of your usual life while carrying around a baby who is no longer living, and studies show that a mother is much more likely to suffer severe depression after the delivery of a stillborn if the delivery is delayed more than 3 days after the death is diagnosed. For this reason, your emotional state will be taken into account while your practitioner decides what to do next. If labor is imminent, or has already started, your stillborn baby will be delivered. If labor isn't clearly about to start, the decision of whether to induce labor immediately or to allow you to return home until it begins spontaneously will depend on how far you are from your due date, your physical condition, and how you're doing emotionally. Most practitioners recommend inducing labor within 1 to 2 days.

After delivery, the fetus, placenta, and umbilical cord are examined carefully to help determine why the baby died. ACOG recommends that genetic testing be performed in all stillbirths, with parental permission. Also with parental permission, an autopsy may be performed. Your practitioner may also suggest some testing for you, but in up to half of all cases, testing can't ultimately determine the cause of stillbirth.

ALL ABOUT:

Coping with Pregnancy Loss

No matter how or when you lose a pregnancy, it can hurt, deeply. Everyone deals with a pregnancy loss differently, but here are some ways of coping.

Coping with First Trimester Loss

Just because it often takes place very early in pregnancy doesn't mean that miscarriage can't be painful for expectant parents. Even though you never saw your baby, except perhaps on ultrasound, you knew that a new life was growing inside of you, and you may have already formed a bond, however abstract. Then, just as it was beginning, that life abruptly ends, and the promise of the months and years ahead is broken. Understandably, you'll be sad, but you may also experience other, less expected emotions. You may be angry at your body for letting you down, or resentful of friends and family who are pregnant or have babies. You may have trouble eating or sleeping, or even accepting the loss. You may cry a lot, or not at all. These are among the many natural, healthy responses to a pregnancy loss. Remember your reaction is what's normal for you.

Some couples approach an early loss matter-of-factly, easily accepting that this pregnancy wasn't meant to be, ready to move on, and eager to try again. Others find it much harder—and in some cases, coping with the early loss ends up being, in certain ways, as difficult as coping with a loss later on. One reason why: Because so many couples hold off on spreading the word about their pregnancy until the first trimester has passed, even close friends and family may not have been told yet, which can mean that support may be hard to come by. Even those who knew about the pregnancy and/or are told about the miscarriage may offer less support than they would have if the pregnancy had been further along. They may try to minimize the significance of the loss with a "Don't worry, you can try again" or "You're lucky it happened so early," not realizing that the loss of a baby, no matter how early in pregnancy it occurs, can be devastating.

Still, if you've suffered a miscarriage (or an ectopic or molar pregnancy), remember that you have the right to grieve as much—or as little—as you need to. Do this in any way that helps you heal and eventually move on, in your way and in your time.

A Personal Process

When it comes to dealing with a miscarriage or other pregnancy loss, there's no single emotional formula that must be followed. Different couples confront, cope with, and process their feelings in completely different ways. You may find yourself deeply saddened, even devastated by the loss—and discover that healing comes surprisingly slowly. Or you may handle the loss more matter-of-factly, seeing it as a bump in the road to having a baby. You may find that after some momentary sadness, you're able to put the experience behind you more quickly than you might have expected, and instead of lingering over the loss, you may choose to look ahead to trying again.

There are a number of factors that may contribute to your sense of loss: how long it took you to conceive (often, the longer it took, the more painful the loss may feel), if you conceived with the help of assisted reproduction (sometimes the more advanced the technology used to become pregnant, the greater the emotional investment in the pregnancy and the greater the loss may feel), your age (if you feel the pressure of your biological clock, you may also feel the loss more intensely as you worry if "time will run out"), the length of the pregnancy (the longer you were pregnant, the more time you had to connect to your baby), and how many losses you've had (grief often builds with each loss or may contribute to a sense of hopelessness or even numbness). Dads may grieve as much, but in a different way (see page 600).

Just remember: The normal reaction to a pregnancy loss is the reaction that's normal for you. Allow yourself to feel whatever you need to feel in order to heal.

Saying goodbye—which, for many parents, is a vital step in the recovery process—is in some ways harder when there's nothing tangible left to say goodbye to. Perhaps you'll find closure in a private ceremony with close family members or just you and your spouse. Or by sharing your feelings—individually, through a support group, or online—with others who have experienced early miscarriage. Since so many women suffer a miscarriage at least once during their reproductive years, you may be surprised to find how many others you know have had the same experience as you but never talked about it with you, or maybe even talked about it at all. (If you don't feel like sharing your feelings—or don't feel you need to—don't. Do only what's right for you.) Some of the tips for those who have later pregnancy losses may be helpful for you, too.

Accept that you may always have a place in your heart for the pregnancy you lost, and you may feel sad on the anniversary of the due date of your lost baby or on the anniversary of the miscarriage itself, even years later. If you find it helps, plan on doing something special at that time to commemorate: planting some new flowers or a tree, having a quiet picnic in the park.

While it's normal to mourn your loss—and important to come to terms with it your way—you should also start to gradually feel better as time passes (for many women it could take 6 months before feeling better, for others it could be up to 2 years). If you don't, or if you have continued trouble coping with everyday life—you're not eating

Postpartum Depression and Pregnancy Loss

Every parent who loses a baby has reason to feel sad. But for some, the sadness can be deepened by postpartum depression and/or anxiety, triggered in part by the same inevitably precipitous drops in pregnancy hormones, acutely heightened by the abrupt end of the pregnancy and tragic loss of the baby. Untreated, PPD can prevent you from experiencing the stages of grief that are essential to healing. Though it might be hard to distinguish PPD from the depression brought on by the loss of your baby, any kind of depression requires help. If you're exhibiting signs of depression (loss of interest in everyday activities, inability to sleep, loss of appetite, extreme sadness that interferes with your ability to function), don't hesitate to get the help you need. Speak to your prenatal practitioner or your regular doctor, and ask to be referred to a mental health professional. Therapy—and, if necessary, medication—can help you feel better.

or sleeping, you're not able to focus at work, you're becoming isolated from family and friends—or if you continue to feel very anxious (anxiety is an even more common symptom after miscarriage than depression is), professional counseling and possibly other therapies can help you recover. For more tips on coping with pregnancy loss, see the box on page 596.

Try to remind yourself that you can—and most likely will—become pregnant again and give birth to a healthy baby, if that's what you decide you want. For the vast majority of women, a miscarriage is a onetime event—and actually, an indication of future fertility.

Coping with Second Trimester Loss

The word "miscarriage" is nearly always associated with pain and sadness—after all, the loss of a baby at any time is something to grieve over. But it's also nearly always associated with the early weeks of a pregnancy, a time when the new life growing deep within feels especially vulnerable, abstract, far from palpable, a time when couples often stay guarded in their joy for fear of loving and losing that new life. Are you ever prepared for a miscarriage? No, but it's something you're more likely to expect, if not accept, when it takes place in the first trimester.

And that's why a second trimester loss can hit so hard. By then, you're off your guard—beginning to see and possibly feel tangible proof of the life within. What was once a blob of cells, then a tiny tadpole, has miraculously transformed into a baby—and if you didn't dare to dream about that baby's future before, those dreams have almost certainly started by the second trimester. Everything is normal, everything is as it should be, you can breathe easily.

Then, suddenly it isn't normal—something is terribly wrong. The pain and the shock may take your breath away, leaving you wondering whether you'll ever breathe easily again—and leaving you asking, of course, why? If something was so wrong, why didn't this loss happen when you were in your first trimester, when you were at least prepared for the possibility? Why did it happen after you'd spent so many weeks and months bonding with your baby and your blossoming baby bump, and maybe even feeling those flutters of life? Why did it have to happen at all?

And as if the news that you lost your baby isn't heartbreaking enough, you may also have to go to the hospital to endure labor and delivery. Going through the motions of delivering a baby you won't be going home with is, understandably, a terrible burden to bear. As is being, most likely, in a wing of the hospital devoted to delivering joy—where happy parents welcome healthy babies, celebrating the beginning of a lifetime while you're faced with a tragic ending. What's more, when you return home, with your arms empty and your heart broken, you'll have the physical recovery to cope with, in addition to the emotional healing. This can be true even if you didn't have to go through labor but had a D&C or D&E instead.

If the option of holding and seeing your baby is possible, consider it carefully. While it may feel unnatural to hold the tiny baby you've just lost, it will likely give you comfort later, when you're able to look back at your loss and remember the brief time you had together. It may also help make the loss more real—and though that painful reality may be exactly what you'd like to avoid facing, it will help you begin the grieving process that's a necessary part of healing. Consider, too, making a keepsake folder or memory box with your baby's footprint, handprint, lock of hair, and pictures, if these are options for you. Use your baby's name when you talk about him or her—and if you hadn't chosen a name before, consider naming your baby now. And be sure to talk to the doctors, nurses, and grief counselors about your options for burying or cremating your baby if you'd like to do so. But remember, as always, what's right for you and your partner during this devastating time is what's

right—don't feel obligated to follow a formula that anyone else suggests.

Just how much pain will you experience, and how long will it last? There is no time limit on grief, no minimum or maximum. Everyone is different, and you'll need to heal in your own way, at your own pace. Use whatever is necessary to find solace—a retreat with your partner, talking online with other women who've also experienced similar loss, a memorial service for your baby, joining a support group, reaching out to a grief counselor, or trying to get pregnant again soon, if that's an option. Comfort might come quickly, or it might take a long time. Either way, it's completely normal. See the box on page 596 for more on the difficult process of coping.

Finally, remember—and keep reminding yourself—that you did nothing wrong. You didn't let your baby down, and the loss is not your fault. Keep that in mind whether or not you find out the cause of the miscarriage.

Coping with Repeat Miscarriages

Suffering a single pregnancy loss can be hard enough to cope with. But if you've suffered more than one, you may find it infinitely harder—with each loss hitting you a little harder than the last. You may be discouraged, depressed, angry, irritable, and/or unable to focus on everyday life (or on anything beyond your losses). The healing of your psyche may not only take a lot longer than the healing of your body, but the sadness can be debilitating. What's more, the emotional pain may lead to physical symptoms, including headaches, appetite loss or overeating, insomnia, and overwhelming fatigue. (Some couples handle even repeat losses more matter-of-factly, and that's completely normal, too.)

The Difficult Process of Coping

When you experience a pregnancy loss you're not only grieving for a baby, but for the hopes, dreams, and potential of what you believed was to come—a life not yet lived. The grieving process, though difficult, is a tribute to that life, and to the connection you made to your baby during the time in your womb—so allow it to happen. The following may help you cope:

- Take the time you need. The grieving process usually has many steps (including denial and isolation, anger, depression, and acceptance), but everyone experiences grief differently and recovers differently. Don't rush the process, but don't prolong it either, once you feel it's time to move on.

- Feel the way you need to. Maybe you'll feel irritable and short-tempered, anxious, depressed. Or lonely and empty, even if you're surrounded with people who love you. Or maybe, you'll feel fleeting sadness, then hopeful to try again. All of this is normal.

- Cry if you need to, for as long and as often as you feel you need to. If you don't feel like crying, that can be just as valid—and just as normal.

- Write about it. Journal your feelings —the sad ones, the anxious ones, the angry ones, the ones you don't feel you can share with anyone else.

- Let go of the guilt. Just about every mom who has lost a baby, no matter how early or how late, looks for a way to blame herself. Maybe you'll look back at everything you ate or drank, every time you threw up your prenatal vitamins or forgot to take them— or you'll wonder whether it was the workout you did or the sex you had or the heavy box you lifted or the stress at work. Maybe you'll agonize over whether it was the mixed feelings you had about being pregnant, especially if you didn't plan the pregnancy. Those self-blaming feelings are understandable, they're normal, they're all too common among women. But the truth is: Your baby's loss was in no way your fault. You are not responsible. If you have a hard time letting go of guilt, turn to professional support.

- Recognize that fathers grieve, too. Dads who have lost a baby are likely to feel as much grief as moms—only they may express and process it differently. Not only for the obvious reason: You carried the baby, the baby was lost in your body. But also because he is likely trying to be strong for you (remember, for better or worse, that's how men are hormonally wired, culturally programmed, and traditionally raised). His feelings of pain may be compounded by frustration, even anger over not being able to do two of the things men often feel they're meant to do (again, for better or worse): protect and fix. He couldn't protect you and the baby you both created, and he can't fix what happened, ever. He may not cry or he may try not to cry in front of you, he may be stoic or he may withdraw or he may try to distract himself with work or other activities—none of which means that he doesn't feel the same pain you feel, that the heartache isn't as real. If you sense that's the case with your partner, and when you feel you're able, encourage him to share what he's feeling with you. He may also find it helpful to talk with another father who's been through a loss. But understand if he doesn't want to talk about his feelings at all. Let him grieve in his way, as you are in yours.

- Take care of each other. Grief can be very self-absorbing. You and your spouse may find yourselves so consumed by your own pain that you don't have the emotional reserves left to comfort each other. But remember, you made this baby together, you lost this baby together, and you'll heal best if you grieve for this baby together. Although there will almost certainly be times when you'll want to be alone with your thoughts, also make time for sharing them with your spouse. Consider seeking grief counseling together, too, which is often more beneficial than individual counseling. Or join a couples' support group. It may not only help you both find comfort but also help preserve—and even deepen—your relationship.

- Don't face the world alone. If you're dreading the friendly faces asking about the baby, take a friend who can field questions the first few times you face the world. Be sure that those at work, and at other places you go frequently, are told about your loss, so you don't have to do any more explaining than necessary.

- Realize that some friends and family may not know what to do or say. Some may be so uncomfortable that they withdraw. Others may say things that hurt more than help (like "Oh, you can have another baby"). Though they certainly mean well, they may not understand that another baby can never take the place of the one you lost and that parents can become attached to a baby long before birth. If you're frequently hearing comments that hurt, ask a close friend or relative to let others know that you would rather they just say they are sorry about your loss.

- Look for support from those who've been there. You may find comfort in a local or online support group for parents who have lost infants (try compassionatefriends.org or national share.org). But try not to let such a group become a way of holding on to—rather than letting go of—your grief.

- Take care of yourself. In the face of emotional pain, your physical needs may be the last thing on your mind. They shouldn't be. Eating right, getting enough sleep, and exercising are vital not just to maintaining your health but also in aiding your recovery. So is taking a break from grieving once in a while to see a movie or have dinner out. If you feel that getting your life back to normal would somehow be disloyal, it may help to ask your baby, in spirit, for permission to enjoy life again. You might try doing it in a "letter" to your baby. For life to go on, after all, you need to go on living.

- Turn to religion, if you find it comforting. For some grieving parents, faith is a great solace. For others, a tragedy can have them questioning their faith. And for still others, religion is not the answer, but spirituality may be. Again, it is your grief, your choice.

- Expect the pain to lessen over time. At first, there may be only bad days, then a few good days mixed in—eventually, there will be more good days than bad. But remember that the grieving process (which may include nightmares and fleeting flashbacks) has no fixed timetable. It may not be fully complete for 2 years, but the worst is usually over after 3 to 6 months (and for some, it may take only a matter of weeks). If after 6 to 9 months your grief remains the center of your life, if you're having trouble functioning or focusing, or have little interest in anything else, seek help. And remember that postpartum depression can cloud the healing process, too; see the box on page 594.

A Surrogate Pregnancy, a Personal Loss

Surrogacy is often referred to as "the gift of life" for couples who can't conceive a baby together and/or aren't able to carry a pregnancy. But just as pregnancies conceived the traditional way sometimes end in miscarriage or stillbirth (or the loss of one twin), so do surrogate pregnancies. If you've experienced the loss of a surrogate pregnancy, it can be just as real, just as deeply painful as if you'd lost a baby you were carrying—and if you've lost pregnancies before turning to surrogacy, it may seem like an extra cruel twist of fate. Surrogacy was the miracle that was finally going to bring you the baby (or babies) you and your partner longed for but couldn't have naturally. The financial investment may have been large, but the emotional investment far larger.

Though the loss didn't happen in your body—and even if the pregnancy wasn't conceived with your egg (or with your partner's sperm)—you are entitled to feel all the same emotions any couple experiencing a loss might feel, from heartbreak to anger and resentment (even toward the surrogate) to guilt. And you are entitled to grieve in any way you need to. Use this chapter to help you through the process.

Time may not heal all—there will always be a little piece of your heart that's been taken—but it will definitely help tremendously, eventually. In the meantime, knowledge can be powerful (finding out as much as you can about what may have caused your miscarriages and what you and your practitioner might be able to do to prevent another; see page 28), but patience and support may be your best remedies. Sharing with others who have suffered through pregnancy losses, especially multiple losses, can help you feel less alone, as well as more hopeful. Most of all, try to let go of any feelings of guilt or self-blame. Too often moms who've suffered multiple miscarriages see it as a failure of their bodies to accomplish the most fundamental of female functions. But miscarriages are not your fault. Instead, try to focus on how strong you've been (even if you haven't always felt that strong) and how determined you are to have a baby.

Coping with Loss During or After Birth

Sometimes the loss of a baby occurs during labor or delivery, sometimes just after delivery. Either way, your world comes crashing down. You've waited for, prepared for, anticipated and expected this baby for months—and now you're going home without your baby.

There's probably no greater pain than that inflicted by the loss of a child. And though nothing can completely heal the hurt you're feeling, there are steps you can take now to lessen the inevitable sadness that follows such a tragedy:

- See your baby, hold your baby, name your baby. Grieving is a vital step in accepting and recovering from your loss, and it's difficult to grieve for a nameless baby you've never seen. Even if your baby has malformations, experts advise that it is better to see him or her than not to, because what is imagined is usually worse than the reality. Holding your baby will make the death more real to you and ultimately easier to accept. So will doing some of those simple firsts that otherwise would never be: giving a bath, putting on a diaper, dressing and swaddling your baby, combing his or her hair, cuddling, kissing. Take time to focus on the details you'll want to remember later: big eyes and long lashes, a button nose, beautiful hands and delicate fingers, a headful of hair. If you have chosen a name for your baby, use it. If you haven't, consider doing that now, so you'll have a name for the baby you'll want to remember always.

- Get the support you need. There are bereavement doulas who specialize in helping grieving parents cope. Hospitals also have grief counselors who can help you, too. Ask for the help you need.

- Don't rush the good-bye if you don't want to. Ask for and take the time you need. Some hospitals may offer CuddleCots, cooling systems that allow parents more time to spend with their babies and say their goodbyes.

- Collect mementos of your baby. Take photos or consider having portraits taken (NowILayMeDownToSleep.org can help with that), and consider preserving baby's handprint and footprint and a lock of hair, so you'll have some tangible reminders to cherish in the future.

- You will be asked for permission to conduct genetic tests and possibly an autopsy on your baby. If you opt to go ahead with these, try not to avoid the facts, as hard as they are to hear. Discuss autopsy findings and other medical reports with your practitioner to help you accept the reality of what happened and to help you in the grieving process, as well as to help you make decisions about future pregnancies.

- Ask friends or relatives to leave the preparations you made for baby at home. Coming home to a house that looks as though a baby was never expected will only make it more difficult to accept the reality of what has happened. It's better if you pack away those things yourselves.

- Remember your baby as privately or publicly as you need to. Arrange for a funeral, and for burial or cremation, which will give you another important opportunity to say good-bye. But when it comes to a memorial service, do whatever feels right to you. That might be a completely private ceremony—which allows you and your spouse to share your feelings alone—or one that surrounds you with the love and support of family, friends, and community.

- Honor your child's memory in a way that has meaning to you, if that helps. Plant a tree or a new flower bed in your backyard or in a local park. Buy books for a childcare center that serves kids in need, or donate to an organization or clinic that helps at-risk expectant and new moms or one that builds playgrounds.

Coping with the Loss of One Twin

Parents who lose one twin (or more babies, in the case of triplets or quads) face celebrating a birth (or births) and mourning a death (or deaths) at the same time. If this happens, you may feel too conflicted to either mourn your lost baby or enjoy your living one—both vitally important processes. Understanding why you feel the way you do may help you better cope with your feelings, which may include all or just some of these:

You're Grieving, Too

You conceived a baby together. You celebrated the positive pregnancy test together. You watched ultrasound images together, checked your pregnancy app for weekly updates on your baby's size and development, from blueberry to peach and maybe well beyond that. Together, you planned and hoped and dreamed and imagined your life as parents, as a family of 3, or more. You guessed (and maybe discovered) baby's gender together, picked out names together, sorted through birth options, maybe even signed up for childbirth classes or baby registries.

And then, in a moment, those plans and hopes and dreams were over. Whether it happened early or late in pregnancy, or whether it happened just before birth or just after, the baby you made together was gone. Leaving both of you to grieve, together—but probably in your own way.

Grief over the loss of a baby takes many shapes and forms and levels of intensity, depending on so many factors (from how far along a pregnancy was to how long it took to conceive to whether the pregnancy was planned), but also on a parent's gender. Moms, it could easily be argued, grieve not only for the loss of the abstract (those visions and daydreams of life with baby) but also for the physically palpable loss. The baby you made together, after all, was growing inside her. Understandably, predictably, sympathy will be centered on her—the hugs, the condolences, the offers of help, even the medical care. The network of support will focus on holding her up, and you'll likely be part of it. Yes, she'll need that support, of course. But what about you? When do you get your chance to grieve?

Here are some things to remember as you try to move forward:

It's your loss, too. People will probably say, "I'm so sorry she lost the baby." You may even find yourself calling the loss of the baby you made together "her loss." For you to grieve and mend, though, you'll need to acknowledge that just as you made the baby together and planned to parent the baby together, you lost the baby together. You may have different ways of expressing and processing your grief, but it's your loss, too.

Your grief is your own. Everyone grieves differently after a pregnancy loss or a stillbirth, and that goes for moms and dads (which, by the way, those who've lost a pregnancy or a baby always will be—loss can't take that away). Maybe you'll process it quickly, or maybe it will be slower in resolving. Maybe it'll be surprisingly intense, or far less so than you might have expected. There are no rules about how you should feel or how long you should feel it—and that goes for your partner, too.

You can be strong and still be sad. Hormones wire men differently from women, but so do cultural expectations, and both of those can affect how you react to loss. You may find yourself shifting automatically into "protector" role, to be as strong as you need to be—stronger still, if your partner is especially vulnerable. The more she cries, the more you may feel compelled to hold in your tears, to put on a brave front. But as much as you can, try not to let that front keep your emotions from surfacing. By all means, be her rock, but crumble every now and then if you need to. Mostly, do what feels right. If you're sad, that's okay. If you need to cry, that's okay. If you're stoic, that's okay, too.

You can grieve more effectively together. Sometimes couples drift apart when they're mourning the loss of a pregnancy, but that isn't at all inevitable. Often, it's a matter of mixed signals and miscommunication—he's trying to be strong, and she takes that as a sign that the loss doesn't really mean much to him. She turns to others for support, and no one offers it to him. Or she gets so caught up in her own grief (and in the physical aftermath of the loss), she doesn't even realize that he's grieving, too. But research shows that couples heal faster when they heal together—that the most effective way of conquering grief is to share it, not divide it. Even if you're finding face-to-face is hard at first, try to grieve side by side. Couples' grief counseling can be especially effective. Know, too, that often grief brings couples closer to each other, and being in pain together can help you both better cope with and heal from your loss.

You'll need to find your way. You're in this together, as you've been from the start. But you may need to find different outlets for your grief, too. Maybe you'll find it in your work, or in volunteer activities, or in exercise, or sports, or music, or nature. Maybe you'll find it in support from friends, especially those who know what you've been through. Or online from other fathers who've lost a pregnancy. Or maybe you'll find it in solitude. One place grieving fathers sometimes turn to is alcohol or recreational drugs—but while that can mask pain, remember that it won't ever resolve it, and that should be your ultimate goal. If you're experiencing signs of addiction or depression, get the help you need right away.

- You may feel heartbroken. You've lost a baby, and the fact that you have another doesn't minimize your loss. Realize that you're entitled to mourn the baby you've lost, even as you're celebrating your other baby's birth. In fact, mourning that loss is an important part of the healing process. Taking the steps for grieving parents described in the previous sections can help you accept your baby's death as a reality.

- You may be happy, too, but ambivalent about showing it. It may seem somehow inappropriate to be excited about the arrival of your surviving baby or even disloyal to the one who didn't live. That's a natural feeling but one you'll need to try to let go of. Loving and nurturing the sibling is a wonderful way of honoring your lost baby—besides, it's essential to your living baby's wellbeing.

- You may want to celebrate but not know if it's okay to. A new baby is always something to celebrate, even when the happy news comes with sadness. If you're uncomfortable holding a baby-welcoming event without acknowledging your loss, consider first holding a memorial ceremony or farewell for the baby who has passed away.

- You may view your baby's death as punishment, perhaps because you really weren't sure you wanted or could handle parenting multiples or because you wanted a girl more than you wanted a boy (or vice versa). Though this kind of guilt is common among parents who experience a pregnancy loss of any kind, it's completely unwarranted. Nothing you did—or thought or imagined or wished for—could have caused the loss.

Palliative Care for Your Baby

There are many hospitals, hospices, and clinics that provide hospice and palliative care support programs for families who wish to continue their pregnancies with babies who likely will be stillborn or not live long after birth. They offer care to the mother and the father, and honor the baby with dignity and compassion. To find a list of these kinds of programs by state, go to perinatalhospice.org.

If you've been told your baby may not live very long after birth, it may also be possible, once all lifesaving efforts have been exhausted, to donate one or more healthy organs to a baby in need—and doing so may bring you some consolation for your own devastating loss. A neonatologist may be able to provide helpful information in such a situation and help you prepare physically and emotionally for it.

- You may feel disappointed that you won't be a parent of multiples. It's normal to be sad over the loss of this excitement, especially if you've been imagining and planning for the arrival of multiples for months. You may even feel twinges of regret when seeing sets of multiples. Don't feel guilty about feeling that way—it's completely understandable.

- You may be afraid that explaining your situation to family and friends will be awkward and difficult, especially if they've been eagerly awaiting the twins. To make facing the world a little easier, enlist a friend or close relative to spread the word so you won't have to. In the first few weeks, try to take someone with you when you go out with your baby, so they can anticipate and answer the inevitable—and possibly painful—questions.

- You may have trouble handling the reactions and comments of family and friends. In trying to help, friends and family may overdo the excitement when welcoming your living child without acknowledging the one you've lost. Or they may urge you to forget your lost baby and appreciate your living one. As well intentioned as their actions and words may be, they can hurt. So don't hesitate to tell people—especially the ones who are closest to you—how you feel.

- You may feel too depressed over your loss to care for your new baby—or, if you're still pregnant, to care for your baby by taking the best possible care of yourself. Don't beat yourself up over your unhappy or conflicted feelings. They're normal, and completely understandable. But do make sure that you get the help you need so you can start meeting your baby's needs—both physical and emotional. Support groups may help, and so can counseling.

- You may feel that you're alone in your pain. Getting support from others who know what you're going through can help more than you can imagine. Find that support in a local support group or online. You can contact Centers for Loss in Multiple Births (CLIMB), at climb-support.org.

No matter what you're feeling—and given your situation, your feelings may be all over the emotional map—give yourself time. Chances are you'll feel progressively better—and better about feeling better.

Trying Again After Pregnancy Loss

Making the decision to try again for a new pregnancy—and a new baby (often referred to as a "rainbow baby")—after a loss isn't always easy, and definitely is not as easy as those around you might think. It's an intensely personal decision, and it can also be a painful one. Here are some things that you might want to consider when deciding when (or whether) to try again:

- Trying again for another baby after losing one (or more) takes courage. Give yourself the credit you deserve—and the pat on the back you need—as you embark on this process.

- The right time is the time that's right for you. It may take just a short time for you to feel emotionally ready to try for another baby—or it may take a much longer time. Don't push yourself (or let others push you) into trying too soon. And don't second-guess yourself (or paralyze yourself) into waiting longer than you have to. Listen to your heart, and you'll know when you're emotionally healed and when you're ready to contemplate a new pregnancy.

- You'll need to be physically ready, too. Check with your practitioner to see whether a waiting period will be necessary in your case. Often, you can try as soon as you feel up to it (and as soon as your cycle begins cooperating). In fact, studies have shown that women actually have a higher than normal fertility rate in the first 3 cycles after a miscarriage. If there's a reason why you have to wait longer than you want to (as may be the case after a molar pregnancy), use the time to get yourself into the best physical condition possible for conception, if you're not already.

- A new pregnancy may be less innocent. Now you know that not all pregnancies end happily, which means you probably won't take anything about your new pregnancy for granted. You may feel more nervous than you did the first time, especially until you've passed the anniversary of the week you lost your last pregnancy (and if you lost your baby at or just before or after birth, you may worry more the entire time). You may try to keep your excitement in check, and you may find that your joy is tempered by trepidation—so much so that you may even hesitate to attach yourself to your new baby until that fear of loving and losing again has dissipated. You may be extra tuned in to every pregnancy symptom: the ones that give you hope (swollen breasts, morning sickness, those frequent runs to the bathroom) and those that trigger anxiety (those pelvic twinges, those crampy feelings). All of this is completely understandable and completely normal, as you'll find out if you reach out to others who've carried a new pregnancy to term after experiencing a loss. Just make sure that if these kinds of feelings keep you from nurturing and nourishing your new pregnancy, you quickly get some help working them out.

Looking forward to the ultimate reward—that baby you're so eager to cuddle—instead of looking back on your loss will help you stay positive. Remember, the vast majority of women who have experienced a pregnancy loss or the loss of a baby go on to have completely normal pregnancies and completely healthy babies. For more about trying again after pregnancy loss, see *What to Expect Before You're Expecting.*

Index

A

M

O